Pathophysiology

made Incredibly Easy!

Seventh Edition

Pathophysiology

made Incredibly Easy!

Seventh Edition

Clinical Editor

Theresa Capriotti, DO, MSN, CRNP, RN
Clinical Professor
M. Louise Fitzpatrick College of Nursing
Villanova University
Villanova, Pennsylvania

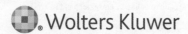
Wolters Kluwer

Philadelphia • Baltimore • New York • London
Buenos Aires • Hong Kong • Sydney • Tokyo

Vice President and Segment Leader, Health Learning & Practice: Julie K. Stegman
Director, Nursing Education and Practice Content: Jamie Blum
Senior Acquisitions Editor: Joyce Berendes
Senior Development Editor: Meredith L. Brittain
Editorial Coordinator: Varshaanaa SM
Marketing Manager: Amy Whitaker
Editorial Assistant: Sara Thul
Manager, Graphic Arts & Design: Stephen Druding
Art Director, Illustration: Jennifer Clements
Production Project Manager: Matthew West
Manufacturing Coordinator: Bernard Tomboc
Prepress Vendor: TNQ Tech

7th edition

Library of Congress Cataloging-in-Publication Data

ISBN-13: 978-1-975236-05-2

Cataloging in Publication data available on request from publisher.

shop.lww.com

QUADM0624

Dedication

To my mother and father, who still make me laugh when I think of them. And for my aunt, Rose Verno, who has seen incredible changes in the world over her 90 years, has always faced her health challenges with courage, and has been there for me throughout my life.

Preface

Each chapter in *Pathophysiology Made Incredibly Easy!* starts by briefly listing the topics that will be covered in the chapter, which lets readers quickly determine where they should focus. Questions at the end of each chapter challenge readers, allowing them to see how much information they absorbed. Colorful illustrations and cartoons make learning fun, which is the surest way to keep readers interested!

In addition, icons draw the reader's attention to important issues:

Now I get it! explains difficult concepts using illustrations and flowcharts.

Battling illness provides the latest treatments for diseases and disorders.

The genetic link connects genetics to many common disorders.

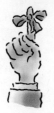

Memory joggers offer mnemonics and other aids to help you understand and remember difficult concepts.

However, the most important thing to remember is that pathophysiology is about people, not just disease. That is, pathophysiology is experienced by people; it's not just about changes that occur in cells, tissues, and organs. Pathophysiology is the study of human challenges and suffering. If you're studying this subject to become a health care provider, always remember that you are treating *people, not disease*—people who have a life with aspirations, loved ones, and responsibilities that are turned upside down by disease. I hope this book allows you to better understand the plight of those who are affected by disease during a time of uncertainty and vulnerability in their lives so that you can *help* them.

Fundamentals of Nursing Made Incredibly Easy! is a helpful addition to the *Made Incredibly Easy* series, serving as a handy reference for newly graduated and experienced nurses and also as a valuable guide for nursing students as they prepare for their nursing careers.

Theresa Capriotti, DO, MSN, CRNP, RN
Clinical Professor
M. Louise Fitzpatrick College of Nursing
Villanova University
Villanova, Pennsylvania

Contents

1 Pathophysiology basics 1

2 Infection, inflammation, immunity, cancer, and genetics 17

3 Cardiovascular system 39

4 Hematologic system 91

5 Respiratory system 129

6 Neurologic system 183

7 Gastrointestinal system 241

8 Endocrine system 299

9 Renal system 337

10 Immune system 377

11 Integumentary system 405

12 Sensory system 423

13 Reproductive system 453

Appendices and index

Practice makes perfect 496

Glossary 533

Index 539

Chapter 1

Pathophysiology basics*

Just the facts

In this chapter, you'll learn:

◆ the structure of cells and how cells reproduce, adapt, age, and die

◆ the concept of homeostasis and how it affects the body

◆ the causes of disease

◆ the process of disease development.

Understanding cells

The cell is the body's basic building block. It's the smallest living component of an organism. Many organisms are made up of one independent, microscopically tiny cell. Other organisms, such as humans, consist of millions of cells grouped into highly specialized units that function together throughout the organism's life.

Large groups of individual cells form tissues, such as muscle, blood, and bone. Tissues form the organs (such as the brain, heart, and liver), which are integrated into body systems (such as the central nervous system [CNS], cardiovascular system, and digestive system).

Cell components

Cells are composed of various structures, or *organelles*, each with specific functions. (See *Just your average cell*, page 2.) The organelles are contained in the *cytoplasm*—an aqueous mass—that's surrounded by the cell membrane. The largest organelle, the *nucleus*, controls cell activity and stores deoxyribonucleic acid (DNA), which carries genetic material and is responsible for cellular reproduction or division.

---

*Note: In this chapter, the term "male" refers to a person assigned male at birth, and the term "female" refers to a person assigned female at birth.

More components

The typical human cell is characterized by several additional elements:

- Adenosine triphosphate (ATP), the energy that fuels cellular activity, is made by the mitochondria.
- Mitochondrion is an organelle known as the powerhouse of the cell that utilizes oxygen in cellular aerobic metabolism to yield ATP (energy).
- Ribosomes and the endoplasmic reticulum synthesize proteins and metabolize fat within the cell; ribosomes can be likened to protein "factories" in the cell.
- The Golgi apparatus is an organelle that contains enzyme systems that package cellular proteins for secretion.
- Lysosomes are organelles that contain enzymes, which allow cytoplasmic digestion of cellular waste products.

Just your average cell

The illustration below shows cell components and structures. Each part has a function in maintaining the cell's life and homeostasis.

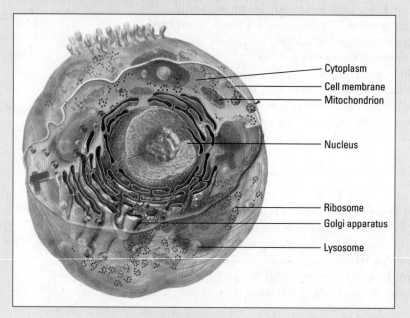

Cytoplasm
Cell membrane
Mitochondrion

Nucleus

Ribosome
Golgi apparatus
Lysosome

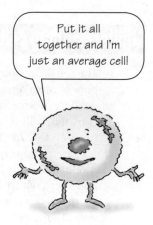

Put it all together and I'm just an average cell!

Cell division and reproduction

Individual cells are subject to wear and tear and must replicate themselves when they need to be replaced. Mitosis is the process of cell division.

Cell division occurs in two stages. In the first stage, *mitosis*, the nucleus and genetic material divide. In the second stage, *cytokinesis*, the cytoplasm divides, beginning during late anaphase or telophase. At the end of cytokinesis, the cell produces two genetically identical daughter cells. (See *Replicate and divide*, page 4.)

The great divide

Before mitotic division, a cell must duplicate its contents. This occurs during *interphase*, which is a growth phase that prepares the cell for the processes of mitosis and cytokinesis. During interphase, chromosomes, which are in the form of a mass of chromatin, make duplicates of themselves.

Interphase can be divided into four steps:
1. **Gap 0 (G0):** The cell is resting.
2. **Gap 1 (G1):** The cellular contents, excluding the chromosomes, are duplicated.
3. **S phase (Synthesis):** Chromatin (which consists of all chromosomes) duplicates itself.
4. **Gap 2 (G2):** The cell "double-checks" the duplicated chromosome pairs for error, making any needed repairs; this is sometimes called the cell's **"checkpoint."** The chromosomes then coil up and become a mass of chromatin again. Next, mitosis begins.

Mitosis is divided into four major phases:
1. Prophase
2. Metaphase
3. Anaphase
4. Telophase

The below subsections describe each phase.

Prophase

During prophase, the chromatin separates into chromosomes, and the nuclear membrane dissolves. Each chromosome pair is made up of two strands called *chromatids*, which are connected by a spindle of fibers called a *centromere*.

Metaphase

During metaphase, the centromeres divide, pulling the chromosome pairs apart. The centromeres then align themselves in the middle of the spindle.

Replicate and divide

These illustrations show the different phases of cell reproduction, or *mitosis.*

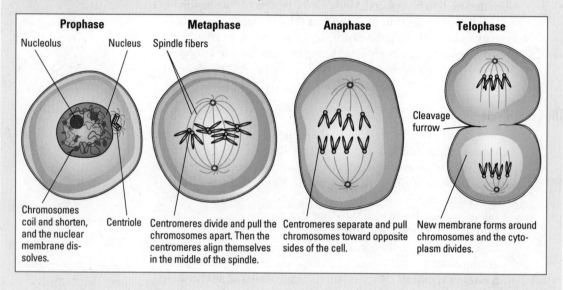

Prophase

Nucleolus   Nucleus   Spindle fibers   **Metaphase**

Anaphase

Telophase

Cleavage furrow

Chromosomes coil and shorten, and the nuclear membrane dissolves.

Centriole

Centromeres divide and pull the chromosomes apart. Then the centromeres align themselves in the middle of the spindle.

Centromeres separate and pull chromosomes toward opposite sides of the cell.

New membrane forms around chromosomes and the cytoplasm divides.

Anaphase

At the onset of anaphase, the centromeres begin to separate and pull the newly replicated chromosomes toward opposite sides of the cell. By the end of anaphase, 46 chromosomes are present on each side of the cell.

Telophase

In the final phase of mitosis—*telophase*—a new membrane forms around each set of 46 chromosomes. The spindle fibers disappear, cytokinesis occurs, and the cytoplasm divides, producing two identical new daughter cells.

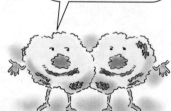

Now that all the work is done, there's two of us where there once was one!

Pathophysiologic concepts

The cell faces a number of challenges throughout its life. Both extrinsic and intrinsic factors can alter normal functioning of a cell; these stressors can include changes in the cell's s environment, attack of pathogens (e.g., bacteria, viruses), and injurious forces, among others.

Adaptation

Cells generally continue functioning despite challenging conditions or stressors. However, severe or prolonged stress or changes may injure or destroy cells. When cell integrity is threatened, the cell reacts by drawing on its reserves to keep functioning, by adaptive changes or by cellular dysfunction. If cellular reserve is insufficient, the cell dies. If enough reserve is available and the body doesn't detect abnormalities, the cell adapts by atrophy, hypertrophy, hyperplasia, metaplasia, or dysplasia. (See *Adaptive cell changes.*)

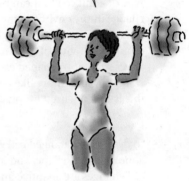

Wait 'til you see my biceps after this!

Atrophy

Atrophy is a reversible reduction in the size of the cell. It results from disuse, insufficient blood flow, malnutrition, denervation, or reduced endocrine stimulation. For example, after stroke, the muscle cells in a paralyzed arm that has lost sensory and motor function will be diminished in size.

Hypertrophy

Hypertrophy is an increase in the size of a cell due to an increased workload. It can result from normal physiologic conditions or abnormal pathologic conditions. For example, in bodybuilding an athlete lifts heavier and heavier weights to build the arm muscles; muscle cells increase in size, creating an enlarged biceps muscle.

Adaptive cell changes

When cells are stressed, they can undergo a number of changes.

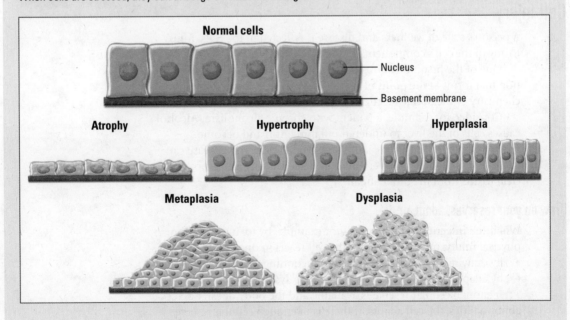

Hyperplasia

Hyperplasia, an increase in the number of cells, is caused by increased workload, hormonal stimulation, or lack of degeneration of cells. For example, as the older adult male ages into his 60s and 70s, the prostate gland undergoes hyperplasia and enlarges, which inhibits urinary flow.

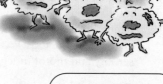

With hyperplasia, it sure can get crowded!

Metaplasia

Metaplasia is the replacement of one adult cell with another type of adult cell that can better endure the stress or the change in the environment. It's usually a response to chronic inflammation or irritation. For example, in chronic gastroesophageal reflux of stomach acid into the esophagus, the lower squamous-shaped esophageal epithelial cells can change to look more like columnar-shaped stomach cells; this is called Barrett esophagus.

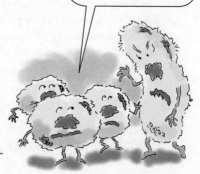

You look like you don't belong!

Dysplasia

In dysplasia, deranged cell growth of specific tissue results in abnormal size, shape, and appearance. Although dysplastic cell changes are adaptive and potentially reversible, they usually proceed to cancerous changes (also called neoplasia). For example, chronic human papilloma viral infection of the cervix can lead to cervical cancer.

Cell injury

A person's state of wellness and disease is reflected in the cells. Injury to any of the cell's components can lead to illness.

One of the first indications of cell injury is an area of inflammation that forms at the point of tissue injury. This lesion changes the chemistry of metabolic reactions within the cells of the tissue.

Consider, for example, a patient with chronic alcoholism. Alcohol causes cells of the liver to undergo inflammation and become replaced by fat cells; this is called fatty liver disease. This disease can cause dysfunction of the liver and diminished ability of the body to clear toxins from the bloodstream.

Draw on your reserves, adapt, or die

When cell integrity is threatened—for example, by toxins, infection, physical injury, or deficit injury—the cell reacts in one of two ways:
- by drawing on its reserves to keep functioning
- by adapting through changes or cellular dysfunction.

If enough cellular reserve is available and the body doesn't detect abnormalities, the cell adapts. If there isn't enough cellular reserve, cell death (*necrosis*) occurs. Necrosis is usually localized and easily identifiable.

Toxic injury

Toxic injuries may be caused by factors inside the body (called *endogenous factors*) or outside the body (called *exogenous factors*). Common endogenous factors include genetically determined metabolic errors, gross malformations, and hypersensitivity reactions. Exogenous factors include alcohol, cigarette smoke, ingested toxins, carbon monoxide, and drugs that alter cellular function. Examples include chemotherapeutic agents used for cancer treatment and immunosuppressive drugs that prevent rejection in organ transplant recipients.

Infectious or inflammatory injury

Viral, fungal, protozoan, and bacterial agents can cause inflammation, cell injury, or death. These organisms affect cell integrity, usually by interfering with cell synthesis, producing inflamed or infected cells. For example, human immunodeficiency virus infects the white blood cell (WBC). The virus takes over the cell's DNA, which programs WBCs to manufacture more HIV.

Physical injury

Physical injury results from a disruption in the cell or in the relationships of the intracellular organelles. Two major types of physical injury are thermal (electrical or radiation) and mechanical (trauma or surgery). Causes of thermal injury include radiation therapy for cancer, X-rays, and ultraviolet radiation of the sun. Causes of mechanical injury include motor vehicle accidents, gunshot wounds, falls, sports trauma, and frostbite.

Deficit injury

When a deficit of water, oxygen, blood flow, or nutrients occurs, or if constant temperature, pH, and adequate waste disposal aren't maintained, cellular function can't take place. A lack of just one of these basic requirements can cause cell disruption or death. The term for lack of blood flow to tissue or organ is *ischemia*. If ischemia is prolonged, this can lead to more permanent tissue death, termed *infarction*. Infarcted cells can then become necrotic.

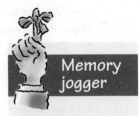

Memory jogger

To remember the four causes of cell injury, think of how the injury tipped (or **TIPD**) the scale of homeostasis:

Toxin or other lethal (cytotoxic) substance

Infection or Inflammation

Physical insult or injury

Deficit, or lack of water, oxygen, blood flow, or nutrients.

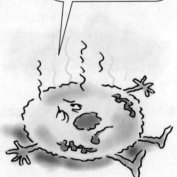

Without enough water, oxygen, blood flow, and nutrients, a cell will die.

Cell degeneration

A type of nonlethal cell damage known as *programmed degeneration*, also called *apoptosis*, generally occurs in specific cells in the body. Degeneration can occur in the cells of bone, ovaries, thymus gland, muscle, heart valves, blood vessels, skin, and nerves, and it can be caused by various processes:

- increased water in the cell or cellular swelling
- fatty or collagen infiltrates
- atrophy
- aging
- autophagocytosis, during which the cell absorbs some of its own parts
- calcification
- hyaline or amyloid infiltration

Talkin' 'bout degeneration

When changes within cells are identified, cell death can be prevented or reversed through prompt treatment. An electron microscope makes the identification of changes within cells easier. When a disease is diagnosed before the patient reports symptoms, it's termed *subclinical identification*. Unfortunately, many cell changes remain unidentifiable even under a microscope, making early detection impossible.

Cellular aging

During the normal process of cellular aging, cells may lose structure and function or control of cellular replication. Lost cell structure may cause a decrease in size or wasting away, a process called *atrophy*. Loss of control of cellular replication can cause *hyperplasia*. Two characteristics of lost cell function are:

- atrophy, loss of cell bulk and function (examples include ovarian degeneration in female menopausal people and decreased muscle mass in the older adult)
- hyperplasia, an increase in the number of cells (examples include benign prostatic hyperplasia [enlarged prostate gland] in the older adult male; pigmented skin lesions [age spots] in older adults).

Warning: This cell will self-destruct

Signs of aging occur in all body systems. Examples of the effects of cell aging include decreases in elasticity of blood vessels, bowel motility, muscle mass, and subcutaneous fat. The cell aging process limits the human life span.

Cell death may be caused by internal (intrinsic) factors that limit the cells' life span or external (extrinsic) factors that contribute to cell damage and aging. (See *In's and out's of cell aging.*)

In's and out's of cell aging

Factors that affect cell aging may be intrinsic or extrinsic, as outlined here.

Intrinsic factors
- Psychogenic
- Inherited
- Congenital
- Metabolic
- Degenerative
- Neoplastic
- Immunologic
- Nutritional

Extrinsic factors
Physical agents
- Force (trauma)
- Temperature
- Humidity
- Radiation
- Electricity
- Chemicals

Infectious agents
- Viruses
- Bacteria
- Fungi
- Parasites
- Prions

Homeostasis

The body is constantly striving to maintain a dynamic, steady state of internal balance called *homeostasis*. Every cell in the body is involved in maintaining homeostasis, on the cellular level and as part of an organism.

Any change or damage at the cellular level can affect the entire body. When an external stressor disrupts homeostasis, illness may occur. Examples of external stressors include injury, lack of nutrients, psychological stress, and invasion by parasites or other organisms. Throughout the course of a person's life, many external stressors affect the body's internal equilibrium.

Maintaining the balance

Three structures in the brain are responsible for maintaining homeostasis:
1. the medulla oblongata, the part of the brain stem that's associated with vital functions, such as consciousness, respiration, and circulation
2. the hypothalamus and pituitary gland, which regulate the function of endocrine glands and a person's growth, maturation, and reproduction
3. the reticular formation, a group of nerve cells or nuclei that form a large network of connected tissues that help control vital reflexes, which includes consciousness, cardiovascular function, and respiration.

Feedback mechanisms

Homeostasis is maintained by self-regulating feedback mechanisms of the endocrine system. These mechanisms have three components:
1. a sensor mechanism that senses disruptions in homeostasis
2. a control center that regulates the body's response to disruptions in homeostasis (CNS)
3. an effector mechanism that acts to restore homeostasis.

An endocrine (hormone-secreting) gland usually controls the sensor mechanism. A signal is sent to the control center in the CNS, which initiates the effector mechanism.

There are two types of feedback mechanisms:
1. a negative feedback mechanism, which works to restore homeostasis by decreasing hormone secretion within the system
2. a positive feedback mechanism, which triggers additional hormone secretion.

For negative feedback mechanisms to be effective, the body senses an excess level in the system and sends a signal to the CNS to decrease the effector mechanism. For example, when the body senses in the blood a high level of cortisol—which is secreted by the adrenal gland—it signals the pituitary gland to decrease stimulation of the adrenal gland in an attempt to return body functions to normal. Homeostasis of the blood cortisol level is then restored.

A positive feedback mechanism senses a deficit in the system and sends a signal to the CNS to stimulate the effector mechanism. For example, when blood glucose is too low, the body senses this, triggering the pancreas to secrete the hormone glucagon, which breaks down stored sugar in the liver to increase blood glucose. Homeostasis of the blood glucose level is then restored.

Disease and illness

Although disease and illness aren't synonymous, they're commonly used interchangeably. Disease occurs when homeostasis isn't maintained. The patient has subjective concerns, a specific medical history, and signs, symptoms, and laboratory or radiologic findings characteristic of that disease. Illness occurs when a person is no longer in their state of normal health. It's highly individualized and subjectively personal.

Consider a person who has coronary artery disease, diabetes, or asthma. This person may feel ill all the time because their body has adapted to the disease. In this situation, a person can still participate in life activities and perform necessary activities of daily living.

Genetic factors plus

Genetic factors (such as a tendency toward obesity), unhealthy behaviors (such as smoking), stress, and even the patient's perception of the disease (such as acceptance or denial) influence the course and outcome of a disease. Diseases are dynamic and may manifest in various ways, depending on the patient and the environment.

Cause

One aspect of disease is its cause (*etiology*). The cause of disease may be intrinsic (caused from within the body) or extrinsic (influenced from the outside). Diseases with no known cause are called *idiopathic*.

Intrinsic or extrinsic

The cause of disease is intrinsic when the disease occurs because of a malfunction or change within the body. Intrinsic factors include inherited traits, the patient's age, ethnicity, and sex assigned at birth.

Extrinsic causes of disease come from outside the body. These include infectious agents, mechanical trauma, smoking, chemical exposure, nutritional problems, drug use, temperature extremes, radiation exposure, and psychological stress.

Development

A disease's development is called its *pathogenesis*. Unless identified and successfully treated, most diseases progress according to a typical pattern of symptoms. Some diseases are self-limiting or resolve quickly with little to no intervention; others are chronic and never fully resolve. Patients with chronic diseases may undergo periods of remission and exacerbation. During remission, the patient's symptoms lessen in severity or disappear. During exacerbation, the patient experiences an aggravation of symptoms or an increase in the severity of the disease.

Telltale signs

Usually, a disease is discovered because of an increase or decrease in metabolism or cell division. Signs and symptoms may include hypofunction, such as constipation, and hyperfunction, such as increased mucus production.

How the cells respond to disease depends on the causative agent and the affected cells, tissues, and organs. Resolution of disease depends on many factors that occur over time.

Disease stages

Typically, diseases progress through these stages:

- *Exposure* or *injury.* Target tissue is exposed to a causative agent or is injured.
- *Incubation period.* The causative agent is exerting its mechanism, but no signs or symptoms are evident yet.
- *Prodromal period.* Signs and symptoms are usually very mild and nonspecific. This is the most contagious phase of an infectious disease.
- *Acute phase.* The disease reaches its full intensity, and the full extent of symptoms is evident.
- *Remission.* This second latent phase, in which symptoms are suppressed, occurs in only some chronic diseases.
- *Convalescence.* In this stage of rehabilitation, the patient progresses toward recovery after the termination of a disease.
- *Recovery.* In this stage, the patient regains health or normal functioning. No signs or symptoms of the disease occur.

Stress and disease

When a stressor such as a life change occurs, a person can respond in one of two ways: by adapting successfully or by failing to adapt. A maladaptive response to stress may result in disease. The underlying stressor may be real or perceived.

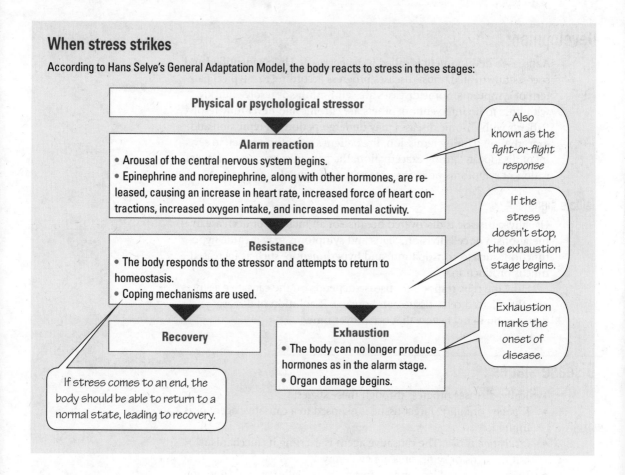

When stress strikes

According to Hans Selye's General Adaptation Model, the body reacts to stress in these stages:

Physical or psychological stressor

Alarm reaction
• Arousal of the central nervous system begins.
• Epinephrine and norepinephrine, along with other hormones, are released, causing an increase in heart rate, increased force of heart contractions, increased oxygen intake, and increased mental activity.

Also known as the fight-or-flight response

Resistance
• The body responds to the stressor and attempts to return to homeostasis.
• Coping mechanisms are used.

If the stress doesn't stop, the exhaustion stage begins.

Recovery

Exhaustion
• The body can no longer produce hormones as in the alarm stage.
• Organ damage begins.

Exhaustion marks the onset of disease.

If stress comes to an end, the body should be able to return to a normal state, leading to recovery.

Stressful stages

Hans Selye, a pioneer in the study of stress and disease, described stages of adaptation to a stressful event: alarm, resistance, and exhaustion or recovery. (See *When stress strikes*.) In the alarm stage, the body senses stress, and the CNS is aroused. The body releases chemicals to mobilize the fight-or-flight response. This release is the adrenaline rush associated with panic or aggression. In the resistance stage, the body either adapts and achieves homeostasis or fails to adapt and enters the exhaustion stage, resulting in disease.

Everything is under control

The stress response is controlled by actions taking place in the nervous and endocrine systems. These actions try to redirect energy to the organ—such as the heart, lungs, or brain—that is most affected by the stress.

Mind–body connection

Physiologic stressors may elicit a harmful response, leading to an identifiable illness or set of symptoms. Psychological stressors, such as the death of a loved one, may also cause a maladaptive response. Stress, whether physiologic or psychological, causes the adrenal gland to secrete excessive cortisol levels. Excessive cortisol levels decrease the function of white blood cells (WBCs), which are the major defenders in our immune system. Therefore, excessive stress can lead to decreased WBC function and, as a result, lowered immunity. Stressful events can also exacerbate some chronic diseases, such as diabetes, heart disease, and multiple sclerosis. Effective coping strategies can reduce the harmful effects of stress.

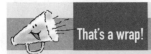 That's a wrap!

Pathophysiology basics review

Understanding cell components
• Organelles—specialized cell structures that perform different functions; they are contained in the cytoplasm and surrounded by the cell membrane
• Nucleus—responsible for cellular reproduction and division; stores DNA (the genetic material that's the blueprint for making all the structure and function of the organism)
• Other cell components:
  – Adenosine triphosphate (ATP): energy used by the cell
  – Mitochondrion: organelle that uses oxygen in aerobic metabolism to create energy
  – Ribosomes and endoplasmic reticulum: protein "factories" of the cell
  – Golgi apparatus: packages and releases proteins made by the cell
  – Lysosomes; organelle containing enzymes that break down cellular waste

Cell reproduction
• Stage 1—mitosis (nucleus and genetic material replicate and divide)
• Stage 2—cytokinesis (cytoplasm divides into two daughter cells)

Cell division phases
• Prophase—chromosomes coil and shorten, the nuclear membrane dissolves, and chromatids connect to a centromere
• Metaphase—centromeres divide, pulling the chromosomes apart, and align in the spindle
• Anaphase—centromeres separate and pull new replicated chromosomes to the opposite sides of the cell, resulting in 46 chromosomes on each side of the cell
• Telophase—final phase; new membrane forms around 46 chromosomes through cytokinesis, producing two identical new cells

Cell adaptation
• Atrophy—reversible reduction in size of cell
• Hypertrophy—increase in size of cell due to an increased workload
• Hyperplasia—increase in the number of cells
• Metaplasia—replacement of one adult cell type with another adult cell type that can better endure change or stress

(Continued)

Pathophysiology basics review *(continued)*

• Dysplasia—deranged cell growth of specific tissue results in abnormal size, shape, and appearance—usually precedes cancerous changes

Types of cell injury
• Toxic injury—endogenous (metabolic errors, gross malformations, hypersensitivity reactions, chemical injury), exogenous (alcohol, cigarette smoke, toxin ingestions, carbon monoxide, drugs)
• Infectious or inflammatory injury—viruses, fungi, parasites, bacteria, prions
• Physical injury—thermal (electrical, radiation), mechanical (trauma, surgery)
• Deficit injury—lack of a basic requirement such as oxygen, blood flow, or nutrients

Maintaining homeostasis
• Medulla, pituitary gland, reticular formation are regulators.
• Two types of feedback mechanisms maintain homeostasis:
 – Negative mechanism senses deficits of hormones and increases stimulation of endocrine organ to return the body to normal.
 – Positive mechanism senses excesses of hormones and decreases stimulation of the endocrine organ to return body to normal.

Differentiating disease and illness
Disease
• Occurs when homeostasis isn't maintained
• Influenced by age, ethnicity, sex assigned at birth, genetic factors, unhealthy behaviors, personality type, and perception of the disease
• Manifests in various ways depending on patient's environment

Illness
• Occurs when a person is no longer in a state of "normal" health
• Enables a person's body to adapt to the disease
• Is subjective

Causes of disease
• Intrinsic—hereditary traits, age, sex assigned at birth
• Extrinsic—infectious agents or behaviors, such as:
 – inactivity
 – smoking
 – drug use
• Stressors, such as:
 – physiologic
 – psychological

Disease development
Signs and symptoms
• Increase or decrease in metabolism or cell division
• Hypofunction such as constipation
• Hyperfunction such as increased mucus production

Disease stages
• Exposure or injury
• Incubation period
• Prodromal period
• Acute phase
• Remission
• Convalescence
• Recovery

Quick quiz

1. The organelle that contains the cell's DNA is the:
   A. mitochondria.
   B. Golgi apparatus.
   C. ribosome.
   D. nucleus.

   Answer: D. The nucleus, the largest organelle, stores DNA and is responsible for cellular reproduction.

2. When a cell gets injured, the first sign is:
   A. a biochemical lesion.
   B. an area of hyperplasia.
   C. a chromatid.
   D. cellular necrosis.

   Answer: A. Chemical reactions in the cell occur as a result of injury and form a biochemical lesion.

3. An extrinsic factor that can cause cell aging and death is:
   A. Down syndrome.
   B. sickle cell anemia.
   C. ultraviolet radiation.
   D. person's advanced age.

   Answer: C. An extrinsic factor, such as ultraviolet radiation, comes from an outside source.

4. Homeostasis can be defined as:
   A. a steady, dynamic state.
   B. a state of flux.
   C. an unbalanced state.
   D. an exaggeration of an original response.

   Answer: A. Homeostasis is a steady, dynamic state that may also be defined as a balancing act performed by the body to prevent illness.

Scoring

★★★ If you answered all four items correctly, fantastic! Your intrinsic and extrinsic understanding of pathophysiology basics is excellent.

★★ If you answered three items correctly, wonderful! Your test-taking skills have achieved a nice homeostasis!

★ If you answered fewer than three items correctly, no sweat! Review this material, and remember that there are many more Quick quizzes to go!

Suggested references

Norris T. (2025). *Porth's pathophysiology: Concepts of altered health states*. 11th ed. Wolters Kluwer.

Strayer D. S., Saffitz J. E. (2020). *Rubin's pathology: Mechanisms of human disease*. 8th ed. Wolters Kluwer.

Chapter 2

Infection, inflammation, immunity, cancer, and genetics*

Just the facts

In this chapter, you'll learn:

◆ the body's defense mechanisms: inflammation and immunity

◆ the four types of infective microorganisms and how they invade the body

◆ the pathophysiology of common infectious diseases

◆ classifications of cancer

◆ pathophysiology of neoplastic (cancer) cell growth

◆ the warning signs of cancer

◆ the process of cancer metastasis

◆ the role of genes and chromosomes and how cells divide

◆ the types of genetic abnormalities and how they are inherited.

Understanding infection, inflammation, immunity, cancer, and genetics

Inflammation and the immune response are the critical defense mechanisms of the body. These are the major mechanisms involved in fighting infection and cancer. A person's genetics influences the body's response to disease. Inflammation, the immune reaction, infection, cancer, and genetics all affect the cell and the cell cycle in different ways. Having a basic understanding of these topics will serve as an introduction to the diseases they cause. Chapter 1 illustrated how cells react in typical and atypical circumstances. In this chapter, we will discuss basic mechanisms of defense that apply to cell pathophysiology. The specific diseases these irregularities cause will then be discussed in future chapters.

*Note: In this chapter, the term "male" refers to a person assigned male at birth, and the term "female" refers to a person assigned female at birth.

Infection, inflammation, and immunity

Understanding infection, inflammation, and immunity

Infection is the process that occurs when a *pathogen*, a disease-causing microorganism, invades the body. Inflammation is the body's response to any type of cell injury, particularly cell injury caused by an invading microorganism. Immunity is the body's higher level of defense after the inflammation response. Immunity involves specific kinds of white blood cells called *lymphocytes*. Infection results when tissue-destroying microorganisms enter and multiply in the body. Some infections take the form of minor illnesses, such as colds and ear infections. Others result in sepsis, a life-threatening organ dysfunction caused by a dysregulated host response to infection.

Infection-causing microbes

Four types of microorganisms can enter the body and cause infection:
- Viruses
- Bacteria
- Fungi
- Parasites.

Viruses
Viruses are microscopic parasites that contain genetic material, such as deoxyribonucleic acid (DNA) or ribonucleic acid (RNA). They have no metabolic capability and need a host cell to replicate.

Viral hide-and-seek

Viral infections occur when normal inflammatory and immune responses fail. The virus develops in the cell and "hides" there. After it's introduced into the host cell, the inner capsule releases genetic material, causing the infection. Some viruses surround the host cell and preserve it; others kill the host cell on contact.

Bacteria
Bacteria are one-celled microorganisms that have no true nucleus and reproduce by cell division. Pathogenic bacteria contain cell-damaging proteins that cause infection. These proteins come in two forms:
- Exotoxins—released during cell growth
- Endotoxins—released when the bacterial cell wall decomposes. These toxins cause fever and aren't affected by antibiotics.

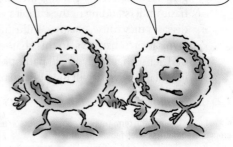

Viruses contain genetic material and need a host cell to replicate.

Bacteria are single-celled organisms that reproduce by cell division and may contain harmful proteins.

Bacteria are classified several other ways, such as by their shape, growth requirements, motility, and whether they're aerobic (requiring oxygen) or anaerobic (don't require oxygen to survive).

Fungi

Fungi are nonphotosynthetic plantlike microorganisms that reproduce asexually (by division) and live in the air, water, and soil. They are large compared to other microorganisms and contain a true nucleus. Some fungi live on the skin as part of the body's normal flora. Normal floras are microorganisms that live on or in the body without causing disease. However, some fungi can invade the body and are classified as:

- yeasts—round, single-celled, facultative anaerobes, which can live with or without oxygen
- molds—filament-like, multinucleated, aerobic microorganisms.

There's a fungus among us

Although fungi are part of the human body's normal flora, they can overproduce, especially when the normal flora is compromised. For example, vaginal yeast infections can occur with antibiotic treatment because normal floras are killed by the antibiotic, allowing yeast to reproduce. Infections caused by fungi are called *mycotic infections* because pathogenic fungi release mycotoxin. Most of these infections are mild unless they become systemic or the patient's immune system is compromised.

Parasites

Parasitic infections are more common in rural or developing areas than industrialized areas. *Parasites* are organisms that live on or inside another organism (the host), depend on the host for food and protection, and harm the host. Most common parasitic infections, such as pinworm and tapeworm, occur in the intestines.

A pathway for parasites

Parasites typically enter the body through the mouth or skin. Ingestion of parasites in contaminated food or water is the most common pathway for infection. Parasites, such as the microorganism that causes malaria, can enter the body by a mosquito bite. Parasites can also enter through the soles of the feet of a person walking barefoot; others can also enter through the skin or mouth of a person who swims or bathes in water that contains parasites.

Barriers to infection

A healthy person can usually ward off infections with the body's own defense mechanisms. The body has many built-in infection barriers, such as the skin and secretions from the eyes, nasal passages, prostate gland, testicles, stomach, and vagina. Most of these secretions contain bacteria-killing particles called *lysozymes*. Other body structures, such as cilia in the pulmonary airways that sweep foreign material from the breathing passages, also provide infection protection. Inflammation is the body's reaction to infection. Inflammation attempts to wall off the infection and allows white blood cells to get to the area of cell injury. Immunity is the mechanism by which white blood cells (specifically *lymphocytes*) attack microorganisms to defend the body.

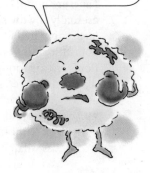

The body has built-in defense mechanisms against pathogens.

Trillions of harmless inhabitants

Normal floras are harmless microorganisms that reside on and in the body. They're found on the skin and in the nose, mouth, pharynx, distal intestine, colon, distal urethra, and vagina. The skin contains 10,000 microorganisms per square centimeter. Trillions of microorganisms are secreted from the GI tract daily.

Many of these microorganisms provide useful, protective functions. For example, the intestinal floras help synthesize vitamin K, which is an important part of the body's blood-clotting mechanism.

The infection process

Infection occurs when the body's defense mechanisms break down or when certain properties of microorganisms, such as virulence or toxin production, override the defense system.

Other factors that create a climate for infection include:
- poor nutrition.
- low immunity (immunosuppression).
- stress.
- humidity.
- poor sanitation.
- crowded living conditions.
- pollution.
- dust.
- medications.
- hospitalization (healthcare-associated infection).

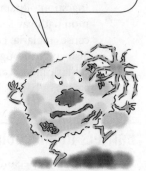

A pathogen may attach itself to a cell and release enzymes that destroy the cell's protective membrane.

Enter, attach, and spread

Infection results when a pathogen enters the body through direct contact, inhalation, ingestion, or an insect or animal bite. The pathogen then attaches itself to a cell and releases enzymes that destroy the cell's protective membrane. If not kept localized by defense mechanisms, it can spread through the bloodstream and lymphatic system, causing a bodywide infection called *sepsis*.

Striking while there's opportunity

Infections that strike people with weakened immune systems (termed *immunosuppression*) are called *opportunistic infections*. For example, patients with acquired immunodeficiency syndrome (AIDS) are plagued by opportunistic infections such as *Pneumocystis carinii* pneumonia.

Cancer

Understanding the impact of cancer

Cancer ranks second to cardiovascular disease (see Chapter 3) as the leading cause of death in the United States. One out of four deaths is due to cancer. In 2022, there were 1.9 million people diagnosed with cancer and more than 600,000 deaths. The four most common forms of cancer are lung, breast, colon, and prostate cancer. Over 50% of cancers are diagnosed in people over age 65.

The importance of early detection

In most cases, early detection of cancer or cardiovascular disease enables treatment that is more effective and a better prognosis for the patient. A careful assessment, beginning with history, is critical. In gathering assessment information, you need to ask the patient about risk factors, such as cigarette smoking, family history, exercise pattern, diet, and exposure to potential hazards, such as asbestos.

Abnormal cell growth in cancer

Cancer cells first develop from a mutation in a single cell. This cell grows without the control that characterizes normal cell growth. At a certain stage of development, the cancer cell fails to mature into the type of normal cell from which it originated. (See *Histologic characteristics of cancer cells.*) In addition to this uncontrolled localized growth, cancer cells can spread from the site of origin, a process called *metastasis*. (See *How cancer metastasizes*, page 22.)

Cancer classifications

Cancer is classified by the tissues or blood cells in which it originates. Most cancers originate from epithelial tissues and are called *carcinomas*. Others arise from the following tissues and cells:
- Glandular tissues (adenocarcinomas)
- Connective, muscle, and bone tissues (sarcomas)
- Tissue of the brain and spinal cord (gliomas)

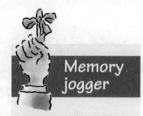

Memory jogger

When asking assessment questions, remember the American Cancer Society's mnemonic device, **CAUTION**.

Change in bowel or bladder habits

A sore that doesn't heal

Unusual bleeding or discharge

Thickening or lump

Indigestion or difficulty swallowing

Obvious changes in a wart or mole

Nagging cough or hoarseness

Histologic characteristics of cancer cells

Cancer is a destructive (malignant) growth of cells, which invades nearby tissues and may metastasize to other areas of the body. Dividing rapidly, cancer cells tend to be extremely aggressive.

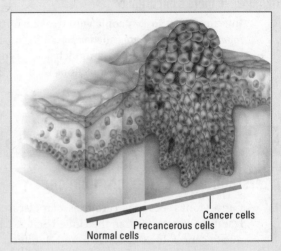

Cancer cells
Precancerous cells
Normal cells

 Now I get it!

How cancer metastasizes

Cancer cells may invade nearby tissues or metastasize (spread) to other organs. They may move to other tissues by any or all of the three routes described below.

Seeding

Cancer may penetrate the wall of an organ, move into a body cavity, and spread throughout that area.

Venous system

Cancer cells may travel through the veins, commonly to the liver and the lungs.

Lymphatic system

Cancer cells may move through this series of channels from the tissues to lymph nodes and eventually, via the circulatory system, to distant sites in the body.

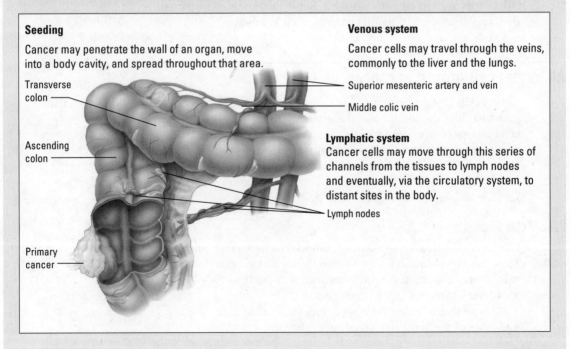

Transverse colon

Ascending colon

Primary cancer

Superior mesenteric artery and vein

Middle colic vein

Lymph nodes

- Pigment skin cells (melanomas)
- Plasma cells (myelomas)
- Lymphatic tissue (lymphomas)
- Leukocytes (leukemia).
    Cancer cells metastasize through three mechanisms:
1. By directly spreading by invasion of other body tissues and organs
2. By circulation through the blood and lymphatic system
3. By direct transportation of cells from one site to another (for example, cells can accidentally be carried to another site on instruments or gloves during surgery or another procedure).

What causes cancer?

All cancers involve the malfunction of genes that control cell growth and division. A cell's transformation from normal to cancerous is called *carcinogenesis*. Carcinogenesis has no single cause but probably results from complex interactions between viruses, physical and chemical carcinogens, and genetic, dietary, immunologic, metabolic, and hormonal factors.

The virus factor

Clinical studies show that some viruses can cause genetic changes in cells that allow development of cancerous changes. The Epstein–Barr virus that causes infectious mononucleosis is associated with Burkitt lymphoma, Hodgkin disease, and nasopharyngeal cancer. Human papillomavirus, cytomegalovirus, and herpes simplex virus type 2 are linked to cancer of the cervix. Human papilloma virus is also linked to vulvar, anorectal, oropharyngeal, and penile cancers. The hepatitis B and hepatitis C viruses cause hepatocellular carcinoma, the human T-cell lymphotropic virus causes adult T-cell leukemia, and the human immunodeficiency virus is associated with Kaposi sarcoma.

Overexposed cells

The relationship between excessive exposure to the sun's ultraviolet (UV) rays and skin cancer is well established. Damage caused by UV light and subsequent sunburn are linked to skin cancers, such as squamous cell carcinoma, basal cell carcinoma, and melanoma. Tanning beds and booths and sunlamps should be avoided because they are another source of UV radiation.

Radiation exposure may induce tumor development. Other factors, such as the patient's tissue type, age, length of exposure, and hormonal status, also contribute to the carcinogenic effect.

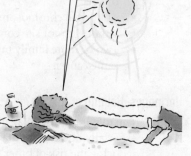

Always use a broad-spectrum sunscreen with an SPF of 30 or higher to help protect against the sun's ultraviolet rays.

Something in the air

Substances in the environment can cause cancer by damaging DNA in the cells. Examples of common carcinogens and related cancers are:

- tobacco (lung, pancreatic, kidney, bladder, mouth, and esophageal cancer)
- asbestos and airborne aromatic hydrocarbons (lung cancer)
- alkylating agents (leukemia).

Immune factor

Evidence suggests that a severely compromised immune system can lead to the development of certain cancers. Transplant recipients receiving immunosuppressant drugs and those with AIDS have an increased risk of certain cancers, such as Kaposi sarcoma, non-Hodgkin lymphoma, and skin cancer.

Danger at the diner

Colorectal cancer is associated with low-fiber and high-fat diets, diets high in red or processed meat, heavy alcohol consumption, and long-term smoking. Food additives, such as nitrates, and food preparation methods, such as charbroiling, may also contribute to the development of cancer.

The genetic factor

About 5% of all cancers are strongly hereditary. An inherited genetic alteration confers a very high risk of developing one or more specific types of cancer. These cancers may be autosomal recessive, X-linked, or autosomal dominant disorders. (See the "Genetics" section later in this chapter.) Such cancers share these characteristics:

- Early onset
- Increased incidence of bilateral cancer in paired organs (breasts, adrenal glands, and kidneys)
- Increased incidence of multiple primary cancers in nonpaired organs
- Abnormal chromosomes in tumor cells
- Unique tumor site combinations
- Two or more family members in the same generation with the same cancer.

Hormones: Helping or hurting?

The role hormones play in cancer is variable. Excessive hormone use, especially of estrogen, may contribute to certain forms of cancer while reducing the risk of other forms.

The best defense

One theory suggests that the body develops cancer cells continuously but that the immune system recognizes them as foreign and destroys them. According to the theory, this defense mechanism, called *immunosurveillance*, promotes antibody production, cellular immunity, and immunologic memory. Therefore, an interruption in immunosurveillance could lead to the overproduction of cancer cells and, possibly, a tumor.

Genetics

Understanding genetics

Genetics is the study of heredity, the passing of traits from biological parents to their children. Physical traits, such as hair and eye color, are hereditary. Biochemical and physiologic traits such as the tendency to develop certain syndromes and diseases are also inherited.

Transmitting an inheritance

Inherited traits are transmitted from biological parents to offspring through genes in germ cells, or gametes. Human gametes are eggs, or ova, and sperm. A person's genetic makeup is determined at fertilization, when ovum and sperm are united.

In the nucleus of each germ cell are structures called *chromosomes*, which are made up of DNA. Chromosomes are usually depicted as pairs; each individual chromosome is termed a *chromatid*. Each chromatid contains a strand of genes. DNA is a long molecule that's made up of thousands of segments called *genes*. Each of the traits that a person inherits—from blood type to toe shape and a myriad of others in between—is coded in their genes.

Counting chromosomes

A human ovum contains 23 chromosomes. A sperm also contains 23 chromosomes, each similar in size and shape to a chromosome in the ovum. When ovum and sperm unite, the corresponding chromosomes pair up. The result is a fertilized cell called a *zygote*, which has 46 chromosomes (23 pairs) in the nucleus.

The fertilized cell soon undergoes cell division (*mitosis*). In mitosis, each of the 46 chromosomes produces an exact duplicate of itself. The cell then divides, and each new cell receives one set of 46 chromosomes. Each of the two cells that result likewise divides, and so on, eventually forming a many-celled human body. Therefore, each cell in a person's body (except the ova or sperm) contains 46 identical chromosomes.

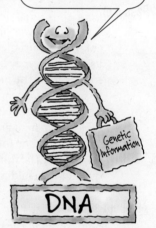

I'm two strands of DNA that can be separated into 23 pairs of chromosomes, which are made up of genes.

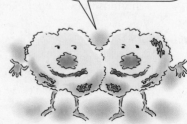

In mitosis, DNA duplicates, and then the cell divides into two equal cells.

A different division

The ova and sperm are formed by a different cell division process called *meiosis*. In meiosis, there are two cell divisions, and each new cell (an ovum or sperm) receives one set of 23 chromosomes.

Location, location, location

The location of a gene on a chromosome is called a *locus*. There are thousands of genes. The locus of each gene is specific and doesn't vary from person to person. All human gene loci have been numbered by the Human Genome Project. Each of the thousands of genes in an ovum pairs up with the corresponding gene from a sperm cell at fertilization. Therefore, everyone has chromosomes that consist of gene pairs; one gene from their biological mother (from the ovum) and one gene from their biological father (from the sperm cell).

Pass it on

A person receives one set of chromosomes and genes from each parent. This means there are two genes for each trait that a person inherits. One gene may be more influential than the other in developing a specific trait. The more influential gene is said to be *dominant*, and the less influential gene is *recessive*.

For example, a child may receive a gene for brown eyes from one biological parent and a gene for blue eyes from the other biological parent. The gene for brown eyes is dominant; the gene for blue eyes is recessive. The dominant gene is more likely to be expressed; consequently, the child is more likely to have brown eyes.

All about alleles

A variation of a gene and the trait it controls—such as brown, green, or blue eye color—is called an *allele*. When two different alleles are inherited, they're said to be *heterozygous*. When the alleles are identical, they're termed *homozygous*.

If the allele is dominant, only one copy may be necessary for expression of the trait, so a dominant allele may be expressed in both the homozygous and heterozygous states. A recessive allele is incapable of expression unless recessive alleles are carried by both chromosomes in a pair.

Gen XX (or XY)

Of the 23 pairs of chromosomes in each living human cell, 22 pairs are *not* involved in controlling a person's sex assigned at birth; they're called *autosomes*.

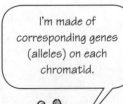

I'm made of corresponding genes (alleles) on each chromatid.

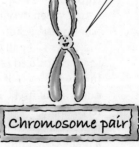

Chromosome pair

The two sex chromosomes of the 23rd pair determine a person's sex assigned at birth. In a person assigned female at birth, both chromosomes are relatively large, and each is designated by the letter X; people assigned female at birth have two X chromosomes. In a person assigned male at birth, one sex chromosome is an X chromosome, and one is a smaller chromosome, designated by the letter Y. (As noted on the first page of this chapter, in this chapter, the term "male" refers to a person assigned male at birth, and the term "female" refers to a person assigned female at birth.)

Each gamete (sperm cell) produced by a male contains either an X or a Y chromosome. When a sperm with an X chromosome fertilizes an ovum, the offspring is female. When a sperm with a Y chromosome fertilizes an ovum, the offspring is male.

An explanation of mutation

A mutation is a permanent change in genetic material. When a gene mutates, it may produce a trait that's different from its original trait. Gene mutations in a gamete may be transmitted during reproduction. Some mutations cause serious or deadly disorders that occur in three different forms:
- Single-gene disorders
- Chromosomal disorders
- Multifactorial disorders.

Single-gene disorders

Single-gene disorders are inherited in clearly identifiable patterns. Two important inheritance patterns are called *autosomal dominant* and *autosomal recessive*. Because there are 22 pairs of autosomes and only one pair of sex chromosomes, most hereditary disorders are caused by autosomal defects.

In a third inheritance pattern, sex-linked inheritance, single-gene disorders are passed through the sex chromosome, usually the X chromosome.

Parent patterns

Keep the definitions of the terms *dominant* and *recessive* in mind. Dominant genes produce abnormal traits in offspring even if only one biological parent has the gene; recessive genes don't produce abnormal traits unless both biological parents have the gene and pass them to their offspring.

Autosomal dominant inheritance
The autosomal dominant inheritance pattern has these characteristics:
- Male and female offspring are affected equally.

- One of the biological parents is also usually affected.
- If one biological parent is affected, their biological children have a 50% chance of being affected.
- If both biological parents are affected, all of their biological children will be affected.

Marfan syndrome is an example of an autosomal dominant disorder. (See *Understanding autosomal dominant inheritance*, page 29.)

Autosomal recessive inheritance

The autosomal recessive inheritance pattern has these characteristics:

- Male and female offspring are affected equally.
- If both biological parents are unaffected but heterozygous for the trait (carriers), each of their biological offspring has a one in four chance of being affected.
- If both biological parents are affected, all of their biological offspring will be affected.
- If one biological parent is affected and the other is not a carrier, all of their biological offspring will be unaffected but will carry the altered gene.

Memory jogger

Remember:
Dominant genes **dominate** any situation—even if only one biological parent carries the gene.

Recessive genes **recede** into the background, unless both biological parents carry the gene.

Now I get it!

Understanding autosomal dominant inheritance

This diagram (called a Punnett square) shows the possible offspring of a biological parent with recessive normal genes (aa) and a biological parent with an altered dominant gene (Aa). Note that with each pregnancy, there is a 50% chance that the offspring will be affected.

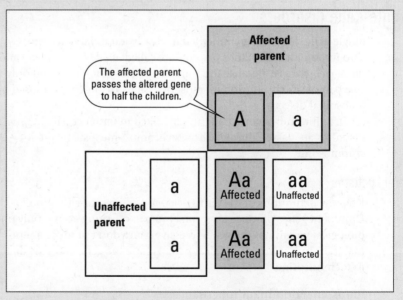

Note: In this figure, "parent" means "biological parent," and "children" means "biological children."

- If one biological parent is affected and the other is a carrier, each of their biological offspring will have a one in two chance of being affected and a one in two chance of being a carrier.
- Certain autosomal recessive conditions are more common in specific ethnic groups; for example, cystic fibrosis is more common in White individuals, and sickle cell anemia is more common in African Americans individuals. (See *Understanding autosomal recessive inheritance*, page 29.)

Negative history

In many cases, no evidence of the trait appears in past generations. In clinical jargon, you can say the patient has a "negative family history."

Now I get it!

Understanding autosomal recessive inheritance

This Punnett square shows the possible offspring of two unaffected biological parents, each with an altered recessive gene (a) on an autosome. Each offspring will have a one in four chance of being affected and a two in four chance of being a carrier.

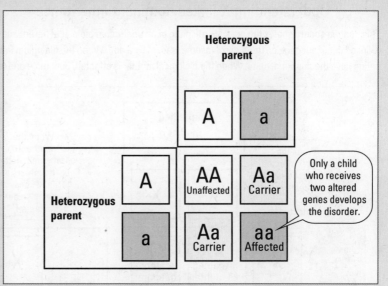

Note: In this figure, "parent" means "biological parent," and "child" means "biological child."

Sex-linked inheritance

Some genetic disorders are caused by genes located on the sex chromosomes and are termed *sex linked*. The Y chromosome carries relatively few disease-causing genes, so the term *sex linked* usually refers to *X-linked* disorders.

Because females receive two X chromosomes (one from the biological father and one from the biological mother), they can be homozygous for a disease allele, homozygous for a normal allele, or heterozygous.

Because males have only one X chromosome, a single X-linked recessive gene can cause disease in a male. In comparison, a female needs two copies of the diseased gene. Therefore, males are more commonly affected by X-linked recessive diseases than females. (See *Understanding X-linked dominant inheritance* and *Understanding X-linked recessive inheritance*, pages 30 and 31.)

> A single X-linked recessive gene can cause disease in a male. In a female, two copies of the diseased gene are needed.

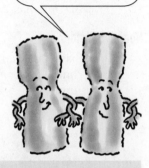

 Now I get it!

Understanding X-linked dominant inheritance

This Punnett square shows the possible offspring of an unaffected biological parent and a biological parent with an X-linked dominant gene on the X chromosome (shown by a dot). When the biological father is affected, only female offspring have the abnormal gene. When the biological mother is affected, both male and female offspring may be affected.

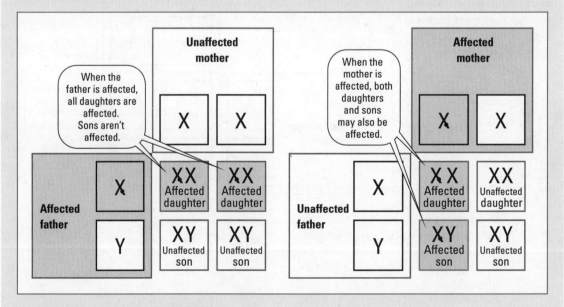

Note: In this figure, "parent" means "biological parent," "child" means "biological child," "son" means offspring assigned male at birth, and "daughter" means offspring assigned female at birth.

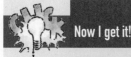

Understanding X-linked recessive inheritance

This Punnett square shows the possible offspring of an unaffected biological parent and a biological parent with a recessive gene on the X chromosome (shown by an open dot). All of the female offspring of an affected biological father will be carriers. The male offspring of a biological mother may inherit a recessive gene on the X chromosome and be affected by the disease.

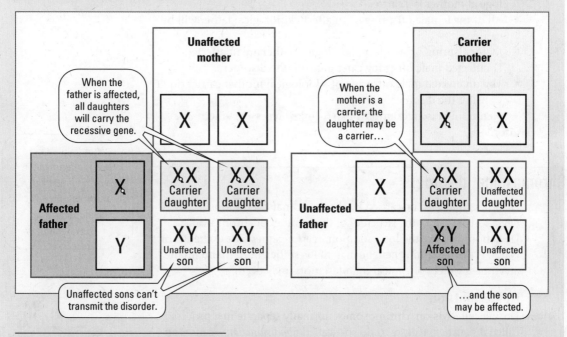

Note: In this figure, "parent" means "biological parent," "child" means "biological child," "son" means offspring assigned male at birth, and "daughter" means offspring assigned female at birth.

Dominant facts

Characteristics of X-linked dominant inheritance include the following:

- A person with the abnormal trait typically will have one affected biological parent.
- If a biological father has an X-linked dominant disorder, all of the female offspring and none of the male offspring will be affected.
- If a biological mother has an X-linked dominant disorder, there's a 50% chance that each child will be affected.
- Evidence of the inherited trait most commonly appears in the family history.

- X-linked dominant disorders are commonly lethal in male off-spring (prenatal or neonatal deaths). The family history may show miscarriages and the predominance of female offspring.

A recessive reading

Here are the basic facts about the X-linked recessive inheritance pattern:

- In most cases, affected people are males with unaffected biological parents. In rare cases, the biological father is affected, and the biological mother is a carrier.
- All of the female offspring of an affected biological father will be carriers.
- Male offspring of an affected biological father are unaffected. Unaffected male offspring can't transmit the disorder.
- The unaffected male offspring of a biological mother carrier don't transmit the disorder.
  Hemophilia is an example of an X-linked recessive inheritance disorder.

Chromosomal disorders

Disorders may also be caused by chromosomal aberrations—deviations in either the structure or the number of chromosomes. Deviations involve the loss, addition, rearrangement, or exchange of genes. If the remaining genetic material is sufficient to maintain life, an endless variety of clinical manifestations may occur.

Nondisjunction

During cell division, chromosomes normally separate in a process called *disjunction*. Failure to do so—called *nondisjunction*—causes an unequal distribution of chromosomes between the two resulting cells. Gain or loss of chromosomes is usually due to nondisjunction of autosomes or sex chromosomes during meiosis.

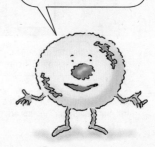

Nondisjunction is a malfunction in which some of my chromosomes fail to separate as they should.

One fewer or more

When chromosomes are gained or lost, the name of the affected cell contains the suffix "-somy." A cell that's missing a chromosome is called a *monosomy*. If the monosomy involves an autosome, the cell will be nonviable. However, monosomy X can be viable and result in a female who has Turner syndrome. A cell that contains one extra chromosome is called a *trisomy*. (See *Understanding nondisjunction of chromosomes*.)

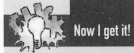

Understanding nondisjunction of chromosomes

This illustration shows normal disjunction and nondisjunction of an ovum. The result of nondisjunction is one trisomic cell and one monosomic (nonviable) cell.

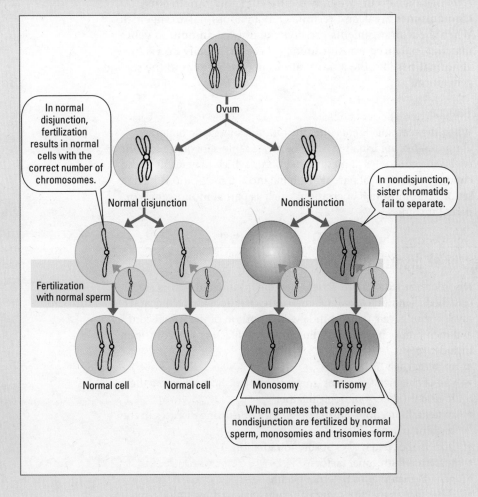

Mixed results

Nondisjunction may occur during very early cell divisions after fertilization and may or may not involve all the resulting cells. A mixture of cells, some with a specific chromosome aberration and some with normal cells, results in *mosaicism*. The effect on the offspring depends on the percentage of normal cells.

The incidence of nondisjunction increases with the age of the biological parents, especially maternal age. Also, miscarriages can result from chromosomal aberrations. Fertilization of an ovum with a chromosome aberration by a sperm with a chromosome aberration usually doesn't occur.

Translocation

A *translocation* occurs when two different (nonhomologous) chromosomes break and reconnect in an abnormal arrangement. When the rearrangements preserve the normal amount of genetic material (balanced translocations), there are usually no visible abnormalities, but the abnormalities may be present in the second generation.

A shift in balance

When the rearrangements alter the amount of genetic material, abnormalities are usually visible or measurable. Unequal separation of the chromosomes at meiosis can occur, which may result in the children of biological parents with balanced translocations having serious chromosomal aberrations, such as partial monosomies or partial trisomies.

Multifactorial disorders

Disorders caused by both genetic and environmental factors are classified as multifactorial. Examples are cleft lip, cleft palate, and myelomeningocele (spina bifida with a portion of the spinal cord and membranes protruding). Environmental factors that contribute include:
- maternal age
- use of chemicals (such as drugs, alcohol, or hormones) by the biological mother or biological father
- maternal infections during pregnancy or existing diseases in the birthing parent
- maternal or paternal exposure to radiation
- maternal nutritional factors
- general maternal or paternal health
- other factors including high altitude, maternal-fetal blood incompatibility, maternal smoking, and poor-quality prenatal care.

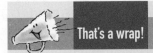
That's a wrap!

Infection, inflammation, immunity, cancer, and genetics review

Infection facts
- Infection is a host's response to a pathogen.
- Viruses, bacteria, fungi, and parasites cause infection.
- Infection results when a pathogen enters the body; the pathogen attaches to a cell and destroys the cell's protective membrane, spreads through blood and lymph nodes, multiplies, and causes infection in target organ or tissue.

Understanding infection
- Results when a host organism responds to a pathogen or disease-causing substance
- Develops when tissue-destroying microorganisms enter and multiply in the body
- Takes the form of minor illnesses, such as colds and ear infections, or results in a life-threatening condition called *sepsis*, which causes widespread vasodilation and multiple organ dysfunction syndrome
- Caused by four types of microorganisms:
  - Viruses
  - Bacteria
  - Fungi
  - Parasites

Infection development
Infection occurs when the body's defense mechanisms break down or when microorganisms override the defense system. Other factors include:
- poor nutrition
- low immunity (immunosuppression)
- stress
- humidity
- poor sanitation
- crowded living conditions
- pollution
- dust
- medications

  Infection results when a pathogen enters the body through direct contact, inhalation, ingestion, or an insect or animal bite.

Cancer facts
- Second leading cause of death
- Classified by tissues or blood cells of origin
- No single cause identified

Understanding cancer
Abnormal cell growth
Cancer is characterized by the abnormal growth of cells that develop from tissues or blood. Most cancers originate from epithelial tissues and are called *carcinomas*. Others arise from these tissues and cells:
- Glandular tissues (adenocarcinoma)
- Connective, muscle, and bone tissues (sarcomas)
- Tissue of the brain and spinal cord (gliomas)
- Pigment cells (melanomas)
- Plasma cells (myelomas)
- Lymphatic tissue (lymphomas)
- Leukocytes (leukemia)

Uncontrolled cell growth
Cancer cells develop without the control that normal cells have, and they spread from the site of origin in three ways:
- Circulating through the blood and lymphatic system
- Accidentally transplanted during surgery
- Spreading invasively to adjacent organs and tissues

Causes
All cancers involve malfunction of genes that control growth and division of cells. Carcinogenesis, the cell's transformation from normal to cancerous, has no single cause but may result from complex interactions between:
- viruses
- physical and chemical carcinogens
- genetic, dietary, immunologic, metabolic, and hormonal factors

Genetic facts
- Ova and sperm each contain 23 chromosomes.
- A fertilized cell, termed a *zygote*, has 46 chromosomes.
- Each chromosome contains genes.

(Continued)

Infection, inflammation, immunity, cancer, and genetics review *(continued)*

- Genes are segments of DNA.
- A person receives one set of chromosomes and genes from each biological parent.
- The more influential gene is dominant.
- The less influential gene is recessive.

Types of disorders
- Single gene—inherited in clearly identifiable patterns; two important inheritance patterns are:

– autosomal dominant
– autosomal recessive
- Chromosomal—deviations in either the structure or the number of chromosomes involving the loss, addition, rearrangement, or exchange of genes
- Multifactorial—caused by genetic and environmental factors

Quick quiz

1. The four types of microorganisms that cause infection are:
   A. bacteria, flora, microbes, and viruses.
   B. bacteria, viruses, fungi, and parasites.
   C. fungoids, spirochetes, mycoplasma, and parasites.
   D. bacteria, yeast, flora, and parasites.

Answer: B. Bacteria, viruses, fungi, and parasites are pathogens that enter the body and cause infections.

2. An opportunistic infection occurs because:
   A. the host has an altered, weak immune system.
   B. the pathogen is especially persistent.
   C. a large number of pathogens attack the host cells.
   D. the host has a fever.

Answer: A. Opportunistic infections occur in AIDS patients and others whose immune systems aren't functioning effectively.

3. The transformation of a cell from normal to cancerous is called:
   A. metastasis.
   B. carcinogenesis.
   C. proliferation.
   D. progression.

Answer: B. Carcinogenesis is a cell's transformation from normal to cancerous.

4. A person who has two different alleles is considered:
   A. heterozygous.
   B. codominant.
   C. homozygous.
   D. recessive.

Answer: A. When two different alleles of a gene are inherited, they are heterozygous.

Scoring

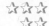 If you answered all four items correctly, awesome!

If you answered three items correctly, that's terrific!

If you answered fewer than three items correctly, don't worry! Remember that early detection is key, and you still have time to assess your learning skills, review the chapter again, and improve your knowledge.

Suggested references

American Cancer Society. (2023). *Cancer facts and figures 2022*. https://www.cancer.org/research/cancer-facts-statistics/all-cancer-facts-figures/cancer-facts-figures-2022.html

Centers for Disease Control and Prevention. (2021). *Genetics basics*. https://www.cdc.gov/genomics/about/basics.htm

Centers for Disease Control and Prevention. (2022). *U.S. cancer statistics: Highlights from 2019 incidence*. https://www.cdc.gov/cancer/uscs/about/data-briefs/no29-USCS-highlights-2019-incidence.htm

National Institutes of Health (NIH). National Human Genome Research Institute. (2022). *Human genome project fact sheet*. https://www.genome.gov/about-genomics/educational-resources/fact-sheets/human-genome-project

National Institutes of Health (NIH). U.S. National Library of Medicine. National Center for Biotechnology Information (NCBI). (2022). *Human genome resources at NCBI*. https://www.ncbi.nlm.nih.gov/projects/genome/guide/human/index.shtml

Norris, T. (2025). *Porth's pathophysiology: Concepts of altered health states*. 10th ed. Wolters Kluwer.

Strayer, D. S., & Saffitz, J. E. (2020). *Rubin's pathology: Mechanisms of human disease*. 8th ed. Wolters Kluwer.

Chapter 3

Cardiovascular system*

Just the facts

In this chapter, you'll learn:

♦ the relationship between oxygen supply and demand

♦ risk factors for cardiovascular disease

♦ causes, pathophysiology, diagnostic tests, and treatments for several common cardiovascular disorders.

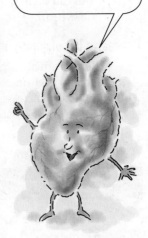

My function is so vital that it defines the very presence of life.

Understanding the cardiovascular system

The cardiovascular system begins its activity when the fetus is barely 1 month old, and it's the last system to cease activity at the end of life.

The heart, arteries, veins, and lymphatics make up the cardio-vascular system. These structures transport life-supporting oxygen and nutrients to cells, remove metabolic waste products, and carry hormones from one part of the body to another. Circulation requires normal heart function because the heart's continuous rhythmic con-tractions propel blood through the system.

Still the leading cause of death

Despite advances in disease detection and treatment, cardiovascu-lar disease remains the leading cause of death in the United States, accounting for about 700,000 deaths annually—that's one in every five deaths. Furthermore, it's estimated that 121 million US adults are living with at least one type of cardiovascular disease. Heart attack, or myocardial infarction (MI), is the primary cause of cardiovascular-related deaths. In the United States, someone has an MI every 40 sec-onds. MI may occur with little or no warning.

---

*Note: In this chapter, the term "male" refers to a person assigned male at birth, and the term "female" refers to a person assigned female at birth.

Oxygen balancing act

A critical balance exists between myocardial oxygen supply and demand. A decrease in oxygen supply or an increase in the heart muscle's oxygen demand can disturb this balance and threaten myocardial function. Coronary arteries supply blood flow, which contains the oxygen that travels to the myocardium.

The four major determinants of myocardial oxygen demand are:

- heart rate
- contractile force
- muscle mass
- ventricular wall tension

Cardiac workload and oxygen demand increase if the heart rate speeds up or if the force of contractions becomes stronger. This can occur in hypertension, ventricular dilation, or heart muscle hypertrophy or as a result of the action of some medications.

The heart's law of supply and demand

If myocardial oxygen demand increases, so must oxygen supply. To effectively increase oxygen supply, coronary artery perfusion must also increase. Tissue hypoxia—the most potent stimulus—causes coronary arteries to dilate and increase coronary blood flow.

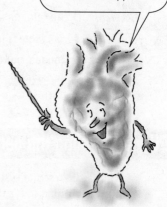

If myocardial oxygen demand increases, so must oxygen supply.

Now I get it!

How the coronary arteries supply the heart muscle

The right and left coronary arteries arise off the aorta. The left coronary artery supplies blood to the left ventricle—the main pump of the heart. The left anterior descending (LAD) artery is the most common site of MI.

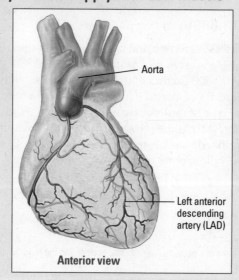

Aorta

Left anterior descending artery (LAD)

Anterior view

Normal coronary vessels can dilate and increase blood flow five to six times above resting levels. However, stenotic (narrowed), atherosclerotic coronary arteries can't dilate, so oxygen deficit may result.

One-way ticket

Normally, blood flows unimpeded across the heart valves in one direction. The valves open and close in response to a pressure gradient. When the pressure in the chamber proximal to the valve exceeds the pressure in the chamber beyond the valve, the valves open. When the pressure beyond the valve exceeds the pressure in the proximal chamber, the valves close. The valve leaflets, or cusps, are so responsive that even a pressure difference of less than 1 mm Hg between chambers will open and close them.

How low can you flow?

Valvular disease is the major cause of low blood flow. A diseased valve allows blood to flow backward across leaflets that haven't closed securely. This phenomenon is called *regurgitation* (or insufficiency). The backflow of blood through the valves forces the heart to pump more blood, increasing cardiac workload. The valve opening may also become restricted by calcium buildup and impede the forward flow of blood. This is referred to as *stenosis*.

Now I get it!

Cardiac valves

There are four cardiac valves that keep the flow of blood through the heart moving in the correct direction: the mitral valve and tricuspid valve are between the atria and ventricles; the pulmonary valve is at the opening of the pulmonary artery; and the aortic valve is at the opening of the aorta.

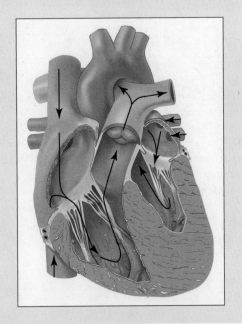

The heart may fail to meet the tissues' metabolic requirements for blood and fail to function as a pump. Eventually, the circulatory system may fail to perfuse body tissues, and blood volume and vascular tone may be altered.

Inner awareness

The body closely monitors both blood volume and vascular tone. Blood flow to each tissue is monitored by microvessels, which measure how much blood each tissue needs and control the local blood flow. The nerves that control circulation also help direct blood flow to tissues.

How the heart responds

The heart pays attention to the tissues' demands. It responds to the return of blood through the veins and to nerve signals that make it pump the required amounts of blood.

Under pressure

Arterial pressure is carefully regulated by the body: if it falls below or rises above its normal mean level, immediate circulatory changes occur.

If arterial pressure falls below normal, then an increase occurs in:
- heart rate
- force of contraction
- constriction of arterioles

If arterial pressure rises above normal, these changes occur:
- reflex slowing of heart rate
- decreased force of contraction
- vasodilation

Risk factors

Risk factors for cardiovascular disease fall into two categories: those that are modifiable and those that are nonmodifiable.

Modifiable risk factors

Some risk factors can be avoided or altered, potentially slowing the disease process or even reversing it. These factors include:
- elevated serum lipid levels
- hypertension
- cigarette smoking
- uncontrolled diabetes
- sedentary lifestyle
- stress

- obesity—especially abdominal (waist measurement greater than 40″ [101.6 cm] in males and greater than 35″ [88.9 cm] in females)
- excessive intake of saturated fats, carbohydrates, and salt

Nonmodifiable risk factors

Four nonmodifiable factors increase a person's risk of cardiovascular disease:

- Age
- Being male, or being a postmenopausal female
- Family history
- Ethnicity

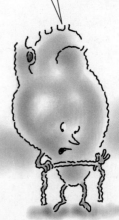

Oh no! If my waist measurement increases, I may be at increased risk for heart disease!

Better to be young at heart

Susceptibility to cardiovascular disease increases with age. Disease before age 40 is unusual; however, the age–disease correlation may simply reflect the longer duration of exposure to other risk factors.

An estrogen effect?

Females are less susceptible to heart disease until after menopause; then they become as susceptible as males. It is theorized that estrogen has a protective effect on the cardiovascular system. More recent research has shown that premenopausal people less than 50 years old have significantly better coronary endothelial function compared to those who are postmenopausal. This may account for the increase in cardiovascular disease risks for postmenopausal people. However, acute coronary syndrome (ACS) is pathologically distinct in females and can present differently than in males. Persistent disparities in mortality from ACS between males and females may be the result of failure to recognize and intervene emergently, especially in the case of females aged less than 55 years.

Nature vs. nurture

A positive family history also increases a person's chance of developing premature cardiovascular disease. For example, genetic factors can cause pronounced, accelerated forms of atherosclerosis such as familial hypercholesterolemia (also called *hyperlipidemia*); this disease is caused by lack of sufficient lipid receptors in the liver, which causes cholesterol accumulation in the blood and arteries (such as coronary arteries). Risk factors—such as obesity, hypertension, and diabetes—recur in families. Although this disease affects all ethnicities, African American people are most susceptible to cardiovascular disease.

Now I get it!

Artery filled with atherosclerotic lipid plaque

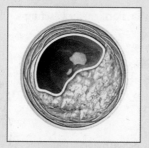

Cardiovascular disorders

The disorders discussed in this section include:
- aneurysm
- cardiac tamponade
- cardiogenic shock
- coronary artery disease (CAD)
- ACS (unstable angina, non–ST elevation myocardial infarction [NSTEMI], ST elevation myocardial infarction [STEMI])
- cardiomyopathy (dilated, hypertrophic, restrictive)
- deep vein thrombophlebitis
- heart failure (HF)
- hypertension
- pericarditis
- rheumatic fever and rheumatic heart disease (RHD)

Aneurysm

An aneurysm is an abnormal dilation or outpouching in an arterial wall or cardiac chamber. It is a weakened area that can rupture, causing hemorrhage. Aneurysms most commonly occur in the cerebral arteries (brain) or aorta. Aortic aneurysms can form in the thoracic area or in the abdominal area, with most occurring abdominally between the renal arteries and the aortic bifurcation.

Aneurysms are four times more common in males than in females and are most prevalent in White people over 65 years (CDC, 2016).

How it happens

The most common cause of abdominal aortic aneurysms (AAAs) is atherosclerosis, with hypertension, smoking, diabetes, and diet all being contributing factors. Additionally, Marfan syndrome or infections that affect arterial walls can lead to aneurysms. Many aneurysms develop slowly over time and go undetected until they become large enough to cause symptoms.

It begins locally

First, a local weakness in the muscular layer of the aorta (tunica media), due to degenerative changes, allows the inner layer (tunica intima) and outer layer (tunica adventitia) to stretch outward. Blood pressure within the aorta progressively weakens the vessel walls and enlarges the aneurysm. Aneurysms can dissect or rip when bleeding into the weakened artery, causing the arterial wall to split. (See *Dissecting aneurysm.*)

Now I get it!

Dissecting aneurysm

Aneurysms can dissect or rip when bleeding into the weakened artery, causing the arterial wall to split.

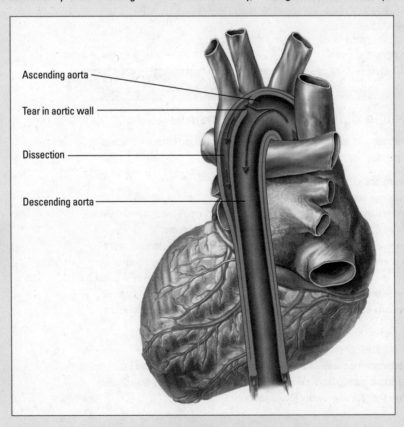

Ascending aorta

Tear in aortic wall

Dissection

Descending aorta

What to look for

Although AAAs usually don't produce symptoms, larger aneurysms may be evident (unless the patient has obesity) as a pulsating mass in the periumbilical area, accompanied by a systolic bruit over the aorta.

Reaching the breaking point

A large aneurysm may continue to enlarge and eventually rupture. If the aneurysm is in the thoracic aorta, it causes a tearing or ripping sensation of pain in the chest. If the aneurysm is in the abdominal aorta, it causes abdominal pain and ruptures into the peritoneal cavity. Aortic aneurysm rupture causes internal hemorrhage and sudden and severe chest, abdominal, or back pain.

Other signs and symptoms of aortic aneurysm enlargement and rupture include:

- sudden, severe, hypotension
- pain (chest, abdominal, or back depending on site of aneurysm)
- weakness
- sweating
- tachycardia or dysrhythmias
- loss of consciousness

Battling illness

Treating abdominal aortic aneurysm

Treatments for abdominal aortic aneurysm are few. They include invasive interventions and drug therapy.

Invasive interventions

Usually, an abdominal aortic aneurysm requires resection of the aneurysm and replacement of the damaged aortic section with a Dacron or polytetrafluoroethylene graft. Surgery is advised when the aneurysm is 5 to 6 cm in diameter.

Another invasive treatment option is a procedure known as endoluminal stent grafting. In this procedure, the physician inserts a catheter through the femoral artery, guided by angiography, and advances the catheter to the aneurysm. A balloon within the catheter is then inflated, pushing the stent open. The stent attaches with tiny hooks above and below the aneurysm. This creates a path for blood flow that bypasses the aneurysm.

Drug options

If the patient's aneurysm is small and produces no symptoms, surgery may be delayed. Beta-adrenergic blockers, which reduce blood pressure, may be administered to decrease the rate of growth of the aneurysm.

What tests tell you

An AAA rarely produces symptoms, and in many cases, it's detected accidentally as the result of an x-ray or a routine physical examination. Because of this and the increased incidence of AAA in aging males, any male aged 65 to 75 years old who has ever smoked should be screened for AAA by abdominal ultrasonography (U.S. Preventive Task Force, 2019). Several tests can confirm suspected AAA:

- Computed tomography (CT) with contrast can visualize the aneurysm's effect on nearby organs, particularly the position of the renal arteries in relation to the aneurysm.
- Serial ultrasonography allows accurate determination of aneurysm size, shape, and location.
- Anteroposterior and lateral x-rays of the abdomen can detect aortic calcification, which outlines the mass at least 75% of the time.
- Angiography, a specialized x-ray that uses radiopaque dye to outline the aorta, shows the condition of vessels proximal and distal to the aneurysm and the extent of the aneurysm.

Cardiac tamponade

In cardiac tamponade, progressive accumulation of fluid in the pericardial sac causes compression of the heart chambers. This obstructs blood flow into the ventricles, or diastolic filling, and reduces the amount of blood that can be pumped out of the heart with each contraction, reducing the cardiac output. As little as 50 to 100 mL of fluid can create an emergency if it accumulates rapidly. If the condition is left untreated, cardiogenic shock and death can occur.

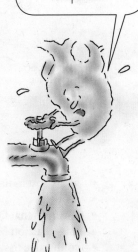

As little as 50 to 100 mL of fluid can cause cardiac tamponade.

Stretching it out

If fluid accumulates slowly and pressure rises—such as in pericardial effusion caused by cancer—signs and symptoms may not be evident immediately. This is because the fibrous wall of the pericardial sac can stretch to accommodate a large amount of fluid.

How it happens

Cardiac tamponade may result from:

- a pericardial effusion, mostly idiopathic, but also from neoplasms or infections
- trauma, such as a gunshot or stab wound in the chest, cardiac surgery, or perforation by a catheter during cardiac or central venous catheterization and pacemaker insertion
- hemorrhage from nontraumatic causes, such as rupture of the heart or great vessels and anticoagulant therapy in a patient with pericarditis

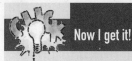

Now I get it!

Cardiac tamponade

Pericardial fluid surrounds the heart and constricts its function.

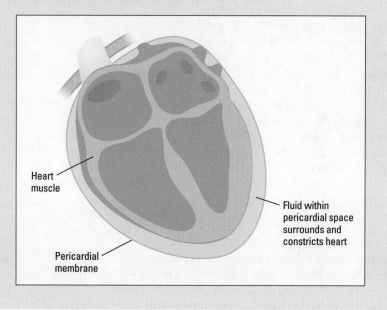

Heart muscle

Fluid within pericardial space surrounds and constricts heart

Pericardial membrane

- viral, post radiation therapy, or idiopathic pericarditis
- acute MI
- chronic renal failure during dialysis
- drug reaction
- connective tissue disorders, such as rheumatoid arthritis, systemic lupus erythematosus, rheumatic fever, vasculitis, and scleroderma

What to look for

Cardiac tamponade has three classic features known as *Beck's triad:*
- Hypotension with narrowing pulse pressure
- Elevated central venous pressure (CVP) with neck vein distention
- Muffled heart sounds
  Other signs and symptoms include:
- orthopnea
- diaphoresis
- anxiety
- restlessness

- pulsus paradoxus (inspiratory drop in systolic blood pressure greater than 15 mm Hg)
- cyanosis
- weak, rapid peripheral pulse

What tests tell you

These tests are used to diagnose cardiac tamponade:
- Chest x-ray shows a slightly widened mediastinum and enlargement of the cardiac silhouette.
- Electrocardiography (ECG) rules out other cardiac disorders. The QRS amplitude may be reduced, and electrical alternans of the P-wave, QRS complex, and T-wave may be present. Generalized ST segment elevation is noted in all leads.
- Pulmonary artery pressure (PAP) monitoring reveals increased right atrial pressure or CVP and right ventricular diastolic pressure.
- Transthoracic or transesophageal echocardiography demonstrates pericardial effusion with signs of ventricular and atrial compression. (See *Treating cardiac tamponade.*)
- Cardiac CT scan can also demonstrate pericardial effusion surrounding the heart.

Battling illness

Treating cardiac tamponade

The goal of treatment for cardiac tamponade is to relieve intrapericardial pressure and cardiac compression by removing the accumulated blood or fluid. This can be done in three different ways:
- Pericardiocentesis or needle aspiration of the pericardial cavity
- Surgical creation of an opening, commonly called a *pericardial window*
- Insertion of a drain into the pericardial sac to drain the effusion

Hypotensive patients

In the hypotensive patient, cardiac output is maintained through trial volume loading with IV normal saline solution, albumin, and, perhaps, an inotropic drug such as dopamine or a vasopressor medication.

Additional treatment

Depending on the cause of tamponade, additional treatment may be required, for example:
- in traumatic injury, blood transfusion or a thoracotomy to drain reaccumulating fluid or to repair bleeding sites
- in heparin-induced tamponade, the heparin antagonist protamine
- in warfarin-induced tamponade, vitamin K, and infusion of fresh frozen plasma, if necessary

Cardiogenic shock

Sometimes called *pump failure*, cardiogenic shock is a condition of diminished cardiac output that severely impairs tissue perfusion as well as oxygen delivery to the tissues. It reflects severe left-sided HF and occurs as a serious complication in some patients hospitalized with acute MI.

Cardiogenic shock typically affects patients whose area of infarction exceeds 40% of the heart's muscle mass. In these patients, mortality exceeds 50%. Most patients with cardiogenic shock die within 24 hours of onset. The prognosis for those who survive is extremely poor. Cardiogenic shock most often occurs after an MI, but can also occur as a result of left-sided HF, dysrhythmias, valvular dysfunction, cardiac and pericardial infections, cardiac tamponade, and drug toxicity, to name a few.

How it happens

Regardless of the underlying cause, left ventricular dysfunction triggers a series of compensatory mechanisms that attempt to increase cardiac output and, in turn, maintain vital organ function.

As cardiac output falls, baroreceptors in the aorta and carotid arteries initiate responses in the sympathetic nervous system. These responses, in turn, increase heart rate, left ventricular filling pressure, and peripheral resistance to flow to enhance venous return to the heart. In addition, in response to low circulation, the kidney releases renin, which stimulates the renin–angiotensin–aldosterone system (RAAS). Angiotensin II causes peripheral arterial vasoconstriction, which further increases blood pressure and workload against the ventricle. Aldosterone enhances sodium and water reabsorption into the bloodstream, which increases blood volume. Although it's a compensatory mechanism, the RAAS raises blood volume and blood pressure, which puts further strain on the weakened left ventricle.

A vicious cycle

These compensatory responses initially stabilize the patient but later cause the heart to further deteriorate. These events comprise a vicious cycle of low cardiac output, sympathetic compensation, increased sodium and water volume in the bloodstream, increased myocardial strain, and even lower cardiac output. (See *Cycle of decompensation*, page 51.)

Now I get it!

Cycle of decompensation

The cycle of decompensation in cardiogenic shock is caused by:
- Stimulation of baroreceptors that trigger the sympathetic nervous system
- Stimulation of RAAS caused by decreased circulation to the kidney

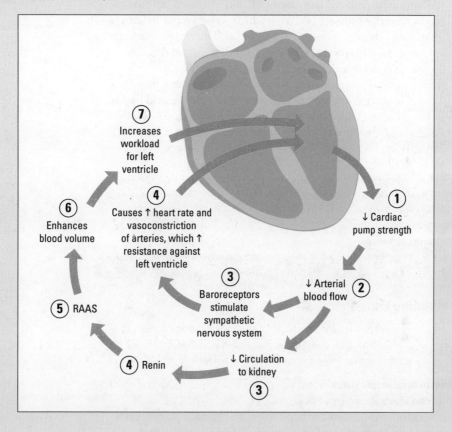

⑦ Increases workload for left ventricle

① ↓ Cardiac pump strength

④ Causes ↑ heart rate and vasoconstriction of arteries, which ↑ resistance against left ventricle

⑥ Enhances blood volume

② ↓ Arterial blood flow

③ Baroreceptors stimulate sympathetic nervous system

⑤ RAAS

④ Renin

③ ↓ Circulation to kidney

What to look for

Cardiogenic shock produces signs of poor tissue perfusion, such as:
- restlessness or confusion
- marked hypotension
- weak peripheral pulses
- tachycardia
- rapid, shallow respirations

- oliguria (urine output less than 20 mL/hour)
- systemic venous and pulmonary edema
- narrowing pulse pressure
- cyanosis
- S_3 and S_4 heart sounds

What tests tell you

These tests help diagnose cardiogenic shock:
- PAP monitoring shows increased PAP and increased pulmonary capillary wedge pressure (PCWP), which reflects a rise in left ventricular end-diastolic pressure (preload) and increased resistance to left ventricular emptying (afterload). Cardiac output measured by thermodilution reveals a diminished cardiac output.
- Invasive arterial pressure monitoring shows hypotension.
- Arterial blood gas analysis reveals metabolic acidosis and hypoxia.
- ECG may reveal evidence of an acute MI or other cause of HF
- Cardiac enzymes and troponin levels are elevated if there is MI. Elevated levels of cardiac troponin is the preferred test to diagnose MI.
- Echocardiography reveals left ventricular dysfunction. (See *Treating cardiogenic shock.*)

Battling illness

Treating cardiogenic shock

The aim of treatment is to enhance cardiovascular status by increasing cardiac output, improving myocardial perfusion, and decreasing cardiac workload. Treatment combines various cardiovascular drugs and mechanical assist techniques.

Management of cardiogenic shock
- Careful fluid and vasopressor drug administration. Drug therapy may include IV dopamine to increase blood pressure and blood flow to the kidneys, inotropic agents to increase myocardial contractility and cardiac output, or vasoconstrictors or vasodilators, if indicated.
- Intra-aortic balloon pump (IABP) placement: a mechanical assist device that attempts to improve coronary artery perfusion and decrease cardiac workload. The balloon pump is inserted through the femoral artery into the descending thoracic aorta, where it inflates during diastole to increase coronary artery perfusion pressure and deflates before systole to reduce resistance to ejection (afterload), thereby lessening cardiac workload and improving cardiac output.
- Early revascularization via percutaneous intervention or bypass surgery.
- Ventricular assist device or cardiac transplantation, if the patient is a candidate.

Coronary artery disease

CAD causes the loss of oxygen and nutrients to myocardial tissue because of poor coronary blood flow. This disease is nearly epidemic in the Western world; in 2020, approximately 380,000 people died of CAD in the United States, and approximately 20.1 million adult Americans over age 20 have CAD. CAD is most prevalent in White, middle-age males, and risk for development of coronary heart disease increases in males starting at age 45 and in females starting at age 55.

How it happens

Atherosclerosis is the most common cause of CAD. The most common predisposing condition to atherosclerosis is hyperlipidemia (high cholesterol in the bloodstream). The lipids deposit onto the arterial walls throughout the body. Coronary arteries develop lipid deposition in their walls in CAD. Lipid-rich atherosclerotic plaque (see *Artery filled with atherosclerotic lipid plaque* earlier in this chapter) progressively narrows the coronary artery lumens, reducing the volume of blood that can flow through them. This can lead to myocardial ischemia (a lack of circulation to the heart muscle) and if prolonged can lead to MI (heart tissue death).

What you can and can't control

Many risk factors are associated with atherosclerosis and CAD. Some are modifiable and some are nonmodifiable.

Nonmodifiable risk factors include age (older than age 45), sex assigned at birth (male), ethnicity, and having a family history or genetic predisposition to CAD. African Americans have a 30% greater chance of dying from heart disease than non-Hispanic Whites.

Modifiable risk factors include:

- hypertension, which is systolic blood pressure greater than 130 mm Hg or diastolic blood pressure greater than 80 mm Hg
- increased low-density lipoprotein (LDL) and decreased high-density lipoprotein (HDL) cholesterol levels
- elevated homocysteine levels (usually associated with low folic acid levels)
- smoking (risk dramatically drops within 1 year of quitting)
- stress
- obesity, which increases the risk of diabetes, hypertension, and high cholesterol
- inactivity
- uncontrolled diabetes

Other risk factors that can be modified include increased levels of serum fibrinogen and uric acid, elevated hematocrit, reduced vital capacity, high resting heart rate, thyrotoxicosis, and the use of hormonal contraceptives.

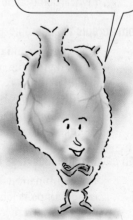

Quitting smoking, reducing stress, and lowering blood pressure and cholesterol can help prevent CAD.

Serum markers for inflammation and thrombosis

Several serum markers for inflammation and thrombosis have been linked to the development of CAD, which include the following:
• High-sensitivity C-reactive protein (hs-CRP)—although this is a nonspecific marker for inflammation, an elevated hs-CRP is strongly linked to increased risk for development of CAD.
• Troponin I—serum protein used to diagnose myocardial infarction.
• Adipokines—these are hormones released from adipose cells and are implicated in hypertension, diabetes, and endothelial cell damage.
• Air pollution—inhalation of toxins known as "free radicals" present in air pollution has been correlated with increased risk for heart disease. This may be due to activation by macrophages, oxidation of LDL, thrombosis, and inflammation of vessels when exposed to toxins in the air.

More blood flow blockers

Coronary artery spasms—referred to as variant or Prinzmetal angina—can impede blood flow. These spontaneous, sustained contractions of one or more coronary arteries occlude the vessel, reduce blood flow to the myocardium, and cause angina pectoris (chest pain). Without treatment, ischemia and, eventually, MI can result.

A precarious balance

As atherosclerosis progresses, luminal narrowing is accompanied by vascular changes that impair the diseased vessel's ability to dilate. This causes an imbalance between myocardial oxygen supply and demand, threatening the myocardium beyond the lesion. When oxygen demand exceeds what the diseased vessels can supply, localized myocardial ischemia results. If ischemia is prolonged; MI occurs.

From aerobic to anaerobic

Transient ischemia causes reversible changes at the cellular and tissue levels, depressing myocardial function. Untreated, it can lead to tissue infarction. Oxygen deprivation forces the cells in the myocardium to shift from aerobic to anaerobic metabolism. As a result, lactic acid (the end product of anaerobic metabolism) accumulates. This reduces cellular pH and causes chest pain.

With each contraction, less blood

The combination of hypoxia, reduced energy availability, and acidosis rapidly impairs left ventricular function. The strength of contractions in the affected myocardial region is reduced as the fibers shorten inadequately with less force and velocity. In addition, the ischemic section's wall motion is abnormal. This generally results in less blood being ejected from the heart with each contraction.

Haphazard hemodynamics

Because of reduced contractility and impaired wall motion, the hemodynamic response becomes variable. It depends on the ischemic segment's size and the degree of reflex compensatory response by the autonomic nervous system.

Depression of left ventricular function may reduce stroke volume and thereby lower cardiac output. This weakened left ventricular function can cause HF. Reduction in systolic emptying increases ventricular volumes. As a result of left ventricular volume overload, backward hydrostatic pressure builds in the left atrium, then backward into the pulmonary veins, then into the pulmonary capillaries. This backward pressure in the pulmonary capillaries (termed *pulmonary capillary wedge pressure* [PCWP]) can lead to pulmonary edema, which is fluid accumulation in the lung tissue, causing dyspnea and crackles heard through the stethoscope.

Compliance counts

These increases in left-sided heart pressures and PCWP are magnified by changes in wall compliance induced by ischemia. Compliance is reduced, magnifying the elevation in pressure.

What to look for

Angina (cardiac chest pain) is the classic sign of CAD. The patient may describe a burning, squeezing, or crushing tightness in the substernal or precordial area that radiates to the arms, neck, jaw, or shoulder blades. The patient may report chest heaviness or pressure. The pain is commonly accompanied by shortness of breath, dizziness, fainting, sweating, and cool extremities. The pain can seem like indigestion, particularly if accompanied by nausea and vomiting.

Angina commonly occurs after physical exertion but may also follow emotional excitement, exposure to cold, or the consumption of a large meal. Sometimes, it develops during sleep and awakens the patient.

When to label it stable or unstable

If the pain is predictable and relieved by rest or nitrates, it's called *stable angina*. If it increases in frequency and duration and is more easily induced, it's called *unstable angina*. Unstable angina is classified as an *acute coronary syndrome* and is much more likely to progress to an MI. Unstable angina is thought to result from unstable plaque rupture that can lead to thrombus formation with an MI. (See *Treating CAD*, page 56.)

Treating CAD

Because coronary artery disease (CAD) is so widespread, controlling risk factors is important. Other treatment may focus on one of two goals: reducing myocardial oxygen demand or increasing the oxygen supply and alleviating pain. Interventions may be noninvasive or invasive.

Controlling risk

Patients should limit calories and their intake of salt, fats, and cholesterol as well as stop smoking. Regular exercise is important, although it may need to be done more slowly to prevent pain. If stress is a known pain trigger, patients should learn stress reduction techniques.

Other preventive actions include controlling hypertension, controlling elevated serum cholesterol or triglyceride levels, and minimizing platelet aggregation and blood clot formation with antiplatelet or anticoagulant drugs.

Invasive measures

Various invasive treatments are commonly used such as coronary artery bypass graft (CABG) surgery, percutaneous coronary intervention (PCI), and atherectomy.

Coronary artery bypass graft

Critically narrowed or blocked arteries may need CABG surgery to alleviate uncontrollable angina and prevent myocardial infarction (MI). In this procedure, the patient's own venous or arterial blood vessels or synthetic grafts are used to bypass the occluded coronary artery. In this type of surgery, the surgeon opens the patient's sternum and spreads the ribs apart to gain access to the heart and coronary arteries.

Minimally invasive CABG requires a shorter recovery period and has fewer complications postoperatively. Instead of opening the patient's sternum, several small cuts are made in the torso through which small surgical instruments and fiber-optic cameras are inserted. This procedure was designed to correct blockages in one or two easily reached arteries and may not be appropriate for more complicated cases.

Percutaneous coronary intervention

Percutaneous coronary intervention (PCI) is an invasive but nonsurgical technique performed as quickly as possible with an MI diagnosis, ideally within 90 minutes of diagnosis. PCI is also called *cardiac catheterization*. The interventional cardiologist inserts an arterial catheter into a peripheral artery (commonly the femoral artery) and threads the catheter up through the aorta into the coronary arteries. The cardiologist performs this procedure using angiography under fluoroscopy and can accomplish coronary artery clot retrieval (atherectomy), percutaneous transluminal coronary angioplasty (PTCA), stent placement, and instillation of intracoronary medications.

A PTCA (also called an *angioplasty*) can reduce the obstruction by pressing the plaque against the vessel wall, thereby decreasing the narrowing in the vessel.

PTCA causes fewer complications than open chest surgery, but it does have risks, such as circulatory insufficiency, restenosis, MI, retroperitoneal bleeding, vasovagal response, arrhythmias, hematoma formation, or, rarely, death.

PTCA is a good alternative to CABG in people who can't tolerate cardiac surgery, such as some older adults. Stenting is commonly done in conjunction with PTCA. A stent is an expandable metal mesh device that is introduced into the artery and placed in the area where the vessel has narrowed to keep the artery open. Without stent placement after PTCA, arteries often reocclude. Drug-eluting stents may help prevent restenosis. Patients often receive anticoagulants during the procedure.

Laser angioplasty corrects occlusion by vaporizing fatty deposits with a laser device. Percutaneous myocardial revascularization (PMR) is a procedure that uses a laser to create channels in the heart muscle to improve perfusion to the myocardium. A carbon dioxide laser is used to create transmural channels from the epicardial layer to the myocardium, extending into the left ventricle. This technique is also known as transmyocardial revascularization and appears to be up to 90% effective.

Rotational ablation, or rotational atherectomy, removes plaque with a high-speed, rotating burr covered with diamond crystals.

What tests tell you

These diagnostic tests confirm CAD:

- ECG during an episode of angina shows ischemia, as demonstrated by T-wave inversion, ST segment depression, and possibly arrhythmias, such as premature ventricular contractions. Results may be normal during pain-free periods. Arrhythmias may occur without infarction, secondary to ischemia.
- Treadmill or bicycle exercise stress test may provoke chest pain and ECG signs of myocardial ischemia. Monitoring of electrical rhythm may demonstrate T-wave inversion or ST segment depression in the ischemic areas.
- Coronary angiography reveals the location and extent of coronary artery stenosis or obstruction, collateral circulation, and the arteries' condition beyond the narrowing.
- Myocardial perfusion imaging with thallium during treadmill exercise detects ischemic areas of the myocardium, visualized as "cold spots."

Acute Coronary Syndrome

Acute coronary syndrome (ACS) is an umbrella term that covers a range of thrombotic CADs, including unstable angina, variant or Prinzmetal angina, NSTEMI (or non–Q-wave MI), and STEMI (or Q-wave MI).

In ACS, it is thought that a complicated atherosclerotic lesion or plaque ruptures, followed by platelet aggregation to the area, and thrombus formation. Additionally, vasoconstrictors are released, which, in combination with the other factors, cause a pronounced decrease in blood supply to the myocardium. The effect is an imbalance of myocardial oxygen and demand. ACS includes unstable angina, variant or Prinzmetal angina, NSTEMI, and STEMI.

- Unstable angina: This occurs when an atherosclerotic plaque progresses into an MI. The pain associated with unstable angina may be poorly relieved by nitroglycerin and rest and can last 10 to 20 minutes. The patient will not have changes in cardiac enzyme levels, but will have ST changes on a 12-lead ECG during the pain. At this point, myocardial ischemia is reversible. The patient with unstable angina should be treated in the hospital with oxygen; aspirin and nitrates (if not contraindicated); morphine, if needed; and rest.
- Variant or Prinzmetal angina: This type of angina is due to coronary artery vasospasm, with or without CAD. The patient may have transient ST wave changes on the 12-lead ECG during the pain. This type of angina is often treated with a calcium channel blocker.

- NSTEMI: If smaller vessels infarct, the patient is at higher risk for MI, which may progress to an NSTEMI. With an NSTEMI, the patient experiences myocardial ischemia and infarction; however, the infarction does not extend through the entire myocardium; it is subendocardial.
- STEMI: If a thrombus lodges in a coronary artery and completely blocks the blood flow through one of the coronary arteries, the patient will experience myocardial ischemia and infarction. Marked STEMI will develop. The damage extends through all layers of the myocardium, also known as a transmural MI.
- NSTEMI: If a thrombus lodges in a coronary artery and causes only subendocardial injury, this often causes an NSTEMI. This is a non-transmural MI, less serious than STEMI.

In North America and Western Europe, MI is one of the leading causes of death. In the United States, approximately 800,000 people endure an MI each year. That is, every 40 seconds, someone has a heart attack (MI). The average age for a first MI for males is 65.3 years, and for females, it is 71.8 years.

Now I get it!

Understanding MI

In myocardial infarction (MI), blood supply to the myocardium is interrupted. Here's what happens:

1. Injury to the endothelial lining of the coronary arteries causes platelets, white blood cells, fibrin, and lipids to converge at the injured site, as shown to the right. Foam cells, or resident macrophages, congregate under the damaged lining and absorb oxidized cholesterol, forming a fatty streak that narrows the arterial lumen.

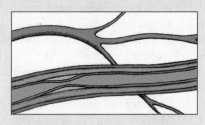

3. When myocardial demand for oxygen is more than the collateral circulation can supply, myocardial metabolism shifts from aerobic to anaerobic, producing lactic acid (represented by "A"), which stimulates nerve endings, as shown above.

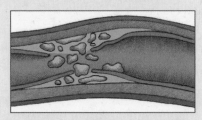

2. If the arterial lumen narrows gradually, collateral circulation develops and helps maintain myocardial perfusion distal to the obstruction. The illustration to the right shows collateral circulation.

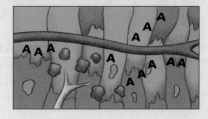

Understanding MI *(continued)*

4. Lacking oxygen, the myocardial cells die (as shown to the right). This decreases contractility, stroke volume, and blood pressure.

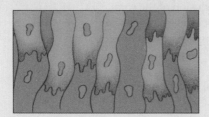

5. Hypoperfusion stimulates baroreceptors, which, in turn, stimulate the sympathetic nervous system and adrenal glands to release epinephrine and norepinephrine. This cycle is shown to the right. These catecholamines increase heart rate and cause peripheral vasoconstriction, further increasing myocardial workload and oxygen demand.

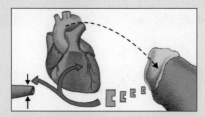

Damaged cell membranes in the infarcted area allow intracellular contents into the vascular circulation, as shown to the right. Ventricular arrhythmias can develop with elevated serum levels of potassium (■), CK-MB (▲), cardiac troponin (●), and lactate dehydrogenase (○).

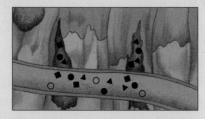

6. All myocardial cells are capable of spontaneous depolarization and repolarization, so the electrical conduction system may be affected by infarct, injury, and ischemia. The illustration to the right shows an injury site. The injury site becomes an area susceptible to rhythm disturbance.

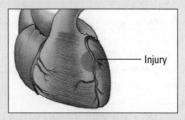

Injury

7. Extensive damage to the left ventricle may impair its ability to pump, causing heart failure, which allows hydrostatic pressure to back up into the left atrium and, eventually, into the pulmonary veins and capillaries, as shown in the illustration to the right. Crackles may be heard in the lungs on auscultation. Pulmonary capillary wedge pressure increases. This is pulmonary edema that occurs with heart failure.

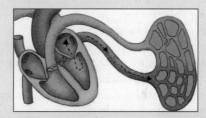

8. As back pressure rises, fluid crosses the alveolocapillary membrane, impeding diffusion of oxygen (O_2) and carbon dioxide (CO_2) (as shown to the right). Arterial blood gas measurements may show decreased partial pressure of arterial oxygen and arterial pH and increased partial pressure of arterial carbon dioxide.

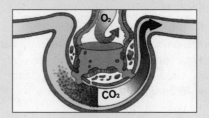

Males are more susceptible to MI than premenopausal females; however, the incidence in postmenopausal females is similar to that in males.

How it happens

MI results from occlusion of one or more of the coronary arteries. The coronary artery obstruction decreases blood flow to the myocardium, which results in ischemia (and, if prolonged, MI). Occlusion of the coronary arteries can be due to atherosclerosis, thrombosis, platelet aggregation, or coronary artery stenosis or spasm. Predisposing factors include:
- aging
- uncontrolled diabetes
- elevated serum triglyceride, LDL, total cholesterol, and homocysteine levels and decreased serum HDL levels
- excessive intake of saturated fats, carbohydrates, or salt
- hypertension; BP > 130/80 mm Hg
- obesity
- positive family history of CAD
- sedentary lifestyle
- smoking
- stress

Susceptibility increases with age

Older adults are more prone to complications and death. The most common complications after an acute MI include:
- arrhythmias
- cardiogenic shock
- HF causing pulmonary edema
- pericarditis
  Other complications include:
- rupture of the atrial or ventricular septum, ventricular wall, or valves
- ventricular aneurysms
- mural thrombi causing cerebral or pulmonary emboli
- extensions of the original infarction
- post-MI pericarditis (Dressler syndrome), which occurs days to weeks after an MI and causes residual pain, malaise, and fever
- psychological problems caused by fear of another MI or organic brain disorder from tissue hypoxia

Heavy reductions

MI results from prolonged ischemia to the myocardium with irreversible cell damage and muscle death. Functionally, MI causes:
- reduced contractility with abnormal wall motion
- altered left ventricular compliance
- reduced stroke volume
- reduced ejection fraction
- elevated left ventricular end-diastolic pressure. (See *Treating MI*, page 61.)

Treating MI

Arrhythmias, the most common problem during the first 48 hours after myocardial infarction myocardial infarction (MI), require antiarrhythmics, a pacemaker (possibly), and cardioversion (rarely). Treatment for MI has three goals:

- To relieve chest pain
- To stabilize heart rhythm
- To reduce cardiac workload

Drug therapy

Drugs are the mainstay of therapy. Typical drugs include the following:

- Aspirin: 325 mg chewed immediately with new-onset angina, suspected or confirmed MI to inhibit platelet aggregation and vasoconstriction (Ignatavicius & Workman, 2016)
- Thrombolytic agents (such as tissue plasminogen activator [tPA] and streptokinase [Streptase]) to dissolve thrombi and restore myocardial blood flow
- Antiarrhythmic drugs for ventricular arrhythmias
- Glycoprotein IIb/IIIa inhibitor (such as *abciximab* [ReoPro]) to minimize platelet aggregation
- Intravenous (IV) atropine for heart block or bradycardia
- Sublingual, topical, transdermal, or IV nitroglycerin and calcium channel blockers (such as diltiazem), given by mouth or IV to relieve angina
- IV morphine (drug of choice) for pain and sedation
- Positive inotropic drugs that increase myocardial contractility (such as dobutamine and milrinone)
- Beta-adrenergic blockers (such as propranolol [Inderal] and metoprolol [Lopressor]) after acute MI to help prevent reinfarction by decreasing myocardial workload and oxygen demand
- Antilipemic to reduce elevated serum cholesterol or triglyceride levels
- Angiotensin-converting enzyme (ACE) inhibitor to reduce afterload and preload and prevent remodeling

Other therapies

Other therapies include:

- temporary pacemaker for heart block or bradycardia
- oxygen administered by nasal cannula at 2 to 4 L/min, or titrated to keep the arterial oxygen saturation at 95% or higher, or at a lower concentration if the patient has chronic obstructive pulmonary disease
- bed rest to decrease cardiac workload
- pulmonary artery catheterization to detect left-sided or right-sided heart failure and to monitor the patient's response to treatment (not routinely done)
- intra-aortic balloon pump for cardiogenic shock
- cardiac catheterization, percutaneous transluminal coronary angioplasty, stent placement, and coronary artery bypass grafting
- intravenous intracoronary or systemic thrombolytic therapy (also called *clot buster*) to dissolve the occlusive clot and reperfuse the coronary arteries. Certain patients with risk for bleeding are not eligible for thrombolytic treatment. Thrombolytic therapy is for patients who don't have a history of stroke, bleeding, GI ulcers, marked hypertension, recent surgery, or chest pain lasting longer than 6 hours. It must begin within 6 hours after the onset of symptoms, ideally with treatment that begins within 1 hour after symptoms first appear.

Tissue destruction in MI

All MIs have a central area of necrosis or infarction surrounded by an area of injury. The area of injury is surrounded by a ring of ischemia. Tissue regeneration doesn't occur after an MI because the affected myocardial muscle is dead.

A compensatory kick

Scar tissue that forms on the necrotic area may inhibit contractility. When this occurs, the compensatory mechanisms are triggered; these include the baroreceptor–sympathetic reflex and the RAAS. These compensatory mechanisms lead to vascular constriction, increased heart rate, and renal retention of sodium and water to try to maintain cardiac output. With high amounts of scar tissue, ventricular dilation also may occur, which decreases contractility and strength of the heart pump. The patient may develop HF or cardiogenic shock.

Siting the infarctions

The infarction site depends on the vessels involved:
- Occlusion of the circumflex coronary artery causes lateral wall infarctions.
- Occlusion of the left anterior coronary artery causes anterior wall infarctions.
- Occlusion of the right coronary artery or one of its branches causes posterior and inferior wall infarctions and right ventricular infarctions.

What to look for

The cardinal symptom of MI is persistent, substernal pain that may radiate to the arms, jaw, neck, or shoulder blades. The pain is commonly described as heavy, squeezing, or crushing and may persist for 12 hours or more. However, in up to 40% of patients—particularly females, older adults, or people with diabetes—chest pain may be mild or not occur at all. In others, it may be mild and confused with indigestion and may include anxiety, diaphoresis, and nausea and vomiting. Females often endure *anginal equivalents* when enduring myocardial ischemia. These are symptoms of myocardial ischemia that differ from chest pressure and radiation. Such anginal equivalents may include feelings of epigastric pressure, dizziness (feeling faint), shoulder pain, or shortness of breath without chest pain. There is increasing evidence that many females experience microvascular angina, which does not cause ST segment changes on ECG or apparent coronary artery obstruction on cardiac catheterization. Microvascular angina is currently under intense study.

An infarction on the horizon?

In patients with CAD, angina of increasing frequency, severity, or duration (especially if not provoked by exertion, a heavy meal, or cold and wind) may signal an impending infarction.

Other associated symptoms that can occur during an MI include:

- a feeling of impending doom
- fatigue
- nausea and vomiting
- chest pressure or heaviness
- shortness of breath
- cool extremities
- diaphoresis
- anxiety
- restlessness

Fever is unusual at the onset of an MI, but a low-grade fever may develop during the next few days. Blood pressure varies. Hypotension or hypertension may occur.

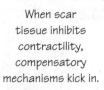

When scar tissue inhibits contractility, compensatory mechanisms kick in.

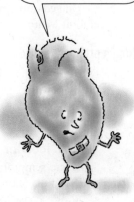

What tests tell you

These tests help diagnose MI:

- Serial 12-lead ECG may be normal or inconclusive during the first few hours after an MI. Abnormalities include serial ST segment depression in NSTEMI and ST segment elevation and Q-waves, representing scarring and necrosis, in STEMI.
- Serum creatine kinase (CK) levels are elevated, especially the CK-MB isoenzyme, the cardiac muscle fraction of CK.
- Troponins, very specific structural proteins found in cardiac muscle, are elevated in the bloodstream. These are the key diagnostic markers indicating MI.
- Echocardiography shows ventricular wall dyskinesia with an STEMI and is used to evaluate the left ventricular ejection fraction.
- Nuclear ventriculography (multiple-gated acquisition scanning or radionuclide ventriculography) can show acutely damaged muscle by picking up accumulations of radionuclide, which appear as a "hot spot" on the film. Myocardial perfusion imaging with thallium-201 or Cardiolite reveals a "cold spot" in most patients during the first few hours after an STEMI.

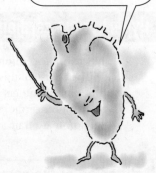

These are all possible signs of MI.

Cardiomyopathy

Cardiomyopathy is a group of diseases that primarily affect the myocardium and can be subacute or chronic. Cardiomyopathies are classified according to abnormalities in structure and physiologic effects on the myocardium. Etiology for development of cardiomyopathies may include infectious disease, uncontrolled diabetes, renal failure, pregnancy complications, alcohol or drug toxicity, ischemia, hypertension, systemic inflammatory disorders, nutritional disorders, genetic predisposition, or idiopathic causes.

Dilated Cardiomyopathy

Dilated cardiomyopathy results from extensively damaged myocardial muscle fibers. This disorder interferes with myocardial metabolism, the ventricular walls thicken, and the ventricles dilate, giving the heart a globular shape.

Dilated cardiomyopathy can lead to intractable HF, arrhythmias, and emboli. Ventricular arrhythmias may lead to syncope and sudden death.

Taking a pregnant pause

Dilated cardiomyopathy may develop during the last trimester of pregnancy or a few months after delivery. Its cause is unknown, but it's most common in multiparous people older than age 30, particularly those with malnutrition or preeclampsia.

What to look for

Signs and symptoms of dilated cardiomyopathy include:
- shortness of breath
- poor exercise tolerance
- fatigue
- palpitations
- peripheral edema
- pulmonary congestion

Hypertrophic cardiomyopathy

Hypertrophic cardiomyopathy is a primary disease of the cardiac muscle. The course of this disorder varies. Some patients have progressive deterioration; others remain stable for years. About 50% of the time, hypertrophic cardiomyopathy is transmitted genetically as an autosomal dominant trait.

A stiffening of the septum

Hypertrophic cardiomyopathy is characterized by left ventricular hypertrophy and an unusual cellular hypertrophy of the upper ventricular septum. The septum is so enlarged that it encroaches onto the aorta and interrupts blood flow from the left ventricle into the aorta. These changes result in obstruction of blood outflow into the aorta. The lack of blood flow also causes lack of blood flow into the coronary arteries that can lead to myocardial ischemia. The left ventricle is also so stiff that it has decreased elasticity and is less able to fill with blood volume during diastole (when the heart relaxes). Pressure can build in the left atrium and cause dilation that can lead to atrial

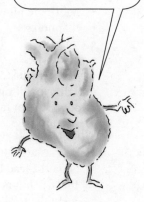

Elevated cardiac troponins in the bloodstream are key in the diagnosis of MI.

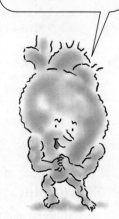

I'm in good shape now, but damage to my muscle fibers will leave me rounded and weak.

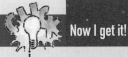

Now I get it!

Hypertrophic septum in the heart

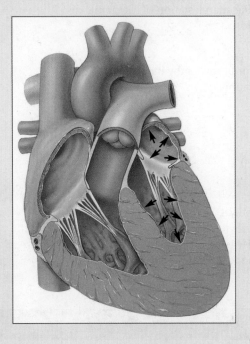

rhythm disruption. This disruption can cause three major problems: decreased flow into the aorta, decreased filling of the left ventricle, and dilation of the left atrium. These problems can cause sudden hypotension, shock, and death. Sudden death is also possible due to ventricular arrhythmias in the left ventricle, such as ventricular tachycardia and ventricular fibrillation.

What to look for

Signs and symptoms of hypertrophic cardiomyopathy include:

- atrial fibrillation or heart palpitations
- angina (due to decreased blood flow into the aorta and coronary arteries)
- dyspnea on exertion
- sudden syncope (fainting)
- dizziness
- sudden death (more common in athletes)
- **OR** there may be no symptoms at all.

Restrictive cardiomyopathy

With restrictive cardiomyopathy, the ventricles may have normal or near-normal systolic function and wall function; however, the ventricles are stiff and restrict filling during diastole. The disease may be primary, be idiopathic, or be a cardiac manifestation of a systemic disease such as sarcoidosis or amyloidosis.

What to look for

Signs and symptoms of restrictive cardiomyopathy include:
- atrial fibrillation or heart palpitations
- systemic venous congestion
- dyspnea on exertion
- right-sided HF
- murmur
- cardiomegaly

What tests tell you

No single test confirms cardiomyopathy. Diagnosis requires elimination of other possible causes of HF and arrhythmias. These tests are used:
- ECG and angiography rule out ischemic heart disease.
- Chest x-ray may demonstrate moderate to marked cardiomegaly.

Battling illness

Treating cardiomyopathy

The goals of treatment for dilated cardiomyopathy are to correct the underlying causes and to improve the heart's pumping ability, initially the same as with heart failure. Drug therapy includes cardiac glycosides (e.g., digoxin), diuretics, oxygen, anticoagulants, vasodilators, angiotensin-converting enzyme (ACE) inhibitors, beta-adrenergic blockers, and a low-sodium diet supplemented by vitamin therapy. Antiarrhythmics may be used to treat arrhythmias.

Therapy may also include prolonged bed rest and selective use of corticosteroids, particularly when myocardial inflammation is present. If the cardiomyopathy is the result of alcohol or drug misuse, the patient must abstain from the use of these.

The goals of treatment for hypertrophic cardiomyopathy are to relax the ventricles and relieve outflow obstruction. Drugs such as beta-adrenergic blockers and calcium channel blockers are the first line of treatment. Heparin may be used if the patient develops atrial fibrillation. Amiodarone is used if heart failure occurs. Diuretics may help decrease diastolic pressure. Surgical treatment of a ventricular septal myectomy may be performed, which involves excision of part of the hypertrophied ventricular septum. Most patients experience long-term improvement in activity tolerance after this surgery. Implantable defibrillators may be inserted in patients with a family history of sudden death. With hypertrophic cardiomyopathy, vasodilators, sympathetic stimulators, and inotropic drugs are contraindicated.

Final option
When these treatments fail, heart transplantation may be the only option for some patients with cardiomyopathy.

- Echocardiography and cardiac catheterization are used to help diagnose and differentiate cardiomyopathies.
- Transvenous endomyocardial biopsy may be useful in some patients to determine the underlying disorder.

Deep vein thrombophlebitis: A potentially lethal venous disease

Deep vein thrombophlebitis (DVT) develops when a thrombus, or blood clot, forms in a vein, usually in the lower extremities. It is important to recognize that DVT is a venous disease that most commonly occurs in a deep vein in the thigh or calf. It is sometimes referred to as *deep venous thromboembolism*. The "thrombo" portion of the word refers to the clot formation, and "phlebitis" means inflammation of a vein. Embolism, or embolus, means that the clot is traveling in the bloodstream. There are three factors that promote venous thrombosis. These three factors, known as *Virchow's triad*, include (1) venous stasis (for example, immobility, age), (2) venous endothelial injury (for example, surgery, trauma, IV medications), and (3) hypercoagulability (oral contraceptives, inherited disorders, pregnancy, any type of cancer).

How did it get there?

A thrombus can form when platelets and clotting factors accumulate in a vein because of the pooling of the blood, vein endothelial injury, or a state of hypercoagulability. As the thrombus grows from more platelet aggregation and inflammation, the area can get edematous. DVTs are often with symptoms; however, they can also cause redness and pain, along with swelling. Often, the thrombus will resolve on its own, undetected and without treatment.

So then, what's all the fuss about?

A DVT can become a medical emergency quickly if the thrombus dislodges and travels through the body. The thrombus then becomes known as an *embolus*. Most commonly, an embolus in a leg vein travels up into the inferior vena cava, then into the right atrium, into the right ventricle, and into the pulmonary artery. In the pulmonary artery, the embolus is called a *pulmonary embolus* (PE) and it is potentially lethal. A pulmonary embolus occludes the pulmonary arterial vessels, causing a medical emergency. Occlusion of the pulmonary artery or a pulmonary arteriole obstructs circulation within the lungs.

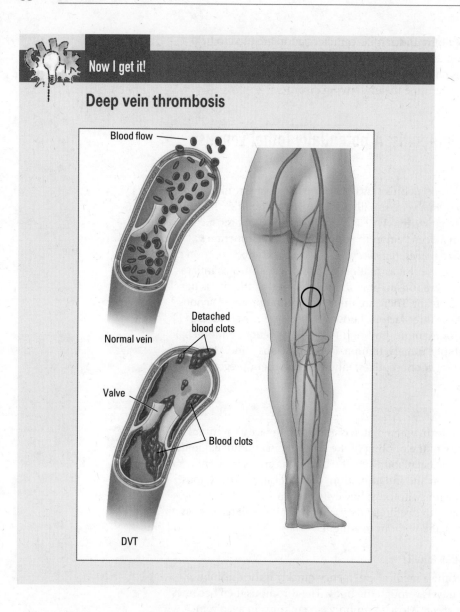

Now I get it!

Deep vein thrombosis

Blood flow

Normal vein

Detached blood clots

Valve

Blood clots

DVT

Patients with a pulmonary embolus usually have a sudden onset of pleuritic chest pain, shortness of breath, tachycardia, tachypnea, and anxiety.

Let's treat this!

DVTs are usually treated with rest and anticoagulant medications. When the patient is in bed or in a chair, they are encouraged to elevate the affected extremity. Compression stockings may be worn to decrease venous insufficiency. Warm, moist soaks to the extremity may also be used. It is very important to avoid massaging the affected extremity, because this could cause the thrombus to dislodge and become an embolus.

Let's get thin

Anticoagulants are the first-line medication used for patients with known DVT or who are at risk for development of DVT. These will help prevent the clot from enlarging and decrease the likelihood of more clots forming by inhibiting clotting factors and decreasing the platelet count. First-line treatment of DVT to prevent PE consists of direct oral anticoagulants: dabigatran, rivaroxaban, apixaban, or edoxaban.

Other treatment

Surgery for a DVT is rare; however, if the thrombus does not respond to the medication regimen, the patient may have to undergo thrombectomy to remove the clot. If the patient has recurrent DVTs, they may be a candidate for an inferior vena cava filtration device. This is a filter or umbrella-type device that is passed through the femoral vein to the inferior vena cava to catch any emboli so they will not travel to the lungs.

An ounce of prevention is worth a pound of cure! If a patient is at risk for thrombus formation, there are several precautions that should be taken. The following should be implemented:

- Avoiding oral contraceptives or hormone therapy
- Staying adequately hydrated
- Performing leg exercises and foot pumps frequently if on prolonged bed rest or immobile states
- Early ambulation after surgery
- Use of compression stockings or intermittent sequential compression devices
- Prophylactic anticoagulation therapy if indicated

Heart failure

HF, often called *congestive HF*, occurs when the heart muscle (myocardium) is weakened by a sudden event or gradually due to strain over time. The ventricle cannot pump enough blood out to the peripheral tissues. When the myocardium can't pump effectively enough to meet the body's metabolic needs, HF occurs. Pump failure usually occurs in a damaged left ventricle, but it may also happen in the right ventricle.

Usually, left-sided HF develops first. HF is often described in terms of *ejection fraction*, which is the percentage of blood volume pumped out of the left ventricle. The healthy heart can pump greater than 60% of its blood volume out of the left ventricle with each contraction. HF is most commonly diagnosed when less than or equal to 40% of blood volume is pumped out of the left ventricle with each contraction.

HF can be described in different ways:
- HFrEF (HF with reduced ejection fraction)
- HFpEF (HF with preserved ejection fraction)
- acute or chronic
- left sided or right sided (See *Understanding left-sided and right-side heart failure*, page 70.)

It's easiest to understand the mechanisms of HF by breaking it down into left-sided heart failure vs. right-sided heart failure. Each side causes specific types of consequences.

HF affects over 6 million people in the United States, and of those diagnosed with HF, over 50% will die within 5 years of diagnosis. HF affects approximately 10% of those individuals aged 65 and over and is the most common reason for hospital admission among this age group. Symptoms of HF may restrict a person's ability to perform activities of daily living and severely affect quality of life.

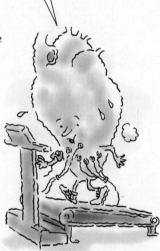

I could fail... gasp... if my myocardium can't pump enough to meet the body's metabolic needs.

Now I get it!

Understanding left-sided and right-sided heart failure

These illustrations show how myocardial damage leads to heart failure.

Left-sided heart failure

1. A myocardial infarction of the left ventricle leaves an area of injury and cell death. Part of the left ventricular muscle is dead, so the left ventricle weakens. The weakened left ventricle cannot optimally pump blood out into the aorta and to the peripheral organs. The area of injury does not contract, and the body will attempt to compensate. The conductive tissue in the area of infarction is dysfunctional, which can cause rhythm disturbances (arrhythmias). In terms of compensatory mechanisms, the patient experiences an increased heart rate due to baroreceptors sensing a lack of arterial circulation and reflex stimulation of the sympathetic nervous system. The patient is pale and has cool skin due to lack of circulation to the extremities. There is decreased cardiac output because part of the left ventricle muscle has died. Also, arrhythmias often occur because part of the conduction tissue is affected by the infarction.

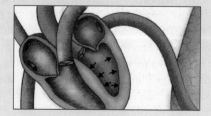

Understanding left-sided and right-sided heart failure *(continued)*

2. Diminished left ventricular function allows blood to pool in the left ventricle; consequently, there is a backup of hydrostatic pressure into the left atrium and eventually a backup into the pulmonary veins and capillaries, as shown below. At this stage, the patient may experience dyspnea on exertion, confusion, dizziness, orthostatic hypotension, decreased peripheral pulses and pulse pressure, cyanosis, and an S_3 gallop.

Simultaneously, another compensatory mechanism is triggered. Due to the left ventricle not pumping adequate blood volume out to the organs, the kidney receives less arterial circulation. This lack of renal circulation causes the kidney to release renin. This then triggers the compensatory mechanism known as the renin–angiotensin–aldosterone system (RAAS). This system increases the amount of sodium and water reabsorbed into the bloodstream at the nephrons, which increases blood volume. It also causes peripheral arterial vasoconstriction, thereby increasing resistance against the left ventricle. The increased blood volume and increased peripheral resistance put further strain on the weakened left ventricle. Therefore, in summary, the compensatory mechanisms of the body actually worsen and further weaken the left ventricle.

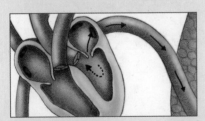

3. The left ventricle has blood that is not ejected and pools in the chamber. This increases backward pressure up into the left atrium, pulmonary veins, and pulmonary capillaries. As the pulmonary capillaries become engorged, rising hydrostatic pressure causes edema; water from the bloodstream is pushed into the interstitial space (as shown at right), causing *pulmonary edema*. The patient demonstrates this pulmonary edema by coughing, severe shortness of breath, and crackles that can be heard in the lungs with the stethoscope. The patient has elevated pulmonary capillary pressure, diminished pulmonary compliance, and increased partial pressure of carbon dioxide. Crackles heard over the lungs are the key sign of pulmonary edema.

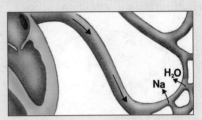

4. When the patient lies down, the change in position causes fluid to spread out within the lungs instead of remaining in the bases as in the sitting position. Also, venous return increases from the extremities into the heart. Because the left ventricle can't handle the increased venous return and fluid impacts the lung tissue from pulmonary edema, the patient has more difficulty breathing. You may note decreased breath sounds, dullness on percussion, crackles, and orthopnea. Orthopnea is difficulty breathing when lying supine (flat). Sitting the patient up (called *high Fowler position*) can help them breathe easier. In the seated position, fluid moves down into the bases of the lungs and allows the patient easier expansion of the chest for breathing.

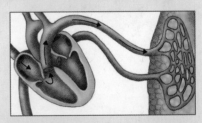

5. The right ventricle may now become stressed because it's pumping against greater pulmonary vascular resistance and left ventricular pressure (see illustration at right). When this occurs, the right ventricle begins to fail, and the patient's symptoms worsen.

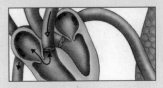

(Continued)

Understanding left-sided and right-sided heart failure *(continued)*

Right-sided heart failure

6. The stressed right ventricle enlarges with the formation of stretched tissue (see illustration below).

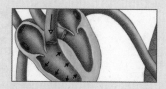

7. Blood pools in the right ventricle, and there is a backup of hydrostatic pressure into the right atrium. The backed-up pressure causes further backup of pressure into the superior and inferior vena cava and venous circulation (see illustration below). The patient has elevated central venous pressure due to right atrial pressure, jugular vein distention due to high pressure in the superior vena cava, and hepatojugular reflux due to venous congestion in the liver.

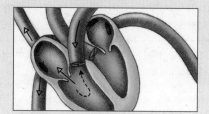

8. Backed-up blood also distends the visceral veins, especially the hepatic vein. As the liver and spleen become engorged (see illustration below), their function is impaired. The peritoneal cavity becomes edematous and abdominal distention occurs; this is referred to as ascites. The patient may develop anorexia, nausea, abdominal pain, palpable liver and spleen, weakness, and dyspnea secondary to abdominal distention.

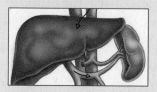

9. Rising capillary pressure forces excess fluid from the capillaries into the interstitial space (see illustration below). This causes tissue edema, especially in the lower extremities at the ankle region. The patient may experience weight gain, pitting ankle edema, and nocturia due to the increased fluid.

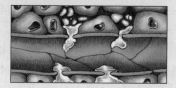

Classifying heart failure

Heart failure may be classified in different ways according to its pathophysiology.

Right sided or left sided

Right-sided heart failure is a result of ineffective right ventricular contractile function. This may be caused by an acute right ventricular infarction or pulmonary embolus. However, the most common cause is profound backward flow due to left-sided heart failure.

Left-sided heart failure is the result of ineffective left ventricular contractile function. This may lead to pulmonary congestion or pulmonary edema and decreased cardiac output. Left ventricular MI, hypertension, and aortic and mitral valve stenosis or insufficiency are common causes.

As the decreased pumping ability of the left ventricle persists, fluid accumulates, backing up into the

Classifying heart failure *(continued)*

left atrium and then into the lungs. If this worsens, pulmonary edema and right-sided heart failure may also result.

HF with reduced ejection fraction or HF with preserved ejection fraction

Heart failure is defined in terms of ejection fraction. The ejection fraction measures how much blood inside the ventricle is pumped out with each contraction. The left ventricle squeezes and pumps some (but not all) of the blood in the ventricle out to the body. A healthy ejection fraction is approximately 60%. This means that 60% of the total blood in the left ventricle is pumped out with each heartbeat.

Heart failure with reduced ejection fraction (**HFrEF**) occurs when the left ventricle loses its ability to contract normally. The heart can't pump with enough force to push enough blood into circulation. The ejected blood volume out of the left ventricle is too low to meet the needs of the tissues. This is an ejection fraction of less than 40% of the blood volume pumped out of the left ventricle. Heart failure with preserved ejection fraction (**HFpEF**) is defined as heart failure with a left ventricular ejection fraction, or LVEF, of 50% or greater. This is usually because the left ventricle cannot fill with sufficient blood volume due to its lack of elasticity.

Acute or chronic

"Acute" refers to the timing of the onset of symptoms and whether compensatory mechanisms kick in. In acute heart failure, there are sudden symptoms due to lack of pumping action of the heart. The patient commonly demonstrates sudden shortness of breath, and coarse crackles are heard in the lungs due to pulmonary edema. In chronic heart failure, the heart slowly weakens over time. Signs and symptoms occur gradually, compensatory mechanisms slowly take effect, and fluid volume overload slowly occurs over time. Drugs, diet changes, and activity restrictions usually control symptoms.

But the good news is…

Advances in diagnostic and therapeutic techniques have greatly improved the outlook for these patients. However, the prognosis still depends on the underlying cause and its response to treatment.

How it happens

The most common causes of HF are chronic hypertension and MI. In hypertension, the high pressure in the arteries causes high pressure in the aorta. The high aortic pressure causes high resistance against the left ventricle, and the heart muscle weakens over time due to the high workload. HF can also result from a primary abnormality of the heart muscle such as MI. Because the MI weakens the heart muscle, it acts as a poor pump. The dead region of the heart muscle impairs ventricular function, which in turn leads to decreased circulation to the body. MI is a common cause of a weakened left ventricle, with consequent HF.

Factors favorable to failure

Certain conditions or diseases can predispose a patient to HF, especially if the person has underlying heart disease. These include:
- cardiomyopathies (see *discussion on cardiomyopathies*)
- substance misuse, including but not limited to excessive alcohol use, smoking, and tobacco use

- congenital heart defects
- uncontrolled diabetes
- family history
- severe lung disease
- obesity
- sleep apnea
- arrhythmias, such as tachyarrhythmias, which can reduce ventricular filling time; arrhythmias that disrupt the normal atrial and ventricular filling synchrony; and bradycardia, which can reduce cardiac output
- pregnancy, which increases circulatory blood volume
- thyrotoxicosis, which increases the force of myocardial contractions
- pulmonary embolism, which elevates pulmonary arterial pressure, causing right-sided HF
- infections, which increase metabolic demands and further burden the heart
- anemia, in which less oxygen is delivered to the heart muscle by the coronary arteries; severe anemia results in decreased cardiac output as the heart muscle is deprived of oxygen
- increased salt or water intake, emotional stress, or failure to adhere with the prescribed treatment regimen for the underlying heart disease

What to look for

The most common signs and symptoms of HF include:
- fatigue
- orthopnea
- exertional dyspnea
- paroxysmal nocturnal dyspnea
- neck vein engorgement (jugular vein distention)
- hepatomegaly and splenomegaly
- ascites (peritoneal edema causing abdominal distention)_
- ankle edema
- hypotension and decreased peripheral pulses
- water weight gain

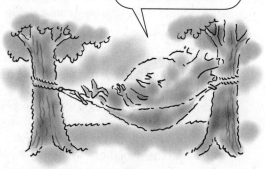

Look what happens if I'm laid up and can't do my job!

What tests tell you

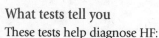

These tests help diagnose HF:
- ECG reveals ischemia, tachycardia, and extrasystole.
- Echocardiogram identifies the underlying cause as well as the type and severity of the HF. Echocardiogram can demonstrate left ventricular ejection fraction.
- Laboratory studies, such as B-type natriuretic peptide (BNP), confirm the presence of heart failure. A highly elevated BNP confirms HF.

- Chest x-ray shows increased pulmonary vascular markings, interstitial edema, or pleural effusion and cardiomegaly.
- PAP, also called *hemodynamic* or *Swan–Ganz catheter monitoring*, shows elevated PCWP, and elevated left ventricular end-diastolic pressure in left-sided HF and elevated right atrial pressure or CVP in right-sided HF. (See *Treating heart failure*, page 75.)

 Battling illness

Treating heart failure

The goal of treatment for heart failure is to improve pump function, thereby reversing the compensatory mechanisms that produce or intensify the clinical effects.

Heart failure can usually be controlled quickly with treatment, including:

- diuretics (such as furosemide [Lasix], metolazone, hydrochlorothiazide, ethacrynic acid [Edecrin], bumetanide, spironolactone [Aldactone] combined with a loop or thiazide diuretic, or triamterene [Dyrenium]) to reduce total blood volume and circulatory congestion
- angiotensin-converting enzyme inhibitor (ACEI) or angiotensin receptor blocker (ARB) to counteract the renin–angiotensin–aldosterone cycling mechanism
- bed rest balanced with prescribed activity and low-sodium diet
- oxygen administration to increase oxygen delivery to the myocardium and other vital organs
- inotropic drugs (such as digoxin) to strengthen myocardial contractility, sympathomimetics (such as dopamine and dobutamine) in acute situations, or milrinone to increase contractility and cause arterial vasodilation
- vasodilators to decrease peripheral arterial resistance
- antiembolism stockings to prevent venostasis and thromboembolism formation

Acute pulmonary edema

As a result of decreased contractility and elevated fluid volume and pressure, fluid may be driven from the pulmonary capillary beds into the alveoli, causing pulmonary edema. Treatment for acute pulmonary edema includes:
- morphine

- nitroglycerin or nitroprusside to diminish blood return to the heart
- dobutamine, dopamine, or milrinone to increase myocardial contractility and cardiac output
- diuretics to reduce fluid volume
- supplemental oxygen
- placement of the patient in high Fowler position

Continued care

After recovery, the patient must continue medical care and will usually continue taking digoxin, an ACEI or ARB, beta-adrenergic blockers, diuretics, and potassium supplements. It is important to inform the patient of diet modifications, including limiting sodium intake, activity instructions, monitoring weight daily, and signs and symptoms of worsening heart failure. Additionally, if the patient has been a smoker, it is important to encourage smoking cessation. The patient with valve dysfunction who has recurrent, acute heart failure may need surgical valve replacement.

What's left?

A cardiac pacemaker alone or in combination with an implantable cardioverter/defibrillator may be implanted to electrically stimulate more synchronous ventricular contractions, thereby improving the patient's cardiac output, ejection fraction, and mean arterial pressure. The only option for some patients is heart transplantation. A left ventricular assist device (VAD) may be necessary either as "short-term" use as a bridge until a heart is available for transplantation or as a "long-term" option, for those who are not candidates for heart transplantation.

Hypertension

Hypertension is an intermittent or sustained elevation of diastolic or systolic blood pressure. Generally, a sustained systolic blood pressure of 130 mm Hg or higher or a diastolic blood pressure greater than 80 mm Hg indicates hypertension.

Hypertension affects about 116 million adults in the United States, which is about one in every three adults. Of those affected, only about one in four adults have their blood pressure treated to within normal limits. Ethnicity also is also an important factor, in that African American people have a higher incidence of hypertension and at earlier ages than White people and Hispanic people, with the highest incidence among African American females.

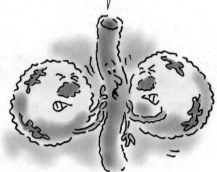

Stop pushing so hard! I don't need all this pressure.

This is essential...

The two major types of hypertension are essential (also called *primary*) and secondary. The etiology of essential hypertension, the most common type, is complex. It involves several interacting homeostatic mechanisms. Hypertension is classified as secondary if it's related to a systemic disease that raises peripheral vascular resistance. Malignant hypertension is a severe type of elevated BP that progresses rapidly and requires emergency treatment.

How it happens

Hypertension most commonly occurs because of increased pressure within the arteries due to a combination of factors. Arteriosclerosis is a common cause of narrowing of the arteries, thereby increasing blood pressure and resistance in the arteries. High fat in the diet contributes to the development of arteriosclerosis. High sodium in the diet increases blood pressure. Smoking can increase blood pressure because nicotine is a vasoconstrictor. Lack of exercise, chronic stress, and genetics also play a role in causing hypertension. Physiologically as one ages, the blood vessels become less elastic; therefore, aging is also a risk factor for hypertension.

Do you get the picture? Essential hypertension is sneaky. It may begin benign, but it will slowly get nasty.

Sly as a fox

Essential hypertension usually begins insidiously as a benign disease. If left untreated, even mild cases can cause major complications and death. Carefully managed treatment, which may include lifestyle modifications and drug therapy, improves prognosis.

Why? Why? Why?

Several theories help to explain the development of hypertension. For example, it's thought to arise from:

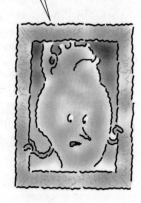

- changes in the arteriolar bed, causing increased resistance
- abnormally increased tone in the sensory nervous system that originates in the vasomotor system centers, causing increased peripheral vascular resistance
- increased blood volume resulting from renal or hormonal dysfunction
- an increase in arteriolar thickening caused by genetic factors, leading to increased peripheral vascular resistance
- abnormal renin release resulting in the formation of angiotensin II, which constricts the arterioles and increases blood volume (See *Understanding hypertension.*)

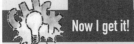

Now I get it!

Understanding hypertension: Constant cycling of the renin–angiotensin–aldosterone system

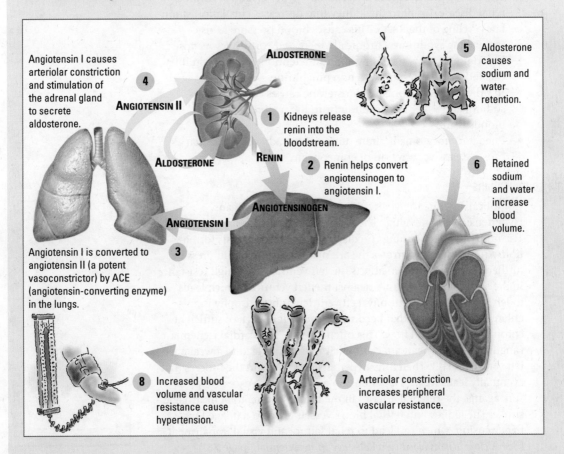

Angiotensin I causes arteriolar constriction and stimulation of the adrenal gland to secrete aldosterone.

4 ANGIOTENSIN II

ALDOSTERONE

ALDOSTERONE

RENIN

5 Aldosterone causes sodium and water retention.

1 Kidneys release renin into the bloodstream.

2 Renin helps convert angiotensinogen to angiotensin I.

ANGIOTENSINOGEN

6 Retained sodium and water increase blood volume.

ANGIOTENSIN I

Angiotensin I is converted to angiotensin II (a potent vasoconstrictor) by ACE (angiotensin-converting enzyme) in the lungs.

3

8 Increased blood volume and vascular resistance cause hypertension.

7 Arteriolar constriction increases peripheral vascular resistance.

Secondary hypertension

Secondary hypertension may be caused by:
- renal disease
- pheochromocytoma (rare adrenal tumor)
- primary hyperaldosteronism
- Cushing syndrome
- uncontrolled diabetes
- dysfunction of the thyroid, pituitary, or parathyroid gland
- coarctation of the aorta; congenital heart defects
- pregnancy
- neurologic disorders
- various drugs such as hormone therapy, cold medications, amphetamines, and illicit drugs

Underneath it all

The pathophysiology of secondary hypertension is related to the underlying disease. For example, consider these points:
- The most common cause of secondary hypertension is chronic renal disease. Insult to the kidney that decreases circulation stimulates cycling of the RAAS. This causes blood pressure to rise.
- In Cushing syndrome, chronically increased cortisol levels raise blood pressure by increasing sodium retention, angiotensin II levels, and vascular response to norepinephrine.
- In primary aldosteronism, aldosterone causes constant excess sodium and water reabsorption from the nephrons into the bloodstream.
- Pheochromocytoma is a rare tumor of the adrenal gland that causes excessive secretion of epinephrine.

Late complications

Complications due to hypertension can affect many organs. Hypertension creates a high shearing force against the arterial linings. The injury to arterial linings predisposes to arteriosclerosis formation. Arteriosclerosis narrows the arteries, increasing blood pressure further. Hypertension also affects the left ventricle. The high resistance in the aorta causes resistance against the left ventricle, which leads to left ventricular hypertrophy. Left ventricular hypertrophy is an enlarged heart muscle that becomes vulnerable to lack of sufficient coronary artery blood flow. This often leads to myocardial ischemia (angina) and MI (heart attack), which in turn can lead to a weakened left ventricle (HF). Therefore, hypertension can begin the process that eventually leads to HF. Hypertension can also cause excessive pressure against the cerebral arteries in the brain, leading to hemorrhagic stroke. The kidney and retinal blood vessels are also damaged by hypertension, which can lead to renal failure and visual impairment. (See *A close look at blood vessel damage in hypertension*, page 78.)

A close look at blood vessel damage in hypertension

Sustained hypertension damages the lining of arterial blood vessels. The endothelial cells that line the arteries become damaged by high blood pressure. Vascular injury causes white blood cells and platelets to rush to the area of injury, and a clot (thrombus) is formed. The clot can attract platelets to enlarge and then obstruct blood flow through the artery.

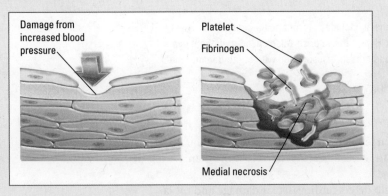

Damage from increased blood pressure

Platelet

Fibrinogen

Medial necrosis

What to look for

Hypertension usually doesn't produce signs and symptoms until vascular changes occur in the heart, brain, or kidneys. Severely elevated blood pressure damages the intima of small vessels, resulting in fibrin accumulation in the vessels, local edema, and, possibly, intravascular clotting.

Location, location, location

Symptoms depend on the location of the damaged vessels, for example:

- *brain*—stroke, transient ischemic attacks
- *retina*—blindness
- *heart*—MI
- *kidneys*—proteinuria, edema, and, eventually, renal failure

What tests tell you

The following tests may reveal predisposing factors and help identify the cause of hypertension:

- Urinalysis may show protein, red blood cells, or white blood cells (WBCs), indicating renal disease, or glucose, indicating diabetes.

Treating hypertension

Although essential hypertension has no cure, drugs and modifications in diet and lifestyle can control the effects. Generally, lifestyle modification is the first treatment used, especially in early, mild cases. Lifestyle modification includes sodium restriction, weight reduction if overweight, regular exercise, use of relaxation techniques, avoidance of caffeine and tobacco, and limiting alcohol intake. If this doesn't work, the healthcare provider may prescribe various types of antihypertensives.

A secondary approach
Treatment of secondary hypertension includes correcting the underlying cause and controlling hypertensive effects. Hypertensive crisis (also called *malignant hypertension*) is severely elevated blood pressure associated with organ damage that may be fatal.

- Blood urea nitrogen levels that are elevated to more than 20 mg/dL and serum creatinine levels that are elevated to more than 1.5 mg/dL suggest renal disease.

  These tests may help detect cardiovascular damage and other complications:
- ECG may show left atrial and ventricular hypertrophy or ischemia.
- Chest x-ray may demonstrate enlarged heart (termed *cardiomegaly*). (See *Treating hypertension*.)

Pericarditis

The pericardium is the fibroserous sac that envelops, supports, and protects the heart. Inflammation of this sac is called *pericarditis*.

This condition occurs in acute and chronic forms. The acute form can be fibrinous or effusive, with serous, purulent, or hemorrhagic exudate. The chronic form, called *constrictive pericarditis*, is characterized by dense, fibrous pericardial thickening. The prognosis depends on the underlying cause but is typically good in acute pericarditis, unless constriction occurs.

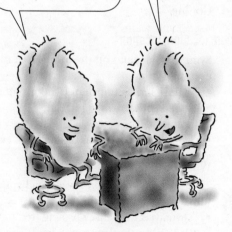

How it happens

Common causes of pericarditis include:

- bacterial, fungal, or viral infection (infectious pericarditis)
- neoplasms (primary or metastatic from the lungs, breasts, or other organs)
- high-dose radiation to the chest
- uremia
- hypersensitivity or autoimmune disease, such as systemic lupus erythematosus, rheumatoid arthritis, or acute rheumatic fever (most common cause of pericarditis in children)
- drugs, such as hydralazine or procainamide
- idiopathic factors (most common in acute pericarditis)
- postcardiac injury, such as MI (which later causes an autoimmune reaction in the pericardium), trauma, and surgery that leaves the pericardium intact but allows blood to leak into the pericardial cavity
- aortic aneurysm with pericardial leakage (less common)
- myxedema with cholesterol deposits in the pericardium (less common)

The effusion conclusion

Pericardial effusion is the major complication of acute pericarditis. If fluid accumulates rapidly, cardiac tamponade may occur. This may lead to shock, cardiovascular collapse, and, eventually, death.

A scarred heart

As the pericardium becomes inflamed, it may become thickened and fibrotic. If it doesn't heal completely after an acute episode, it may calcify over a long period and form a firm scar around the heart. This scarring interferes with diastolic filling of the ventricles.

What to look for

In acute pericarditis, a sharp, sudden pain usually starts over the sternum and radiates to the neck, shoulders, back, and arms. However, unlike the pain of MI, this pain is commonly pleuritic, increasing with deep inspiration and decreasing when the patient sits up and leans forward, pulling the heart away from the diaphragmatic pleurae of the lungs. A friction rub (a distinct sound heard when two dry surfaces rub together) is audible on auscultation.

Pericardial effusion, the major complication of acute pericarditis, may produce symptoms of HF, such as dyspnea, orthopnea, and tachycardia. Pleural effusion may also produce ill-defined substernal chest pain and a feeling of chest fullness.

If the fluid accumulates rapidly, cardiac tamponade may occur, causing pallor, clammy skin, hypotension, pulsus paradoxus, neck vein distention, and, eventually, cardiovascular collapse and death.

Treating pericarditis

The goal of treatment for pericarditis is to relieve symptoms, prevent or treat pericardial effusion and cardiac tamponade, and manage the underlying disease.

Bed rest and drug therapy

In idiopathic pericarditis, postmyocardial infarction pericarditis, and postthoracotomy pericarditis, treatment is twofold: bed rest as long as fever and pain persist and nonsteroidal anti-inflammatory drugs, such as aspirin and indomethacin, to relieve pain and reduce inflammation.

If symptoms continue, the healthcare provider may prescribe corticosteroids. Although they provide rapid and effective relief, corticosteroids must be used cautiously because pericarditis may recur when drug therapy stops.

More involved treatment

When infectious pericarditis results from disease of the left pleural space, mediastinal abscesses, or septicemia, the patient requires antibiotics, surgical drainage, or both. If cardiac tamponade develops, the doctor may perform emergency pericardiocentesis and may inject antibiotics directly into the pericardial sac.

Heavy-duty treatment

Recurrent pericarditis may require partial pericardiectomy, which creates a window that allows fluid to drain into the pleural space. In constrictive pericarditis, total pericardiectomy may be necessary to permit the heart to fill and contract adequately.

What tests tell you

These laboratory test results reflect inflammation and may identify the disorder's cause:

- History and physical examination: pericardial friction rub and pulsus paradoxus (a decrease in systolic BP during inspiration exaggerated in cardiac tamponade).
- WBC count may be normal or elevated, especially in infectious pericarditis.
- Erythrocyte sedimentation rate (ESR) is elevated.
- Troponin levels may be elevated with acute pericarditis.
- Pericardial biopsy and pericardial fluid culture to identify a causative organism with infectious pericarditis.
- ECG shows characteristic changes in acute pericarditis. This includes widespread ST segment elevations, indicative of abnormal repolarization. Rhythm changes may also occur, including atrial ectopic rhythms, such as atrial fibrillation and sinus arrhythmias.
- Echocardiography diagnoses pericardial effusion or cardiac tamponade (Lewis et al., 2014).

Rheumatic fever and RHD

A systemic inflammatory disease of childhood, acute rheumatic fever develops after infection of the upper respiratory tract with group A beta-hemolytic streptococci. Group A beta-hemolytic streptococci often causes pharyngitis (strep throat). If antibiotic treatment is not obtained, rheumatic fever can occur. This disorder involves the heart, joints, central nervous system, skin, and subcutaneous tissues. If rheumatic fever isn't treated, deformity of the cardiac valves can occur, resulting in RHD.

Group A beta-hemolytic streptococci infection is mainly a pediatric disease in regions with poor medical resources. It is estimated that 1% to 3% of patients with this untreated disease, typically pharyngitis (strep throat), will develop rheumatic fever, and of these, up to 60% of cases will result in chronic RHD.

How it happens

Rheumatic fever appears to be a hypersensitivity reaction. For some reason, antibodies produced to combat streptococci react and produce characteristic lesions at specific tissue sites, particularly the heart valves.

Getting complicated

The mitral and aortic valves are commonly destroyed by rheumatic fever's long-term effects. Their malfunction leads to severe heart inflammation (called *carditis*) and, occasionally, produces pericardial effusion and fatal HF.

Rheumatic carditis develops in up to 50% of patients with rheumatic fever and may affect the endocardium, myocardium, or pericardium during the early acute phase (Burke, 2015). Later, the heart valves may be damaged, causing chronic valvular disease. (See *Sequelae of rheumatic heart disease.*)

Follow the infection

The extent of heart damage depends on where the infection strikes and whether or not the disease is self-limiting or chronic:

- Myocarditis produces characteristic lesions called *Aschoff bodies* in the interstitial tissue of the heart as well as cellular swelling and fragmentation of interstitial collagen. These lesions lead to formation of progressively fibrotic nodules and interstitial scars.
- Endocarditis causes valve leaflet swelling, erosion along the lines of leaflet closure, and blood, platelet, and fibrin deposits, which form beadlike vegetation. Endocarditis strikes the mitral valve most commonly in females and the aortic valve in males. It affects the tricuspid valves in both males and females and, rarely, can affect the pulmonic valve.

Now I get it!

Sequelae of rheumatic heart disease

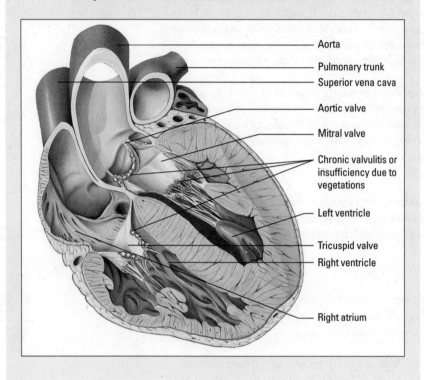

- Aorta
- Pulmonary trunk
- Superior vena cava
- Aortic valve
- Mitral valve
- Chronic valvulitis or insufficiency due to vegetations
- Left ventricle
- Tricuspid valve
- Right ventricle
- Right atrium

What to look for

Acute rheumatic fever can only follow a streptococcal pharyngeal infection. This infection usually occurred a few days to 6 weeks prior.

Most patients report migratory joint pain or polyarthritis. Swelling, redness, and signs of effusion usually accompany such pain, which most commonly affects the knees, ankles, elbows, and hips.

Rash talk

About 5% of patients (usually those with carditis) develop a nonpruritic, macular, transient rash called *erythema marginatum*. This rash gives rise to red lesions with blanched centers. These same patients may also develop firm, movable, nontender subcutaneous nodules about 3 mm to 2 cm in diameter, usually near tendons or bony prominences of joints. These nodules persist for a few days to several weeks.

What tests tell you

No specific laboratory tests can determine the presence of rheumatic fever, but these test results support the diagnosis:

- WBC count and ESR may be elevated during the acute phase; blood studies show slight anemia caused by suppressed erythropoiesis during inflammation.
- C-reactive protein is positive, especially during the acute phase.
- Cardiac enzyme levels may be increased in severe myocarditis.
- Antistreptolysin O titer is elevated in 95% of patients within 2 months of onset.
- Throat cultures may continue to show group A beta-hemolytic streptococci; however, they usually occur in small numbers and isolating them is difficult.
- ECG reveals delayed AV conduction, as evidenced by a prolonged PR interval.
- Chest x-ray shows normal heart size, except with myocarditis, HF, and pericardial effusion.
- Echocardiography helps evaluate valvular damage, chamber size, ventricular function, and the presence of a pericardial effusion.
- Cardiac catheterization evaluates valvular damage and left ventricular function in severe cardiac dysfunction. (See *Treating rheumatic fever and rheumatic heart disease.*)

Battling illness

Treating rheumatic fever and rheumatic heart disease

Effective treatment for rheumatic fever and rheumatic heart disease aims to eradicate the streptococcal infection, relieve symptoms, and prevent recurrence, thus reducing the chance of permanent cardiac damage.

Acute phase

During the acute phase, treatment includes appropriate antibiotic therapy to treat the infection. Salicylates and NSAIDS are used to relieve fever, joint pain, and other symptoms. Corticosteroids may be used if salicylates fail to relieve pain and inflammation.

Patients with active carditis require strict bed rest for about 5 weeks during the acute phase, followed by a progressive increase in physical activity. The increase depends on clinical and laboratory findings and the patient's response to treatment.

Long-term treatment

After the acute phase subsides, lifelong prophylactic antibiotic therapy before any invasive procedure (e.g., dental treatment) is recommended to prevent infective endocarditis.

Complications

Heart failure requires continued bed rest and diuretics. Severe mitral or aortic valvular dysfunction that causes persistent heart failure will require corrective surgery, such as commissurotomy (separation of the adherent, thickened leaflets of the mitral valve), valvuloplasty (inflation of a balloon within a valve), or valve replacement (with a prosthetic valve). However, this surgery is seldom necessary before late adolescence.

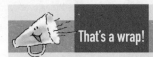

Cardiovascular system review

Understanding the cardiovascular system
The cardiovascular system is made up of the heart, arteries, veins, and lymphatics.
• Organs transport life-supporting oxygen and nutrients to cells, remove metabolic waste products, and carry hormones from one part of the body to another.

Myocardial function
• Increase in oxygen demand must be met by increase in oxygen supply.
• Blood normally flows in one direction across heart valves.
• Pressure gradient causes the valves to open and close.

Response to blood pressure drop
• Heart rate increases.
• Force of contraction increases.
• Arterioles constrict.

Response to blood pressure increase
• Heart rate decreases.
• Force of contraction decreases.
• Vasodilation occurs.

Cardiovascular disorders
• *Aneurysm*—an abnormal dilation or outpouching in an arterial wall or cardiac chamber
• *Cardiogenic shock*—condition of diminished cardiac output that severely impairs tissue perfusion as well as oxygen delivery to the tissues
• *Cardiac tamponade*—condition caused by blood or fluid accumulation in the pericardium, which leads to compressed heart chambers and decreased cardiac output

• *Coronary artery disease*—most commonly due to arteriosclerotic plaque, which narrows coronary arteries. This leads to lack of sufficient coronary artery blood supply to the myocardium, which can cause myocardial ischemia (angina) or myocardial infarction (heart attack).
• *Cardiomyopathy*—disorder that's caused by extensive damage to the heart's muscle fibers, which results in dilated heart chambers
• *Deep vein thrombophlebitis* (DVT)—develops when a thrombus, or blood clot, attaches to a vessel wall, usually in the lower extremities. The clot can dislodge and travel as a thromboembolism up to the inferior vena cava into the right atrium, into the right ventricle, and then into the pulmonary artery in the lungs.
• *Heart failure*—impaired ventricular function due to a heart muscle abnormality that prevents the heart from pumping enough blood
• *Hypertension*—intermittent or sustained elevation of diastolic or systolic blood pressure
• *MI*—myocardial cell death caused by blockage of one or more coronary arteries. Myocardial infarction begins with myocardial ischemia, which is prolonged and results in irreversible cell damage and muscle death.
• *Pericarditis*—acute or chronic condition that's caused by an attack of bacteria or other substances that results in fibrosis and scar tissue after the infection ceases
• *Rheumatic fever and heart disease*—systemic inflammatory disease of childhood that develops after infection of the upper respiratory tract with group A beta-hemolytic streptococci

Quick quiz

1. Which factor is a major modifiable risk factor for CAD?
    A. High cholesterol
    B. Genetic predisposition
    C. Age
    D. Family history

Answer: A. High cholesterol is a risk factor that can be modified.

2. Which cause accounts for 50% of all cases of hypertrophic cardiomyopathy?
    A. Autoimmune disease
    B. Genetic predisposition
    C. Malnutrition
    D. MI

Answer: B. Genetic predisposition accounts for 50% of all cases of hypertrophic cardiomyopathy. The other 50% have unknown causes.

3. Which of the following is the major pathophysiologic effect of cardiac tamponade?
    A. Atelectasis
    B. Hypertension
    C. Compressed heart
    D. Distended pericardium

Answer: C. Cardiac tamponade is the progressive accumulation of fluid in the pericardium and causes compression of the heart chambers.

4. When a thrombus completely occludes the blood flow through one of the coronary arteries, causing myocardial ischemia, injury, and necrosis through all layers of the myocardium, it is known as a:
    A. nontransmural MI.
    B. NSTEMI.
    C. STEMI.
    D. Prinzmetal angina.

Answer: C. If a thrombus lodges in a coronary artery and completely blocks the blood flow through one of the coronary arteries, the patient will experience myocardial ischemia, injury, and necrosis. Marked ST segment elevation MI will develop. The damage extends through all layers of the myocardium, also known as a transmural MI.

Scoring

☆☆☆   If you answered all four items correctly, hats off! There's only one way to say it: You're all heart!

☆☆   If you answered three items correctly, great job! Your heart is in the right place and so is your nose (your nose is in this book).

☆   If you answered fewer than three items correctly, don't fret! You may want to review a little more.

Suggested references

Aguilar-Salinas, C. A., Gómez-Díaz, R. A., & Corral, P. (2022). New therapies for primary hyperlipidemia. *The Journal of Clinical Endocrinology and Metabolism, 107*(5), 1216–1224. https://doi.org/10.1210/clinem/dgab876

Al Ghorani, H., Götzinger, F., Böhm, M., & Mahfoud, F. (2022). Arterial hypertension—clinical trials update 2021. *Nutrition, Metabolism, and Cardiovascular Diseases : NMCD, 32*(1), 21–31. https://doi.org/10.1016/j.numecd.2021.09.007

Aldiwani, H., Mahdai, S., Alhatemi, G., & Bairey Merz, C. N. (2021). Microvascular angina: Diagnosis and management. *European Cardiology, 16*, e46. https://doi.org/10.15420/ecr.2021.15

American Heart Association (AHA). (2019). *Cardiovascular diseases affect nearly half of American adults, statistics show.* https://www.heart.org/en/news/2019/01/31/cardiovascular-diseases-affect-nearly-half-of-american-adults-statistics-show

Andreis, A., Imazio, M., Casula, M., Avondo, S., & Brucato, A. (2021). Recurrent pericarditis: An update on diagnosis and management. *Internal and Emergency Medicine, 16*(3), 551–558. https://doi.org/10.1007/s11739-021-02639-6

Atwood, J. (2022). Management of acute coronary syndrome. *Emergency Medicine Clinics of North America, 40*(4), 693–706. https://doi.org/10.1016/j.emc.2022.06.008

Bouriche, F., Toro, A., Negre, V., & Yvorra, S. (2021). Acute pericarditis: Aetiologic diagnosis and practical aspect of the management. *Current Problems in Cardiology, 46*(4), 100769. https://doi.org/10.1016/j.cpcardiol.2020.100769

Brown, R. M. (2022). Acute coronary syndrome in women. *Emergency Medicine Clinics of North America, 40*(4), 629–636. https://doi.org/10.1016/j.emc.2022.06.003

Centers for Disease Control and Prevention (CDC). (2022). *Heart disease facts.* https://www.cdc.gov/heartdisease/facts.htm

Centers for Disease Control and Prevention (CDC). 2023. *Facts about hypertension.* https://www.cdc.gov/bloodpressure/facts.htm

Chen, J., & Aronowitz, P. (2022). Congestive heart failure. *The Medical Clinics of North America, 106*(3), 447–458. https://doi.org/10.1016/j.mcna.2021.12.002

Duffett, L. (2022). Deep venous thrombosis. *Annals of Internal Medicine, 175*(9), ITC129–ITC144. https://doi.org/10.7326/AITC202209200

Fan, J., & Watanabe, T. (2022). Atherosclerosis: Known and unknown. *Pathology International, 72*(3), 151–160. https://doi.org/10.1111/pin.13202

Ford, T. J., Ong, P., Sechtem, U., Beltrame, J., Camici, P. G., Crea, F., Kaski, J. C., Bairey Merz, C. N., Pepine, C. J., Shimokawa, H., Berry, C., & COVADIS Study Group.

(2020). Assessment of vascular dysfunction in patients without obstructive coronary artery disease: Why, how, and when. *JACC. Cardiovascular Interventions*, *13*(16), 1847–1864. https://doi.org/10.1016/j.jcin.2020.05.052

Govea, A., Lipinksi, J., & Patel, M. P. (2021). Prehospital evaluation, ED management, transfers, and management of inpatient STEMI. *Interventional Cardiology Clinics*, *10*(3), 293–306. https://doi.org/10.1016/j.iccl.2021.03.002

Harding, D., Chong, M. H. A., Lahoti, N., Bigogno, C. M., Prema, R., Mohiddin, S. A., & Marelli-Berg, F. (2023). Dilated cardiomyopathy and chronic cardiac inflammation: Pathogenesis, diagnosis and therapy. *Journal of Internal Medicine*, *293*(1), 23–47. https://doi.org/10.1111/joim.13556

Health and Human Services Office of Minority Health. (2023). *Heart Disease and African Americans*. https://minorityhealth.hhs.gov/omh

Kearns, M. J., & Walley, K. R. (2018). Tamponade: Hemodynamic and echocardiographic diagnosis. *Chest*, *153*(5), 1266–1275. https://doi.org/10.1016/j.chest.2017.11.003

Kumar, R. K., Antunes, M. J., Beaton, A., Mirabel, M., Nkomo, V. T., Okello, E., Regmi, P. R., Reményi, B., Sliwa-Hähnle, K., Zühlke, L. J., Sable, C., & American Heart Association Council on Lifelong Congenital Heart Disease and Heart Health in the Young; Council on Cardiovascular and Stroke Nursing; and Council on Clinical Cardiology. (2020). Contemporary diagnosis and management of rheumatic heart disease: Implications for closing the gap—A scientific statement from the American Heart Association. *Circulation*, *142*(20), e337–e357. https://doi.org/10.1161/CIR.0000000000000921

Lahiri, S., & Sanyahumbi, A. (2021). Acute rheumatic fever. *Pediatrics in Review*, *42*(5), 221–232. https://doi.org/10.1542/pir.2019-0288

de Loizaga, S. R., & Beaton, A. Z. (2021). Rheumatic fever and rheumatic heart disease in the United States. *Pediatric Annals*, *50*(3), e98–e104. https://doi.org/10.3928/19382359-20210221-01

Maron, B. J., Desai, M. Y., Nishimura, R. A., Spirito, P., Rakowski, H., Towbin, J. A., Rowin, E. J., Maron, M. S., & Sherrid, M. V. (2022). Diagnosis and evaluation of hypertrophic cardiomyopathy: JACC state-of-the-art review. *Journal of the American College of Cardiology*, *79*(4), 372–389. https://doi.org/10.1016/j.jacc.2021.12.002

Mateo-Rodríguez, I., Danet, A., Bolívar-Muñoz, J., Rosell-Ortriz, F., Garcia-Mochón, L., & Daponte-Codina, A. (2022). Gender differences, inequalities and biases in the management of Acute Coronary Syndrome. *Journal of Healthcare Quality Research*, *37*(3), 169–181. https://doi.org/10.1016/j.jhqr.2021.10.010

Meyers, H. P., Bracey, A., Lee, D., Lichtenheld, A., Li, W. J., Singer, D. D., Kane, J. A., Dodd, K. W., Meyers, K. E., Thode, H. C., Shroff, G. R., Singer, A. J., & Smith, S. W. (2021). Comparison of the ST-elevation myocardial Infarction (STEMI) vs. NSTEMI and Occlusion MI (OMI) vs. NOMI paradigms of acute MI. *The Journal of Emergency Medicine*, *60*(3), 273–284. https://doi.org/10.1016/j.jemermed.2020.10.026

Murphy, S. P., Ibrahim, N. E., & Januzzi, J. L. Jr. (2020). Heart failure with reduced ejection fraction: A review. *JAMA*, *324*(5), 488–504. https://doi.org/10.1001/jama.2020.10262

Norris, T. (2025). *Porth's pathophysiology: Concepts of altered health states*. 11th ed. Wolters Kluwer.

Ono, M., Serruys, P. W., Hara, H., Kawashima, H., Gao, C., Wang, R., Takahashi, K., O'Leary, N., Wykrzykowska, J. J., Sharif, F., Piek, J. J., Garg, S., Mack, M. J., Holmes, D. R., Morice, M. C., Head, S. J., Kappetein, A. P., Thuijs, D. J. F. M., Noack, T., … SYNTAX Extended Survival Investigators. (2021). 10-Year follow-up after revascularization in elderly patients with complex coronary artery disease. *Journal of the American College of Cardiology, 77*(22), 2761–2773. https://doi.org/10.1016/j.jacc.2021.04.016

Samsky, M. D., Morrow, D. A., Proudfoot, A. G., Hochman, J. S., Thiele, H., & Rao, S. V. (2021). Cardiogenic shock after acute myocardial infarction: A review. *JAMA, 326*(18), 1840–1850. https://doi.org/10.1001/jama.2021.18323

Savarese, G., Stolfo, D., Sinagra, G., & Lund, L. H. (2022). Heart failure with mid-range or mildly reduced ejection fraction. *Nature Reviews Cardiology, 19*(2), 100–116. https://doi.org/10.1038/s41569-021-00605-5

Shah, A. H., Puri, R., & Kalra, A. (2019). Management of cardiogenic shock complicating acute myocardial infarction: A review. *Clinical Cardiology, 42*(4), 484–493. https://doi.org/10.1002/clc.23168

Shaw, P. M., Loree, J., Gibbons, R. C. (2023, January). *Abdominal aortic aneurysm.* In: *StatPearls* [Internet]. StatPearls Publishing. Available from: https://www.ncbi.nlm.nih.gov/books/NBK470237/

Sinnenberg, L., & Givertz, M. M. (2020). Acute heart failure. *Trends in Cardiovascular Medicine, 30*(2), 104–112. https://doi.org/10.1016/j.tcm.2019.03.007

Skeik, N., Smith, J. E., Jensen, J. D., Nowariak, M. E., Manunga, J. M., Mirza, A. K. (2021). Literature review of distal deep vein thrombosis. *Journal of Vascular Surgery, Venous and Lymphatic Disorders, 9*(4), 1062–1070.e6. https://doi.org/10.1016/j.jvsv.2021.01.018

Skotsimara, G., Antonopoulos, A., Oikonomou, E., Papastamos, C., Siasos, G., & Tousoulis, D. (2022). Aortic wall inflammation in the pathogenesis, diagnosis and treatment of aortic aneurysms. *Inflammation, 45*(3), 965–976. https://doi.org/10.1007/s10753-022-01626-z

Waheed, N., Elias-Smale, S., Malas, W., Maas, A. H., Sedlak, T. L., Tremmel, J., & Mehta, P. K. (2020). Sex differences in non-obstructive coronary artery disease. *Cardiovascular Research, 116*(4), 829–840. https://doi.org/10.1093/cvr/cvaa001

Chapter 4

Hematologic system*

Just the facts

In this chapter, you'll learn:

♦ about blood and its components

♦ the function of blood

♦ pathophysiology, signs and symptoms, diagnostic tests, and treatments for common blood disorders.

Understanding blood

Blood is one of the body's major fluid tissues. Pumped by the heart, it continuously circulates through the blood vessels, carrying vital elements to every part of the body. Blood is made of:
- a liquid component—plasma
- cellular components—erythrocytes, leukocytes, and thrombocytes (platelets) suspended in plasma

A component list

Each of blood's components performs specific vital functions:
- Plasma carries antibodies and nutrients to tissues and carries wastes away.
- Erythrocytes, also called *red blood cells* (RBCs), carry oxygen to the tissues and remove carbon dioxide from them.
- Leukocytes, or *white blood cells* (WBCs), participate in the inflammatory and immune response.
- Thrombocytes, or *platelets*, along with the coagulation factors in plasma, are essential to normal blood clotting.
  A problem with any of these components may have serious and even deadly consequences.

---

*Note: In this chapter, the term "male" refers to a person assigned male at birth, and the term "female" refers to a person assigned female at birth.

Plasma

Plasma is a clear, straw-colored fluid that consists mainly of the proteins, albumin, globulin, and fibrinogen held in aqueous suspension. Plasma's fluid characteristics, including its osmotic pressure, viscosity, and suspension qualities, depend on its protein content.

Other components in plasma include glucose, lipids, amino acids, electrolytes, pigments, hormones, oxygen, and carbon dioxide. These components regulate acid–base balance and immune responses as well as carry nutrients to tissues and help to mediate coagulation.

Don't forget to digest this bit of info

Important products of metabolism that circulate in plasma include urea, uric acid, creatinine, and lactic acid.

Red blood cells

RBCs in adults are produced in the bone marrow. In the fetus, the liver and spleen also participate in RBC production. The RBC production process is called *erythropoiesis*.

All aboard

RBCs transport oxygen to body tissues and carbon dioxide away from them. Hemoglobin (Hgb), an oxygen-carrying substance, gives RBCs this ability. Synthesis of hemoglobin requires iron (Fe^{++}).

RBC production is regulated by the tissues' demand for oxygen and the blood cells' ability to deliver it. A lack of oxygen in the tissues (hypoxia) stimulates the formation and release of erythropoietin, a hormone that activates the bone marrow to produce RBCs. About 80% to 90% of erythropoietin is made in the kidneys; the remainder comes from the liver. The lifespan for the typical RBC is 120 days.

The making of an erythrocyte

Erythrocyte formation begins with a precursor, called a *stem cell*. All precursor cells in the bone marrow are termed *stem cells*—they have the potential to become RBC, WBC, or platelet depending on the body's needs. The kidney secretes erythropoietin when it senses hypoxia. Erythropoietin goes to the bone marrow to stimulate stem cells to become mature RBCs. RBC development requires vitamin B_{12}, folic acid, and minerals, such as copper, cobalt, and—especially—*iron*.

Ironclad facts

Iron (Fe^{++}) is a component of hemoglobin and is vital to the blood's oxygen-carrying capacity. Iron is found in food and, when consumed, is absorbed in the duodenum and upper jejunum. The most absorbable sources of iron are meats and some fish. Some plants contain iron such as legumes (beans) and spinach. After iron is absorbed, it is transported to the bone marrow for hemoglobin synthesis. Iron may also be transported to needy tissues such as muscle for myoglobin synthesis.

Unused iron is temporarily stored as ferritin and hemosiderin in specialized cells called *reticuloendothelial cells* (most commonly in the liver) until it's released for use in the bone marrow to form new RBCs.

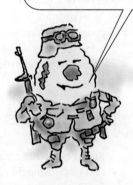

White blood cells protect the body by phagocytosis of pathogens and producing antibodies and antitoxins against foreign invaders.

White blood cells

WBCs protect the body against harmful bacteria and infection. They're classified in one of the two ways as:
1. granular leukocytes (granulocytes), such as neutrophils, eosinophils, and basophils
2. nongranular leukocytes, such as monocytes and lymphocytes
   Most WBCs are produced in bone marrow. Lymphocytes complete their maturation in the lymph nodes.

Running the gamut

WBCs have a wide range of lifespans; some granulocytes circulate for less than 6 hours, some monocytes may survive for weeks or months, and some lymphocytes last for years. Normally, the number of WBCs ranges from 5,000 to 10,000/µL.

It takes all types

Types of granulocytes include the following:
- Neutrophils, the predominant form of granulocyte, make up about 60% of WBCs. They surround and digest invading organisms and other foreign matter by phagocytosis.
- Eosinophils, minor granulocytes, defend against parasites, participate in allergic reactions, and fight lung and skin infections.
- Basophils, also minor granulocytes, release histamine into the blood and participate in delayed allergic reactions. They also contain heparin, an anticoagulant.

Types of nongranular leukocytes include the following:
- Monocytes, along with neutrophils, devour invading organisms by phagocytosis. They also migrate to tissues where they develop into cells called *macrophages* that participate in immunity.
- Lymphocytes occur mostly in two forms: B cells and T cells. B cells produce antibodies, while T cells regulate cell-mediated immunity.

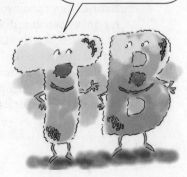

Call me T cell, and this is my fellow lymphocyte, B cell. We're just a couple of WBCs working hard to bolster your immunity.

Platelets

Platelets are small (2 to 4 μm in diameter), colorless, disk-shaped cytoplasmic cells split from cells in bone marrow. They have a lifespan of 7 to 10 days.

Platelets perform three vital functions to help minimize blood loss:
1. They help constrict damaged blood vessels.
2. They form hemostatic plugs in injured blood vessels by becoming swollen, spiky, sticky, and secretory.
3. They provide substances that accelerate blood clotting, such as factors III and XIII and platelet factor III.

It's a team effort

In a complex process called *hemostasis*, platelets, plasma, and coagulation factors interact to control bleeding. When tissue injury occurs, blood vessels at the injury site constrict and platelets mesh or clump to help prevent hemorrhage. (See *Understanding clotting*, page 95.)

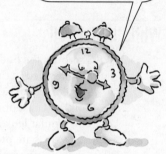

Clotting begins within minutes when a blood vessel is injured or severed.

Blood dyscrasias

Blood elements are prone to various types of dysfunction. An abnormal or pathologic condition of the blood is called a *dyscrasia*.

Erythrocytes, leukocytes, and platelets are manufactured in the bone marrow. Bone marrow cells and their precursors are especially vulnerable to physiologic changes that can affect cell production. Why? Because bone marrow cells reproduce rapidly and have a short lifespan. In addition, storage of circulating cells in the bone marrow is minimal.

Bringing some order to blood disorders

Blood disorders may be primary or secondary and quantitative or qualitative. They may involve some or all blood components.

A primary bleeding disorder occurs because of a problem within the blood itself. A secondary bleeding disorder results from a cause other than a defect in the blood.

Qualitative blood disorders stem from intrinsic cell abnormalities or plasma component dysfunction. Quantitative blood disorders result from increased or decreased cell production or cell destruction.

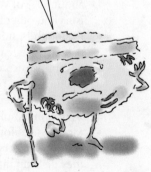

As a bone marrow cell, I can have it rough—my rapid reproduction coupled with a short life leaves me vulnerable to dysfunction.

Now I get it!

Understanding clotting

When a blood vessel is severed or injured, clotting begins within minutes to stop loss of blood. Coagulation factors are essential to normal blood clotting. Absent, decreased, or excess coagulation factors may lead to a clotting abnormality. Coagulation factors are commonly designated by Roman numerals.

Arriving at clotting through two pathways

Clotting may be initiated through two different pathways, the intrinsic pathway or the extrinsic pathway. The intrinsic pathway is activated when plasma comes in contact with damaged vessel surfaces. The extrinsic pathway is activated by tissue injury when tissue thromboplastin, a substance released by damaged endothelial cells, comes in contact with one of the clotting factors.

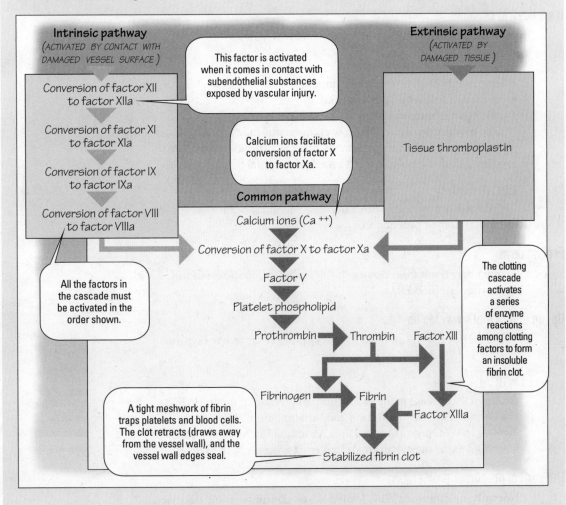

These can all end in bad blood

Blood disorders may be caused by:
- trauma
- cancer (infiltration of bone marrow)
- chemotherapy
- chronic disease such as cirrhosis
- surgery
- malnutrition
- drugs
- toxins
- radiation
- genetic and congenital defects
- sepsis

It's a no-win situation

Depressed bone marrow production or increased destruction of mature blood cells can result in:
- decreased RBCs (anemia)
- decreased platelets (thrombocytopenia)
- decreased leukocytes (leukopenia)
- all three components being decreased (pancytopenia)

The production of bone marrow components may increase. This results in myeloproliferative disorders, such as chronic myeloid leukemia, myelofibrosis, polycythemia vera, and essential thrombocytosis.

RBC disorders

RBC disorders may occur with a decrease (anemia) or increase (polycythemia) in their production.

Feeling down

Anemia may result from decreased RBC production, increased RBC destruction, or blood loss.

Up, up and…that's way too up

Polycythemia may result from hypoxia, tumors that secrete erythropoietin, kidney disease, or genetic defects.

WBC disorders

A temporary increase in the production and release of mature WBCs is a normal response to infection and inflammation. However, an increase in WBC precursors and their accumulation in bone marrow or lymphoid tissue signal leukemia. Leukemia is cancer of the WBCs.

The peril of precursor proliferation

Not only are cancerous WBC (called *blasts*) nonfunctioning, because they don't protect against infection—they can be harmful as well:

- They take over the bone marrow, crowding out other vital components, such as RBCs, platelets, and mature healthy WBCs.
- They spill into the bloodstream, sometimes infiltrating organs and impairing their function.

Running at a deficit

The most common types of WBC deficiencies are neutropenia (decrease in the number of neutrophils in the blood) and lymphocytopenia (reduction in the number of lymphocytes in the blood). The latter is less common.

WBC deficiencies may result from:
- inadequate cell production
- drug reactions
- ionizing radiation
- infiltrated bone marrow (cancer)
- congenital defects
- aplastic anemias
- folic acid deficiency
- hypersplenism

Platelet disorders

Disorders may occur with platelets when they're:
1. too few (thrombocytopenia)
2. too many (thrombocytosis)
3. dysfunctional (thrombocytopathy)

> Decrease, excess, dysfunction...it all leads to disorder.

Too few...

Thrombocytopenia may result from a congenital deficiency, or it may be acquired through one of the following:
- exposure to drugs such as heparin
- cancerous infiltration of bone marrow
- abnormal sequestration (blood accumulation and pooling) in the spleen
- infection
- exposure to ionizing radiation

Too many...

Thrombocytosis occurs as a result of certain diseases such as cancer.

Too much trouble...

Thrombocytopathy usually results from disease, such as uremia or liver failure, or adverse effects of medications, such as salicylates and nonsteroidal anti-inflammatory drugs (NSAIDs). It can also be caused by some herbs, such as alfalfa, chamomile, clove, evening primrose oil, garlic, ginger, ginseng, and red clover.

Blood disorders

The disorders discussed in this section include:
- acid–base imbalances
- anemia
- disseminated intravascular coagulation (DIC)
- hemophilia
- idiopathic thrombocytopenic purpura (ITP)
- iron deficiency anemia
- leukemia
- lymphomas
- multiple myeloma
- thrombocytopenia

Acid–base imbalances

Normally, the body's pH control mechanism is so effective that blood pH stays within a narrow range—7.35 to 7.45. Acid–base balance is maintained by buffer systems and by the lungs and kidneys, which neutralize and eliminate acids as rapidly as the acids are formed. (See *Maintaining acid–base balance*).

Now I get it!

Maintaining acid–base balance

The chemical reaction that is a buffer system occurring in the bloodstream at all times is:

$$CO^2 + H_2O \leftrightarrow H_2CO_3 \leftrightarrow H^+ \text{ and } HCO_3^-$$

(This chemical reaction is constantly moving left to right and also right to left, to maintain equilibrium.)

The lungs can cause an increase or a decrease in CO_2. The kidneys can excrete H^+ or retain HCO_3^-, or they can retain H^+ and excrete HCO_3^-. H^+ is a very strong acid, and HCO_3^- is a weak base.
- Too much acid (H^+) in the blood is called *acidosis*.
- Too much base (HCO_3^-) in the blood is called *alkalosis*.
  When lungs hypoventilate (breathe more slowly than normal), CO_2 accumulates in the bloodstream.
- If CO_2 increases, this pushes the chemical reaction above to the right, which increases the production of H^+ (causing acidosis) and HCO_3^- (weak base). Therefore, hypoventilation causes acidosis.
- CO_2 can be blown off and out of the lungs by hyperventilation (breathing faster than normal). If CO_2 decreases, this pulls the chemical reaction to the left, pulling H^+ out of the solution. This causes the bloodstream to become deficient in H^+, and too basic. Therefore, hyperventilation causes alkalosis.

Buffer balancing act

The lungs influence acid–base balance by regulating carbon dioxide ($PaCO_2$). The kidneys exert their effect by regulating bicarbonate (HCO_3^-) and acid (H^+). Dysfunction or interruption of a buffer system can cause an acid–base imbalance.

To understand acid–base balance in the blood, you have to know the normal values of arterial blood gases—that is, carbon dioxide ($PaCO_2$) and oxygen (PaO_2)—as well as blood pH and bicarbonate ion. (See *Acid–base balance: normal values and abnormal values.*)

How acid–base imbalance happens

Disturbances in acid–base balance can be caused by respiratory dysfunction or metabolic dysfunction. In respiratory dysfunction, the lungs are the cause of the problem—this could be retention of too much CO_2 or elimination of too much CO_2. In metabolic dysfunction, any of the following could be the cause of the problem: renal disorders, gastrointestinal problems (vomiting or diarrhea), toxin ingestion, drug overdose, uncontrolled diabetes (ketoacidosis), or other metabolic disturbance.

There are four states of acid–base imbalance: **respiratory acidosis, respiratory alkalosis, metabolic acidosis,** and **metabolic alkalosis.** (See *Understanding acid–base disorders*, page 100.)

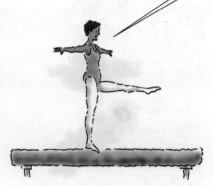

It's all about balance…acid–base balance is maintained by buffer systems and by the lungs and kidneys, which neutralizes and eliminates acids as rapidly as the acids are formed.

Acid–base balance: normal values and abnormal values

Normal values

Item measured	*Normal value*
Blood pH	7.35–7.45
$PaCO_2$	35–45 mm Hg
PaO_2	90–100 mm Hg
HCO_3^-	22–26 mEq/L
SaO_2 (saturation of blood with oxygen)	95%–100%

Abnormal values

Issue	*Abnormal value*
Hypoventilation causes CO_2 retention	$PaCO_2 > 45$ mm Hg
Hyperventilation causes a loss of CO_2	$PaCO_2 < 35$ mm Hg
Acidosis	Blood pH decreases to <7.35
Alkalosis	Blood pH increases to >7.45

The body usually attempts to compensate for acid–base imbalances via the lungs or the kidneys. The lungs can increase the rate of breathing or slow the rate of breathing to compensate. The kidneys can conserve or excrete acid or base, depending on which is necessary, to compensate. However, because such compensation can take many hours to days to compensate for acid–base imbalances, medical treatment is often necessary to reverse an acid–base imbalance.

Now I get it!

Understanding acid–base disorders

This chart provides an overview of the four states of acid–base imbalance.

Disorder	ABG findings	Possible causes
Respiratory acidosis (excess carbon dioxide [CO_2] retention)	• pH < 7.35 • HCO_3^- > 26 mEq/L (if compensating) • $PaCO_2$ > 45 mm Hg	• Central nervous system depression from drugs, injury, or disease, causing hypoventilation • Asphyxia • Hypoventilation from pulmonary, cardiac, musculoskeletal, or neuromuscular disease
Respiratory alkalosis (excess CO_2 excretion)	• pH > 7.45 • HCO_3^- < 22 mEq/L (if compensating) • $PaCO_2$ < 35 mm Hg	• Hyperventilation from anxiety, pain, or improper ventilator settings • Respiratory stimulation due to drugs, disease, hypoxia, or fever
Metabolic acidosis (bicarbonate [HCO_3^-] loss, acid retention)	• pH < 7.35 • HCO_3^- < 22 mEq/L • $PaCO_2$ < 35 mm Hg (if compensating)	• Bicarbonate depletion from diarrhea • Excess production of organic acids from diabetic ketoacidosis, hepatic disease, endocrine disorders, shock, or drug intoxication • Inadequate excretion of acids from renal disease
Metabolic alkalosis (HCO_3^- retention, acid loss)	• pH > 7.45 • HCO_3^- > 26 mEq/L • $PaCO_2$ > 45 mm Hg (if compensating)	• Loss of hydrochloric acid from prolonged vomiting or gastric suctioning • Loss of potassium from increased renal excretion (as in diuretic therapy) or steroids • Excessive alkali ingestion (toxicity)

Respiratory acidosis

When a patient hypoventilates, carbon dioxide ($PaCO_2$) builds up in the bloodstream. Retained carbon dioxide combines with water to form carbonic acid, which dissociates to release free hydrogen (H^+) and bicarbonate ions (HCO_3^-) (see the chemical equation in *Maintaining acid–base balance*, above). Increased partial pressure of arterial carbon dioxide ($PaCO_2$) and free hydrogen ions stimulate the medulla to increase respiratory drive and expel carbon dioxide.

Hefty hemoglobin

As pH falls, 2,3-diphosphoglycerate accumulates in RBCs, where it alters hemoglobin to release oxygen. The hemoglobin picks up hydrogen ions and carbon dioxide and removes them from the serum.

As respiratory mechanisms fail, rising $PaCO_2$ stimulates the kidneys to retain bicarbonate and sodium ions and excrete hydrogen ions.

As the hydrogen ion concentration overwhelms compensatory mechanisms, hydrogen ions move into the cells and potassium ions move out. Without enough oxygen, anaerobic metabolism produces lactic acid.

Respiratory alkalosis

As pulmonary ventilation increases, excessive carbon dioxide is exhaled. Resulting hypocapnia leads to reduction of carbonic acid, excretion of hydrogen and bicarbonate ions (see the chemical equation in *Maintaining acid–base balance*, above), and rising serum pH.

Against rising pH, the hydrogen–potassium buffer system pulls hydrogen ions out of cells and into blood in exchange for potassium ions. Hydrogen ions entering blood combine with bicarbonate ions to form carbonic acid, and pH falls.

Hypocapnia causes an increase in heart rate, cerebral vasoconstriction, and decreased cerebral blood flow. After 6 hours, kidneys conserve bicarbonate and less hydrogen.

Continued low $PaCO_2$ and vasoconstriction increase cerebral and peripheral hypoxia. Severe alkalosis inhibits calcium ionization, increasing nerve and muscle excitability.

Metabolic acidosis

As hydrogen ions begin accumulating in the body, chemical buffers (bicarbonate and proteins) in cells and extracellular fluid bind them. Excess hydrogen ions decrease blood pH and stimulate chemoreceptors in the medulla to increase respiration. Consequent fall in $PaCO_2$ frees hydrogen ions to bind with bicarbonate ions. Respiratory compensation occurs but isn't sufficient to correct acidosis.

Lots of movin' goin' on

Healthy kidneys compensate, excreting excess hydrogen ions, buffered by phosphate or ammonia. For each hydrogen ion excreted, renal tubules reabsorb and return to the blood one sodium ion and one bicarbonate ion.

Excess hydrogen ions in the extracellular fluid passively diffuse into cells. To maintain balance of charge across the cells' membrane, cells release potassium ions. Excess hydrogen ions change the normal balance of potassium, sodium, and calcium ions, impairing neural excitability.

Metabolic alkalosis

Chemical buffers in the extracellular fluid and intracellular fluid bind with bicarbonate in the body. Excess unbound bicarbonate raises blood pH, depressing chemoreceptors in the medulla, inhibiting respiration, and raising $PaCO_2$. Carbon dioxide combines with water to form carbonic acid. Low oxygen levels limit respiratory compensation.

When blood bicarbonate rises to 28 mEq/L, the amount filtered by the renal glomeruli exceeds the reabsorptive capacity of the renal tubules. Excess bicarbonate is excreted in the urine, and hydrogen ions are retained. To maintain electrochemical balance, sodium ions and water are excreted with bicarbonate ions.

When hydrogen ion levels in the extracellular fluid are low, hydrogen ions diffuse passively out of cells and extracellular potassium ions move into cells. As intracellular hydrogen levels fall, calcium ionization decreases, and nerve cells become permeable to sodium ions. Sodium ions moving into cells trigger neural impulses in the peripheral and central nervous systems.

What to look for

Each disturbance in acid–base balance has its own distinct signs and symptoms. (See *Treating disorders of acid–base balance*, page 103.)

Respiratory acidosis

Possible signs and symptoms of respiratory acidosis include:

- restlessness
- confusion
- diaphoresis
- bounding pulse
- apprehension
- somnolence
- asterixis (fine or flapping tremor)
- coma
- headaches
- dyspnea and tachypnea

Treating disorders of acid–base balance

The goal of treating all acid–base imbalances is reversing the underlying cause. In addition, each imbalance has its own individualized treatment plan.

Respiratory acidosis

Treatment of respiratory acidosis focuses on improving ventilation and lowering the partial pressure of arterial carbon dioxide. If hypoventilation can't be corrected, the patient should have an artificial airway inserted and be placed on mechanical ventilation.

Treatment for respiratory acidosis with a pulmonary cause also includes:
• a bronchodilator to open constricted airways
• supplemental oxygen as needed
• drug therapy to treat hyperkalemia
• an antibiotic to treat infection
• chest physiotherapy to remove secretions from the lungs
• removal of a foreign body from the patient's airway if needed

If respiratory acidosis stems from nonpulmonary conditions, such as neuromuscular disorders or a drug overdose, the underlying cause must be corrected.

Respiratory alkalosis

Treatment varies, depending on the cause.
• Treating the underlying condition may include removing the causative agent, such as a salicylate or other drugs, or taking steps to reduce fever and eliminate the source of sepsis.
• If acute hypoxemia is the cause, oxygen therapy is initiated. If anxiety is the cause, the patient may receive a sedative or an anxiolytic.
• Hyperventilation can be counteracted by having the patient breathe into a paper bag, which forces the patient to breathe exhaled carbon dioxide (CO_2), thereby raising the CO_2 level. A CO_2 rebreather mask can also be used in the clinical setting to allow the patient to raise CO_2 levels.

• If a patient's respiratory alkalosis is *iatrogenic* (caused by the effects of treatment), mechanical ventilator settings may be adjusted by decreasing the tidal volume or the number of breaths delivered per minute.

Metabolic acidosis

Treatment aims to correct the acidosis as quickly as possible by addressing both the symptoms and the underlying cause.
• Respiratory compensation is usually the first line of therapy, including mechanical ventilation if needed.
• For patients with diabetes, expect to administer rapid-acting insulin to reverse diabetic ketoacidosis and drive potassium back into the cell.
• For any patient with metabolic acidosis, monitor serum potassium levels. Even though high serum levels exist initially, serum potassium levels will drop when the acidosis is corrected, possibly resulting in hypokalemia. Any other electrolyte imbalances are evaluated and checked.
• Sodium bicarbonate is administered IV to neutralize blood acidity in patients with a pH lower than 7.1 and bicarbonate loss. Fluids are replaced parenterally as needed.
• Dialysis may be initiated in patients with renal failure or a toxic reaction to a drug. Such patients may receive an antibiotic to treat sources of infection or an antidiarrheal to treat diarrhea bicarbonate loss.

Metabolic alkalosis

Treatment for metabolic alkalosis may involve these interventions:
• Rarely, ammonium chloride is administered IV over 4 hours in severe cases.
• Diuretics and nasogastric suctioning are discontinued.
• An antiemetic may be administered to treat underlying nausea and vomiting.
• Acetazolamide may be administered to increase renal excretion of bicarbonate.

- papilledema
- depressed reflexes
- hypoxemia
- tachycardia
- hypertension
- atrial and ventricular arrhythmias
- hypotension with vasodilation

Respiratory alkalosis

Possible signs and symptoms of respiratory alkalosis include:
- deep, rapid respirations
- light-headedness or dizziness
- agitation
- circumoral and peripheral paresthesia
- carpopedal spasms, twitching, and muscle weakness

Metabolic acidosis

Possible signs and symptoms of metabolic acidosis include:
- headache and lethargy progressing to drowsiness
- Kussmaul respirations
- hypotension
- stupor and, if condition is severe and untreated, coma and death
- anorexia
- nausea and vomiting
- diarrhea
- dehydration
- warm, flushed skin
- fruity-smelling breath

Metabolic alkalosis

Possible signs and symptoms of metabolic alkalosis include:
- irritability
- carphology (picking at bedclothes)
- twitching
- confusion
- nausea and vomiting
- diarrhea
- cardiac arrhythmias
- slow, shallow respirations
- diminished peripheral blood flow
- carpopedal spasm in the hand
- Trousseau sign (spasm of the wrist elicited by applying a blood pressure cuff to the upper arm and inflating it to a pressure 20 mm Hg above the patient's systemic blood pressure)

What tests tell you

Arterial blood gas results are the most commonly used laboratory tests to help diagnose acid–base imbalances.

Respiratory acidosis

These test results help diagnose respiratory acidosis:

- Chest x-ray may reveal the cause, such as heart failure, pneumonia, pneumothorax, or chronic obstructive pulmonary disease.
- Serum potassium level is greater than 5 mEq/L.
- Serum chloride level is low.
- Urine pH is acidic.

Respiratory alkalosis

These test results indicate respiratory alkalosis:

- Electrocardiogram (ECG) may reveal cardiac arrhythmias.
- Serum chloride level is low.
- Urine pH is basic.

Metabolic acidosis

These test results help confirm the diagnosis of metabolic acidosis:

- Urine pH is less than 4.5 in the absence of renal disease.
- Serum potassium level is greater than 5.5 mEq/L.
- Blood glucose level is greater than 150 mg/dL.
- Serum ketone bodies are present if the patient has diabetes.
- Plasma lactic acid is elevated, if lactic acidosis is present.
- Anion gap is greater than 14 mEq/L in high anion gap metabolic acidosis, lactic acidosis, ketoacidosis, aspirin overdose, alcohol poisoning, renal failure, or other conditions characterized by accumulation of organic acids, sulfates, or phosphates. (The anion gap is calculated by adding the chloride level and the bicarbonate level and then subtracting that total from the sodium level. The value normally ranges from 8 to 14 mEq/L and represents the level of unmeasured anions [negatively charged ions] in extracellular fluid.)
- Anion gap is 12 mEq/L or less in normal anion gap metabolic acidosis from bicarbonate loss, GI or renal loss, increased acid load (from total parenteral nutrition fluids), rapid IV saline administration, or other conditions characterized by bicarbonate loss.

Metabolic alkalosis

The following findings suggest metabolic alkalosis:

- Serum potassium level is less than 3.5 mEq/L.
- Serum calcium level is less than 8.9 mg/dL.
- Serum chloride level is less than 98 mEq/L.

- Urine pH is 7; then, alkaline urine after renal compensatory mechanism begins to excrete bicarbonate.
- ECG may reveal depressed T wave, merging with a P wave, and atrial or sinus tachycardia.

Anemia

In anemia, because of an insufficient number of RBCs, the oxygen-carrying capacity in the body is reduced, resulting in a diminished amount of oxygen being delivered to the tissues and organs. The manifestations of anemia are caused by the body's reaction to tissue hypoxia. A deficiency in any of the following may result in anemia:

- The quantity of erythrocytes
- The amount of hemoglobin
- The volume of packed RBCs (hematocrit)

What tests tell you

As previously mentioned, anemia is diagnosed if a CBC shows both low hemoglobin and low hematocrit when compared with the normal values, which are ≥12 g/dL for females and ≥13 g/dL for males.

Now I get it!

Diagnosis of anemia

Anemia is diagnosed if a complete blood count (CBC) shows low hemoglobin and low hematocrit, keeping in mind the following normal values:

Normal Hgb for females[*]: >12 g/dL

Normal Hgb for males[*]: >13 g/dL

---

[*]Note: In this box, the term "male" refers to a person assigned male at birth, and the term "female" refers to a person assigned female at birth.

Now I get it!

Causes of anemia

Anemia is caused by:

- Blood loss
  - Acute hemorrhage
  - Chronic slow blood loss (most commonly from GI blood loss or excessive menstrual blood loss)
- Decreased erythrocyte production
  - Inadequate nutrients, decreased availability of iron, vitamin B_{12}, or folic acid
  - Insufficient amount of erythropoietin from the kidneys
- Increased erythrocyte destruction
  - Hemolysis
  - Hemoglobin levels help determine severity of anemia

Anemia caused by blood loss

	Acute blood loss	Chronic blood loss
Examples of causes:	Sudden hemorrhage (surgery, trauma)	Bleeding ulcers Excessive monthly menstrual blood loss
Treatment focus:	Replace blood volume, locate source of hemorrhage, and stop bleeding	Identify the source of bleeding, stop the bleeding, and supplemental iron administration

Anemia caused by decreased erythrocyte production

Anemia type	Aplastic anemia	Anemia of chronic disease	Iron deficiency anemia	Vitamin B$_{12}$ deficiency anemia	Folic acid deficiency anemia	Thalassemia
Pathophysiology	Peripheral blood pancytopenia. All blood cells are decreased (erythrocytes, leukocytes, and platelets) from depressed stem cell proliferation. • **Congenital** from chromosome abnormalities • **Acquired** from radiation, chemicals, autoimmune disorders, or infection Half of all cases are idiopathic (cause is unknown).	• Decreased erythrocyte lifespan, failure of erythrocyte proliferation, and limited iron availability • Associated with chronic infections, chronic inflammatory conditions, and malignancies	• Slow, chronic blood loss such as that occurs in people with excessive monthly menstrual blood loss or those with slow bleeding peptic ulcer or colon cancer	• Vitamin B$_{12}$ is needed for health of neurons in the spinal cord and brain. Lack of vitamin B$_{12}$ causes paresthesias and gait disturbances, and can lead to concentration problems, and confusion. Severe deficiency can cause dementia. • Vitamin B$_{12}$ is also needed for folic acid metabolism. • Vegans can have inadequate dietary intake of vitamin B$_{12}$ (e.g., best sources of vitamin B$_{12}$ are meat and dairy products). • Alcohol interferes with metabolism of vitamin B$_{12}$. • Pernicious anemia (a type of vitamin B$_{12}$ anemia most prevalent in people over 60 years old) is an autoimmune disease that destroys intrinsic factor in the stomach so that it no longer absorbs vitamin B$_{12}$.	• Lack of folic acid leads to accumulation of homocysteine, which is an amino acid that causes endothelial injury and increases risk of arteriosclerosis. • During pregnancy, the fetus needs folic acid for development of spinal cord and brain.	Group of inherited blood disorders in which the body has defective hemoglobin synthesis followed by homolyses causing anemia. • **Alpha-thalassemia**—There is a defect with the alpha-globulin protein gene. • **Beta-thalassemia**—There is a defect with the beta-globulin protein gene.

Anemia type	Aplastic anemia	Anemia of chronic disease	Iron deficiency anemia	Vitamin B_{12} deficiency anemia	Folic acid deficiency anemia	Thalassemia
Risk Factors	• Chromosomal abnormalities • Autoimmune disorders • Cancer	• Chronic inflammatory conditions (rheumatoid arthritis) • Chronic infections (AIDS) • Malignancies	• People with heavy monthly menstrual blood loss • Slow, chronic GI blood loss from peptic ulcer or colon cancer • Vegans • Patients with malabsorption • Malnourished adults • Children on solely cow's milk • Teens going through a growth spurt	• Vegans • Older adults with pernicious anemia • People who misuse alcohol	• Inadequate intake of green vegetables or whole grains • Inadequate intake of folic acid by pregnant people can cause neurologic defects in the fetus (e.g., spina bifida, meningocele, anencephaly).	• People of Mediterranean, Asian, Chinese, and African descent • Family history of the disorder
Treatment	• Treatment consists of identifying and removing the cause if possible, blood product transfusions, immunosuppressive therapy, and bone marrow transplant.	• Treatment consists of treating the underlying disorder. If anemia is severe or the patient is symptomatic, blood transfusions or erythropoietin therapy may be administered.	• Treatment focuses on what is causing the anemia (malabsorption, dependence on alcohol, reduced intake of iron) • Replacement of iron through nutritional therapy, oral iron supplements, or transfusions of packed red blood cells	• Replacement of vitamin B_{12}, preferably by intramuscular injection or nasal spray	• Increase folic acid sources in diet • Folate supplements	• Treatment includes blood transfusions with chelation therapy (to remove excess iron), bone marrow transplant, and splenectomy.

Anemia caused by increased erythrocyte destruction

Anemia type	Hemolytic anemia (acquired)	Sickle cell anemia (inherited)
Pathophysiology	Premature hemolysis of mature erythrocytes in the circulation. Hemolysis of erythrocytes caused by infection, systemic disease, liver disease, kidney disease, drugs, or toxins.	An inherited, autosomal, recessive disorder characterized by abnormal hemoglobin synthesis and irregularly shaped erythrocytes. When the patient has hypoxia or excessive stress, RBCs start to change and take on a sickle shape. Sickled RBCs are stiff and clog small capillaries, causing tissue ischemia, hypoxia, and pain. Over time, all body systems may become affected, causing end organ damage.
Treatment	Treatment focuses on identifying and eliminating the cause. Reduce risk of kidney tubule injury from built up hemoglobin with hydration and electrolyte replacement.	Treatment focuses on preventing organ damage, alleviating symptoms, and treating life-threatening conditions. Hospitalization for sickle cell crisis includes oxygen therapy, fluid and electrolyte administration to reduce viscosity of blood, and anticoagulation therapy to prevent deep vein thrombosis. Pain medication (e.g., opioid). Hydroxyurea is an oral medicine that has been shown to reduce or prevent several complications of sickle cell disease. Multiple other drugs (L-glutamine, crizanlizumab, and voxelotor) have recently been approved for the treatment.

Disseminated intravascular coagulation

In DIC (also called *consumption coagulopathy*), clotting and hemorrhage occur at the same time in the vascular system. DIC is complete dysfunction of the coagulation system.

A look at the DIC disaster area

DIC causes small blood vessel blockage, organ tissue damage (necrosis), depletion of circulating clotting factors and platelets, and activation of a clot-dissolving process called *fibrinolysis*. This, in turn, can lead to severe hemorrhage.

How it happens
There are five major precipitating causes of DIC:
- sepsis—gram-negative or gram-positive bacterial septicemia; viral, fungal, rickettsial, or protozoal infection
- obstetric complications—abruptio placentae, amniotic fluid embolism, retained dead fetus, eclampsia, septic abortion, postpartum hemorrhage
- neoplastic disease—acute leukemia, metastatic carcinoma, lymphomas
- disorders that produce necrosis—extensive burns and trauma, brain tissue destruction, transplant rejection, liver necrosis, anorexia
- other disorders and conditions associated with massive insult to the body—heatstroke, shock, cirrhosis, fat embolism, incompatible

blood transfusion, drug reactions, cardiac arrest, surgery necessitating cardiopulmonary bypass, severe venous thrombosis, adrenal disease, acute respiratory distress syndrome, diabetic ketoacidosis, pulmonary embolism, multiple trauma, and sickle cell anemia

DIC—a BIG mystery in many ways

No one knows why these conditions and disorders lead to DIC. Furthermore, whether they lead to it through a common mechanism is also uncertain. In many patients, DIC may be triggered by the entrance of foreign protein into the circulation or by vascular endothelial injury.

DIC usually develops in association with three pathologic processes:
1. damage to the endothelium
2. release of tissue thromboplastin
3. activation of factor X

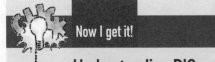

Now I get it!

Understanding DIC

The simplified illustration below shows the pathophysiology of disseminated intravascular coagulation (DIC). Circulating thrombin activates both coagulation and fibrinolysis, leading to paradoxical bleeding and clotting.

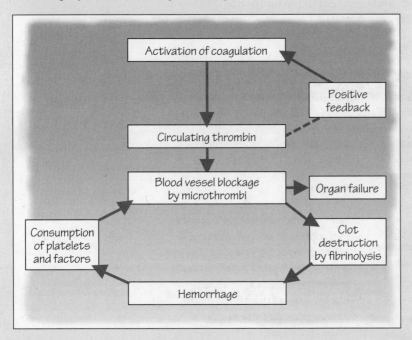

The play-by-play

DIC arises from the series of events described below:

- One of DIC's many causes triggers the coagulation system.
- Excess fibrin is formed (triggered by the action of thrombin, an enzyme) and becomes trapped in the microvasculature along with platelets, causing clots.
- Blood flow to the tissues decreases, causing acidemia, blood stasis, and tissue hypoxia; organ failure may result.
- Both fibrinolysis and antithrombotic mechanisms lead to anticoagulation.
- Platelets and coagulation factors are consumed and massive hemorrhage may ensue. (See *Understanding DIC*, page 111.)

What to look for

The most significant clinical feature of DIC is abnormal bleeding without a history of serious hemorrhagic disorder. Other signs and symptoms include:

- cutaneous oozing
- petechiae (microhemorrhages on the skin)
- bleeding from surgical or IV sites
- bleeding from the GI tract, urinary tract, or vagina
- cyanosis of the extremities

DIC is usually acute, although it may be chronic in cancer patients. The prognosis depends on the timeliness of detection, severity and site of the hemorrhage, and treatment of the underlying disease or condition. (See *Treating DIC*, page 112.)

Battling illness

Treating DIC

Successful management of disseminated intravascular coagulation (DIC) requires prompt treatment of the underlying disorder.

Support

Treatment may be highly specific or supportive. Supportive care is appropriate if the underlying disorder is self-limiting or if the patient isn't actively bleeding.

In case of bleeding

Active bleeding may require administration of fresh-frozen plasma, platelets, cryoprecipitate, or packed red blood cells to support hemostasis.

Drug therapy

Heparin therapy is controversial; it may be used early in the disease to prevent microclotting or as a last resort in a patient who's actively bleeding. If thrombosis occurs, heparin therapy is usually mandatory. In most cases, it's administered along with transfusion therapy. Aminocaproic acid may be given to inhibit fibrinolysis.

What tests tell you

Abnormal bleeding with no other blood disorder suggests DIC. These test results support the diagnosis:

- Platelet count is decreased, usually to less than 100,000/μL, because platelets are consumed during thrombosis.
- Fibrinogen levels are decreased to less than 150 mg/dL because fibrinogen is consumed in clot formation. Levels may be normal if elevated by hepatitis or pregnancy.
- Prothrombin time (PT) is prolonged to more than 15 seconds.
- Partial thromboplastin time (PTT) is prolonged to more than 60 to 80 seconds.
- Fibrin degradation products are increased, usually to greater than 45 μg/mL. Increases are produced by excess fibrin clots broken down by plasmin.
- D-dimer test is positive at less than 1:8 dilution.
- Other blood test results include positive fibrin monomers, diminished levels of factors V and VIII, fragmentation of RBCs, and hemoglobin levels decreased to less than 10 g/dL.
- Renal status test results demonstrate reduced urine output (less than 30 mL/hour), elevated blood urea nitrogen levels (greater than 25 mg/dL), and elevated serum creatinine levels (greater than 1.3 mg/dL).

Confirmation can prove complicated

Final confirmation of the diagnosis may be difficult because similar test results also occur in other disorders such as primary fibrinolysis. However, fibrin degradation products and D-dimer tests are considered specific and diagnostic of DIC. Additional tests may determine the underlying cause.

Hemophilia

Hemophilia is an X-linked recessive disorder resulting in defective clotting factors. Hemophilia is classified as A, B, or von Willebrand depending on the type of defective clotting factor. The disease can range from mild to severe.

- Hemophilia A
  - Classic hemophilia
  - Factor VIII (clotting protein) deficiency
  - Most common form of hemophilia
  - Recessive sex linked
- Hemophilia B
  - "Christmas disease"
  - Factor IX (clotting protein) deficiency
  - Recessive sex linked
- von Willebrand disease
  - Deficiency of von Willebrand clotting protein
  - Most common congenital bleeding disorder
  - Autosomal dominant

What to look for

Clinical manifestations of hemophilia relate to bleeding: spontaneous bleeding, recurrent bleeding, prolonged bleeding after small cuts, hematuria, epistaxis, easy bruising, and hemarthrosis (bleeding in the joints).

What tests tell you

Laboratory studies are used to determine the type of hemophilia.
- PTT—prolonged due to deficiency in intrinsic clotting system factor
- Bleeding time—prolonged in von Willebrand disease because platelets in this disease are defective

Treatment for hemophilia

Treatment for hemophilia consists of replacing missing clotting factors, replacement therapy as a prophylaxis for surgery and dental procedures, desmopressin acetate to proliferate von Willebrand factor, and antifibrinolytic therapy.

Idiopathic thrombocytopenic purpura

Thrombocytopenia that results from immunologic platelet destruction is known as *ITP*. It occurs in two forms:
1. Acute ITP, also called *postviral thrombocytopenia*, usually affects children between ages 2 and 6.
2. Chronic ITP, also called *Werlhof disease*, *purpura hemorrhagica*, *essential thrombocytopenia*, or *autoimmune thrombocytopenia*, affects adults younger than age 50, especially females between ages 20 and 40.

How it happens

ITP is an autoimmune disorder. Antibodies that reduce the lifespan of platelets appear in nearly all patients.

One follows infection, the other doesn't

Acute ITP usually follows a viral infection, such as rubella or chickenpox, and can result from immunization with a live vaccine.

Chronic ITP seldom follows infection and is commonly linked with immunologic disorders, such as systemic lupus erythematosus and human immunodeficiency virus infection. Chronic ITP affects females more commonly than males.

A plague on platelets

ITP occurs when circulating immunoglobulin G (IgG) molecules react with host platelets, which are then destroyed by phagocytosis in the spleen and, to a lesser degree, in the liver. Normally, the lifespan of platelets in circulation is 7 to 10 days. In ITP, platelets survive 1 to 3 days or less.

Getting complicated

Hemorrhage can severely complicate ITP. Potentially fatal purpuric lesions (caused by hemorrhage into tissues) may occur in vital organs, such as the brain and kidneys. ITP is usually a precursor of lymphoma.

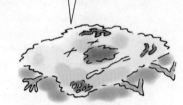

What hit me? It looked like my own immune system!

What to look for

Signs and symptoms that indicate decreased platelets include:
- nosebleed
- oral bleeding
- purpura (large hemorrhages under the skin)
- petechiae (tiny hemorrhages under the skin)
- excessive menstruation

Sudden bleeding here; creeping over there

In the acute form, sudden bleeding usually follows a recent viral illness, although it may not occur until 21 days after the virus strikes. In the chronic form, the onset of bleeding is insidious.

The prognosis for acute ITP is excellent; nearly four of five patients recover completely without specific treatment. The prognosis for chronic ITP is good; transient remissions lasting weeks or even years are common, especially in females. (See *Treating ITP*.)

 Battling illness

Treating ITP

Acute idiopathic thrombocytopenic purpura (ITP) may be allowed to run its course without intervention. Alternatively, it may be treated with glucocorticoids or immunoglobulin (IVIG). Treatment with plasmapheresis or plateletpheresis with transfusion has met with limited success.

For chronic ITP, corticosteroids may be used to suppress phagocytic activity, promote capillary integrity, and enhance platelet production.

Splenectomy

Patients who don't respond spontaneously to treatment within 1 to 4 months or who require high doses of corticosteroids to maintain platelet counts require splenectomy. This procedure is up to 85% successful in adults when splenomegaly accompanies the initial thrombocytopenia.

Looking at alternatives

Alternative treatments include immunosuppressants, such as cyclophosphamide or vincristine, and high-dose IV immunoglobulin, which is effective in 85% of adults.

Immunosuppressant use requires weighing the risks against the benefits. Immunoglobulin has a rapid effect, raising platelet counts within 1 to 5 days, but this effect lasts only about 1 to 2 weeks. Immunoglobulin is usually administered to prepare severely thrombocytic patients for emergency surgery.

Thrombopoiesis-stimulating agents, such as romiplostim (Nplate) and eltrombopag olamine (Promacta), have been used as a second-line treatment in adults with insufficient response to corticosteroids, immunoglobulins, or splenectomy.

What tests tell you

These tests help diagnose ITP:

- Platelet count less than 20,000/µL and prolonged bleeding time suggest ITP. Platelet size and appearance may be abnormal, and anemia may be present if bleeding has occurred.
- Bone marrow studies show an abundance of megakaryocytes (platelet precursors) and a circulating platelet survival time of only several hours to a few days.
- Humoral antibody blood tests that measure platelet-associated IgG may help establish the diagnosis. However, they're nonspecific, so their usefulness is limited. One-half of patients with thrombocytopenia show an increased IgG level.

Iron deficiency anemia

Iron deficiency anemia is a disorder of oxygen transport in which the production of hemoglobin is inadequate. A common disease worldwide, iron deficiency anemia affects 10% to 30% of the adult population in the United States. Iron deficiency anemia occurs most commonly in premenopausal females, infants (particularly premature or low birth weight infants), children, and adolescents (especially females).

How it happens

Iron deficiency anemia can result from:

- inadequate dietary intake of iron; vegans often do not get sufficient iron (because the best absorbable iron comes from meat and dairy products, which vegans don't eat)
- excessive monthly menstrual blood loss
- colon cancer: tumors of GI tract often have slow, chronic blood loss
- blood loss secondary to GI bleeding from peptic ulcer (chronic use of certain drugs can cause GI ulcer and bleeding. These include: aspirin, NSAIDs, or steroids)
- blood loss from esophageal varices (commonly accompanies cirrhosis of liver)
- Adolescents growing rapidly in growth spurt
- Infants being weaned from breast milk to cow's milk (cow's milk lacks iron)
- conditions resulting in iron malabsorption, such as chronic diarrhea from inflammatory bowel disease (Crohn disease and ulcerative colitis); malabsorption syndromes such as celiac disease
- pregnancy, which diverts iron from the pregnant person to the fetus for RBC production

In short supply

Iron deficiency anemia occurs when the supply of iron is too low for optimal RBC formation. This results in smaller (microcytic) cells that contain less color (hypochromic) when they're stained for visualization under a microscope.

When the body's stores of iron, including plasma iron, become used up, the concentration of transferrin, which binds with and transports iron, decreases. Insufficient iron stores lead to smaller than normal RBCs that have a lower than normal hemoglobin concentration. In turn, the blood carries less oxygen.

What to look for

Iron deficiency anemia usually develops slowly, and therefore many patients have no symptoms at first. By the time they develop symptoms, anemia is usually severe. These signs and symptoms include:

- generalized weakness and fatigue
- light-headedness and inability to concentrate
- palpitations
- dyspnea on exertion
- pica (craving for nonnutritive substances), especially for clay, cornstarch, and ice
- pallor, especially of the conjunctiva
- tachycardia
- dry, brittle, ridged nails with concave contours
- dry, brittle hair and hair loss
- tender, pale, atrophic tongue (glossitis)
- cracking at the edges of the lips (angular stomatitis or cheilitis) (See *Treating iron deficiency anemia.*)

Battling illness

Treating iron deficiency anemia

The first priority of treating iron deficiency anemia is determining the cause. After that's determined, replacement therapy can begin.

Drug options

If the cause was inadequate dietary intake, the treatment of choice is an oral preparation of iron or a combination of iron and ascorbic acid (vitamin C) (which enhances iron absorption). In some cases, the iron may have to be administered parenterally; for example, if the patient is nonadherent to the oral preparation or in the case of malabsorption conditions.

Because total dose IV infusion of supplemental iron is painless and requires fewer injections, it's usually preferred over IM (which must be given by Z-track injection) administration.

What tests tell you

As iron deficiency anemia develops, it causes a predictable sequence of abnormalities in laboratory tests:

- In early stages, the total iron binding capacity (TIBC) may be elevated, and serum iron (Fe++) levels are decreased.
- Serum ferritin level (stored iron) is low.
- Complete blood count shows a low hemoglobin level (males, less than 13 g/dL; females, less than 12 g/dL) and low hematocrit (males, less than 47%; females, less than 42%).
- Red cell indices reveal microcytic (smaller in size than normal) and hypochromic (contain less color than normal) cells.
- Bone marrow biopsy demonstrates depleted or absent iron stores and reduced production of precursors to RBCs. (See *Peripheral blood smear in iron deficiency anemia*, page 118.)

Now I get it!

Peripheral blood smear in iron deficiency anemia

This peripheral blood smear shows the microcytic hypochromic RBCs of iron deficiency anemia. These RBCs are small and pale.

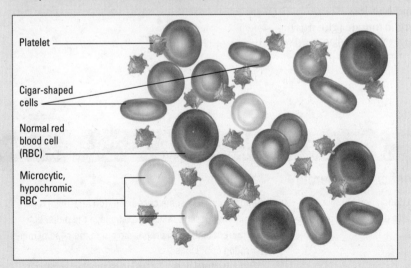

Leukemia

Leukemia is cancer of the WBCs. It begins in the bone marrow with abnormal production of cancerous WBCs that infiltrate different organs. In the bone marrow, the cancerous WBCs overtake the bone marrow and inhibit normal synthesis of WBCs, RBCs, and platelets (hematopoiesis). This causes many complications including:

- Lack of healthy WBCs, which in turn causes low immune defense and increased risk of infection
- Lack of RBC production leading to anemia, which results in decreased oxygen delivery to tissues
- Lack of platelet production leading to thrombocytopenia, which causes spontaneous bleeding and bruising

Leukemias are classified as acute vs. chronic (cell maturation at disease onset), by type of leukocyte involved, and by whether its origin is myelogenous (arising in the bone marrow) or lymphocytic (arising from lymphocytes).

Characteristics of different types of leukemia

Type of leukemia	Onset and symptoms	Lab test results
Acute myelogenous leukemia (AML)	Onset is sudden. Patients may experience serious infection and bleeding from disease onset.	Low RBC, Hgb, Hct, platelets.
Acute lymphocytic leukemia (ALL)	Most common type of leukemia in children. Signs and symptoms may appear suddenly or develop as the disease progresses and include bleeding, fatigue fever, weakness, and bone pain.	Low RBC, Hgb, Hct, platelets. Lymphoblasts present in cerebrospinal fluid. 20% of patients present with Philadelphia chromosome.
Chronic myelogenous leukemia (CML)	No symptoms noted in early stage of disease. Symptoms develop as the disease progresses and include fever, weakness, joint pain/bone pain, and weight loss. CML presents initially with a stable chronic phase which develops into an acute, destructive phase. This acute phase requires more aggressive treatment than the chronic phase.	Low RBC, Hgb, Hct, and high platelet count at disease onset and then platelets decrease as the disease progresses. 90% of patients present with Philadelphia chromosome.
Chronic lymphocytic leukemia (CLL)	Patients frequently present with no symptoms. As the disease progresses, symptoms include lymph node enlargement, fatigue, anorexia, enlarged liver and spleen, and infections.	Initially no symptoms may be present and treatment may not be required. Anemia and thrombocytopenia occur as the disease progresses.

What to look for

Leukemia has various clinical manifestations related to bone marrow suppression and leukemic cell infiltration. These manifestations include anemia, bleeding (purpura, petechiae, ecchymosis, and hemorrhage), infection, bone pain, liver, spleen, and lymph node enlargement.

What tests tell you

Tests used to diagnosis and classify the type of leukemia include the following:

- Lab studies include analysis of the bone marrow biopsy or bone marrow aspirate, which show the extent of invasion of cancerous WBCs and suppression of RBCs and platelets.
- Immunohistochemistry studies show what abnormal WBCs are present and what surface antigens and enzymes these abnormal WBCs are producing.
- Cytogenetic analysis demonstrates the exact genetic defects that are causing the cancerous changes in the WBCs.

All of these types of studies are important for making a specific diagnosis of the cancer, deciding which targeted treatment is best, and ascribing a prognosis.

Treatments for leukemia

(See the subsection *Treatments for leukemia and lymphomas* in the next section.)

Lymphomas

Lymphomas are cancers of lymphatic tissue that cause the overproduction of cancerous lymphocytes. Cancerous lymphocytes do not function, which causes decreased immunity. Cancerous lymphocytes grow in the bone marrow, lymph nodes, and other organs.

Comparison of Hodgkins lymphoma and non-Hodgkins lymphoma

Lymphoma type	Hodgkin lymphoma	Non-Hodgkin lymphoma (NHL)
Comparing and contrasting	Large, multinucleated Reed–Sternberg cells are found in the lymph nodes. The lymph nodes are destroyed by the increased growth of monocytes and macrophages. Extranodal involvement is rare. The disease is local. It is more common in White individuals than in African American individuals.	A proliferation of malignant lymphocytes. There are many subtypes of NHL including large B-cell lymphoma and Burkitt lymphoma. Extranodal involvement is common. The disease is disseminated in its extent.

Lymphoma type	Hodgkin lymphoma	Non-Hodgkin lymphoma (NHL)
Causes	The cause is unknown but infection with Epstein–Barr virus, a genetic tendency, and contact with environmental and occupational toxins are thought to have roles in the development of Hodgkin lymphoma.	The cause is unknown, but chromosomal translocations, infections, environmental factors, immunodeficiency states (AIDS), or patients who have received chemotherapy or radiation.
Clinical manifestations	There is a slow and subtle onset of the disease. Enlargement of lymph nodes, weight loss, fever, fatigue, weakness, chills, tachycardia, and night sweats can all be seen with Hodgkin lymphoma. B symptoms (weight loss, night sweats, and fever over 100.4°F) are commonly seen in Hodgkin lymphoma.	NHL can develop slowly or rapidly. The most common manifestation is a painless, enlarged lymph node. Other symptoms are based on dissemination of the disease. B-cell origin lymphoma symptoms occur in 40% of patients in North America.
Diagnostic testing	Biopsy of lymph tissue will show the presence of Reed–Sternberg cells. Radiologic studies can determine which lymph nodes are involved.	Biopsy of lymph node for identification of cell type. MRI and CT scan to visualize other organ involvement.
Treatment	Early stages may be difficult to detect as asymptomatic lymphadenopathy may advance several years unnoticed. Chemotherapy and radiation are two treatment methods that are used. Other treatments are based on alleviating symptoms including pain, pancytopenia, and protecting the patient from infection.	Chemotherapy, immunotherapy, and radiation are the main treatment modalities.

Source: National Institutes of Health: National Cancer Institute. (2023). *Hodgkin Lymphoma Treatment (PDQ®)–Health Professional Version*. (Accessed October 26, 2023) https://www.cancer.gov/types/lymphoma/hp/adult-hodgkin-treatment-pdq#_36; National Institutes of Health: National Cancer Institute. (2023). *Non-Hodgkin Lymphoma Treatment (PDQ®)–Patient Version*. (Accessed October 26, 2023) https://www.cancer.gov/types/lymphoma/patient/adult-nhl-treatment-pdq

Treatments for leukemia and lymphomas

The most common treatments for leukemia and lymphomas have been chemotherapeutic agents and radiation that are designed to attack rapidly multiplying cells. However, chemotherapy can cause collateral damage by attacking normal, rapidly dividing cells. Bone marrow transplants have been successful but require a matching donor, which is often difficult to find. Current research is seeking more precise treatments that can specifically target only the cancer cells. The newest treatments available are:

- Immunotherapy, which involves specifically engineered antibodies that target specific antigens found on the cancer cells
- Targeted therapy, which uses specifically devised medications that attack certain enzymes that are only produced by the rapidly dividing cancer cells
- CAR T-cell therapy, which genetically modifies a patient's own T cells to specifically target an attack on only the cancer cells

Multiple myeloma

Multiple myeloma, also known as plasma cell myeloma, is a disease in which malignant plasma cells penetrate bone marrow and combine to form masses of tumors throughout the skeletal system, destroying bone. In multiple myeloma, an excessive amount of plasma cells are produced. The plasma cells arise from one clone of B cells that produce only one type of antibodies. This is harmful because plasma cells normally produce various antibodies to help fight against various infections. The antibodies produced in multiple myeloma also infiltrate the bone marrow.

What to look for

Multiple myeloma develops slowly with most patients not experiencing symptoms until the disease is far advanced. Skeletal pain is usually the first and most common manifestation. Osteoporosis, vertebral destruction, loss of bone integrity, hypercalcemia, and symptoms of spinal cord compression can be seen in advanced multiple myeloma.

What tests tell you

Diagnosis of multiple myeloma is based upon symptoms, laboratory studies, bone marrow biopsy, and radiologic exams. Laboratory studies of immunoglobulins (IgF, IgM, and IgA) show the M protein (produced by the myeloma cell) significantly increased while the others are suppressed in multiple myeloma. Radiologic studies show bone erosion, thinning of bones and fractures. Bone marrow biopsy shows large numbers of plasma cells.

Treatment for multiple myeloma

First-line treatment for multiple myeloma is chemotherapy with corticosteroids to reduce the amount of plasma cells. Other treatments include bisphosphonates for bone breakdown and pain, targeted therapy, and radiation therapy. Patients rarely experience a cure for multiple myeloma, but treatments can provide relief from symptoms and extend life.

Thrombocytopenia

Thrombocytopenia is characterized by a deficient number of circulating platelets.

How it happens

Thrombocytopenia may be congenital or acquired, but the acquired form is more common. In either case, it usually results from:

- decreased or defective platelet production in the bone marrow
- increased destruction outside the marrow caused by an underlying disorder
- sequestration (increase in the amount of blood in a limited vascular area)
- (See *Factors that decrease platelet count*, page 123.)

Let's meet the mechanisms responsible

In thrombocytopenia, lack of platelets can cause inadequate hemostasis. Four mechanisms are responsible:

1. decreased platelet production
2. decreased platelet survival
3. pooling of blood in the spleen
4. intravascular dilution of circulating platelets

Fe, fi, fo, fum…

Platelets are produced by giant cells in bone marrow called *megakaryocytes*. Platelet production falls when the number of megakaryocytes is reduced or when platelet production becomes dysfunctional.

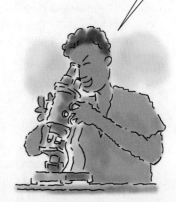

Platelets play a vital role in coagulation… that's why thrombocytopenia threatens the body's ability to control bleeding.

Factors that decrease platelet count

Decreased platelet count may result from diminished or defective platelet production, increased peripheral destruction of platelets, sequestration (separation of a portion of the circulating blood in a specific body part), or blood loss. More specific causes are listed below.

Diminished or defective production
Congenital
- Wiskott–Aldrich syndrome
- Maternal ingestion of thiazides
- Neonatal rubella

Acquired
- Aplastic anemia
- Marrow infiltration (acute and chronic leukemia, tumor)
- Nutritional deficiency (B_{12}, folic acid)
- Myelosuppressive agents
- Drugs that directly influence platelet production (thiazides, alcohol, hormones)

- Radiation
- Viral infections (measles, dengue)

Increased peripheral destruction
Congenital
- Nonimmune (prematurity, erythroblastosis fetalis, infection)
- Immune (drug-induced, especially with quinine and quinidine; posttransfusion purpura; acute and chronic idiopathic thrombocytopenic purpura; sepsis; alcohol)

Acquired
- Invasive lines or devices

- Ventricular assist devices, intra-aortic balloon pump, cardiopulmonary bypass
- Artificial hearts and prosthetic valves
- Heparin administration

Sequestration
- Hypersplenism
- Hypothermia

Blood Loss
- Hemorrhage
- Bleeding

What to look for

Thrombocytopenia typically produces a sudden onset of petechiae in the skin and bleeding into any mucous membrane. Nearly, all patients are otherwise symptom-free, although some may complain of malaise, fatigue, and general weakness.

In adults, large blood-filled blisters usually appear in the mouth. In severe disease, hemorrhage may lead to tachycardia, shortness of breath, loss of consciousness, and death.

Prognosis is excellent in drug-induced thrombocytopenia if the offending drug is withdrawn. Recovery may be immediate. In other cases, the prognosis depends on the patient's response to treatment of the underlying cause. (See *Treating thrombocytopenia*, page 124.)

What tests tell you

These tests help establish a diagnosis of thrombocytopenia:

- Platelet count is decreased, usually to less than 100,000/µL in adults.
- Bleeding time is prolonged.
- PT and PTT are normal.
- Platelet antibody studies can help determine why the platelet count is low and can also be used to select treatment.
- Platelet survival studies help differentiate between ineffective platelet production and platelet destruction as causes of thrombocytopenia.
- Bone marrow studies determine the number, size, and cytoplasmic maturity of megakaryocytes in severe disease. This helps identify ineffective platelet production as the cause and rules out malignant disease at the same time.

Battling illness

Treating thrombocytopenia

When treating thrombocytopenia, withdrawing the offending drug or treating the underlying cause, if possible, is essential. Other treatments include:

- administration of corticosteroids to increase platelet production
- administration of folate to stimulate bone marrow production of platelets
- IV administration of gamma-globulin for severe or refractory thrombocytopenia (still experimental)
- platelet transfusion to stop episodic abnormal bleeding caused by a low platelet count (only minimally effective if platelet destruction results from an immune disorder; may be reserved for life-threatening bleeding)
- splenectomy to correct disease caused by platelet destruction because the spleen acts as the primary site of platelet removal and antibody production

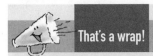
That's a wrap!

Hematologic system review

Plasma
• Consists of proteins, albumin, globulin, and fibrinogen
• Regulates acid–base balance and immune responses
• Mediates coagulation
• Increased number in multiple myeloma

Red blood cells
• Transport oxygen and carbon dioxide to and from body tissues
• Contain hemoglobin
• Decreased number in anemia
• Increased number in polycythemia

White blood cells
• Protect against infection and inflammation
• Produced in bone marrow
• Increase and accumulation of abnormal WBCs in bone marrow or lymphoid tissue indicates leukemia or lymphoma

Platelets
• Interact with plasma and coagulation factors to control bleeding
• Provide factors III and XIII and platelet factor III that accelerate blood clotting
• Decrease (thrombocytopenia), excess (thrombocytosis), or dysfunction (thrombocytopathy) cause platelet disorders

Understanding blood dyscrasias
Dyscrasias are abnormal conditions of the blood that are caused by the rapid reproduction and short lifespan of blood elements, such as:
• bone marrow cells
• erythrocytes
• leukocytes
• platelets

Understanding blood disorders
• *Primary*—occur as a result of a problem within the blood itself
• *Secondary*—result from a cause other than a defect in the blood
• *Quantitative*—result from increased or decreased cell production or cell destruction
• *Qualitative*—stem from intrinsic cell abnormalities or plasma component dysfunction

Blood disorders
• *Acid–base imbalances*—disturbances in acid–base balance can cause respiratory acidosis, respiratory alkalosis, metabolic acidosis, or metabolic alkalosis
• *Anemia*—a deficiency in the quantity of erythrocytes, amount of hemoglobin, or the volume of packed red blood cells (hematocrit) in the blood resulting in decreased capacity to transport oxygen to tissues
• *DIC*—clotting and hemorrhage occur in the vascular system at the same time; blood flow is diminished to tissues and anticoagulation results in possible hemorrhage
• *Hemophilia*—a deficiency in specific clotting proteins (factor) resulting in abnormal bleeding
• *ITP*—antibodies develop against platelets; platelets are destroyed and may result in hemorrhage
• *Iron deficiency anemia*—occurs due to decreased iron supply and leads to blood cells becoming smaller, paler; results in less oxygen carried by blood
• *Leukemia*—a cancer of WBCs that originates in the bone marrow; the abnormal, cancerous WBCs crowd out healthy RBCs and platelets in the bone marrow
• *Lymphomas*—a cancer of the lymph systems involving the overproduction of abnormal lymphocytes
• *Multiple myeloma*—a plasma cell cancer involving the bone marrow and skeletal tumors
• *Thrombocytopenia*—results in a deficient number of platelets; occurs due to decreased platelet production, blood loss, sequestration, or destruction

Quick quiz

1. A vital function of platelets is to:
   A. form hemostatic plugs in injured blood vessels.
   B. regulate acid–base balance and immune responses.
   C. protect the body against harmful bacteria and infection.
   D. carry oxygen to the tissues and remove carbon dioxide from them.

Answer: A. A vital function of platelets is to form hemostatic plugs in injured blood vessels. Platelets also minimize blood loss by causing damaged blood vessels to contract and provide materials that accelerate blood coagulation.

2. Which of the following is the normal lifespan of an RBC?
   A. 90 days
   B. 30 days
   C. 240 days
   D. 120 days

Answer: D. A normal RBC is viable for approximately 120 days.

3. Thrombocytopenia is characterized by:
   A. not enough circulating platelets.
   B. too many circulating platelets.
   C. decreased RBC production.
   D. decreased iron supply.

Answer: A. Platelet deficiency may be due to decreased or defective production of platelets or increased destruction of platelets.

4. The initial response to tissue injury in the extrinsic pathway is the release of which substance?
   A. Prothrombin
   B. Thrombin
   C. Tissue thromboplastin
   D. Fibrinogen

Answer: C. Tissue thromboplastin is also called *factor III*.

5. DIC is characterized by:
   A. clotting deficiency and immune dysfunction.
   B. clotting and hemorrhage.
   C. hemorrhagic and fibrinolytic coagulopathy.
   D. excess carbon dioxide retention.

Answer: B. In DIC, clotting and hemorrhage occur simultaneously in the vascular system.

Scoring

☆☆☆ If you answered all five items correctly, you're golden! Indeed, your knowledge of red and white blood cells has us green with envy!

☆☆ If you answered four items correctly, congrats! You're a connoisseur of liquid and formed components.

☆ If you answered fewer than four items correctly, don't stop circulating. Never give up. Need inspiration? Think of the stem cell precursor that eventually emerges to become a mighty RBC.

Suggested references

Bergamaschi, G., Caprioli, F., Lenti, M. V., Elli, L., Radaelli, F., Rondonotti, E., Mengoli, C., Miceli, E., Ricci, C., Ardizzone, S., Vecchi, M., & Di Sabatino, A. (2022). Pathophysiology and therapeutic management of anemia in gastrointestinal disorders. *Expert Review of Gastroenterology & Hepatology*, 16(7), 625–637. https://doi.org/10.1080/17474124.2022.2089114

Brandow, A. M., & Liem, R. I. (2022). Advances in the diagnosis and treatment of sickle cell disease. *Journal of Hematology & Oncology*, 15(1), 20. https://doi.org/10.1186/s13045-022-01237-z

Candelario, N., & Klein, C. (2022). Megaloblastic anemia due to severe vitamin B12 deficiency. *Cleveland Clinic Journal of Medicine*, 89(1), 8–9. https://doi.org/10.3949/ccjm.89a.21041

Cappellini, M. D., Musallam, K. M., & Taher, A. T. (2020). Iron deficiency anaemia revisited. *Journal of Internal Medicine*, 287(2), 153–170. https://doi.org/10.1111/joim.13004

Craig, W. J., Mangels, A. R., Fresán, U., Marsh, K., Miles, F. L., Saunders, A. V., Haddad, E. H., Heskey, C. E., Johnston, P., Larson-Meyer, E., & Orlich, M. (2021). The safe and effective use of plant-based diets with guidelines for health professionals. *Nutrients*, 13(11), 4144. https://doi.org/10.3390/nu13114144

Ghosh, K., Ghosh, K., Agrawal, R., & Nadkarni, A. H. (2020). Recent advances in screening and diagnosis of hemoglobinopathy. *Expert Review of Hematology*, 13(1), 13–21. https://doi.org/10.1080/17474086.2019.1656525

Kattamis, A., Kwiatkowski, J. L., & Aydinok, Y. (2022). Thalassaemia. *Lancet (London, England)*, 399(10343), 2310–2324. https://doi.org/10.1016/S0140-6736(22)00536-0

Kumar, A., Sharma, E., Marley, A., Samaan, M. A., & Brookes, M. J. (2022). Iron deficiency anaemia: Pathophysiology, assessment, practical management. *BMJ Open Gastroenterology*, 9(1), e000759. https://doi.org/10.1136/bmjgast-2021-000759

Leukemia—Health professional version. (Accessed October 6, 2023). https://www.cancer.gov/types/leukemia/hp

Lewis, M. J. (2020). Alcoholism and nutrition: A review of vitamin supplementation and treatment. *Current Opinion in Clinical Nutrition & Metabolic Care*, 23(2), 138–144. https://doi.org/10.1097/MCO.0000000000000622

Mansour, D., Hofmann, A., & Gemzell-Danielsson, K. (2021). A review of clinical guidelines on the management of iron deficiency and iron-deficiency anemia in women with heavy menstrual bleeding. *Advances in Theraphy, 38*(1), 201–225. https://doi.org/10.1007/s12325-020-01564-y

Mohamed, M., Thio, J., Thomas, R. S., & Phillips, J. (2020). Pernicious anaemia. *BMJ (Clinical Research ed.), 369*, m1319. https://doi.org/10.1136/bmj.m1319

National Institutes of Health: National Cancer Institute. (2023). *Plasma cell neoplasms (including multiple myeloma) treatment (PDQ®)–Health professional version.* (Accessed October 6, 2023). https://www.cancer.gov/types/myeloma/hp/myeloma-treatment-pdq

National Institutes of Health: National Heart Lung and Blood Institute. (2022). *What is anemia?* (Accessed October 6, 2023). https://www.nhlbi.nih.gov/health/anemia#:~:text=Anemia%20is%20a%20condition%20that,you%20feel%20tired%20or%20weak

Newhall, D. A., Oliver, R., & Lugthart, S. (2020). Anaemia: A disease or symptom. *The Netherlands Journal of Medicine, 78*(3), 104–110.

Norris, T. L. (2025). *Porth's pathophysiology: Concepts of altered health states* (11th ed.). Wolters Kluwer.

Onimoe, G., & Rotz, S. (2020). Sickle cell disease: A primary care update. *Cleveland Clinic Journal of Medicine, 87*(1), 19–27. https://doi.org/10.3949/ccjm.87a.18051

Pasricha, S. R., Tye-Din, J., Muckenthaler, M. U., & Swinkels, D. W. (2021). Iron deficiency. *Lancet (London, England), 397*(10270), 233–248. https://doi.org/10.1016/S0140-6736(20)32594-0

Pelcovits, A., & Niroula, R. (2020). Acute myeloid leukemia: A review. *Rhode Island Medical Journal, 103*(3), 38–40.

Petraglia, F., & Dolmans, M. M. (2022). Iron deficiency anemia: Impact on women's reproductive health. *Fertility and Sterility, 118*(4), 605–606. https://doi.org/10.1016/j.fertnstert.2022.08.850

Rai, P., & Ataga, K. I. (2020). Drug therapies for the management of sickle cell disease. *F1000Res, 9*(F1000 Faculty Rev-592), F1000 Faculty Rev-592. https://doi.org/10.12688/f1000research.22433.1

Shulpekova, Y., Nechaev, V., Kardasheva, S., Sedova, A., Kurbatova, A., Bueverova, E., Kopylov, A., Malsagova, K., Dlamini, J. C., & Ivashkin, V. (2021). The concept of folic acid in health and disease. *Molecules (Basel, Switzerland), 26*(12), 3731. https://doi.org/10.3390/molecules26123731

Slywitch, E., Savalli, C., Duarte, A. C. G., & Escrivão, M. A. M. S. (2021). Iron deficiency in vegetarian and omnivorous individuals: Analysis of 1340 individuals. *Nutrients, 13*(9), 2964. https://doi.org/10.3390/nu13092964

Sterner, R. C., & Sterner, R. M. (2021). CAR-T cell therapy: Current limitations and potential strategies. *Blood Cancer Journal, 11*(4), 69. https://doi.org/10.1038/s41408-021-00459-7

Strayer, D., Saffitz, J., & Rubin, E. (2020). *Rubin's pathology: Mechanisms of human disease* (8th ed.). Wolters Kluwer.

Weikert, C., Trefflich, I., Menzel, J., Obeid, R., Longree, A., Dierkes, J., Meyer, K., Herter-Aeberli, I., Mai, K., Stangl, G. I., Müller, S. M., Schwerdtle, T., Lampen, A., & Abraham, K. (2020). Vitamin and mineral status in a vegan diet. Deutsches Ärzteblatt International, *117*(35–36), 575–582. https://doi.org/10.3238/arztebl.2020.0575

Chapter 5

Respiratory system*

Just the facts

In this chapter, you'll learn:

♦ structures of the respiratory system

♦ how the respiratory system functions

♦ pathophysiology, diagnostic tests, and treatments for several respiratory diseases.

Understanding the respiratory system

The respiratory system consists of two lungs, conducting airways, and associated blood vessels.

The major function of the respiratory system is gas exchange. During ventilation, air is taken into the body on inhalation (inspiration) and travels through respiratory passages to the lungs. Oxygen (O_2) inhaled into the lungs diffuses into the bloodstream at the alveolar–capillary membranes. The O_2 is then absorbed by the red blood cells (RBCs) in the arterial blood.

Let's define some of the terms associated with this process:

• **PaO_2 (or PO_2):** The measure of the pressure of the oxygen in the arterial blood.

• **Carbon dioxide (CO_2):** The waste product that diffuses from the blood into the alveoli for expiration by the lungs.

• **$PaCO_2$ (or PCO_2):** The measurement of CO_2 in the arterial blood.

• **Arterial blood gases (ABGs):** A common laboratory test that indicates the patient's ability to ventilate by providing measurements of PaO_2 and $PaCO_2$. ABGs influence the pH of the bloodstream.

• **The pH:** The measure of acidity (acid content) or alkalinity (base content) of the bloodstream. (For more information about pH, see the *Acid–base imbalances* section of Chapter 4.)

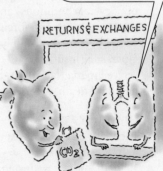

Gas exchange, that's the name of the game.

RETURNS & EXCHANGES

CO_2

---

*Note: In this chapter, the term "male" refers to a person assigned male at birth.

Disease or trauma may interfere with the respiratory system's vital work, affecting any of the following structures and functions:
- conducting airways (nasopharynx, trachea, and bronchioles)
- lungs (alveolar–capillary membranes are the major regions of gas exchange)
- breathing mechanics (mainly involving the thoracic cage and chest muscles)
- neurochemical control of ventilation (central control of breathing by the respiratory center in the brain)

Conducting airways

The conducting airways allow air into and out of structures within the lung that perform gas exchange. The conducting airways include the upper airways and the lower airways.

Upper airways
The upper airway consists of the:
- nose
- mouth
- pharynx
- larynx

Going up

The upper airway allows airflow into and out of the lungs. It warms, humidifies, and filters inspired air and protects the lower airways from foreign matter.

Blocked!

Upper airway obstruction occurs when the nose, mouth, pharynx, or larynx becomes partially or totally blocked, cutting off the O_2 supply. Several conditions can cause upper airway obstruction, including trauma, tumors, and foreign objects.

If not treated promptly, upper airway obstruction can lead to *hypoxemia* (insufficient O_2 in the blood) and then progress quickly to severe *hypoxia* (lack of O_2 available to body tissues), loss of consciousness, and death. (See *The upper and lower airways*, page 131.)

Lower airways
The lower airways consist of the:
- trachea
- right and left mainstem bronchi
- five secondary bronchi
- bronchioles

The lower airways facilitate gas exchange. Each bronchiole descends from a lobule and contains terminal bronchioles, alveolar

The upper and lower airways

The structures of the respiratory system (the airways, lungs, bony thorax, respiratory muscles, and central nervous system) work together to deliver oxygen to the bloodstream and remove excess carbon dioxide from the body.

Upper airways

The upper airways include the nasopharynx (nose), oropharynx (mouth), laryngopharynx, and larynx. These structures warm, filter, and humidify inhaled air.

Lower airways

The lower airways begin with the trachea, or windpipe, which extends from the cricoid cartilage to the carina. The trachea then divides into the right and left mainstem bronchi, which continue to divide all the way down to the alveoli, the gas exchange units of the lungs.

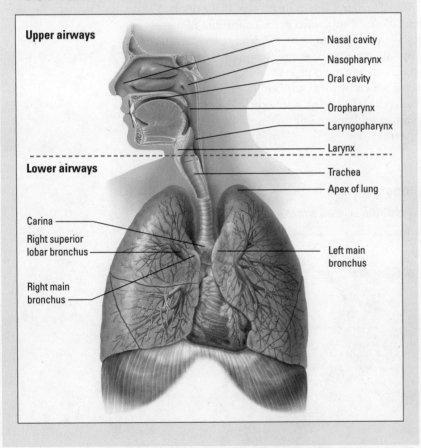

Upper airways

- Nasal cavity
- Nasopharynx
- Oral cavity
- Oropharynx
- Laryngopharynx
- Larynx

Lower airways

- Trachea
- Apex of lung

Carina

Right superior lobar bronchus

Right main bronchus

Left main bronchus

ducts, and alveoli. The alveoli are the chief units of gas exchange. (See *A close look at a pulmonary airway*, page 132.)

On the defense

In addition to warming, humidifying, and filtering inspired air, the lower airways provide the lungs with defense mechanisms, including:

- **irritant reflex, which stimulates cough.** The irritant reflex is triggered when inhaled particles, cold air, or toxins stimulate irritant receptors. Reflex bronchospasm then occurs to limit the exposure, followed by coughing, which expels the irritant.
- **mucociliary system, which traps inhaled debris in mucus and sweeps it away.** The mucociliary system produces mucus, which traps foreign particles. Foreign matter is then swept to the upper airways for expectoration. A breakdown in the epithelium of the lungs or the mucociliary system can cause the defense mechanisms to malfunction. This allows atmospheric pollutants and irritants to enter and cause inflammation to occur in the lungs.
- **secretory immunity, which involves antibodies.** Secretory immunity protects the lungs by releasing an antibody in the respiratory mucosal secretions that initiates an immune response against antigens contacting the mucosa.

A close look at a pulmonary airway

As illustrated below, each lobule or airway contains bronchioles and alveoli.

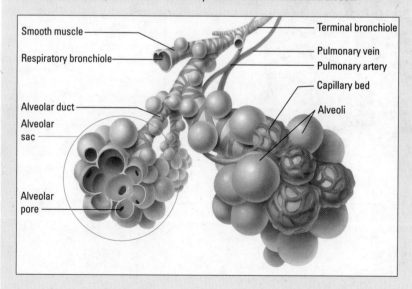

Smooth muscle

Respiratory bronchiole

Alveolar duct

Alveolar sac

Alveolar pore

Terminal bronchiole

Pulmonary vein

Pulmonary artery

Capillary bed

Alveoli

Blocked again!

Like the upper airways, the lower airways can become partially or totally blocked as a result of inflammation, tumors, foreign bodies, bronchospasm, or trauma. This can lead to respiratory distress and failure.

Lungs

The lungs are air-filled, spongelike organs. They're divided into lobes (three lobes on the right, two lobes on the left). Lobes are further divided into lobules and segments.

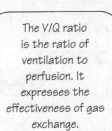

What's my secret? Millions of pulmonary alveoli that perform gas exchange.

Plunging into the lungs

Adult lungs contain about 300 million pulmonary alveoli which are grapelike clusters of air-filled sacs at the ends of the respiratory passages. Here, gas exchange takes place by diffusion (the passage of gas molecules through respiratory membranes) into the capillaries that surround the alveoli.

In diffusion, O_2 is passed to the blood for circulation throughout the body. At the same time, CO_2—a cellular waste product that's gathered by the blood as it circulates—is collected from the blood for exhalation out of the body through the lungs.

All about alveoli

Alveoli consist of type I and type II epithelial cells:
1. Type I cells form the alveolar walls, through which gas exchange occurs.
2. Type II cells produce surfactant, a lipid-type substance that coats the alveoli. During inspiration, the alveolar surfactant allows the alveoli to expand uniformly. During expiration, the surfactant prevents alveolar collapse.

Trading places: O_2 and CO_2

How much O_2 and CO_2 trade places in the alveoli? That depends largely on the amount of air in the alveoli (ventilation) and the amount of blood in the pulmonary capillaries (perfusion). The ratio of ventilation to perfusion is called the V/Q ratio. The V/Q ratio expresses the effectiveness of gas exchange.

For effective gas exchange, ventilation and perfusion must match as closely as possible. (See *Understanding ventilation and perfusion*, page 134.)

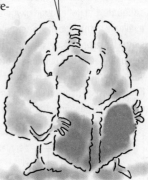

The V/Q ratio is the ratio of ventilation to perfusion. It expresses the effectiveness of gas exchange.

Now I get it!

Understanding ventilation and perfusion

Effective gas exchange depends on the relationship between ventilation and perfusion or the V/Q ratio. The diagrams below show what happens when the V/Q ratio is normal and abnormal.

Normal ventilation and perfusion

When ventilation and perfusion are matched, deoxygenated blood from the venous system returns to the right atrium, goes into the right ventricle, then travels via the pulmonary artery into the lungs, carrying carbon dioxide (CO_2). The pulmonary artery branches into pulmonary arterioles, which then branch into the alveolar capillaries. Gas exchange takes place at the alveolar–capillary membranes.

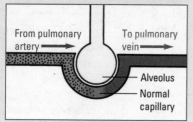

Inadequate ventilation

When the V/Q ratio is low, ventilation is low and pulmonary circulation is adequate, but not enough oxygen (O_2) is available to the alveoli for normal diffusion. The region of low alveolar oxygen stimulates reflexive pulmonary arteriolar vasoconstriction in that region of the lungs. Chronic hypoxia stimulates pulmonary arterial vasoconstriction. This diverts blood away from poorly oxygenated areas and allows more blood to go to the well-ventilated areas of the lungs. *This is a KEY reaction to understand that takes place uniquely in the lungs!*

Inadequate perfusion (dead space ventilation)

When the V/Q < ratio is high, ventilation is normal, but lung perfusion (circulation) is reduced. Note the narrowed blood vessels, indicating poor perfusion. This commonly results from a perfusion or circulation defect, or any cause of decreased pulmonary circulation such as pulmonary embolism. A pulmonary embolism is a clot that blocks a pulmonary arterial vessel.

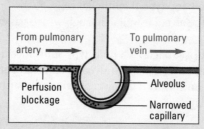

Inadequate ventilation and perfusion (silent unit)

A silent unit indicates an absence of ventilation and perfusion to the lung area.

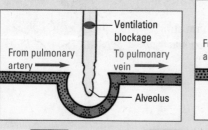

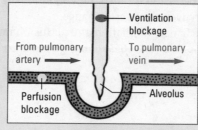

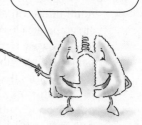

A high V/Q ratio results from reduced or absent alveolar perfusion.

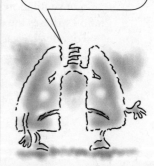

A silent unit can stem from several causes, including pulmonary embolism and chronic alveolar collapse.

Key [illustration] Blood with CO_2 [illustration] Blood with O_2 [illustration] Blood with CO_2 and O_2

Mismatch mayhem

A V/Q mismatch, resulting from ventilation–perfusion dysfunction, accounts for most of the impaired gas exchange in respiratory disorders. Ineffective gas exchange between the alveoli and the pulmonary capillaries can affect all body systems by altering the amount of O_2 delivered to the tissues in the body.

Ineffective gas exchange from an abnormality can cause three outcomes:

1. inadequate ventilation with consequent pulmonary arterial vasoconstriction (e.g., this often occurs in long-term chronic obstructive pulmonary disease [COPD], which causes chronic hypoxia and consequent pulmonary arterial vasoconstriction, termed pulmonary hypertension)
2. inadequate circulation to a lung region, where there is adequate ventilation but no circulation; this will result in dead space ventilation (e.g., this most often occurs with pulmonary embolism, which is a clot that blocks the pulmonary arterial circulation)
3. silent unit, which is a combination of the above—that is, a lack of both ventilation and circulation to an area of lung tissue (e.g., this most often occurs in acute respiratory distress syndrome [ARDS])

Breathing mechanics

The amount of air that reaches the lungs carrying O_2 and then departs carrying CO_2 depends on three factors:

1. lung volume and capacity
2. compliance (the lungs' ability to expand)
3. resistance to airflow

Air apparent

Lung volume and capacity are the amount of air that's moved in and out of the lungs.

No room for expansion

Changes in compliance can occur in either the lung or the chest wall. Destruction of the lung's elastic fibers, which occurs in ARDS, decreases lung compliance. The lungs become stiff, making breathing difficult. The alveolocapillary membrane may also be affected, causing hypoxia. Chest wall compliance is also affected by thoracic deformity, chest muscle spasm, and abdominal distention.

La pièce de résistance

Resistance refers to opposition to airflow. Changes in resistance may occur in the lung tissue, chest wall, or airways. Airway resistance accounts for about 80% of all respiratory system resistance. It's increased in such obstructive diseases as asthma, chronic bronchitis, and emphysema.

With increased resistance, a person has to work harder to breathe, especially during expiration, to compensate for narrowed airways and diminished gas exchange.

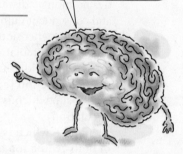

The central nervous system's respiratory center is located in the medulla of the brain stem.

Neurochemical control

The respiratory center of the central nervous system (CNS) is located in the medulla of the brain stem. Impulses travel down the phrenic nerves to the diaphragm and then down the intercostal nerves to the intercostal muscles between the ribs. There, they change the rate and depth of respiration.

Factors of influence

Chemoreceptors respond to the hydrogen ion concentration (pH) of arterial blood, the pressure of arterial carbon dioxide ($PaCO_2$), and the pressure of arterial oxygen (PaO_2).

As mentioned earlier in this chapter, when discussing the dissolved oxygen and carbon dioxide gases in the arterial blood, we use the terms PaO_2, PO_2, $PaCO_2$, and PCO_2, and we can measure the level of dissolved oxygen and carbon dioxide in the arterial blood using the blood tests known as *arterial blood gases*. The ABGs indicate the blood pH, PO_2 or PaO_2, PCO_2 or $PaCO_2$, and HCO_3^- and SaO_2 (saturation of hemoglobin with oxygen). See Chapter 4 for information about acid–base imbalances.

$PaCO_2$ also helps regulate ventilation (by impacting the pH of cerebrospinal fluid [CSF], and it affects brain control of the respiratory rate). If $PaCO_2$ is high, the respiratory rate increases. If $PaCO_2$ is low, the respiratory rate decreases.

On the periphery

The respiratory center also receives information from peripheral chemoreceptors in the carotid and aortic bodies (small neurovascular structures in the carotid arteries and on either side of the aorta). These chemoreceptors respond to decreased PaO_2 and decreased pH. Either change results in increased respiratory drive within minutes.

Respiratory disorders

The respiratory disorders discussed in this section include:
- ARDS
- acute respiratory failure (ARF)
- asthma
- chronic bronchitis
- cor pulmonale
- emphysema
- lung cancer
- pneumonia
- pneumothorax
- pulmonary edema
- pulmonary embolism
- respiratory syncytial virus (RSV)
- tuberculosis

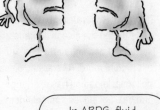

Shock, sepsis, and trauma are the most common causes of ARDS.

Acute respiratory distress syndrome

ARDS represents critical illness involving lung inflammation and injury. It is defined by (1) acute onset of bilateral fluid infiltrates on chest x-ray and (2) a low pressure of arterial oxygen (PaO_2).

ARDS most commonly occurs with shock, severe trauma, severe pneumonia (such as can occur with a COVID-19 infection), or sepsis. It's difficult to diagnose and can prove fatal within 48 hours of onset if not promptly diagnosed and treated. Mortality associated with ARDS is 40% in adults under 60 and is much higher in older adults (age 60 and over).

How it happens

Shock, sepsis, COVID-19 infection, and trauma are the most common causes of ARDS.

An account of fluid accumulation

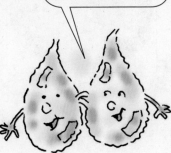

In ARDS, fluid builds up in the lungs, causing them to stiffen.

In ARDS, fluid accumulates in the lungs' interstitial tissues, alveolar spaces, and small airways, causing the lungs to stiffen. A key characteristic of ARDS is decreased compliance or decreased elasticity of the lungs due to fluid accumulation. This impairs ventilation and reduces oxygenation of pulmonary capillary blood. Hypoxemia is another key characteristic of ARDS. (See *Alveolar changes in ARDS*, page 138.)

Now I get it!

Alveolar changes in ARDS

The alveoli undergo major changes in each phase of ARDS.

Phase 1

In *phase 1*, injury reduces normal blood flow to the lungs. Platelets aggregate and release histamine (H), serotonin (S), and bradykinin (B).

Phase 2

In *phase 2*, those substances—especially histamine—inflame and damage the alveolocapillary membrane, increasing capillary permeability. Fluids then shift into the interstitial space.

Phase 3

In *phase 3*, as capillary permeability increases, proteins and fluids leak out, increasing interstitial osmotic pressure and causing pulmonary edema.

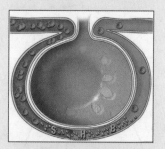

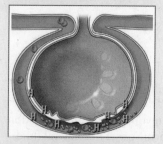

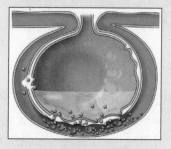

Phase 4

In *phase 4*, decreased blood flow and fluids in the alveoli damage surfactant and impair the cell's ability to produce more. As a result, alveoli collapse, impeding gas exchange and decreasing lung compliance.

Phase 5

In *phase 5*, sufficient oxygen can't cross the alveolocapillary membrane, but carbon dioxide (CO_2) can and is lost with every exhalation. Oxygen (O_2) and CO_2 levels decrease in the blood.

Phase 6

In *phase 6*, pulmonary edema worsens, inflammation leads to fibrosis, and gas exchange is further impeded.

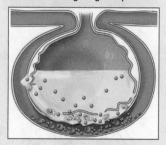

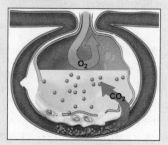

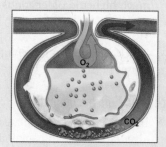

What to look for

ARDS initially produces rapid, shallow breathing and dyspnea within hours to days of the initial injury. As ARDS progresses, look for the following signs and symptoms:

- Hypoxemia develops, causing an increased drive for ventilation. Because of the effort required to expand the stiff lungs, intercostal and suprasternal retractions result.
- Fluid accumulation produces crackles and rhonchi. Worsening hypoxemia causes restlessness, apprehension, mental sluggishness, motor dysfunction, and tachycardia.
- Severe ARDS causes overwhelming hypoxemia. If uncorrected, this results in hypotension, decreased urine output, and respiratory and metabolic acidosis. Eventually, ventricular fibrillation or standstill may occur. (See *Treating ARDS*, page 139.)

Battling illness

Treating ARDS

Therapy focuses on correcting the cause of acute respiratory distress syndrome (ARDS) and preventing progression of hypoxemia and respiratory acidosis. Supportive care consists of administering continuous positive airway pressure. However, this therapy alone seldom fulfills the patient's ventilatory requirements, so several other treatments are used.

Ventilation
The primary treatment for ARDS is intubation and mechanical ventilation to increase lung volume, open airways, and improve oxygenation. Positive end-expiratory pressure is also added to increase lung volume and open alveoli. Patients are often placed in the prone position when on the ventilator because that position has been proven to enhance oxygenation.

Drugs
During mechanical ventilation, sedatives (such as propofol or midazolam), opioids, or neuromuscular blocking agents such as pancuronium may be ordered. These drugs minimize restlessness, O_2 consumption, and CO_2 production and facilitate ventilation. This is sometimes referred to as a "medically induced coma" to allow the patient to be mechanically ventilated.

When ARDS results from fat emboli or a chemical injury, a short course of high-dose corticosteroids may be given. Sodium bicarbonate may reverse severe metabolic acidosis, and fluids and vasopressors help maintain blood pressure. Nonviral infections require treatment with antimicrobial drugs.

Additional support
Supportive measures include vasopressive agents, nutritional support, correction of electrolyte and acid–base imbalances, prone positioning, and fluid restriction (even small increases in capillary pressures from IV fluids can greatly increase interstitial and alveolar edema).

Other therapies may include surfactant replacement, pulmonary antihypertensive medications, and antisepsis agents.

What tests tell you

ABG analysis (see Chapter 4 for a discussion of ABGs) with the patient breathing room air initially shows a reduced PaO_2 (less than 60 mm Hg) and a decreased $PaCO_2$ (less than 35 mm Hg). Hypoxemia despite increased supplemental oxygen indicates the presence of an ARDS characteristic shunt. The resulting blood pH usually reflects respiratory alkalosis.

As ARDS worsens, ABG values show:

- respiratory acidosis—increasing $PaCO_2$ (more than 45 mm Hg)
- metabolic acidosis—decreasing bicarbonate (HCO_3^-) levels (less than 22 mEq/L)
- declining PaO_2 despite oxygen therapy
- declining oxygen saturation (SaO_2)
  Other diagnostic tests include the following
- Pulmonary artery catheterization (also called a Swan–Ganz catheter) identifies the cause of edema by measuring pulmonary capillary wedge pressure (PCWP). It is important to distinguish ARDS from pulmonary edema due to left ventricular failure because they both present with similar findings. However, ARDS is not due to heart failure. The PCWP is normal (12 mm Hg or less) in ARDS, proving that it is not pulmonary edema due to left ventricular failure.
- Serial chest x-rays in early stages show bilateral infiltrates. In later stages, they show lung fields that have the appearance of ground-up glass and, with irreversible hypoxemia, "whiteouts" of both lung fields. This ground-glass appearance on chest x-ray has recently been seen most often in severe COVID-19 pneumonia. ARDS is a major cause of death for people with COVID-19.
- Pulse oximetry shows decreasing SaO_2 (decreased saturation of blood with oxygen).

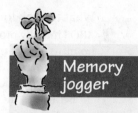

Memory jogger

To remember the progression of **ARDS**, use this mnemonic.

Assault to the pulmonary system

Respiratory distress

Decreased lung compliance

Severe respiratory failure

Differential diagnosis

A differential diagnosis rules out cardiogenic pulmonary edema, pulmonary vasculitis, and diffuse pulmonary hemorrhage. Tests that aid in the diagnosis include:

- sputum analysis, including Gram stain and culture and sensitivity tests, to identify organisms (bacterial pneumonia can cause ARDS)
- blood cultures to identify infectious organisms in blood (sepsis often causes ARDS)
- toxicology tests to screen for drug ingestion (drug toxicity can cause ARDS)
- serum amylase and lipase tests to rule out pancreatitis (pancreatitis can cause ARDS)

Acute respiratory failure

When the lungs can't adequately maintain oxygenation or eliminate CO_2, ARF results, which can lead to tissue hypoxia.

How it happens

In patients with essentially normal lung tissue, ARF usually means a $PaCO_2$ above 50 mm Hg, a PaO_2 below 50 mm Hg, and a pH of less than 7.35. The key finding of respiratory failure is a trend of falling PaO_2 and a trend of rising $PaCO_2$ on serial ABGs over time.

Conditions that can lead to ARF include:

- COPD
- bronchitis
- pneumonia
- bronchospasm
- ventilatory failure
- pneumothorax
- atelectasis
- cor pulmonale
- pulmonary edema
- pulmonary emboli
- ARDS
- influenza
- neuromuscular dysfunction (such as amyotrophic lateral sclerosis, Guillain-Barré syndrome, and myasthenia gravis)
- CNS disease
- CNS depression–head trauma or overuse of sedatives, opioids, tranquilizers, or O_2

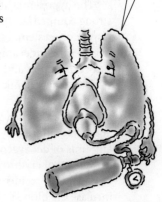

When I can't adequately maintain oxygenation or eliminate carbon dioxide, ARF results.

If it isn't hypoventilation…

ARF results from impaired gas exchange. Conditions associated with alveolar hypoventilation (deficient movement of air into and out of the alveoli) and V/Q (ventilation–perfusion) mismatch can cause ARF if left untreated. Decreased SaO_2 may result from alveolar hypoventilation, in which chronic airway obstruction reduces alveolar ventilation (the volume of air inhaled). PaO_2 levels fall and $PaCO_2$ levels rise, resulting in hypoxemia and hypercapnia.

Hypoventilation can result from a decrease in the respiratory rate or duration or inspiratory signal from the respiratory center, such as with CNS conditions, trauma, or CNS-depressant drugs. The most common cause of alveolar hypoventilation is airway obstruction, commonly seen with COPD (emphysema or bronchitis).

...then it's hypoxemia

Hypoxemia—V/Q imbalance—most commonly occurs when such conditions as pulmonary embolism or ARDS interrupt normal gas exchange in a specific lung region. Too little ventilation with normal blood flow or too little blood flow with normal ventilation may cause the imbalance, resulting in decreased PaO_2 levels and, thus, hypoxemia.

The hypoxemia and hypercapnia characteristic of ARF stimulates strong compensatory responses by all body systems, including the respiratory system, cardiovascular system, and CNS. In response to hypoxemia, for example, the sympathetic nervous system triggers vasoconstriction and increases peripheral resistance and heart rate.

Tissue hypoxemia also occurs in ARF, resulting in anaerobic metabolism and lactic acidosis. Respiratory acidosis is due to hypercapnia (see Chapter 4). Heart rate increases, stroke volume increases, and heart failure may occur. Cyanosis occurs because of increased amounts of deoxygenated blood. Hypoxia of the kidneys results in the release of erythropoietin from renal cells, which in turn causes the bone marrow to increase RBC production—an attempt by the body to increase the blood's O_2-carrying capacity.

The body responds to hypercapnia with cerebral depression, hypotension, circulatory failure, and increased heart rate and cardiac output. Hypoxemia, hypercapnia, or both cause the brain's respiratory control center first to increase respiratory depth (tidal volume) and then to increase the respiratory rate. As ARF worsens, intercostal muscle retractions may also occur, which indicate severe breathing difficulty.

(For more information on acid–base balance, see the *Acid–base imbalances* section of Chapter 4.)

What to look for

Specific symptoms vary with the underlying cause of ARF, and the following body systems may be affected:

• Respiratory system—Rate may be increased, decreased, or normal depending on the cause; respirations may be shallow or deep or alternate between the two. The patient may experience air hunger. Extreme difficulty breathing is indicated by intercostal muscle retractions and cyanosis. Cyanosis occurs when hypoxemia occurs (low blood PaO_2). Auscultation of the chest may reveal crackles, rhonchi, wheezing, or diminished breath sounds.
• CNS—The patient may demonstrate restlessness, confusion, loss of concentration, irritability, tremulousness, diminished tendon reflexes, stupor, or coma.
• Cardiovascular system—Tachycardia, increased cardiac output, and mildly elevated blood pressure occur early in response to low PaO_2. With myocardial hypoxia, arrhythmias may develop. Pulmonary hypertension may cause increased pressure on the right side of the heart, distended neck veins, enlarged liver, and peripheral edema. (See *Treating ARF.*)

What tests tell you

These tests help identify ARF:

- ABG analysis shows deteriorating values and a pH below 7.35 (see the *Acid–base imbalances* section of Chapter 4). Patients with COPD may have a lower-than-normal pH compared with previous levels.
- Chest x-rays identify pulmonary diseases or conditions, such as emphysema, atelectasis, lesions, pneumothorax, infiltrates, and effusions.
- Electrocardiography (ECG) can demonstrate ventricular arrhythmias (indicating myocardial hypoxia) or right ventricular hypertrophy (indicating cor pulmonale).
- Pulse oximetry reveals decreasing SaO_2.
- White blood cell (WBC) count detects an underlying infection.
- Abnormally low hemoglobin level and hematocrit signal blood loss, which indicates decreased O_2-carrying capacity.
- Pulmonary artery catheterization (also called Swan–Ganz catheterization) helps to distinguish pulmonary and cardiovascular causes of ARF and monitors hemodynamic pressures.

Battling illness

Treating ARF

Therapy for acute respiratory failure (ARF) focuses on correcting hypoxemia and preventing respiratory acidosis.

Oxygenation

These measures can be used to improve oxygenation in patients with ARF:

- deep breathing with pursed lips, if the patient isn't intubated and mechanically ventilated, to help keep airway patent
- incentive spirometry to increase lung volume
- oxygen therapy to promote oxygenation and raise partial pressure of arterial oxygen
- mechanical ventilation with an endotracheal or tracheostomy tube, if needed, to provide adequate oxygenation

Drugs

These drugs may be used in the treatment of ARF:

- antibiotics to treat infection
- bronchodilators to open airways
- corticosteroids to decrease inflammation
- positive inotropic agents to enhance cardiac contractility and increase cardiac output
- vasopressors to maintain blood pressure
- diuretics to reduce edema and fluid overload
- opioids such as morphine to reduce respiratory difficulty and to promote comfort by relieving anxiety
- anxiolytics such as lorazepam to reduce anxiety
- sedatives, such as propofol, if the patient requires mechanical ventilation and is having difficulty tolerating it (this is often referred to as a medically induced coma)
- fluid restriction to reduce volume and cardiac workload (for patients with ARF who have cor pulmonale)

Asthma

Asthma is a chronic inflammatory airway disorder that can present as an acute attack. It causes episodic airway obstruction resulting from bronchospasms, increased mucus secretion, and bronchial inflammation. Asthma is a long-term pulmonary disease characterized by airflow obstruction. The three most common signs and symptoms are cough, dyspnea, and wheezing.

It usually strikes early

Cases of asthma continue to rise. It currently affects an estimated 21 million American adults and 4.1 million children.

It's a family affair

Many patients develop asthma as a child and have at least one immediate biological family member with the disease.

How it happens

In asthma, bronchial linings overreact to various triggers, causing episodic smooth muscle spasms that severely constrict the airways. Mucosal edema and thickened secretions further block the airways. (See *Understanding asthma*, page 145.)

This process can be attributed to:
1. genetics
2. environment

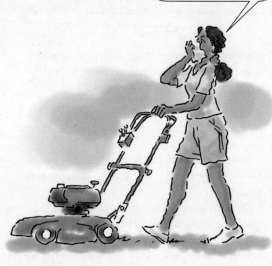

Environmentally induced asthma occurs due to a combination of genetic susceptibility and exposure to allergens.

It's all in the genes

Genetically induced asthma begins in childhood and is commonly accompanied by other hereditary allergies, such as eczema and allergic rhinitis.

Environmentally speaking

Environmentally induced asthma occurs due to a combination of genetic susceptibility and exposure to allergens. Specific environmental allergens include pollen, animal dander, house dust or mold, synthetic or feather pillows, food additives containing sulfites,

Now I get it!

Understanding asthma

During an asthma attack, muscles surrounding the bronchial tubes tighten (bronchospasm), narrowing the air passage and interrupting the normal flow of air into and out of the lungs. Airflow is further interrupted by an increase in mucus secretion, forming mucus plugs, and inflammation of the bronchioles.

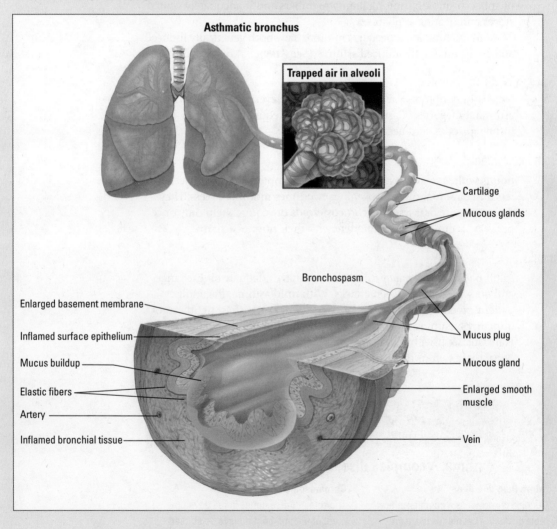

Asthmatic bronchus

Trapped air in alveoli

Cartilage

Mucous glands

Bronchospasm

Enlarged basement membrane

Inflamed surface epithelium

Mucus buildup

Elastic fibers

Artery

Inflamed bronchial tissue

Mucus plug

Mucous gland

Enlarged smooth muscle

Vein

cockroach and rodent droppings, cigarette smoke, urban pollutants (major allergens for inner-city children), and any other sensitizing substances.

However, asthma can be due to a severe respiratory tract infection, such as acute bronchitis, especially in adults. Other predisposing conditions include irritants, pollutants, emotional stress, fatigue, endocrine changes, temperature and humidity variations, and exposure to noxious fumes, such as nitrogen dioxide, which is produced by tobacco smoking among family members and inadequately vented stoves and heating appliances.

Many asthmatics, especially children, have both genetically induced and environmentally induced asthma. (See *Asthma: A complex disease.*)

What to look for

Signs and symptoms vary depending on the severity of a patient's asthma. Categories of asthma are based on frequency of attacks, nocturnal episodes, and need for corticosteroids.

From intermittent...

Adults with *intermittent asthma* experience symptoms 2 days a week or less and have nighttime awakenings two times monthly or less. They do not require oral systemic corticosteroids or require them only once per year. Asthma does not interfere with their normal activity.

To mild...

Adult patients with *mild persistent asthma* have adequate air exchange and no symptoms between attacks. With mild asthma, the adult patient experiences symptoms of cough, wheezing, chest tightness, or difficulty breathing more than twice weekly, but not on a daily basis. Flare-ups are brief but may vary in intensity. Nighttime symptoms occur three to four times monthly.

The genetic link

Asthma: A complex disease

More than one gene
Asthma is known as a complex inheritable disease. That means there are several genes that make a person susceptible to the disease, including genes on chromosomes 5, 6, 11, 12, and 13.

Chromosome 5
The role of these genes in the development of asthma continues to be studied. One of the most evolving sites of study is chromosome 5.

...to moderate...

Patients with *moderate persistent asthma* have normal or below-normal air exchange as well as signs and symptoms that include cough, wheezing, chest tightness, or difficulty breathing daily. Flare-ups may affect the patient's level of activity. Nighttime symptoms occur more than once weekly, but not nightly.

...to worse

Patients with *severe persistent asthma* have below-normal air exchange and experience continual symptoms of cough, wheezing, chest tightness, and difficulty breathing. Their activity level is extremely limited. Nighttime symptoms occur frequently, often nightly.

Patients with any type of asthma may develop status asthmaticus, a severe acute attack that doesn't respond to conventional treatment. The patient will have signs and symptoms that include:

- marked respiratory distress
- marked wheezing or absent breath sounds
- pulsus paradoxus greater than 10 mm Hg
- chest wall contractions (See *Treating asthma*, page 148.)

What tests tell you

These tests are used to diagnose asthma:

- Pulmonary function tests (also called spirometry) reveal signs of obstructive airway disease, low-normal or decreased vital capacity, and increased total lung and residual capacities. Pulmonary function may be normal between attacks. Individuals with asthma are encouraged to test their pulmonary function during attacks. The most common pulmonary function measurements used to diagnose asthma are the forced vital capacity and forced expiratory volume (FEV). FEV is usually prolonged in asthma; the individual takes an increased amount of time to exhale air from the lungs.
- Serum immunoglobulin (Ig) E levels may increase from an allergic reaction.
- Complete blood count (CBC) with differential reveals increased eosinophil count.
- Chest x-rays can diagnose or monitor asthma's progress and may show hyperinflation with areas of atelectasis.
- ABG analysis detects hypoxemia and guides treatment.
- Skin testing may identify specific allergens. Test results are read in 1 to 2 days to detect an early reaction and again after 4 to 5 days to reveal a late reaction.
- Bronchial challenge testing evaluates the clinical significance of allergens identified by skin testing.
- Forced exhalation of nitric oxide (FeNO) testing can demonstrate inflammation in the lungs.
- Pulse oximetry may show a reduced SaO_2 level.

Treating asthma

The best treatment for asthma is prevention by identifying and avoiding precipitating factors, such as environmental allergens or irritants. Usually, such stimuli can't be removed entirely, so desensitization to specific antigens may be helpful, especially in children. Allergen immunotherapy is commonly used to desensitize allergic individuals. Other common treatments are medication and oxygen (O_2).

Medication

These types of drugs are usually given:

Long-acting bronchodilators (salmeterol and formoterol) decrease bronchoconstriction, reduce bronchial airway edema, and increase pulmonary ventilation.

Corticosteroids (budesonide and fluticasone) have anti-inflammatory effects. Inhaled corticosteroids are used in long-term control of asthma.

Combined medications (fluticasone/salmeterol and budesonide/formoterol) have both the bronchodilator and anti-inflammatory effects in one inhaler.

Leukotriene receptor antagonists (montelukast, zafirlukast, and zileuton) are effective in reducing leukotrienes, which are inflammatory mediators that cause airway constriction.

Immunomodulators (e.g., omalizumab) counteract the IgE antibody that causes inflammation in people with allergy-induced asthma. These drugs change how the immune system reacts to asthma triggers and are used in long-term asthma control.

Oxygen

Low-flow humidified O_2 (also called nebulizer treatment) may be needed to treat dyspnea, cyanosis, and hypoxemia. The amount delivered is designed to maintain a partial pressure of arterial oxygen between 65 and 85 mm Hg, as determined by arterial blood gas studies. Mechanical ventilation is necessary if the patient doesn't respond to initial ventilatory support and drugs or develop respiratory failure.

Chronic bronchitis

Chronic bronchitis, a form of COPD, is inflammation of the bronchi caused by irritants or infection. (See *Understanding COPD*, page 148.)

Understanding COPD

Chronic obstructive pulmonary disease (COPD) refers to long-term pulmonary disorders characterized by high airflow resistance. Two such disorders are chronic bronchitis and emphysema. Chronic bronchitis and emphysema are both involved in COPD and occur together.

Predisposing factors

Factors that predispose a patient to COPD include:
• smoking
• recurrent or chronic respiratory infections

• allergies
• hereditary factors such as an inherited deficiency in alpha$_1$-protease inhibitor (an inhibitor to the enzyme protease)

Smoking ranks first

Smoking is the most important predisposing factor of COPD. It impairs ciliary action and macrophage function, causing inflammation in the airway, increased mucus production, alveolar destruction, and peribronchiolar fibrosis.

In chronic bronchitis, hypersecretion of mucus and chronic productive cough last for 3 months of the year and occur for at least two consecutive years. The distinguishing characteristic of bronchitis is obstruction of airflow caused by mucus and inflammation of the bronchioles.

How it happens

Chronic bronchitis occurs when irritants are inhaled for a prolonged period. The result is resistance in the small airways and severe V/Q imbalance that decreases arterial oxygenation.

Patients have a diminished respiratory drive, so they usually hypoventilate. The patient is not well oxygenated; because O_2 is low, cyanosis is evident. (See *Mucus buildup in chronic bronchitis.*)

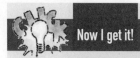

Now I get it!

Mucus buildup in chronic bronchitis

In chronic bronchitis, excessive mucus production obstructs the small airways.

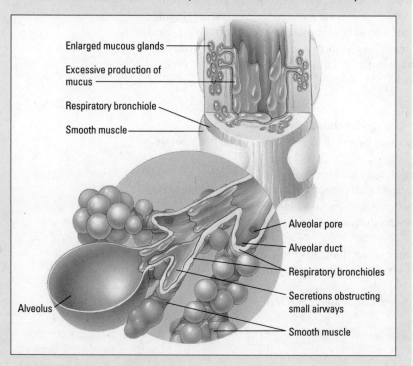

- Enlarged mucous glands
- Excessive production of mucus
- Respiratory bronchiole
- Smooth muscle
- Alveolar pore
- Alveolar duct
- Respiratory bronchioles
- Secretions obstructing small airways
- Smooth muscle
- Alveolus

What to look for

Signs and symptoms of advanced chronic bronchitis include:

- productive cough
- dyspnea
- cyanosis
- use of accessory muscles for breathing
- pulmonary hypertension (due to chronic hypoxia)

The pressure is on

Chronic hypoxia in chronic bronchitis causes areas of low ventilation and oxygenation in the lungs. When there is an area of hypoxia in the lungs, the pulmonary arterial vessels vasoconstrict and decrease the amount of perfusion in that nonventilated area; this is referred to as shunting. As pulmonary arterial vessels constrict, this raises pressure within the pulmonary arterial system. Pulmonary artery pressure becomes high; this is known as pulmonary hypertension. As pulmonary hypertension continues, the right ventricle of the heart hypertrophies in order to deal with the high workload against it. The right ventricle endures undue strain, and eventually right ventricular failure occurs. This is referred to as *cor pulmonale (right ventricular hypertrophy with right-sided heart failure)*. Right ventricular failure causes a backup of pressure from the right atrium into the vena cava, which causes increased venous pressure, jugular venous distension, ascites, liver and spleen venous congestion, and dependent ankle edema. In chronic bronchitis, cor pulmonale can occur, which is right ventricular failure due to lung disease. (See *Treating chronic bronchitis.*)

What tests tell you

These tests are used to diagnose chronic bronchitis:

- Chest x-rays may show hyperinflation and increased bronchovascular markings.
- Pulmonary function tests indicate signs of COPD: increased residual volume, decreased vital capacity, decreased FEV, and decreased forced expiratory volume in 1 second (FEV1).
- ABG analysis displays decreased PaO_2 and normal or increased $PaCO_2$.
- Sputum culture may reveal many microorganisms and neutrophils.
- ECG shows right ventricular hypertrophy and possible arrhythmias.
- Pulse oximetry shows a decreased SaO_2 level.

Treating chronic bronchitis

The most effective treatment for chronic bronchitis is to avoid air pollutants and, if the patient smokes, to stop smoking. Other treatments include:
- antibiotics to treat recurring infections
- bronchodilators to relieve bronchospasm and facilitate mucus clearance
- adequate hydration
- chest physiotherapy to mobilize secretions
- nebulizer treatments to loosen and mobilize secretions
- corticosteroids to combat inflammation
- diuretics for edema
- oxygen for hypoxia

Cor pulmonale

Cor pulmonale is right ventricular failure that is due to a lung disorder characterized by chronic hypoxia. Chronic bronchitis is a key cause of chronic hypoxia. Chronic hypoxia causes reflexive pulmonary arterial vasoconstriction. Pulmonary arterial vasoconstriction leads to pulmonary hypertension, which leads to cor pulmonale. COPD is the most common cause of cor pulmonale.

The core facts about cor pulmonale

Cor pulmonale causes between 10% and 30% of all types of heart failure. Cor pulmonale is most common in older adults with a long history of smoking that caused COPD.

How it happens
Cor pulmonale may result from:
- disorders that affect the pulmonary tissue and causes chronic hypoxia
- pulmonary diseases that affect the airways such as COPD
- chest wall abnormalities, including such thoracic deformities as kyphoscoliosis and pectus excavatum (funnel chest) that cause chronic hypoxia
- neuromuscular disorders, such as muscular dystrophy and poliomyelitis that cause poor ventilation and chronic hypoxia

What to look for
In early stages of cor pulmonale, patients are most likely to report:
- chronic productive cough
- exertional dyspnea
- wheezing respirations
- fatigue and weakness

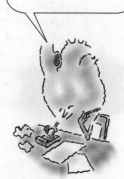

Cor pulmonale causes about 10% to 30% of all types of heart failure.

As the compensatory mechanism begins to fail, larger amounts of blood remain in the right ventricle at the end of diastole, causing ventricular dilation. As cor pulmonale progresses, these additional symptoms occur:

- dyspnea at rest
- tachypnea
- orthopnea (difficulty breathing when lying flat)
- dependent edema
- distended neck veins (jugular vein distension)
- hepatomegaly (enlarged, tender liver)
- hepatojugular reflux (jugular vein distention induced by pressing over the liver)
- tachycardia
- decreased cardiac output
- weight gain

Chest examination reveals characteristics of the underlying lung disease.

(See *Understanding cor pulmonale*, page 153.)

Because cor pulmonale occurs late in the course of COPD and other irreversible diseases, prognosis is poor. (See *Treating cor pulmonale*, page 154.)

What tests tell you

These tests are used to diagnose cor pulmonale:

- Pulmonary artery catheterization (also called a Swan–Ganz catheterization) shows increased right ventricular and pulmonary artery pressures, resulting from increased pulmonary vascular resistance. Both right ventricular systolic and pulmonary artery systolic pressures are greater than 30 mm Hg, and pulmonary artery diastolic pressure is greater than 15 mm Hg.
- Echocardiography or angiography demonstrates right ventricular enlargement.
- Chest x-rays reveal large central pulmonary arteries and right ventricular enlargement.
- ABG analysis detects decreased PaO_2 (usually less than 70 mm Hg).
- Pulse oximetry shows a reduced SaO_2 level.
- ECG shows right ventricular hypertrophy and possible arrhythmias.
- Pulmonary function tests reflect underlying pulmonary disease such as decreased FEV, FEV1, increased RV.
- Magnetic resonance imaging (MRI) measures right ventricular mass, wall thickness, and low right ventricular ejection fraction.
- Elevated liver enzymes if there is liver congestion with decreased liver function.
- Serum bilirubin levels may be elevated if liver dysfunction and hepatomegaly are present.

Now I get it!

Understanding cor pulmonale

Three types of disorders are responsible for cor pulmonale:
1. restrictive pulmonary disorders, such as fibrosis or obesity
2. obstructive pulmonary disorders such as chronic obstructive pulmonary disease
3. primary vascular disorders such as recurrent pulmonary emboli

These disorders share a common pathway to the formation of cor pulmonale. Hypoxic constriction of pulmonary blood vessels and obstruction of pulmonary blood flow lead to increased pulmonary resistance, which progresses to cor pulmonale.

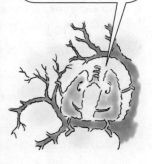

Three different types of disorders may cause cor pulmonale, but all share a common pathway.

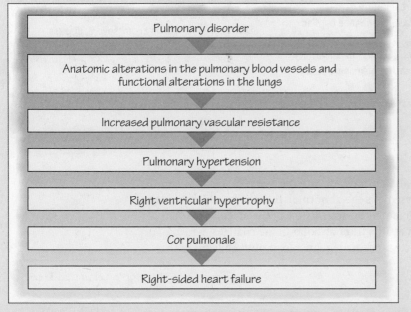

Pulmonary disorder

↓

Anatomic alterations in the pulmonary blood vessels and functional alterations in the lungs

↓

Increased pulmonary vascular resistance

↓

Pulmonary hypertension

↓

Right ventricular hypertrophy

↓

Cor pulmonale

↓

Right-sided heart failure

Treating cor pulmonale

Therapy for the patient with cor pulmonale has three aims:

1. reducing hypoxemia and pulmonary vasoconstriction
2. increasing exercise tolerance
3. correcting the underlying condition when possible

Bed rest, drug therapy, and more
Treatment includes:

- bed rest
- antibiotics for an underlying respiratory tract infection
- cardiac glycosides (e.g., digoxin) to enhance cardiac contractility
- oral calcium channel blockers, such as nifedipine, nicardipine, amlodipine, and diltiazem, for pulmonary artery vasodilation
- potent pulmonary artery vasodilator, such as diazoxide, nitroprusside, or hydralazine, to treat primary pulmonary hypertension
- IV prostacyclin therapy to dilate blood vessels and reduce clotting by stopping platelet aggregation
- endothelin receptor antagonists such as bosentan to reduce pulmonary artery vasoconstriction
- continuous administration of low concentrations of oxygen due to chronic hypoxia
- chest physiotherapy to loosen secretions
- mechanical ventilation in acute, severe, disease
- low-sodium diet with restricted fluid

Emphysema

Chronic bronchitis and emphysema are the two diseases that comprise COPD. Emphysema is the abnormal, permanent enlargement of the alveoli accompanied by destruction of the alveolar membranes. Obstruction results from alveolar tissue changes, which causes lack of elasticity and inadequate recoil of the alveoli with exhalation.

Losing elasticity

The distinguishing characteristic of emphysema is airflow limitation caused by lack of elastic recoil in the lungs. The alveoli are overly distended and filled with air (like over-stretched balloons).

How it happens

Emphysema may be caused by a deficiency of alpha$_1$-protease inhibitor or by cigarette smoking.

In emphysema, recurrent inflammation is associated with the release of proteolytic enzymes (enzymes that breakdown proteins). Alveolar membranes are destroyed, and alveoli become overly distended with weakened membrane walls. There is loss of recoil and compliance in the lungs; lungs retain air and cannot exhale CO_2. (See *Air trapping in emphysema*, page 155.)

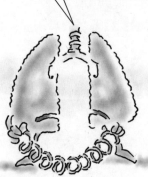

Now that I have emphysema, I seem to lack the spring in my step!

Now I get it!

Air trapping in emphysema

After alveolar walls are damaged or destroyed, they can't support and keep the airways open. The alveolar walls then lose their capability of elastic recoil. Collapse then occurs on expiration, as shown here.

Normal expiration
Note normal recoil and the open bronchiole.

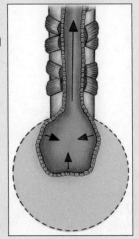

Impaired expiration
Note decreased elastic recoil and a narrowed bronchiole.

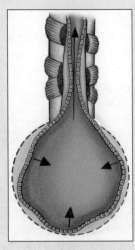

What to look for

Signs and symptoms of emphysema include:
- dyspnea on exertion (initial symptom)
- barrel-shaped chest from lung overdistention, which increases size of thoracic cage
- prolonged expiration because patient cannot get air out of lungs
- decreased breath sounds

What tests tell you

The following tests are used to diagnose emphysema:
- Chest x-rays in advanced disease may show a flattened diaphragm, reduced vascular markings at the lung periphery, overventilation of the lungs, a vertical heart, and enlarged anteroposterior chest diameter (barrel-shaped chest).
- Pulmonary function tests indicate increased residual volume and total lung capacity and decreased FEV.
- ABG analysis usually shows reduced PaO_2 and elevated $PaCO_2$.
- ECG may reveal right ventricular hypertrophy late in the disease.
- Pulse oximetry may show a reduced SaO_2 level.

Battling illness

Treating emphysema

Patients with emphysema need counseling on avoiding smoking and air pollution. Additional treatment includes:
- bronchodilators to reverse bronchospasm and promote mucociliary clearance
- inhaled corticosteroids or short-term oral corticosteroids to decrease inflammation
- mucolytics to thin secretions and aid mucus expectoration
- antibiotics to treat respiratory tract infections
- immunizations to prevent influenza, COVID-19, and pneumococcal pneumonia
- adequate hydration
- chest physiotherapy to mobilize secretions
- oxygen therapy at low concentrations to increase patient's partial pressure of arterial oxygen to 55 to 65 mm Hg
- in severe emphysema, lung volume reduction surgery (LVRS) to excise dead lung tissue and allow more functional lung tissue to expand

Lung Cancer

Bronchogenic carcinomas, known as lung cancer, originate from the epithelium of the respiratory tract with smoking tobacco as the most common cause. Tobacco smoke is rich in carcinogen; therefore, smokers and those who inhale smoke passively (even if they are nonsmokers) are at risk. See Chapter 2 for more information about understanding cancer.

It's in your genes!

Genetics play a large part in lung cancer via:
- gene mutations
- gene amplification
- increase in protein expression
- losses in protein expression
- tumor-suppressing alterations
- tumor-acquired DNA methylation
- chromosomal aberrations

Where you work and play

There are many environmental and occupational risk factors associated with the development of lung cancer. Those who worked in factories and refineries, and military veterans, have found themselves exposed to various materials that have been linked to cancer, including:
- benzopyrene
- radon gas
- metals (chromium, cadmium, arsenic)
- asbestos fibers
- exhaust
- nitrogen and mustard gases
- nickel
- silica
- vinyl chloride
- chloromethyl methyl ether

What's the difference?

Non–small cell lung carcinoma includes:
- squamous cell carcinoma
- adenocarcinoma
- large cell carcinoma (undifferentiated)
Neuroendocrine tumors include:

- small cell bronchial carcinoid tumors
- large cell neuroendocrine carcinoma

See the table below, which indicates differences in tumor type, growth rate, metastasis, diagnosis, clinical signs and symptoms, and treatment.

Tumor type	Rate of growth	Site(s) of metastasis	Diagnosis	Clinical signs and symptoms	Treatment options
Squamous cell carcinoma	Slow	Late, mostly to hilar lymph nodes	Biopsy, sputum analysis, electron microscopy immunohistochemistry	Cough, sputum production, airway obstruction	Surgery, chemotherapy
Adenocarcinoma	Moderate	Early	Radiography, fiber-optic bronchoscopy, electron microscopy	Pleural effusion	Surgery, chemotherapy
Large cell carcinoma	Rapid	Early and widespread	Sputum analysis, bronchoscopy, electron microscopy	Chest wall pain, pleural effusion, cough, sputum production, hemoptysis, airway obstruction resulting in pneumonia	Surgery
Small cell carcinoma	Very rapid	Very early in the mediastinum or distally in lung	Radiography sputum analysis, bronchoscopy, electron microscopy, immunohistochemistry	Cough, chest pain, dyspnea, hemoptysis, localized wheezing, excessive hormone secretion	Chemotherapy or ionizing radiation to the thorax and central nervous system

Small cell carcinoma has the poorest prognosis. Lung cancers tend to secrete inappropriate hormones, which are called paraneoplastic syndromes. Initial symptoms of lung cancer are often related to the inappropriate hormone that is being secreted by the cancer:

- hyponatremia—antidiuretic hormone
- Cushing syndrome—adrenocorticotropic hormone
- hypocalcemia—calcitonin
- gynecomastia—gonadotropins (such as estrogens or progesterone)
- carcinoid syndrome—serotonin

Bronchial carcinoid tumors are rare and usually are not related to a history of smoking. They are slow growing, usually do not metastasize, are easily visualized via bronchoscopy, and often have no symptoms.

Other tumor types include adenoid cystic tumors and mucoepidermoid carcinomas that are rare bronchial gland tumors, found in the trachea and large airways, that cause obstruction. These can be malignant or metastasize early. Mesotheliomas are rare tumors associated with asbestos exposure. These are aggressive and malignant, although the onset of symptoms may not take place until 20 to 40 years following exposure.

How is lung cancer diagnosed?

Diagnosis is made through chest x-ray, CT scans, thoracoscopy, and tumor markers (which are proteins secreted by cancer cells)—osteopontin and mesothelin.

Visualizing lung cancer

In the early stages, patients may experience:
- coughing
- chest pain
- excessive sputum production
- hemoptysis
- pneumonia
- airway obstruction
- pleural effusions
- weight loss

In later stages, particularly when the cancer has metastasized, symptoms may include:
- neurologic deficits
- bone pain
- paraneoplastic syndrome

Pneumonia

Pneumonia is an acute infection of the alveoli that commonly impairs gas exchange.

It occurs in people of all ages. More than 1.5 million cases of pneumonia occur annually in the United States. More deaths result from pneumonia annually. It's the leading cause of death from infectious disease.

The prognosis is good for patients with normal lungs and adequate immune systems. However, bacterial pneumonia is a major cause of death in debilitated patients.

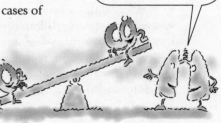

If I don't perform gas exchange properly, the CO_2 in the blood is too high, and the O_2 in the blood is too low.

How it happens

Pneumonia is classified in three ways:

1. *Origin*—Pneumonia may be viral, bacterial, fungal, or protozoal in origin.
2. *Location*—Bronchopneumonia involves distal airways and alveoli; lobar pneumonia involves part of a lobe or an entire lobe.
3. *Type*—Primary pneumonia results from inhalation or aspiration of a pathogen, such as bacteria or a virus, and includes pneumococcal and viral pneumonia; secondary pneumonia may follow lung damage from a noxious chemical or other insult or may result from hematogenous spread of bacteria; aspiration pneumonia results from inhalation of foreign matter from the oropharynx such as vomitus or food particles into the bronchi.

Colonial expansion

In general, the lower respiratory tract can be exposed to pathogens by inhalation, aspiration, vascular dissemination, or direct contact with contaminated equipment such as suction catheters. After pathogens get inside, they begin to colonize and infection develops.

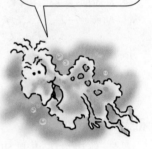

I can sneak into the lower respiratory tract through inhalation, aspiration, or vascular dissemination, or through contaminated equipment.

Stasis report

In bacterial pneumonia, which can occur in any part of the lungs, an infection initially triggers alveolar inflammation and edema. This produces an area of low ventilation with normal perfusion. The infectious exudate between the alveolar membrane and capillaries prevents diffusion of oxygen into the blood.

Virus attack!

In viral pneumonia, the virus first attacks bronchiolar epithelial cells. This causes interstitial inflammation and desquamation. The virus also invades bronchial mucous glands and goblet cells. It then spreads to the alveoli, which fill with inflammatory exudate (sometimes referred to as consolidation). (See *Looking at lobar pneumonia and bronchopneumonia*, page 160.)

Subtracting surfactant

In aspiration pneumonia, inhalation of gastric juices or hydrocarbons triggers inflammatory changes and also inactivates surfactant over a large area. Decreased surfactant leads to alveolar collapse. Acidic gastric juices may damage the airways and alveoli. Particles containing aspirated gastric juices may obstruct the airways and reduce airflow, leading to secondary bacterial pneumonia.

Looking at lobar pneumonia and bronchopneumonia

Pneumonia can involve the distal airways, alveoli, part of a lobe, or an entire lobe.

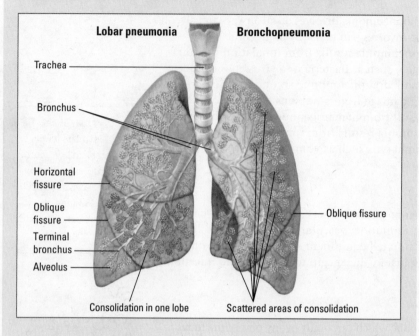

Lobar pneumonia   Bronchopneumonia

Trachea
Bronchus
Horizontal fissure
Oblique fissure
Terminal bronchus
Alveolus

Oblique fissure

Consolidation in one lobe   Scattered areas of consolidation

Risky business

Certain predisposing factors increase the risk of pneumonia. For bacterial and viral pneumonia, these include:
- chronic illness and debilitation
- cancer (particularly lung cancer)
- abdominal and thoracic surgery
- atelectasis
- colds or other viral respiratory infections (particularly COVID-19 infection)
- chronic respiratory disease, such as COPD, bronchiectasis, or cystic fibrosis
- influenza
- smoking

- malnutrition
- alcoholism
- sickle cell disease
- tracheostomy
- exposure to noxious gases
- aspiration
- immunosuppressive therapy
- premature birth

Aspiration pneumonia is more likely to occur in older adults or patients who are debilitated by another illness, those receiving nasogastric tube feedings, and those with an impaired gag reflex, poor oral hygiene, or a decreased level of consciousness. (See *Treating pneumonia*, page 161.)

What to look for

The signs and symptoms of different types of pneumonia vary. (See *Distinguishing among types of pneumonia*, page 161.)

What tests tell you

These tests are used to diagnose pneumonia:

- Chest x-rays confirm the diagnosis by disclosing infiltrates.
- Sputum specimen, Gram stain, and culture and sensitivity tests help differentiate the type of infection and the drugs that are effective in treatment.
- Polymerase chain reaction (PCR) testing: particularly useful to detect viral RNA.
- WBC count indicates leukocytosis in bacterial pneumonia and a normal or low count in viral or mycoplasmal pneumonia.
- Blood cultures reflect bacteremia and are used to determine the causative organism.
- ABG levels vary, depending on the severity of pneumonia and the underlying lung state.
- Bronchoscopy or transtracheal aspiration allows the collection of material for culture (however, this is highly invasive diagnostic testing and not always necessary).
- Pulse oximetry may show a reduced SaO_2 level.

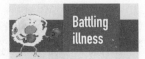
Battling illness

Treating pneumonia

The patient with pneumonia needs antimicrobial or antiviral therapy based on the causative agent. Reevaluation should be done early in treatment.

Supportive measures include:
- humidified oxygen therapy for hypoxia
- bronchodilator therapy
- antitussives (cough suppressants or expectorants)
- mechanical ventilation for respiratory failure
- positive end-expiratory pressure ventilation to maintain adequate oxygenation for patients with severe pneumonia on mechanical ventilation
- high-calorie diet and adequate fluid intake
- bed rest
- analgesic agents to relieve pleuritic chest pain

Distinguishing among types of pneumonia

The characteristics and prognosis of the different types of pneumonia vary.

Type	Characteristics
Viral	
Influenza	• Prognosis is poor even with treatment • High mortality rate from cardiopulmonary collapse • Cough (initially nonproductive; later, purulent sputum), marked cyanosis, dyspnea, high fever, chills, substernal pain and discomfort, moist crackles, frontal headache, myalgia • **Diagnosis:** Rapid flu test on oronasal secretions, PCR testing, pulse oximetry, chest x-ray, ABGs, CBC • **Treatment:** Anti-influenza viral agents (e.g., oseltamivir) • **Prevention:** Flu vaccine annually
Adenovirus	• Insidious onset • Generally affects young adults • Good prognosis; usually clears with no residual effects • Sore throat, fever, cough, chills, malaise, small amounts of mucoid sputum, retrosternal chest pain, anorexia, rhinitis, adenopathy, scattered crackles, and rhonchi • **Diagnosis:** PCR testing, pulse oximetry, chest x-ray, ABGs, CBC • **Treatment:** Supportive care, fluids, acetaminophen or ibuprofen, guaifenesin for cough
Respiratory syncytial virus	• Most prevalent in infants and children • Complete recovery in 1 to 3 weeks; may cause death in premature infants younger than age of 6 months • Listlessness, irritability, tachypnea with retraction of intercostal muscles, slight sputum production, fever, severe malaise, possible cough or croup, and fine, moist crackles • **Diagnosis:** PCR testing, CBC, pulse oximetry, ABGs, chest x-ray • **Treatment:** Palivizumab • **Prevention:** RSV vaccine for older adults

Type	Characteristics
Viral (continued)	
Coronavirus (SARS-CoV2) (COVID-19)	• Spread by droplet infection • Symptoms range from mild upper respiratory infection to life-threatening sepsis and acute respiratory failure. Symptomatic course worse in smokers, older adults, and immunosuppressed people. Cough, headache, fever, sore throat, body aches, chills, and loss of taste or smell. Complications of coagulopathy (clot formation), multiple organ dysfunction, and ARDS possible. • **Diagnosis:** Requires PCR testing, screening with antigen detection test. CBC, ABGs; chest x-ray shows characteristic ground-glass opacities. • **Treatment:** Supportive care, oxygen administration, oral nirmatrelvir and ritonavir, ventilator support in respiratory failure • **Prevention:** COVID-19 vaccine and boosters
Chickenpox (varicella pneumonia)	• Uncommon in children but present in 30% of adults with varicella • Characteristic rash, cough, dyspnea, cyanosis, tachypnea, pleuritic chest pain, and hemoptysis and rhonchi 1 to 6 days after onset of rash • **Diagnosis:** PCR testing, ABGs, CBC, chest x-ray • **Treatment:** Supportive care, oxygen administration (if necessary) • **Prevention:** Varicella vaccine

Distinguishing among types of pneumonia *(continued)*

Type	Characteristics
Viral (continued)	
Cytomegalovirus	• Difficult to distinguish from other non-bacterial pneumonias • In adults with healthy lung tissue, resembles mononucleosis and is generally benign; in neonates, occurs as devastating multisystemic infection; in immunocompromised hosts, varies from clinically inapparent to fatal infection • Fever, cough, shaking chills, dyspnea, cyanosis, weakness, and diffuse crackles • **Diagnosis:** PCR testing, chest x-ray, pulse oximetry, ABGs, CBC • **Treatment:** Supportive care, oxygen administration (if necessary)
Bacterial	
Streptococcus	• Sudden onset of a single, shaking chill and sustained temperature of 102° to 104° F (38.9° to 40° C); commonly preceded by upper respiratory tract infection • **Diagnosis:** Chest x-ray, urine test, sputum culture • **Treatment:** Antibiotic, oxygen administration, supportive care • **Prevention:** Pneumococcal vaccine for older adults

Type	Characteristics
Bacterial (continued)	
Klebsiella	• More likely in patients with chronic alcoholism, pulmonary disease, and diabetes • Fever and recurrent chills; cough producing rusty, bloody, viscous sputum (currant jelly); cyanosis of the lips and nail beds from hypoxemia; shallow, grunting respirations • **Diagnosis:** Chest x-ray, sputum culture, PCR testing, pulse oximetry • **Treatment:** Antibiotic, oxygen administration, supportive care
Staphylococcus	• Commonly occurs in patients with viral illness, such as influenza or measles, and in those with cystic fibrosis • Temperature of 102° to 104° F (38.9° to 40° C), recurrent shaking chills, bloody sputum, dyspnea, tachypnea, and hypoxemia • **Diagnosis:** Chest x-ray, sputum culture, CBC, pulse oximetry, blood cultures • **Treatment:** Antibiotic, oxygen administration, supportive care
Aspiration	
	• Results from vomiting and aspiration of gastric or oropharyngeal contents into the trachea and lungs • Noncardiogenic pulmonary edema possible with damage to respiratory epithelium from contact with gastric acid • Subacute pneumonia possible with cavity formation • Lung abscess possible if foreign body present • Crackles, dyspnea, cyanosis, hypotension, and tachycardia • **Diagnosis:** Chest x-ray, sputum culture • **Treatment:** Antibiotic, oxygen administration, supportive care

Pneumothorax

Pneumothorax is an accumulation of air in the pleural cavity that leads to partial or complete lung collapse. When the amount of air between the visceral and parietal pleurae increases, increasing tension in the pleural cavity can cause the lung to progressively collapse. In some cases, venous return to the heart is impeded, causing a life-threatening condition called *tension pneumothorax*.

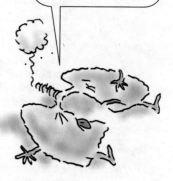

When air accumulates in my pleural cavity, I begin to collapse.

Spontaneous or traumatic?

Pneumothorax is classified as either traumatic or spontaneous. *Traumatic pneumothorax* may be further classified as *open* (sucking chest wound) or *closed* (blunt or penetrating trauma). Note that an open (penetrating) wound may cause closed pneumothorax if communication between the atmosphere and the pleural space seals itself off. *Spontaneous pneumothorax*, which is also considered closed, can be further classified as *primary* (idiopathic) or *secondary* (related to a specific disease).

How it happens

The causes of pneumothorax vary according to classification.

Traumatic pneumothorax

A penetrating injury, such as a stab wound, a gunshot wound, or an impaled object, may cause traumatic open pneumothorax, traumatic closed pneumothorax, or hemothorax (accumulation of blood in the pleural cavity).

Blunt trauma from a car accident, a fall, or a crushing chest injury may also cause traumatic closed pneumothorax or hemothorax.

Traumatic pneumothorax may also result from:
- insertion of a central line that damages the pleural membrane
- thoracic surgery
- thoracentesis
- pleural or transbronchial biopsy

Tension pneumothorax can develop from either spontaneous or traumatic pneumothorax. (See *Understanding tension pneumothorax*, page 164.)

A change in atmosphere

Open pneumothorax results when atmospheric air (positive pressure) flows directly into the pleural cavity (negative pressure). As the air pressure in the pleural cavity becomes positive, the lung collapses on the affected side. Lung collapse leads to decreased total lung capacity. The patient then develops lack of ventilation ability, leading to hypoxia.

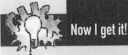

Now I get it!

Understanding tension pneumothorax

In tension pneumothorax, air accumulates intrapleurally and can't escape.

Intrapleural pressure rises, collapsing the ipsilateral lung.

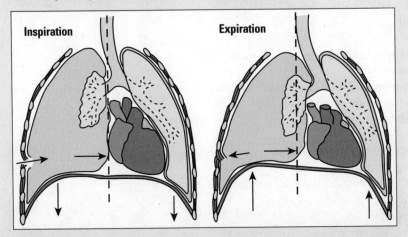

Inspiration

Expiration

On inspiration, the mediastinum shifts toward the unaffected lung, impairing ventilation.

On expiration, the mediastinal shift distorts the vena cava and reduces venous return.

A leak within the lung

Closed pneumothorax occurs when air enters the pleural space from within the lung. This causes increased pleural pressure and prevents lung expansion during inspiration. It may be called *traumatic pneumothorax* when blunt chest trauma causes lung tissue to rupture, resulting in air leakage.

Rupture!

Spontaneous pneumothorax is a type of closed pneumothorax. It's more common in males and in older patients with chronic pulmonary disease. However, it also occurs in healthy young adults. The usual cause is rupture of a subpleural bleb (a small cystic space) at the surface of the lung. This causes air leakage into the pleural spaces; then, the lung collapses, causing decreased total lung capacity, vital capacity, and lung compliance—leading, in turn, to hypoxia. The total amount of lung collapse can range from 5% to 95%.

What to look for

Although the causes of traumatic and spontaneous pneumothorax vary greatly, the effects are similar. The cardinal signs and symptoms of pneumothorax include:

- sudden, sharp, pleuritic pain exacerbated by chest movement, breathing, and coughing
- asymmetric chest wall movement
- absence of lung sounds on affected side
- shortness of breath
- cyanosis
- hyperresonance or tympany heard with percussion
- respiratory distress
  The signs and symptoms of open pneumothorax also include:
- absent breath sounds on the affected side
- chest rigidity on the affected side
- tachycardia
- subcutaneous emphysema (air in the tissues) causing crackling beneath the skin upon palpation
  Tension pneumothorax produces the most severe respiratory symptoms, including:
- decreased cardiac output
- hypotension
- compensatory tachycardia
- tachypnea
- lung collapse due to air or blood in the intrapleural space
- mediastinal shift and tracheal deviation to the opposite side
- cardiac arrest (See *Treating pneumothorax*, page 166.)

What tests tell you

These tests are used to diagnose pneumothorax:

- Chest x-rays confirm the diagnosis by revealing air in the pleural space and, possibly, a mediastinal shift. Sequential chest x-rays show whether thoracostomy was effective in resolving pneumothorax.
- ABG studies may show hypoxemia, possibly with respiratory acidosis and hypercapnia. SaO_2 levels may decrease at first but typically return to normal within 24 hours.
- Pulse oximetry reveals hypoxemia.

Battling illness

Treating pneumothorax

Treatment of pneumothorax depends on its type.

Spontaneous
Treatment is usually conservative for spontaneous pneumothorax when there's:
- no sign of increased pleural pressure
- lung collapse less than 30%
- no dyspnea or indication of physiologic compromise

   Such treatment consists of bed rest; careful monitoring of blood pressure, pulse, and respiratory rate; use of pulse oximetry; oxygen administration; and, possibly, aspiration of air with a large-bore needle attached to a syringe.

   If more than 30% of the lung collapses, a thoracostomy tube (also called a chest tube) is typically placed in the second intercostal space in the midclavicular line to try to reexpand the lung. The tube then connects to low-pressure suction. If blood is present in the pleural space, a second thoracostomy tube is placed in the fourth, fifth, or sixth intercostal space to drain the blood. Treatment for recurring spontaneous pneumothorax is thoracotomy and pleurectomy, which cause the lung to adhere to the parietal pleura.

Traumatic
Traumatic pneumothorax requires thoracostomy tube insertion and chest drainage and may also require surgical repair.

Tension
Tension pneumothorax is a medical emergency. If the tension in the pleural space isn't relieved, the patient will die from inadequate cardiac output or hypoxemia. A large-bore needle is inserted into the pleural space through the second intercostal space. If large amounts of air escape through the needle after insertion, the needle is left in place until a thoracostomy tube can be inserted.

Pulmonary edema

Pulmonary edema is a common complication of cardiac disorders. It's marked by accumulated fluid in the extravascular spaces of the lung. It may occur as a chronic condition or develop quickly and rapidly become fatal.

How it happens
Pulmonary edema may result from left-sided heart failure caused by arteriosclerotic, cardiomyopathic, hypertensive, or valvular heart disease.

Off balance
Normally, pulmonary capillary hydrostatic pressure, capillary oncotic pressure, capillary permeability, and lymphatic drainage are in balance. This prevents fluid infiltration to the lung tissues. When this balance changes, pulmonary edema results. Pulmonary edema most commonly develops from left ventricular failure, which causes an imbalance of pressures in the left ventricle, left atrium, pulmonary veins, and pulmonary capillaries. High hydrostatic pressure in the pulmonary capillaries causes pulmonary edema. Fluid between the alveolar membrane and capillary impairs diffusion of oxygen into the blood.
(See *How pulmonary edema develops,* page 169.)

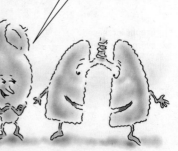

Let's face it: We have to depend on each other.

Now I get it!

How pulmonary edema develops

In pulmonary edema, diminished function of the left ventricle causes blood to pool there; hydrostatic pressure increases in the left atrium, then in the pulmonary veins, then in the pulmonary capillaries.

Increasing capillary hydrostatic pressure pushes fluid into the interstitial spaces and alveoli. Edema forms between the alveoli and capillaries, preventing diffusion of oxygen into the bloodstream. The illustrations below show a normal alveolus and the effects of pulmonary edema.

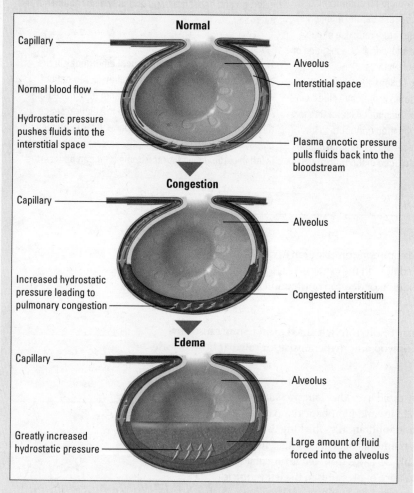

Normal

Capillary

Normal blood flow

Hydrostatic pressure pushes fluids into the interstitial space

Alveolus

Interstitial space

Plasma oncotic pressure pulls fluids back into the bloodstream

Congestion

Capillary

Increased hydrostatic pressure leading to pulmonary congestion

Alveolus

Congested interstitium

Edema

Capillary

Greatly increased hydrostatic pressure

Alveolus

Large amount of fluid forced into the alveolus

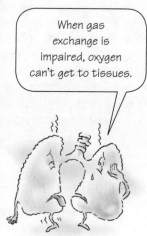

When gas exchange is impaired, oxygen can't get to tissues.

What to look for

Signs and symptoms vary with the stage of pulmonary edema. In the early stages, look for:

- dyspnea on exertion
- paroxysmal nocturnal dyspnea
- orthopnea (difficulty breathing when lying flat)
- cough
- mild tachypnea
- pulmonary crackles (from the fluid accumulation in the lungs)
- diastolic S_3 gallop indicating heart failure
- tachycardia
  As tissue hypoxia and decreased cardiac output occur, you'll see:
- labored, rapid respiration
- more diffuse coarse crackles—this is a KEY finding
- cough producing frothy, pink sputum
- increased tachycardia as compensation for left ventricular failure
- possible arrhythmias
- cold, clammy skin due to lack of peripheral circulation
- diaphoresis
- cyanosis
- falling blood pressure due to left ventricular failure
- thready pulse due to left ventricular failure (See *Treating pulmonary edema.*)

What tests tell you

Clinical features of pulmonary edema permit a working diagnosis. These diagnostic tests are used to confirm the disease:

- ABG analysis usually shows hypoxia with variable $PaCO_2$, depending on the patient's degree of fatigue. Metabolic acidosis may be revealed.
- Chest x-rays show diffuse haziness of the lung fields and, usually, cardiomegaly and pleural effusion.
- Pulse oximetry may reveal decreasing SaO_2 levels.
- Pulmonary artery catheterization identifies left-sided heart failure and helps rule out ARDS.
- ECG may show previous or current myocardial infarction (MI).

Battling illness

Treating pulmonary edema

Treatment for pulmonary edema has three aims:
1. reducing extravascular fluid
2. improving gas exchange and myocardial function
3. correcting the underlying disease, if possible
   Treatments include:
- high concentrations of oxygen (O_2) administered by nasal cannula (the patient usually can't tolerate a mask)
- assisted ventilation to improve O_2 delivery to the tissues and acid–base balance for persistently low arterial oxygen levels
- diuretics (such as furosemide, ethacrynic acid, and bumetanide) decrease excessive fluid in the lungs and increase urination, which helps mobilize extravascular fluid
- positive inotropic agents (such as digoxin), to enhance contractility in myocardial dysfunction
- pressor agents to enhance contractility and promote vasoconstriction in peripheral vessels
- antiarrhythmics for arrhythmias related to decreased cardiac output
- arterial vasodilators (such as nitroprusside) to decrease peripheral vascular resistance, preload, and afterload
- morphine to reduce anxiety and dyspnea and dilate the systemic venous bed, promoting blood flow from pulmonary circulation to the periphery
- B-type natriuretic peptide (BNP) (such as nesiritide) to reduce pulmonary capillary wedge pressure and systemic arterial pressure

Pulmonary embolism

Pulmonary embolism is an obstruction of the pulmonary arterial bed by a dislodged thrombus, heart valve growths, or a foreign substance. It strikes an estimated 900,000 American adults each year in the United States, resulting in 60,000 to 100,000 deaths.

May not produce symptoms or may be fatal

Although pulmonary infarction that results from embolism may be so mild as to produce no symptoms, massive embolism (more than a 50% obstruction of pulmonary arterial circulation) and the accompanying infarction can be rapidly fatal.

How it happens

Pulmonary embolism generally results from dislodged thrombi originating in the leg veins (called venous thromboembolism,

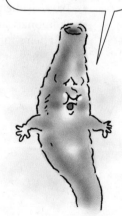

Pulmonary embolism generally results from dislodged thrombi originating in the leg veins or pelvis.

thrombophlebitis, or DVT) or pelvis. More than one-half of these thrombi arise in the deep veins of the legs.

Predisposing factors include:
- long-term immobility
- chronic pulmonary disease
- heart failure
- atrial fibrillation
- thrombophlebitis (DVT)
- polycythemia vera
- thrombocytosis
- autoimmune hemolytic anemia
- sickle cell disease
- varicose veins
- recent surgery
- advanced age
- pregnancy
- lower extremity fractures or surgery
- burns
- obesity
- vascular injury
- cancer
- IV drug misuse
- hormonal contraceptives

The key triad of symptoms of DVT and pulmonary embolism is called *Virchow's triad*:
1. Venous stasis (from any cause of immobility)
2. Vein injury (from trauma or surgery)
3. Hypercoagulability of blood (occurs most often in cancer and high estrogen states)

Floating fragments

Thrombus formation results directly from vascular wall damage, venostasis, or hypercoagulability of the blood (Virchow's triad). Trauma, clot dissolution, sudden muscle spasm, intravascular pressure changes, or a change in peripheral blood flow can cause the thrombus to loosen or fragment. Then the thrombus—now called an *embolus*—travels from the leg veins into the inferior vena cava and then into the right atrium, right ventricle, and pulmonary artery to the lungs. There, the embolus may dissolve, continue to fragment, or grow and obstruct blood flow in the lungs.

A growing problem

By occluding the pulmonary artery, the embolus prevents alveoli from producing enough surfactant to maintain alveolar integrity. As a result, alveoli collapse and atelectasis develop. If the embolus enlarges, it may clog most or all of the pulmonary vessels and cause death. (See *Looking at pulmonary emboli.*)

Now I get it!

Looking at pulmonary emboli

This illustration shows multiple emboli in pulmonary artery branches and a larger embolus that has resulted in an infarcted area in the lung.

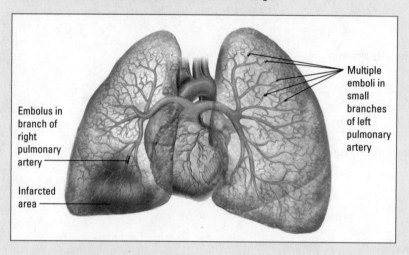

Multiple emboli in small branches of left pulmonary artery

Embolus in branch of right pulmonary artery

Infarcted area

What to look for

Total occlusion of the main pulmonary artery is rapidly fatal; smaller or fragmented emboli produce symptoms that vary with the size, number, and location of the emboli. Usually, the first symptom of pulmonary embolism is dyspnea, which may be accompanied by pleuritic chest pain.

Other clinical features include:

- tachycardia
- "air hunger"
- feeling of impending doom
- productive cough (sputum may be blood-tinged)
- low-grade fever
- pleural effusion

Additionally, pulmonary embolism may cause pleural friction rub, signs of circulatory collapse (weak, rapid pulse and hypotension), and hypoxia (restlessness and anxiety). (See *Treating pulmonary embolism.*)

What tests tell you

The patient history should reveal predisposing conditions for pulmonary embolism as well as risk factors, including long car or plane trips, cancer, pregnancy, hypercoagulability, and previous deep vein thromboses or pulmonary emboli.

These tests support the diagnosis of pulmonary embolism:

- Chest x-rays help to rule out other pulmonary diseases.
- Lung scan shows perfusion defects in areas beyond occluded vessels.
- Pulmonary angiography is the most definitive test.
- D-dimer blood test indicates clotting fragments in the bloodstream.
- ECG is inconclusive but helps distinguish pulmonary embolism from MI.
- Auscultation occasionally reveals a right ventricular S_3 gallop and increased intensity of a pulmonic component of S_2. Also, crackles and a pleural rub may be heard at the embolism site.
- ABG measurements showing decreased PaO_2 and $PaCO_2$ are characteristic but don't always occur.
- If pleural effusion is present, thoracentesis may rule out empyema, which indicates pneumonia.

Battling illness

Treating pulmonary embolism

Treatment of pulmonary embolism is designed to:
- dissolve the clot within the pulmonary arterial system
- maintain adequate cardiovascular and pulmonary function during resolution of the obstruction
- prevent embolus recurrence

Heparin and nonpharmacologic therapies

Treatment consists of oxygen therapy, as needed, and anticoagulation with heparin or enoxaparin (another form of heparin) to inhibit new thrombus formation. Heparin therapy is monitored with daily coagulation studies (international normalized ratio). Nonpharmacologic therapies include pneumatic compression devices or antiembolism stockings.

Fibrinolytic therapy

Patients with massive pulmonary embolism and shock may need fibrinolytic therapy (also called a clot buster) with streptokinase or alteplase to enhance fibrinolysis of the pulmonary emboli and remaining thrombi.

Direct oral anticoagulants

Direct oral anticoagulants are classed as direct thrombin inhibitors and direct factor Xa inhibitors. Apixaban, a factor Xa inhibitor, is commonly used for prophylaxis of, as well as treatment of, venous thromboembolism and pulmonary embolism.

Surgery

Surgery may be performed on patients who can't take anticoagulants (because of recent surgery or blood dyscrasias) or who have recurrent emboli during anticoagulant therapy. Surgery consists of either a mechanical thrombectomy (removal of the clot) or vena caval insertion of a device (umbrella filter) to filter blood returning to the heart and lungs.

Respiratory syncytial virus

RSV is the most commonly associated pathogen that leads to bronchiolitis, an asthma-like syndrome that presents with mild coldlike symptoms. The typical recovery is 1 to 2 weeks, yet this condition can be a serious threat to children under the age of 2. RSV is highly contagious and can lead to croup and pediatric pneumonia.

Symptoms in infants include:

- irritability
- decreased activity
- breathing trouble
- poor appetite
- cough

Other signs and symptoms, often seen in older children, include:

- runny nose
- sneezing
- fever
- wheezing

RSV is often passed from person to person quickly, much like transmission of the common cold. Diagnosis is made through chest x-rays, swab of secretions, and blood tests to check the white cell count. Treatment is often supportive. If hospitalized, a patient may receive humidified oxygen, intravenous fluids, or mechanical ventilation if needed.

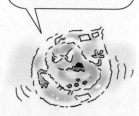

I'm flying in a droplet, looking for someone to land on.

Tuberculosis

Tuberculosis is an infectious disease that primarily affects the lungs but can invade other body systems as well. In tuberculosis, mycobacteria invade the lungs and can cause deterioration of lung tissue, development of round cavities, and the formation of masses of granulated tissue within the lungs. Tuberculosis may occur as an acute infection with active symptoms or can be a latent, asymptomatic, dormant infection. In 2022, there were approximately 8,300 adults with active TB in the United States. However, there are thousands of people with asymptomatic, latent TB.

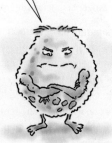

No doubt, the immune system will try to wipe me out.

Too many people, not enough air

Incidence is highest in people who live in crowded, poorly ventilated, unsanitary conditions, such as prisons, tenement houses, and homeless shelters. Others at high risk for tuberculosis include people with alcoholism, those who are IV drug users, older adults, and those who are immunocompromised.

How it happens

Tuberculosis results from exposure to *Mycobacterium tuberculosis* or, sometimes, other strains of mycobacteria. Here's what happens:

- *Transmission*—An infected person coughs or sneezes, spreading infected droplets. When someone without immunity inhales these droplets, the bacilli are deposited in the lungs.
- *Immune response*—The immune system responds by sending leukocytes, and inflammation results. After a few days, leukocytes are replaced by macrophages. Bacilli are then ingested by the macrophages and carried off by the lymphatics to the lymph nodes.
- *Tubercle formation*—Macrophages that ingest the bacilli fuse to form epithelioid cell tubercles, tiny nodules surrounded by lymphocytes. Within the lesion, caseous necrosis develops and scar tissue encapsulates the tubercle. The organism may be killed in the process.
- *Dissemination*—If the tubercles and inflamed nodes rupture, the infection contaminates the surrounding tissue and may spread through the blood and lymphatic circulation to distant sites. This process is called *hematogenous dissemination*. (See *Understanding tuberculosis invasion*, page 175.)

Now I get it!

Understanding tuberculosis invasion

After infected droplets are inhaled, they enter the lungs and are usually deposited in the upper lobe. Leukocytes surround the bacteria in the lungs, which leads to a granulomatous, inflammatory lesion called a tubercle. The leukocytes can't kill the bacteria; the most they can do is isolate and surround the bacteria. Hence, a round cavity (tubercle) is formed. As part of the inflammatory response, some mycobacteria are carried off in the lymphatic circulation by the lymph nodes.

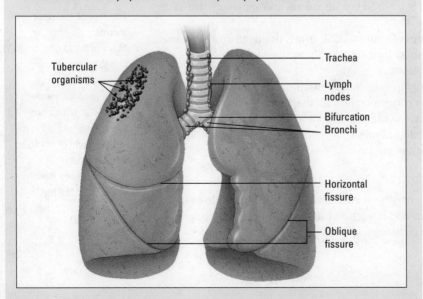

What to look for

After exposure to *M. tuberculosis*, a small percentage of infected people develop active tuberculosis within 1 year. They may report a low-grade fever at night (called night sweats), a productive cough that lasts longer than 3 weeks, weight loss, fatigue, and symptoms of airway obstruction from lymph node involvement.

In other infected people, microorganisms cause a latent infection. This is a dormant infection with reactivation potential. The encapsulated bacilli live within the tubercle. They may lie dormant for years, reactivating later in life to cause active infection.

Adding insult to injury

Tuberculosis can cause massive pulmonary tissue damage, with inflammation and tissue necrosis eventually leading to respiratory failure. Bronchopleural fistulas can develop from lung tissue damage, resulting in pneumothorax. The disease can also lead to hemorrhage, pleural effusion, and pneumonia. Small mycobacterial foci can infect other body organs, including the kidneys, skeleton, and CNS.

With proper treatment, the prognosis for a patient with tuberculosis is usually excellent. (See *Treating tuberculosis*, on the right.)

What tests tell you

These tests are used to diagnose tuberculosis:
- Chest x-rays show nodular lesions, patchy infiltrates (mainly in upper lobes), cavity formation, scar tissue, and calcium deposits.
- A tuberculin skin test reveals infection at some point but doesn't indicate active disease.
- QuantiFERON-TB, a blood test, measures antibodies against TB in the blood.
- Stains and cultures of sputum, CSF, urine, drainage from abscesses, or pleural fluid show heat-sensitive, nonmotile, aerobic, acid-fast bacilli.
- Computed tomography or MRI scans allow the evaluation of lung damage and may confirm a difficult diagnosis.
- Bronchoscopy shows inflammation and altered lung tissue. It may also be performed to obtain sputum if the patient can't produce an adequate sputum specimen.

Ruling out the copycats

Several of these tests may be needed to distinguish tuberculosis from other diseases that mimic it, such as lung cancer, lung abscess, pneumoconiosis, and bronchiectasis.

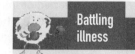
Battling illness

Treating tuberculosis

The usual treatment is daily oral doses of isoniazid or rifampin, with ethambutol added in some cases, for at least 9 months. After 2 to 4 weeks, the disease is no longer infectious, and the patient can resume normal activities while continuing to take medication.

The patient with atypical mycobacterial disease or drug-resistant tuberculosis may require second-line drugs, such as capreomycin, streptomycin, pyrazinamide, and cycloserine.

The rise of resistant strains

Many patients find it difficult to follow this lengthy treatment regimen, so adherence to treatment is sometimes compromised. This has led to the development of resistant strains of tuberculosis in recent years. Remind patients to take the full course of medication.

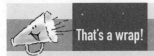
That's a wrap!

Respiratory system review

Understanding the respiratory system
- The major function of the respiratory system is gas exchange.
- Components consist of two lungs, conducting airways, and associated blood vessels.
- During ventilation:
  - air is taken into the body by inhalation (inspiration) and travels through respiratory passages to the lungs.
- During perfusion:
  - O_2 in the lungs replaces CO_2 in the blood
  - CO_2 is expelled from the body on exhalation (expiration).

Conducting airways
Conduction airways allow air into and out of structures within the lung that perform gas exchange. Upper airways consist of the:
- nose
- mouth
- pharynx
- larynx
   Lower airways consist of the:
- trachea
- right and left mainstem bronchi
- five secondary bronchi
- bronchioles

Breathing mechanisms
Three factors regulate the amount of air that reaches the lungs carrying O_2 and departs with CO_2:
- lung volume and capacity
- compliance (the lungs' ability to expand)
- resistance to airflow

Neurochemical control
The respiratory center, located in the lateral medulla oblongata of the brain stem, consists of three different groups of neurons:
- dorsal respiratory neurons
- ventral respiratory neurons
- pneumotaxic center and apneustic center

Chemoreceptors
Factors that influence respiration are called *chemoreceptors* that respond to the:
- hydrogen ion concentration (pH) of arterial blood
- $PaCO_2$
- PaO_2

   Functions of pH, $PaCO_2$, and PaO_2 are as follows:
- $PaCO_2$ regulates ventilation by impacting the pH of cerebrospinal fluid.
- If $PaCO_2$ is high and PaO_2 and pH are low, respiratory rate increases.

Respiratory disorders
- *ARDS*—form of pulmonary edema that can quickly lead to acute respiratory failure
- *ARF*—condition in which the lungs can't adequately maintain oxygenation or eliminate CO_2, which can lead to tissue hypoxia
- *Asthma*—chronic reactive airway disorder that can present as an acute attack
- *Chronic bronchitis*—one of the two components of COPD; it's an inflammation of the bronchi caused by obstruction in small airways from prolonged irritant inhalation
- *Cor pulmonale*—right ventricular failure that occurs secondary to a lung condition that causes chronic hypoxia and pulmonary hypertension
- *Emphysema*—one of the two components of COPD; it's the abnormal, permanent enlargement and lack of recoil of the alveoli accompanied by destruction of the alveolar walls
- *Pneumonia*—acute infection of the lung tissue that causes accumulation of exudate that impairs gas exchange at the alveoli; sometimes referred to as a consolidation in the lungs

(Continued)

Quick quiz

1. In response to chronically low oxygen due to low ventilation, which is the reflexive action that occurs in the lungs?
    A. Pulmonary artery vasodilation
    B. Pulmonary arterial vasoconstriction
    C. Increased capillary permeability, causing edema
    D. Decreased pulmonary artery pressure

Answer: B. Pulmonary arterial vasoconstriction is a reflexive homeostatic mechanism that is intrinsic to the pulmonary arterial vasculature in reaction to alveolar hypoxia. Intrapulmonary arteries constrict in response to low oxygenation, which in turn diverts blood to better-oxygenated lung segments, thereby optimizing ventilation/perfusion matching and systemic oxygen delivery to the body tissues. This reflexive reaction is evident in patients with chronic hypoxia due to lung disease; these patients develop pulmonary hypertension that leads to right ventricular failure (termed cor pulmonale).

2. Asthma is MOST commonly triggered by:
    A. sensitivity to specific allergens.
    B. intense exercise.
    C. emotional stress.
    D. fatigue.

Answer: A. Asthma is most commonly triggered by sensitivity to specific external allergens, including pollen, animal dander, house dust, cockroach allergens, and mold.

3. Tuberculosis is transmitted through:
      A.   the fecal–oral route.
      B.   contact with blood.
      C.   contact with urine.
      D.   inhalation of infected droplets.

Answer: D. Transmission occurs when an infected person coughs or sneezes, spreading infected droplets.

4. Patients with cor pulmonale usually also have which other respiratory disorder?
      A.   Tuberculosis
      B.   Emphysema
      C.   COPD
      D.   Asthma

Answer: C. A large majority of patients with cor pulmonale also have COPD. COPD causes chronic hypoxia, which causes pulmonary arterial vasoconstriction. Eventually this leads to pulmonary hypertension, which is high resistance against the right ventricle. High strain on the right ventricle can eventually cause right ventricular failure, termed cor pulmonale.

5. In COPD (which is a combination of chronic bronchitis and emphysema), one of the major pulmonary function test findings is:
      A.   increased PO_2 in the alveoli.
      B.   decreased residual volume in the lungs.
      C.   prolonged forced expiratory volume (FEV1).
      D.   decreased PCO_2 in the alveoli.

Answer: C. In COPD, the emphysema component causes increased air trapping in the lungs due to inability to exhale all the air in the lungs, so there is a prolonged expiratory volume (FEV1). The thoracic cage enlarges over time to cause a "barrel-shaped" chest. The chest has a high residual volume and high PCO_2 in the alveoli that cannot be expelled. The patient has trouble exhaling all the air and CO_2 in the lungs. The chronic bronchitis component of COPD causes obstructed ventilation (due to inflammation and mucus plugs), which causes hypoxia (because there is low PO_2 in the alveoli).

6. Which type of pneumonia is associated with symptoms of cough, fever, headache, poor taste and smell early in the infection, and the potential complication of ARDS?
      A.   Cytomegalovirus
      B.   Varicella
      C.   SARS-CoV-2 (COVID-19)
      D.   Influenza

Answer: C. Pneumonia caused by SARS-CoV-2 (COVID-19) causes a characteristic loss of taste and smell, cough, fever, and headache early in the infection. Complications can include severe hypoxemia, coagulopathy, and ARDS, requiring mechanical ventilation.

Scoring

⭐⭐⭐ If you answered all six items correctly, excellent! When it comes to understanding the respiratory system, no one can accuse you of being full of hot air.

⭐⭐ If you answered five items correctly, swell up with pride! You inhaled the chapter and exhaled right answers.

⭐ If you answered fewer than five items correctly, review the chapter topics you're unsure of.

Suggested references

Adeloye, D., Song, P., Zhu, Y., Campbell, H., Sheikh, A., Rudan, I., & NIHR RESPIRE Global Respiratory Health Unit. (2022). Global, regional, and national prevalence of, and risk factors for, chronic obstructive pulmonary disease (COPD) in 2019: A systematic review and modelling analysis. *The Lancet Respiratory Medicine, 10*(5), 447–458. https://doi.org/10.1016/S2213-2600(21)00511-7

Celli, B. R., & Wedzicha, J. A. (2019). Update on clinical aspects of chronic obstructive pulmonary disease. *The New England Journal of Medicine, 381*(13), 1257–1266. https://doi.org/10.1056/NEJMra1900500

Centers for Disease Control and Prevention (CDC). (2022a). Pneumonia. https://www.cdc.gov/nchs/fastats/pneumonia.htm

Centers for Disease Control and Prevention (CDC). (2022b). Tuberculosis. https://www.cdc.gov/tb/statistics/default.htm

Centers for Disease Control and Prevention (CDC). (2022c). Symptoms of COVID-19. https://www.cdc.gov/coronavirus/2019-ncov/symptoms-testing/symptoms.html

Centers for Disease Control and Prevention (CDC). (2023a). Deep venous thrombosis and pulmonary embolism. https://wwwnc.cdc.gov/travel/yellowbook/2024/air-land-sea/deep-vein-thrombosis-and-pulmonary-embolism

Centers for Disease Control and Prevention (CDC). (2023b). Asthma. https://www.cdc.gov/asthma/most_recent_national_asthma_data.htm

Centers for Disease Control and Prevention (CDC). (2023c). Chronic obstructive pulmonary disease. https://www.cdc.gov/copd/data.html

Gans, M. D., & Gavrilova, T. (2020). Understanding the immunology of asthma: Pathophysiology, biomarkers, and treatments for asthma endotypes. *Paediatric Respiratory Reviews, 36*, 118–127. https://doi.org/10.1016/j.prrv.2019.08.002

Global Initiative for Asthma Main Report. (2022). Global strategy for asthma management and prevention. https://ginasthma.org/wp-content/uploads/2022/07/GINA-Main-Report-2022-FINAL-22-07-01-WMS.PDF

Gorman, E. A., O'Kane, C. M., & McAuley, D. F. (2022). Acute respiratory distress syndrome in adults: Diagnosis, outcomes, long-term sequelae, and management. *Lancet (London, England), 400*(10358), 1157–1170. https://doi.org/10.1016/S0140-6736(22)01439-8

Halpin, D. M. G., Criner, G. J., Papi, A., Singh, D., Anzueto, A., Martinez, F. J., Agusti, A. A., & Vogelmeier, C. F. (2021). Global initiative for the diagnosis, management, and prevention of chronic obstructive lung disease. The 2020 GOLD

Science Committee report on COVID-19 and chronic obstructive pulmonary disease. *American Journal of Respiratory and Critical Care Medicine, 203*(1), 24–36. https://doi.org/10.1164/rccm.202009-3533SO

Ish, P., Malhotra, N., & Gupta, N. (2021). GINA 2020: what's new and why? *Journal of Asthma, 58*(10), 1273–1277. https://doi.org/10.1080/02770903.2020.1788076

Jung, Y. E. G., & Schluger, N. W. (2020). Advances in the diagnosis and treatment of latent tuberculosis infection. *Current Opinion in Infectious Diseases, 33*(2), 166–172. https://doi.org/10.1097/QCO.0000000000000629

Kaku, S., Nguyen, C. D., Htet, N. N., Tutera, D., Barr, J., Paintal, H. S., & Kuschner, W. G. (2020). Acute respiratory distress syndrome: Etiology, pathogenesis, and summary on management. *Journal of Intensive Care Medicine, 35*(8), 723–737. https://doi.org/10.1177/0885066619855021

Long, B., Carius, B. M., Chavez, S., Liang, S. Y., Brady, W. J., Koyfman, A., & Gottlieb, M. (2022). Clinical update on COVID-19 for the emergency clinician: Presentation and evaluation. *The American Journal of Emergency Medicine, 54*, 46–57. https://doi.org/10.1016/j.ajem.2022.01.028

Machanahalli Balakrishna, A., Reddi, V., Belford, P. M., Alvarez, M., Jaber, W. A., Zhao, D. X., & Vallabhajosyula, S. (2022). Intermediate-risk pulmonary embolism: A review of contemporary diagnosis, risk stratification and management. *Medicina (Kaunas, Lithuania), 58*(9), 1186. https://doi.org/10.3390/medicina58091186

Meyer, N. J., Gattinoni, L., & Calfee, C. S. (2021). Acute respiratory distress syndrome. *Lancet (London, England), 398*(10300), 622–637. https://doi.org/10.1016/S0140-6736(21)00439-6

Najjar-Debbiny, R., Gronich, N., Weber, G., Khoury, J., Amar, M., Stein, N., Goldstein, L. H., & Saliba, W. (2023). Effectiveness of paxlovid in reducing severe coronavirus disease 2019 and mortality in high-risk patients. *Clinical Infectious Diseases,76*(3), e342–e349. ciac443. Advance online publication. https://doi.org/10.1093/cid/ciac443

Peloquin, C. A., & Davies, G. R. (2021). The treatment of tuberculosis. *Clinical Pharmacology & Therapeutics, 110*(6), 1455–1466. https://doi.org/10.1002/cpt.2261

Piraino, T. (2019). Noninvasive respiratory support in acute hypoxemic respiratory failure. *Respiratory Care, 64*(6), 638–646. https://doi.org/10.4187/respcare.06735

Reddel, H. K., Bacharier, L. B., Bateman, E. D., Brightling, C. E., Brusselle, G. G., Buhl, R., Cruz, A. A., Duijts, L., Drazen, J. M., FitzGerald, J. M., Fleming, L. J., Inoue, H., Ko, F. W., Krishnan, J. A., Levy, M. L., Lin, J., Mortimer, K., Pitrez, P. M., Sheikh, A., … Boulet, L. P. (2022). Global initiative for asthma strategy 2021: Executive summary and rationale for key changes. *European Respiratory Journal, 59*(1), 2102730. https://doi.org/10.1183/13993003.02730-2021

Sossen, B., Richards, A. S., Heinsohn, T., Frascella, B., Balzarini, F., Oradini-Alacreu, A., Odone, A., Rogozinska, E., Häcker, B., Cobelens, F., Kranzer, K., Houben, R. M. G. J., & Esmail, H. (2023). The natural history of untreated pulmonary tuberculosis in adults: A systematic review and meta-analysis. *The Lancet Respiratory Medicine, 11*(4), 367–379. https://doi.org/10.1016/S2213-2600(23)00097-8

Swenson, K. E., & Swenson, E. R. (2021). Pathophysiology of acute respiratory distress syndrome and COVID-19 lung injury. *Critical Care Clinics, 37*(4), 749–776. https://doi.org/10.1016/j.ccc.2021.05.003

Vogelmeier, C. F., Román-Rodríguez, M., Singh, D., Han, M. K., Rodríguez-Roisin, R., & Ferguson, G. T. (2020). Goals of COPD treatment: Focus on symptoms and exacerbations. *Respiratory Medicine, 166*, 105938. https://doi.org/10.1016/j.rmed.2020.105938

Wenger, N., Sebastian, T., Engelberger, R. P., Kucher, N., & Spirk, D. (2021). Pulmonary embolism and deep vein thrombosis: Similar but different. *Thrombosis Research, 206*, 88–98. https://doi.org/10.1016/j.thromres.2021.08.015

Wiersinga, W. J., Rhodes, A., Cheng, A. C., Peacock, S. J., & Prescott, H. C. (2020). Pathophysiology, transmission, diagnosis, and treatment of coronavirus disease 2019 (COVID-19): A review. *JAMA, 324*(8), 782–793. https://doi.org/10.1001/jama.2020.12839

Chapter 6

Neurologic system*

Just the facts

In this chapter, you'll learn:

◆ the structures of the neurologic system

◆ how the neurologic system works

◆ causes, pathophysiology, diagnostic tests, and treatments for several common neurologic disorders.

Understanding the neurologic system

The neurologic, or nervous, system is the body's communication network that works to coordinate and organize the functions of all other body systems. This network is made of complex structures that transmit electrical and chemical signals between the body's organs, tissues, and brain. This intricate network has two main divisions:

- The central nervous system (CNS), made up of the brain and spinal cord, is the body's control center.
- The peripheral nervous system (PNS), containing cranial and spinal nerves, provides communication between the CNS and remote body parts.

The fundamental unit

The neuron, or nerve cell, is the nervous system's fundamental unit. This highly specialized conductor cell receives and transmits electrochemical nerve impulses. Delicate, threadlike nerve fibers called *axons* and *dendrites* extend from the central cell body and transmit signals. Axons carry impulses away from the cell body; dendrites carry impulses to the cell body. Most neurons have multiple dendrites but only one axon. Neuroglial cells, which outnumber neurons, provide support, nourishment, and protection for neurons.

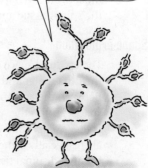

Glad to meet you. I'm a neuron, the basic unit of the nervous system.

---

*Note: In this chapter, the term "male" refers to a person assigned male at birth, and the term "female" refers to a person assigned female at birth.

The body's information superhighway

This intricate network of interlocking receptors and transmitters, along with the brain and spinal cord, forms a living computer that controls and regulates every mental and physical function. From birth to death, the nervous system efficiently organizes the body's affairs, controlling the smallest actions, thoughts, and feelings.

Central nervous system

The CNS consists of the brain and the spinal cord. The fragile brain and spinal cord are protected by the bony skull and vertebrae, cerebrospinal fluid (CSF), and three membranes called the meninges—the dura mater, the arachnoid mater, and the pia mater.

They all "mater"

The *dura mater* (Latin for "tough mother"), which forms the outermost protective layer, is a tough, fibrous, leatherlike tissue composed of two layers, the endosteal dura and the meningeal dura. The endosteal dura forms the periosteum of the skull and is continuous with the lining of the vertebral canal, whereas the meningeal dura, a thick membrane, covers the brain, dipping between the brain tissue and providing support and protection.

The *arachnoid mater* (Latin for "spider mother"), which forms the middle protective layer, is a thin, delicate, weblike structure that loosely hugs the brain and spinal cord. The arachnoid mater is avascular.

The *pia mater* (Latin for "tender mother") is the delicate, innermost protective layer of the connective tissue that covers and contours the spinal tissue and brain. The pia mater is vascular.

Space exploration

The epidural space lies between the skull and the dura mater. Between the dura mater and the arachnoid mater is the subdural space. Between the arachnoid mater and the pia mater is the subarachnoid space. Within the subarachnoid space and the brain's four ventricles is the CSF, a liquid composed of water and traces of organic materials (especially protein), glucose, and minerals. This fluid protects the brain and spinal tissue from jolts and blows.

Cerebrum

The cerebrum, the largest part of the brain, houses the nerve center that controls sensory and motor activities and intelligence. The outer layer, the cerebral cortex, consists of neuron cell bodies (gray matter). The inner layer consists of axons (white matter) plus basal ganglia, which control motor coordination and steadiness.

The right controls the left; the left controls the right

The cerebrum is divided into the right and left hemispheres. Because motor impulses descending from the brain cross in the medulla, the right hemisphere controls the left side of the body and the left hemisphere controls the right side of the body. Several fissures divide the cerebrum into lobes. Each lobe has a specific function. (See *A close look at lobes and fissures*, page 185.)

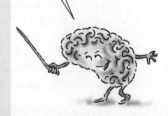

I'm rather proud of my cerebrum and its two cerebral hemispheres. They control sensory and motor activities as well as intelligence.

A close look at lobes and fissures

Several fissures divide the cerebrum into hemispheres and lobes:
• The Sylvian fissure, or the lateral sulcus, separates the temporal lobe from the frontal and parietal lobes.
• The fissure of Rolando, or the central sulcus, separates the frontal lobes from the parietal lobe.
• The parieto-occipital fissure separates the occipital lobe from the two parietal lobes.

To each lobe, a function
Each lobe has a specific function:
• The frontal lobe controls voluntary muscle movements and contains motor areas such as the one for speech (Broca's motor speech area). This is the center for personality, behavioral functions, intellectual functions (such as judgment, memory, and problem solving), autonomic functions, and emotional responses.
• The temporal lobe is the center for taste, hearing, smell, and interpretation of spoken language.
• The parietal lobe coordinates and interprets sensory information from the opposite side of the body.
• The occipital lobe interprets visual stimuli.

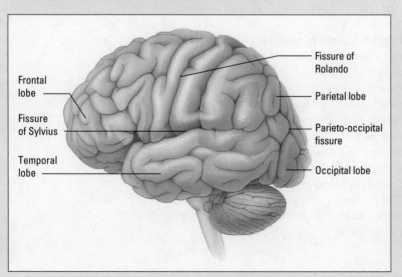

Frontal lobe

Fissure of Sylvius

Temporal lobe

Fissure of Rolando

Parietal lobe

Parieto-occipital fissure

Occipital lobe

A call to order

The thalamus, a relay center in the cerebrum, further organizes cerebral function by transmitting impulses to and from appropriate areas of the cerebrum. The thalamus is also responsible for emotional responses such as fear and for distinguishing pleasant stimuli from unpleasant ones.

The multitasker

The hypothalamus, located beneath the thalamus, is an autonomic center with connections to the brain, spinal cord, autonomic nervous system, and pituitary gland. The hypothalamus regulates temperature control, appetite, blood pressure, breathing, sleep patterns, and peripheral nerve discharges that occur with behavioral and emotional expression. The hypothalamus also partially controls pituitary gland secretion and stress reaction.

Cerebellum and brain stem

Other main parts of the brain are the cerebellum and the brain stem.

Tell 'em about the cerebellum

The cerebellum lies beneath the cerebrum, at the base of the brain. The cerebellum coordinates muscle movements, controls posture, and maintains equilibrium.

A gem of a stem

The brain stem includes the midbrain, pons, and medulla oblongata. Cell bodies for most of the cranial nerves are housed in the brain stem. Along with the thalamus and hypothalamus, it makes up a nerve network called the *reticular formation*, which acts as an arousal mechanism.

The three parts of the brain stem provide two-way conduction between the spinal cord and the brain. In addition, they perform the following functions:
- The midbrain is the reflex center for the third and fourth cranial nerves and mediates pupillary reflexes and eye movements.
- The pons helps regulate respirations and is the reflex center for cranial nerves V through VIII. The pons mediates chewing, taste, saliva secretion, hearing, and equilibrium.
- The myelencephalon, or medulla oblongata, influences reflex activities such as heart rate, blood pressure, respirations, and vasomotor functions. The medulla oblongata is the center for vomiting, coughing, and hiccuping reflexes. Cranial nerves IX through XII emerge from the medulla.

Spinal cord

The spinal cord extends downward from the brain to the second lumbar vertebra. The spinal cord functions as a two-way conductor pathway between the brain stem and the PNS. (See *A look inside the spinal cord*, page 187.)

A gray area

The spinal cord contains a mass of gray matter divided into horns, which consist mostly of neuron cell bodies. The horns of the spinal cord relay sensations and are needed for voluntary or reflex motor activity.

The outside of the horns is surrounded by white matter consisting of myelinated nerve fibers grouped in vertical columns called *tracts*.

Tract record

The sensory, or ascending, tracts carry sensory impulses up the spinal cord to the brain, whereas motor, or descending, tracts carry motor impulses down the spinal cord.

A look inside the spinal cord

This cross section of the spinal cord shows an H-shaped mass of gray matter divided into horns, which consist primarily of neuron cell bodies.

Cell bodies in the posterior or dorsal horn primarily relay information. Cell bodies in the anterior or ventral horn are needed for voluntary or reflex motor activity.

The illustration below shows the major components of the spinal cord.

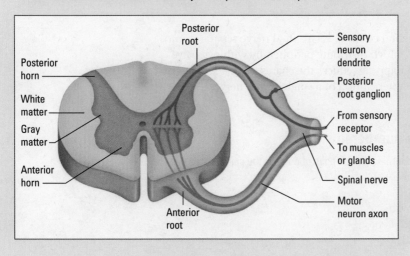

The brain's motor impulses reach a descending tract and continue to the PNS via upper motor neurons (also called *cranial motor neurons*).

Upper motor neurons in the brain conduct impulses from the brain to the spinal cord. Upper motor neurons form two major systems:

- The pyramidal system, or corticospinal tract, is responsible for fine, skilled movements of the skeletal muscle.
- The extrapyramidal system, or extracorticospinal tract, is responsible for the control of gross motor movements.

Lower motor neurons or spinal motor neurons conduct impulses that originate in upper motor neurons to the muscles.

Peripheral nervous system

Messages transmitted through the spinal cord reach outlying areas through the PNS. The PNS originates in 31 pairs of spinal nerves arranged in segments and attached to the spinal cord. (See *How spinal nerves are numbered*, page 188.)

A route with two roots

Spinal nerves are attached to the spinal cord by two roots:

- The anterior, or ventral, root consists of motor fibers that relay impulses from the spinal cord to the glands and muscles.
- The posterior, or dorsal, root consists of sensory fibers that relay information from receptors to the spinal cord.

An enlarged area of the posterior root, the posterior root ganglion, is made up of sensory neuron cell bodies.

Ramifications of rami

After leaving the vertebral column, each spinal nerve separates into branches called *rami*, which distribute peripherally with extensive overlapping. This overlapping reduces the chance of lost sensory or motor function from interruption of a single spinal nerve.

How spinal nerves are numbered

Spinal nerves are numbered according to their point of origin in the spinal cord:
- 8 cervical: C1 to C8
- 12 thoracic: T1 to T12
- 5 lumbar: L1 to L5
- 5 sacral: S1 to S5
- 1 coccygeal

Who's in control here?

The PNS can be divided into the somatic nervous system and the autonomic nervous system. The somatic nervous system regulates voluntary motor control. The autonomic nervous system helps regulate the body's internal environment through involuntary control of organ systems.

Balancing act

The autonomic nervous system controls involuntary body functions, such as digestion, respirations, and cardiovascular function. The autonomic nervous system divided into two antagonistic systems that balance each other to support homeostasis:

- The sympathetic nervous system controls energy expenditure, especially in stressful situations, by releasing the adrenergic catecholamine norepinephrine.
- The parasympathetic nervous system helps conserve energy by releasing the cholinergic neurohormone acetylcholine.

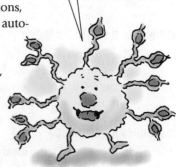

The autonomic nervous system operates without conscious control as the caretaker of the body.

So much to know about the somatic system

The somatic nervous system, composed of somatic nerve fibers, conducts impulses from the CNS to skeletal muscles. The somatic nervous system is typically referred to as the voluntary nervous system because it allows the individual to consciously control skeletal muscles.

Neurologic disorders

In this section, you'll find information on the following neurologic disorders:

- Alzheimer disease (AD)
- Amyotrophic lateral sclerosis (ALS)
- Bell palsy
- Epilepsy
- Guillain-Barré syndrome (GBS)
- Meningitis
- Migraine
- Multiple sclerosis (MS)
- Myasthenia gravis
- Parkinson disease (PD)
- Stroke

Alzheimer disease

Alzheimer disease (AD) is a progressive neurodegenerative disease of the brain that accounts for 60% to 80% of all cases of dementia. Cortical degeneration is most marked in the frontal lobes, but atrophy occurs in all areas of the cortex.

A growing problem

An estimated 6.7 million Americans have AD. This number is projected to more than double to 14 million people by 2060. The number of people living with the disease doubles every 5 years beyond age 65. Because AD is a primary progressive dementia, the prognosis is poor. Most patients die 4 to 8 years after diagnosis, though some can live for 20 years. AD is the fifth leading cause of death for adults aged 65 and older, and the seventh leading cause of death for all adults.

Sometimes it's all in the family

There are two forms of AD: familial and sporadic. In familial AD, genes directly cause the disease. These cases are very rare and have been identified in a relatively small number of families, with many people in multiple generations affected. (See *Genes and AD*, page 190.)

Sometimes it's sporadic

In sporadic AD, the most common form of the disease, there is no familial connection, but genes may influence the risk of developing the disease. The incidence of sporadic AD is less predictable than the familial type and occurs in fewer family members. (See *Tissue changes in AD*, page 191.)

The genetic link

Genes and AD

According to the Alzheimer's Association, two categories of genes—risk genes and deterministic genes—have a direct link to the development of AD.

The researched risk genes that relate to AD are APOE, which are responsible for the production of a protein that transports cholesterol and other fats throughout the body. The protein may also be involved in the structure and function of the outer wall of a brain cell. APOE has three common forms: APOE-epsilon 2, APOE-epsilon 3, and APOE-epsilon 4. A person inherits one form of the gene from each biological parent. The risk gene with the strongest risk for development of AD is APOE-epsilon 4.

Those who carry at least one type of risk gene are at high risk of developing AD. People who have two of the risk genes are at greatest risk.

Deterministic genes directly cause disease, and anyone who inherits these will develop a disease. Scientists have discovered that these rare genes cause AD in only a few hundred extended families across the globe. These genes account for less than 5% of AD cases, and these cause familial early onset where symptoms develop between the ages of 40 and 50. Even though these genes are rare, identifying them has been very helpful in understanding AD.

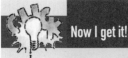

Now I get it!

Tissue changes in AD

The illustrations below show the progressive tissue changes that occur in AD.

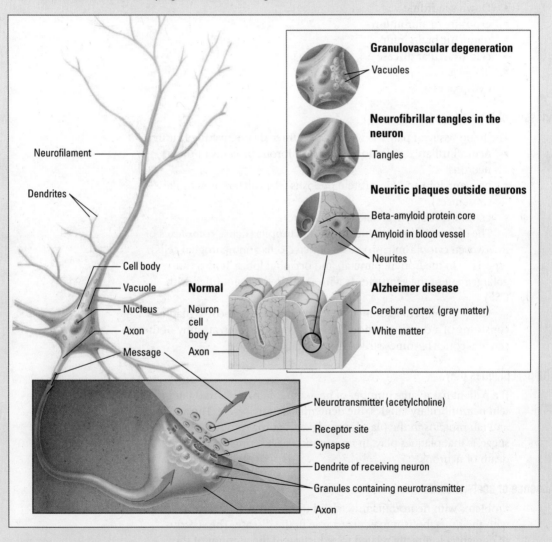

Granulovascular degeneration

Vacuoles

Neurofibrillar tangles in the neuron

Tangles

Neuritic plaques outside neurons

Beta-amyloid protein core

Amyloid in blood vessel

Neurites

Neurofilament

Dendrites

Cell body

Vacuole

Nucleus

Axon

Message

Normal

Neuron cell body

Axon

Alzheimer disease

Cerebral cortex (gray matter)

White matter

Neurotransmitter (acetylcholine)

Receptor site

Synapse

Dendrite of receiving neuron

Granules containing neurotransmitter

Axon

How it happens
The cause of AD is unknown, but the following are the most common
risk factors:
- advanced age; particularly 80+ years
- genetic factors; particularly the APOE-epsilon 4 allele (which
  increases the risk an estimated three to four times)
- Down syndrome
- exposure to aluminum
- traumatic brain injury
- cardiovascular disease
- diabetes
- dyslipidemia

An issue of brain tissue

The brain tissue of patients with AD has three distinguishing features:
- neurofibrillary tangles formed out of fibrous proteins in the
  neurons
- beta-amyloid and tau protein deposits (deposits of proteinlike
  substances)
- granulovacuolar degeneration of neurons

The disease causes degeneration of neuropils (dense complexes of
interwoven cytoplasmic processes of nerve cells and neuroglial cells),
especially in the frontal, parietal, and occipital lobes. It also causes
enlargement of the ventricles (cavities within the brain filled with
CSF).

Early cerebral changes include formation of microscopic plaques,
consisting of a core surrounded by fibrous tissue. Later, atrophy of the
cerebral cortex becomes strikingly evident.

The part plaques play

If a patient has a large number of beta-amyloid plaques and tau protein neurofibrillary tangles, the dementia is more severe. The amyloid
and tau proteins in the plaques may exert neurotoxic effects. Evidence
suggests that plaques play an important part in bringing about the
death of neurons.

Absence of acetylcholine

Problems with neurotransmitters and the enzymes associated
with their metabolism may play a role in the disease. The severity
of dementia is directly related to reduction of the amount of the
neurotransmitter acetylcholine. On autopsy, the brains of patients
with AD may contain as little as 10% of the normal amount of
acetylcholine.

Getting complicated

Complications may include injury resulting from the patient's behavior, wandering, or unsupervised activity. Other complications include pneumonia and other infections, especially if the patient doesn't receive enough exercise; malnutrition and dehydration, especially if the patient refuses or forgets to eat; and aspiration.

What to look for

AD has an insidious onset. At first, changes are barely perceptible, but they gradually lead to serious problems. Patient history is almost always obtained from a family member or caregiver. (See *New developments in AD*, page 193.)

Early changes may include memory loss that affects job skills, difficulty performing familiar tasks, difficulty learning and retaining new information, inability to concentrate, and deterioration in personal hygiene and appearance. As the disease progresses, signs and symptoms indicate a degenerative disorder of the frontal lobe. Symptoms may include:

- difficulty with abstract thinking and activities that require judgment
- progressive difficulty in communicating
- severe deterioration of memory, language, and motor function progressing to coordination loss and an inability to speak or write
- repetitive actions
- restlessness, wandering
- irritability, depression, mood swings, paranoia, hostility, and combativeness
- nocturnal awakenings
- disorientation (See *Treating AD*, page 193.)

New developments in AD

AD is now described as moving through a continuum of stages, each with its own characteristics:
- In *preclinical AD*, measurable changes in biomarkers are seen; these earliest indications of disease occur before such noticeable signs and symptoms as memory loss and confusion about time or place develop.
- In *mild cognitive impairment (MCI) due to AD*, mild changes in memory and thinking ability occur; these changes are measurable, and the patient and family members and friends notice the changes. There may be small personality changes and forgetfulness beyond what is seen in a normal person. The patient's ability to carry out everyday activities may be slightly impacted as there may be a decrease in the ability to plan and organize and forgetfulness of recent events and names of people or things.
- In *dementia due to AD*, thinking impairment, memory impairment, and behavioral changes that impair the patient's ability to function in daily life occur. There is severe impairment in cognitive function and inability to perform self-care activities.

Treating AD

There is no cure for AD, and current drug therapy cannot alter the progression of disease. The following is a list of the drugs that are currently used or in development:

• Cholinesterase inhibitors, such as donepezil, rivastigmine, and galantamine, prevent the breakdown of acetylcholine, a chemical messenger in the brain that's important for memory and other thinking skills. The drugs work to keep levels of acetylcholine high, even while the cells that produce it continue to become damaged or die.

• Memantine, an uncompetitive low-to-moderate affinity *N*-methyl-D-aspartate receptor antagonist, is sometimes prescribed. It appears to work by regulating the activity of glutamate, one of the brain's chemicals that's involved in information processing, storing, and retrieval.

• Monoclonal antibody type agents (mAbs) aducanumab and lecanemab are new drugs that mount an immune response against beta-amyloid proteins. Approved by the FDA in 2021 and 2022 and currently in long-term clinical trials, they are recommended for patients in the early stages of AD.

The proof is in the...

Neurologic examination of the patient with dementia confirms many of the cognitive problems revealed during the history. Common signs of dementia include amnesia (memory loss; particularly short-term memory), anomia (forgetting the names of people and objects), apathy (unconcerned about loss of memory and disability), apraxia (inability to perform simple actions), and agnosia (inability to recognize familiar objects and their purpose).

In the final stages of dementia, the patient is usually mute, disengaged, unable to perform any activities of daily living, and in need of complete nursing care.

What tests tell you

AD can't be confirmed until death, when an autopsy reveals pathologic findings.

The following tests help rule out other disorders:

• Positron-emission tomography (PET) scan measures the metabolic activity of the cerebral cortex and may help confirm early diagnosis.

• Computed tomography (CT) scan may show more brain atrophy than what occurs in normal aging.

• Magnetic resonance imaging (MRI) evaluates the condition of the brain and rules out intracranial lesions as the source of dementia.

• EEG evaluates the brain's electrical activity and may show brain wave slowing late in the disease. It also helps to differentiate

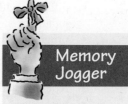

Memory Jogger

Use the "5 A's" to remember the common signs of dementia:

Amnesia

Anomia

Apathy

Agnosia

Apraxia

tumors, abscesses, and other intracranial lesions that might cause symptoms.
- CSF analysis can show beta-amyloid and tau proteins; it helps determine whether signs and symptoms stem from a chronic neurologic infection.
- Cerebral blood flow studies may detect abnormalities in blood flow to the brain.
- Potential diagnostic tools under investigation include blood biomarkers that show the level of beta-amyloid and tau protein accumulation and biomarkers that show injured or actually degenerating nerve cells.

Amyotrophic lateral sclerosis

Commonly called *Lou Gehrig disease,* after the New York Yankee first baseman who died of the disorder in the 1940s, amyotrophic lateral sclerosis (ALS) is a progressive neurodegenerative disease that affects motor nerve cells of the brain and spinal cord. Motor neurons in ALS eventually die and voluntary muscle movement is impacted; people may lose the ability to speak, eat, move, and breathe. There are two types of ALS, sporadic and familial. Sporadic is the most common form accounting for 90% to 95% of all cases. Familial means the disease is inherited, and this type accounts for 5% to 10% of all cases. Onset occurs between the ages of 40 and 70, and there are an estimated 31,000 Americans living with ALS, with 20% more males diagnosed than females. ALS is a progressively debilitating disease and is considered rapidly fatal, with an average survival time of 3 years.

All about ALS

The onset involves muscle weakness (an early symptom), weakness progresses, and muscle wasting and paralysis of muscles are evident affecting the limbs and trunk, impacting speech, swallowing, and breathing.
ALS may result from:
- gene mutation
- chemical imbalance that results in higher than normal levels of glutamate; too much glutamate is toxic to nerve cells
- accumulation of abnormal forms of proteins, which destroy nerve cells
- autoimmune disorders; sometimes the immune system attacks normal cells in the body, which can result in nerve cell death
Precipitating factors for acute deterioration include trauma, viral infection, and physical exhaustion.

The genetic link

ALS breakthrough

The good news...

Although more than 50 potentially causative or disease-modifying genes have been identified, pathogenic variants in *SOD1*, *C9ORF72*, *FUS*, and *TARDBP* occur most frequently in ALS. Such discoveries have contributed to our understanding of the genetic causes of familial ALS, with approximately 40% to 55% of cases accounted for by variants in known ALS-linked genes.

...and the not so good news

In sporadic ALS cases, however, diagnostic advancements have helped in explaining only a fraction of cases, with the etiology remaining unexplained in over 90% of patients.

How it happens

In ALS, the nerve cells that control the muscles, known as *motor neurons*, gradually degenerate. Dead motor neurons cannot produce or transport signals to muscles. Messages from the brain cannot reach the muscles to activate them. The patient's signs and symptoms develop according to the affected motor neurons because specific neurons activate specific muscle fibers.

What to look for

Muscle weakness is the primary or hallmark sign of ALS; some people may have trouble grabbing an item such as a pen or lifting a glass or cup, while others experience changes in speaking. Difficulty walking, clumsiness, muscle twitching, muscle spasms, and falls are some of the first signs of ALS. Other mores advanced signs and symptoms include:

- impaired speech
- difficulty chewing and swallowing
- difficulty breathing
- choking
- excessive drooling
- depression
- inappropriate laughing
- crying spells (See *Treating ALS.*)

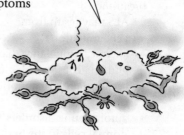

I apologize for lying down on the job, but this ALS hurts us motor neurons! In "amyotrophic," "a" means no, "myo" means muscle, and "trophic" means nourishment; without nourishment, the neurons waste away.

Treating ALS

There is no cure for amyotrophic lateral sclerosis (ALS); treatment aims to control symptoms and provide emotional, psychological, and physical support. Patients who experience difficulty swallowing may require gastric feedings. Depending upon the patient's wishes, tracheotomy and mechanical ventilation may be an option when hypoventilation develops.

Drug therapy

Riluzole inhibits presynaptic glutamate release and enhances glial and neuronal glutamate uptake. Glutamate accumulation causes neuron damage. Edaravone is a strong antioxidant that prevents oxidative stress from inducing motor neuron death in ALS patients. Sodium phenylbutyrate and taurursodiol protect cellular mitochondria from injury. These drugs are neuroprotective agents that can slow the progression of the disease. Baclofen, dantrolene, or diazepam may be given to control spasticity. Quinine therapy may be prescribed for painful muscle cramps.

Future prospects: Stem cells

With the advancement of stem cell technologies, there is hope for their application as novel treatments for ALS. In animal models, mesenchymal stem cells and neural fetal stem cells have emerged as safe and potentially effective cell types in treating ALS, but more research, including appropriately designed experimental studies to verify their long-term safety and possibly efficacy, is needed.

What tests tell you

These tests help confirm the diagnosis:
- Electromyography helps show nerve damage instead of muscle damage.
- Muscle biopsy helps rule out muscle disease.
- CSF analysis reveals increased protein content in one-third of patients.
- A thorough neurologic examination is needed to rule out other diseases of the neuromuscular system.

Bell palsy

Bell palsy (also known as acute peripheral facial paresis) is the most common facial nerve disorder, characterized by inflammation of cranial nerve VII, on one side of the face, in the absence of stroke or other disease.

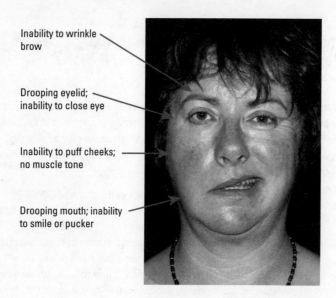

Inability to wrinkle brow

Drooping eyelid; inability to close eye

Inability to puff cheeks; no muscle tone

Drooping mouth; inability to smile or pucker

About Bell palsy

The cause of Bell palsy is unknown, though 40,000 Americans are diagnosed with it every year. This disorder affects all genders, aged 15 to 60 years.

The risk factors...

- Being in the third trimester of pregnancy
- Early postpartum
- Older adults
- People with diabetes or hypothyroidism
- Persons with tick bite (may be linked to Lyme disease)

How it happens

The etiology is unknown, though theories suggest there is acute demyelination of nerves. The strongest supported cause is reactivation of the herpes simplex virus isoform (HSV-1) and/or herpes zoster virus (HZV). It has also been linked to Lyme disease, which is caused by a tick-carrying the bacteria: *Borrelia burgdorferi*. Viral infections can cause inflammation, leading to compression of the nerve that results in facial paralysis. Other causes may be influenza, mumps, and rubella. Noninfectious causes include Hashimoto thyroiditis and genetic factors.

What to look for

- Rapid onset of facial weakness on one side
- Pain around and behind the ear
- Recent viral illness or tick bite
- Numbness of the face, tongue, and ear
- Ringing in the ear (tinnitus)
- Headache
- Hearing deficit in the ear on the affected side
- Drooping of the mouth on the affected side and drooling
- Inability to close the eyelid on the affected side (the trademark sign)
- Other manifestations include inability to smile, frown, and whistle; loss of taste; and altered chewing.

What tests tell you

Diagnosis is made by excluding other conditions:
- MRI and CT may rule out other causes of facial paralysis.
- Blood tests may be used to rule out infections or other diseases, particularly Lyme disease.
  Patients should be referred to a neurologist.

Good news?!

Bell palsy is considered benign, and most patients recover within 3 weeks to 6 months. The extent of damage directly impacts the extent of recovery. Only about one-third of patients report lingering effects such as facial weakness, involuntary movements, and constant tearing of the eye on the affected side.

Epilepsy

Epilepsy, also known as seizure disorder, is a neurologic disorder in which brain activity is abnormal, causing seizures. Epilepsy is diagnosed if a patient has:
- two unprovoked seizures occurring more than 24 hours apart
- a single unprovoked seizure if recurrence risk is high (i.e., >60% over 10 years)
- a diagnosis of an epilepsy syndrome
  Seizures are paroxysmal events associated with abnormal electrical discharges of neurons in the brain. The discharge may trigger a convulsive movement, an interruption of sensation, an alteration in the level of consciousness (LOC), or a combination of these symptoms.

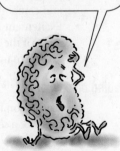

I've got those abnormal electrical discharge blues.

From young to old

This condition affects people of all ages and ethnic backgrounds. About 3.4 million people in the United States have epilepsy, and 1 in 26 people in the United States will develop epilepsy in their lifetime.

How it happens

Epilepsy has no known cause, though seizures are caused by abnormal brain activity.

Don't know why

In about 50% of cases, epilepsy has no known cause. In other cases, however, possible causes of epilepsy include:
- genetic influences; certain genes may cause a person to be more sensitive to environmental conditions that trigger seizure activity
- perinatal injuries
- metabolic abnormalities (such as hyponatremia, hypocalcemia, hypoglycemia, and pyridoxine deficiency)
- brain conditions (such as strokes and brain tumors)
- infections (such as meningitis, encephalitis, or AIDS)
- traumatic brain injury
- ingestion of toxins (such as mercury, lead, or carbon monoxide)

All fired up

This is what happens during a seizure:
- The electronic balance at the neuronal level is altered, causing the neuronal membrane to become susceptible to activation.
- Increased permeability of the cytoplasmic membranes helps hypersensitive neurons fire abnormally. Abnormal firing may be activated by hyperthermia, hypoglycemia, hyponatremia, hypoxia, or repeated sensory stimulation.
- When the intensity of a seizure discharge has progressed sufficiently, it spreads to adjacent brain areas. The midbrain, thalamus, and cerebral cortex are most likely to become epileptogenic.
- Excitement feeds back from the primary focus and to other parts of the brain.
- The discharges become less frequent until they stop.

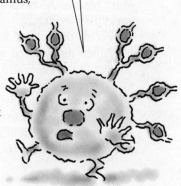

I'm hypersensitive by nature—and a change in my environment can really make me hyperactive.

Getting complicated

Depending on the type of seizure, injury may result from a fall at the onset of a seizure or afterward, when the patient is confused. Injury may also result from the rapid, jerking movements that occur during or after a seizure. Anoxia can occur due to airway occlusion by the tongue, aspiration of vomit, or traumatic injury. A continuous seizure state known as *status epilepticus* can cause respiratory distress and even death. Sudden unexpected death in epilepsy (SUDEP) is one of the main causes of epilepsy-related death and occurs most commonly during sleep. The cause is unknown. SUDEP is preceded by a seizure followed shortly by apnea and then asystole. (See *Understanding status epilepticus* and *Electrical impulses in seizures.*)

What to look for
Signs and symptoms of epilepsy vary depending on the type and cause of the seizure. (See *Understanding types of seizures*, page 203.)

It isn't always clear

Physical findings may be normal if the patient doesn't have a seizure during assessment and the cause is idiopathic. If the seizure is caused by an underlying problem, the patient's history and physical examination should uncover related signs and symptoms.

In many cases, the patient's history shows that seizures are unpredictable and unrelated to activities. Occasionally, a patient may report

Now I get it!

Understanding status epilepticus

Status epilepticus is a continuous seizure state that must be interrupted by emergency measures. It can occur during all types of seizures. For example, generalized tonic-clonic status epilepticus is a continuous generalized tonic-clonic seizure without an intervening return of consciousness. People with status epilepticus have an increased risk of brain damage and death.

Always an emergency
Status epilepticus is accompanied by respiratory distress. It can result from withdrawal of antiepileptic medications, hypoxic or metabolic encephalopathy, acute head trauma, or septicemia secondary to encephalitis or meningitis.

Acting fast
Emergency treatment guidelines are proposed in four phases. The first phase is the stabilization phase, which includes interventions such as stabilizing the patient, timing the seizure, monitoring vital signs, assessing oxygenation, monitoring ECG, and use of a finger stick for blood glucose level monitoring. The initial therapy phase follows. The initial therapy phase is where a benzodiazepine is given intravenously. Medications that may be used in this phase include lorazepam, midazolam, and diazepam. The second therapy phase is initiated if seizures continue. The second therapy phase may include intravenous fosphenytoin, valproic acid, or levetiracetam. If seizures continue, then the third therapy phase is initiated. The third therapy phase may include repeating the second therapy or administration of anesthetic medications such as thiopental, pentobarbital, or propofol.

Electrical impulses in seizures

The spread of electrical impulses is different in each type of seizure.

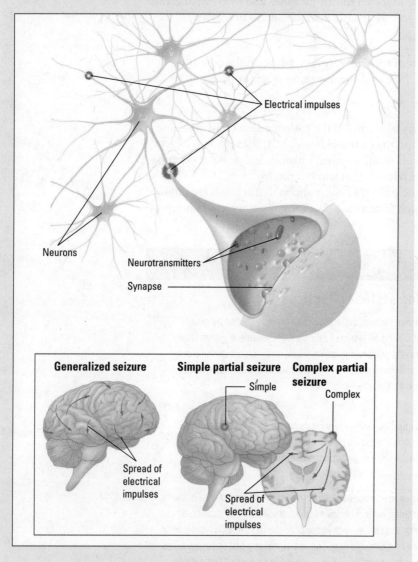

Electrical impulses

Neurons

Neurotransmitters

Synapse

Generalized seizure

Simple partial seizure

Simple

Complex partial seizure

Complex

Spread of electrical impulses

Spread of electrical impulses

precipitating factors. For example, the seizures may always take place at a certain time, such as during sleep, or after a particular circumstance, such as lack of sleep or emotional stress. The patient may also report nonspecific symptoms, such as headache, mood changes, lethargy, and myoclonic jerking up to several hours before a seizure. (See *Treating epilepsy*, page 204.)

Understanding types of seizures

Use these guidelines to understand different seizure types. Remember that patients may be affected by more than one type of seizure.

Partial seizures

Arising from a localized area in the brain, partial seizure activity may spread to the entire brain, causing a generalized seizure. Several types and subtypes of partial seizures exist:
- simple partial, which includes Jacksonian seizures and sensory seizures
- complex partial
- secondarily generalized partial seizure (partial onset leading to generalized tonic-clonic seizure)

Jacksonian seizure

A Jacksonian seizure, also known as a simple partial seizure, is a type of focal partial seizure, caused by unusual electrical activity in a small area of the brain. The patient experiences a stiffening or jerking in one extremity, accompanied by a tingling sensation in the same area.

Sensory seizure

Symptoms of a sensory seizure include hallucinations, flashing lights, tingling sensations, vertigo, déjà vu, and smelling a foul odor.

Complex partial seizure

Signs and symptoms of a complex partial seizure are variable but usually include purposeless behavior, including a glassy stare, picking at clothes, aimless wandering, lip-smacking or chewing motions, and unintelligible speech. An aura may occur first, and seizures may last from a few seconds to 20 minutes. Afterward, mental confusion may last for several minutes, and an observer may mistakenly suspect alcohol or drug intoxication or psychosis. The patient has no memory of their actions during the seizure.

Secondarily generalized seizure

A secondarily generalized seizure can be simple or complex and can progress to a generalized seizure. An aura may occur first, with loss of consciousness occurring immediately or 1 to 2 minutes later.

Generalized seizures

Generalized seizures cause a generalized electrical abnormality within the brain. Types include:
- absence or petit mal
- myoclonic
- generalized tonic-clonic
- akinetic or atonic

Absence seizure

Absence seizure occurs most commonly in children. It usually begins with a brief change in the level of consciousness, signaled by blinking or rolling of the eyes, a blank stare, and slight mouth movements. The patient retains their posture and continues preseizure activity without difficulty. Seizures last from 1 to 10 seconds, and impairment is so brief that the patient may be unaware of it. However, if not properly treated, these seizures can recur up to 100 times per day and progress to a generalized tonic-clonic seizure.

Myoclonic seizure

Myoclonic seizure, also called *bilateral massive epileptic myoclonus*, is marked by brief, involuntary muscular jerks of the body or extremities, which may occur in a rhythmic manner, and a brief loss of consciousness.

Generalized tonic-clonic seizure

Typically, a generalized tonic-clonic seizure begins with a loud cry, caused by air rushing from the lungs through the vocal cords. The patient falls to the ground, losing consciousness. The body stiffens (tonic phase) and then alternates between episodes of muscle spasm and relaxation (clonic phase). Tongue biting, incontinence, labored breathing, apnea, and cyanosis may also occur.

The seizure stops in 2 to 5 minutes, when abnormal electrical conduction of the neurons is completed. Afterward, the patient regains consciousness but is somewhat confused. They may have difficulty talking and may have drowsiness, fatigue, headache, muscle soreness, and arm or leg weakness. They may fall into a deep sleep afterward.

Akinetic seizure

Akinetic seizure, also called *atonic seizure,* is characterized by a general loss of postural tone and a temporary loss of consciousness; akinetic seizure occurs in young children. Sometimes it's called a "drop attack" because the child falls.

Battling illness

Treating epilepsy

Treatment of epilepsy seeks to reduce the frequency of seizures or prevent their occurrence.

Drug therapy

Antiseizure drug therapy is specific to the type of seizure. The goal of therapy is to prevent seizures with minimal side effects and minimal drug toxicity. Drug therapy is based on age and weight, type, frequency, and cause of seizure. Drug therapy for seizure disorders includes carbamazepine, diazepam, levetiracetam, phenytoin, primidone, valproic acid, and clonazepam.

Surgery

If drug therapy fails, some patients are candidates for surgical therapy to prevent the spread of epileptic activity in the brain. The classic surgical treatment has been an anterior temporal lobe resection. However, the current goal of surgical interventions is to carefully remove the precise localized area within the brain. Approximately 70% to 80% of patients are seizure-free after surgery, and 10% to 20% have a marked reduction in seizure activity.

Aura report

Some patients report an aura a few seconds or minutes before a generalized seizure. An aura signals the beginning of abnormal electrical discharges within a focal area of the brain. Typical auras include:
- a pungent smell
- nausea or indigestion
- a rising or sinking feeling in the stomach
- a dreamy feeling
- an unusual taste
- a visual disturbance such as a flashing light

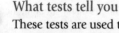

What tests tell you

These tests are used to diagnose epilepsy:
- EEG showing paroxysmal abnormalities may confirm the diagnosis by providing evidence of continuing seizure tendency. A negative EEG doesn't rule out epilepsy because paroxysmal abnormalities occur intermittently. EEG also helps determine the prognosis and can help classify the disorder.
- CT scan and MRI provide density readings of the brain and may indicate abnormalities in internal structures.

    Other tests include serum glucose and calcium studies, skull x-rays, lumbar puncture, brain scan, cerebral angiography, and vagal nerve stimulation, which is an implanted electrode that delivers an impulse to the vagus nerve when a seizure is impending.

Guillain-Barré syndrome

Guillain-Barré syndrome (GBS), also called *acute inflammatory demyelinating polyneuropathy* (AIDP), is a rapidly progressing acute, autoimmune process occurring a few days to weeks following a viral or bacterial infection. Other causes of GBS are immunizations or vaccinations, surgical interventions, trauma, bone marrow transplant, and certain systemic diseases like disseminated lupus erythematosus, sarcoidosis, or Hodgkin lymphoma. It is a potentially fatal syndrome associated with segmented demyelination of peripheral nerves.

This syndrome occurs equally in males and females, usually occurring between ages 30 and 50. It affects about 1 out of every 100,000 people. As a result of blood treatments that include plasma exchange and immunoglobulin therapy, 70% of patients recover with few or no residual symptoms.

Going through the phases

The clinical course of GBS has three phases:
1. The acute phase begins when the first definitive symptom develops and ends 1 to 3 weeks later, when no further deterioration is noted.
2. The plateau phase lasts for several days to 2 weeks.
3. The recovery phase, believed to coincide with remyelination and axonal process regrowth, can last from 4 months to 3 years.

How it happens

The precise cause of GBS is unknown, but it's thought to be a cell-mediated, immunologic attack on peripheral nerves in response to a virus or other cause of cell injury.

Danger! Demyelination!

An immunologic reaction causes segmental demyelination of the peripheral nerves, which prevents normal transmission of electrical impulses along the sensorimotor nerve roots.

The myelin sheath, which covers the nerve axons and conducts electrical impulses along the nerve pathways, degenerates for unknown reasons. With degeneration comes inflammation, swelling, and patchy demyelination. (See *Peripheral nerve demyelination in GBS*, page 206.)

As myelin is destroyed, the nodes of Ranvier, located at the junctures of the myelin sheaths, widen. This causes a delay and impairs impulse transmission along the dorsal and ventral nerve roots. As demyelination occurs, the transmission of nerve impulses slows down or stops, resulting in peripheral nerve damage and atrophy.

We're under attack! Inflammation and degenerative changes in both the sensory and motor nerve roots cause sensory and motor impairment simultaneously!

Now I get it!

Peripheral nerve demyelination in GBS

The illustration below shows the inflammation and degeneration of the myelin sheath.

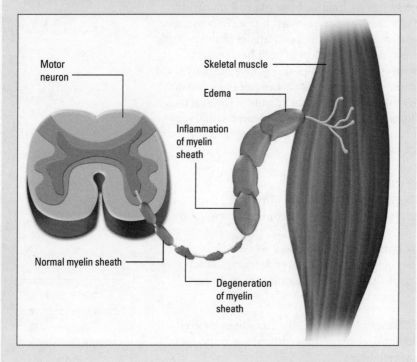

Motor neuron

Skeletal muscle

Edema

Inflammation of myelin sheath

Normal myelin sheath

Degeneration of myelin sheath

What to look for

Impairment of dorsal nerve roots affects sensory function, so the patient may experience tingling and numbness. Impairment of ventral nerve roots affects motor function, causing the patient to experience muscle weakness, immobility, and paralysis.

Other signs and symptoms include muscle stiffness and pain, sensory loss, loss of position sense, and diminished or absent deep tendon reflexes.

Symptoms usually follow an ascending pattern, beginning in the legs and progressing to the arms, trunk, and face. In mild forms, only cranial nerves may be affected. In some patients, muscle weakness may be absent.

Respiratory risk

The disorder commonly affects respiratory muscles. If death occurs with this syndrome, it is likely from respiratory complications. Paralysis of the internal and external intercostal muscles leads to a reduction in functional breathing. Vagus nerve paralysis causes a loss of the protective mechanisms that respond to bronchial irritation and foreign bodies, as well as a diminished or absent gag reflex. (See *Treating GBS*, page 207.)

What tests tell you

These tests are used to diagnose GBS:

- CSF analysis may show a normal white blood cell (WBC) count, an elevated protein count, and, in severe disease, increased CSF pressure. The CSF protein level begins to rise several days after the onset of signs and symptoms, peaking in 4 to 6 weeks, probably because of widespread inflammatory disease of the nerve roots.
- Electromyography may demonstrate repeated firing of the same motor unit instead of widespread sectional stimulation.
- Electrophysiologic testing may reveal marked slowing of nerve conduction velocities.

Battling illness

Treating GBS

Most patients seek treatment when the disease is in the acute stage. Treatment is primarily supportive and may require endotracheal intubation or tracheotomy if the patient has difficulty breathing or clearing secretions.

Continuous electrocardiographic monitoring is necessary to identify symptoms such as cardiac arrhythmias. Atropine may be used for bradycardia. Marked hypotension may require volume replacement and administration of vasopressors, such as dopamine.

A spontaneous recovery

Most patients recover spontaneously. Intensive physical therapy starts as soon as voluntary movement returns to skeletal muscles, to prevent muscle and joint contractures. However, a small percentage of patients are left with some residual disability.

Alternative approaches

High-dose IV immune globulin (to suppress the immune response) and plasmapheresis may shorten recovery time. Plasmapheresis temporarily reduces circulating antibodies through removal of the patient's blood, centrifugation of blood to remove plasma, and subsequent reinfusion. It's most effective during the first few weeks of the disease, and patients need less ventilatory support if treatment begins within 2 weeks of onset. The patient may receive three to five plasma exchanges.

Meningitis

In meningitis, the brain and spinal cord meninges become inflamed. Inflammation may involve all three meningeal membranes: the dura mater, the arachnoid mater, and the pia mater and the underlying cortex. Blood flow to the brain is reduced. Tissues swell, causing increased intracranial pressure (ICP).

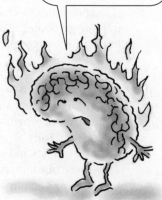

Oh no! In meningitis, my meninges become inflamed.

Knowledge is power

The prognosis for patients with meningitis is good and complications are rare, especially if the disease is recognized early and the infecting organism responds to antibiotics. However, mortality in untreated meningitis is 70% to 100%. The prognosis is poorer for infants and older adults.

How it happens

The origin of meningeal inflammation may be:

- bacterial
- viral
- protozoal
- fungal

The most common causes of meningitis are bacterial and viral. Bacterial infection may be due to *Neisseria meningitidis*, *Haemophilus influenzae*, *Streptococcus pneumoniae*, or *Escherichia coli*. Sometimes, no causative organism can be found.

Blame it on bacteria

Bacterial meningitis is one of the most serious infections that may affect infants and children. In most patients, the infection that causes meningitis is secondary to another bacterial infection, such as bacteremia (especially from pneumonia, empyema, osteomyelitis, and endocarditis), sinusitis, otitis media, encephalitis, myelitis, or brain abscess. Respiratory infections increase the risk of bacterial meningitis. Meningitis may also follow a skull fracture, a penetrating head wound, lumbar puncture, ventricular shunting, or other neurosurgical procedures.

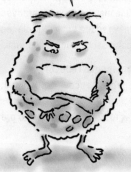

Bacterial meningitis begins when I enter the subarachnoid space.

Sabotage in the subarachnoid space

Bacterial meningitis occurs when bacteria enter the subarachnoid space and cause an inflammatory response. Usually, organisms enter the nervous system after invading and infecting another region of the body. The organisms gain access to the subarachnoid space and the CSF, where they cause irritation of the tissues bathed by the fluid.

The viral version

Meningitis caused by a virus is called *aseptic viral meningitis.* Aseptic viral meningitis may result from a direct infection or secondary to disease, such as mumps, herpes, measles, or leukemia. Usually, symptoms are mild and the disease is self-limiting. (See *Understanding aseptic viral meningitis,* page 209.)

Risky business

Infants, children, and older adults have the highest risk of developing meningitis. Other risk factors include malnourishment, immunosuppression (for example, from radiation therapy), and CNS trauma. (See *Meningeal inflammation in meningitis,* page 209.)

Now I get it!

Understanding aseptic viral meningitis

A benign syndrome, aseptic viral meningitis results from infection with enteroviruses (most common), arboviruses, herpes simplex virus, mumps virus, or lymphocytic choriomeningitis virus.

First, a fever

Signs and symptoms of viral meningitis usually begin suddenly with a temperature up to 104° F (40° C), drowsiness, confusion, stupor, and slight neck or spine stiffness when the patient bends forward. The patient history may reveal a recent illness.

Other signs and symptoms include headache, nausea, vomiting, abdominal pain, poorly defined chest pain, and sore throat.

What virus is this anyway?

A complete patient history and knowledge of seasonal epidemics are key to differentiate among the many forms of aseptic viral meningitis. Negative bacteriologic cultures and cerebrospinal fluid (CSF) analysis showing pleocytosis (a greater than normal number of cells in the CSF) and increased protein suggest the diagnosis. Isolation of the virus from CSF confirms diagnosis.

Begin with bed rest

Treatment for aseptic viral meningitis includes bed rest, maintenance of fluid and electrolyte balance, analgesics for pain, and exercises to combat residual weakness. Careful handling of excretions and good hand-washing technique prevent the spread of the disease, although isolation isn't necessary.

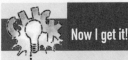

Now I get it!

Meningeal inflammation in meningitis

The illustration below shows normal meninges and how the meninges become inflamed in meningitis.

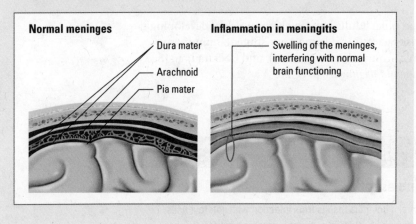

Normal meninges

Dura mater
Arachnoid
Pia mater

Inflammation in meningitis

Swelling of the meninges, interfering with normal brain functioning

Getting complicated

Potential complications of meningitis include:
- vision impairment
- optic neuritis
- cranial nerve palsies
- deafness
- personality changes
- headache
- paresis or paralysis
- endocarditis
- coma
- vasculitis
- cerebral infarction

Complications in infants and children may also include:
- sensory hearing loss
- epilepsy
- mental retardation
- hydrocephalus
- subdural effusions

What to look for

The cardinal signs and symptoms of meningitis are those of infection and increased ICP:
- Headache

- Stiff neck and back
- Malaise
- Photophobia
- Chills
- Fever
- Vomiting
- Twitching
- Seizures
- Altered LOC, such as confusion or delirium
  Signs and symptoms in infants and children may also include:
- fretfulness
- bulging of the fontanels (infants)
- refusal to eat (See *Important signs of meningitis*, page 211.)

Patient history is key

Findings vary depending on the type and severity of meningitis. In pneumococcal meningitis, the patient history may uncover a recent lung, ear, or sinus infection or endocarditis. It may also reveal alcoholism, sickle cell disease, basal skull fracture, recent splenectomy, or organ transplant. In meningitis caused by *H. influenzae*, the patient history may reveal a recent respiratory tract or ear infection. In meningococcal meningitis, you may see a petechial, purpuric, or ecchymotic rash on the patient's lower body.

Important signs of meningitis

A positive response to the following tests helps establish a diagnosis of meningitis.

Brudzinski sign
Place the patient in a dorsal recumbent position; then put your hands behind the patient's neck and bend it forward. Pain and resistance may indicate neck injury or arthritis. But if the patient also involuntarily flexes the hips and knees, chances are they have meningeal irritation and inflammation, a sign of meningitis.

Kernig sign
Place the patient in a supine position. Flex the patient's leg at the hip and knee; then straighten the knee. Pain or resistance suggests meningitis.

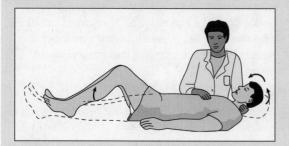

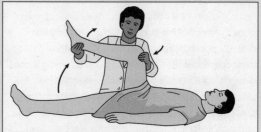

It's so irritating

Signs of meningeal irritation are nuchal rigidity, exaggerated and symmetrical deep tendon reflexes, opisthotonos (a spasm in which the back and extremities arch backward so that the body rests on the head and heels), and positive Brudzinski and Kernig signs. (See *Treating meningitis*, page 212.)

What tests tell you

These tests are used to diagnose meningitis:

- Lumbar puncture shows elevated CSF pressure, cloudy or milky CSF, a high protein level, positive Gram stain and culture that usually identifies the infecting organism (unless it's a virus), and depressed CSF glucose concentration.
- CT scan is performed to look at the brain for signs of swelling, hemorrhage, or abscess.
- MRI is performed to identify brain and spinal cord inflammation, infection, and tumors.
- EEG is performed to identify abnormal brain waves.
- Chest x-rays are important because they may reveal pneumonitis or lung abscess, tubercular lesions, or granulomas secondary to fungal infection.
- Sinus and skull x-rays may help identify the presence of cranial osteomyelitis, paranasal sinusitis, or skull fracture.
- WBC count usually indicates leukocytosis and abnormal serum electrolyte levels.
- CT scan rules out cerebral hematoma, hemorrhage, or tumor.
- Blood cultures identify the causative agent in bacteremia.

Battling illness

Treating meningitis

The ultimate goal of treatment for patients with meningitis is to return neurologic function, control pain, and resolve the infection. Prevention and health promotion through vaccinations are the primary focus. Three kinds of meningococcal vaccines are available in the United States: meningococcal conjugate vaccine (MCV4), meningococcal polysaccharide (MPSV4), and serogroup B meningococcal vaccines. Treatment for patients with meningitis includes codeine for pain relief, phenytoin or levetiracetam if seizures occur, and aspirin or acetaminophen for fever. Note: Aspirin should not be used in children under the age of 12 due to an increased incidence of Reye syndrome.

Antibiotics and more antibiotics

IV antibiotics should be administered after the lumbar puncture; however, if a viral form of meningitis is discovered, antibiotics are discontinued. IV antibiotics include ampicillin, penicillin, cephalosporin, and ceftriaxone. If intercranial pressure increases, then mannitol may be given.

Supportive measures

Supportive measures include bed rest, hypothermia, and fluid therapy to prevent dehydration. Isolation is necessary if nasal cultures are positive.

Migraine

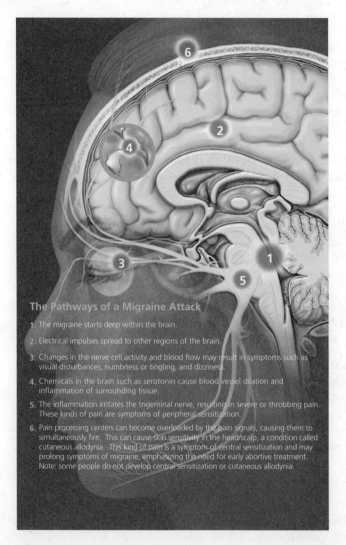

The Pathways of a Migraine Attack

1. The migraine starts deep within the brain.

2. Electrical impulses spread to other regions of the brain.

3. Changes in the nerve cell activity and blood flow may result in symptoms such as visual disturbances, numbness or tingling, and dizziness.

4. Chemicals in the brain such as serotonin cause blood vessel dilation and inflammation of surrounding tissue.

5. The inflammation irritates the trigeminal nerve, resulting in severe or throbbing pain. These kinds of pain are symptoms of peripheral sensitization.

6. Pain processing centers can become overloaded by the pain signals, causing them to simultaneously fire. This can cause skin sensitivity in the head/scalp, a condition called cutaneous allodynia. This kind of pain is a symptom of central sensitization and may prolong symptoms of migraine, emphasizing the need for early abortive treatment. Note: some people do not develop central sensitization or cutaneous allodynia.

Migraine is an episodic neurologic disorder characterized by a headache lasting 4 to 72 hours. Migraines can be classified as migraine with aura (visual, sensory, or motor symptoms) or migraine without aura (the more common type). Migraine occurs in about 12% of people age 12 and older in the United States. It is about three times more common in females (17% of this population) than in males (6% of this population). It is most common in midlife, and rates decrease after age 60.

How it happens

The pathophysiologic basis for migraines is not clearly identified. There may be an association between changes in blood flow to the brain and brain metabolism. Some theories suggest a vascular, hormonal, or neurotransmitter component as cause. People who menstruate may experience migraines more frequently before and during menstruation or report a decrease in occurrence during pregnancy and menopause, indicating a cyclic withdrawal of estrogen and progesterone as a trigger for migraines.

Migraine attacks in phases!

1. *Premonitory phase (also called prodrome)*: Symptoms occur hours to days before the onset of a headache or aura. Symptoms include tiredness, irritability, inability to concentrate, and stiff neck.
2. *Migraine aura*: Aura symptoms occur and may last up to 1 hour. Symptoms include visual, sensory, or motor. Only one-third of people report these symptoms.
3. *Headache phase*: Headache described as throbbing and spreading to the entire head is experienced. Pain may be accompanied by nausea, vomiting, fatigue, and dizziness. Symptoms may last 4 to 72 hours.
4. *Recovery phase (also called postdrome)*: Symptoms include irritability, fatigue, and depression, which can last from hours to days.

Diagnosis and management

Diagnosis is made from medical history and physical examination. EEG and imaging may be used to rule out other diagnoses. Management of migraines may include avoiding triggers, using pharmacologic management, and using transcutaneous electrical stimulation devices providing trigeminal nerve stimulation.

Multiple sclerosis

Multiple sclerosis (MS) results from progressive demyelination of the white matter of the brain and spinal cord, leading to widespread neurologic dysfunction. The structures usually involved are the optic and oculomotor nerves and the spinal nerve tracts.

The ups and downs of MS

The National MS Society identifies MS as a major cause of chronic neurological disability, characterized by exacerbations and remissions. MS is commonly diagnosed in people between the ages of 20 and 40.

The incidence is highest in females, in northern urban areas, in higher socioeconomic groups, and in people with a family history of the disease.

    The prognosis varies. Life expectancy has increased, likely due to treatment breakthroughs and improved health care and lifestyle changes. There are rare instances where the progression of MS is rapid and the disease can be fatal.

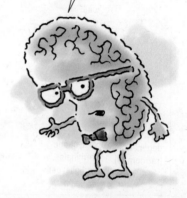

Demyelination is the loss of myelin sheath that is essential in nerve impulse transmission.

How it happens

The exact cause of MS is unknown. MS is most commonly defined as an autoimmune disorder in which antibodies destroy the myelin sheaths around sensory and motor neurons. The trigger for the development of the antibodies is unknown. Genetic factors may also play a part.

Dots of demyelination

MS affects the white matter of the brain and spinal cord by causing scattered demyelinated lesions that prevent normal neurologic conduction. After the myelin is destroyed, neuroglial tissue in the white matter of the CNS proliferates, forming hard yellow plaques of scar tissue. Proliferation of neuroglial tissue is called *gliosis*. (See *Understanding myelin breakdown*, page 216.)

Interrupting an impulse

Scar tissue damages the underlying axon fiber so that nerve conduction is disrupted. The symptoms of MS caused by demyelination become irreversible as the disease progresses. However, remission may result from healing of demyelinated areas by sclerotic tissue.

What to look for

Signs and symptoms of MS depend on four factors:
1. the extent of myelin destruction
2. the site of myelin destruction
3. the extent of remyelination
4. the adequacy of subsequent restored synaptic transmission

There just aren't words

Symptoms may be unpredictable and difficult for the patient to describe. They may be transient or may last for hours or weeks. Usually, the patient history reveals two initial symptoms: vision problems (caused by an optic neuritis) and sensory impairment such as paresthesia. After the initial episode, findings may vary. Double vision

Understanding myelin breakdown

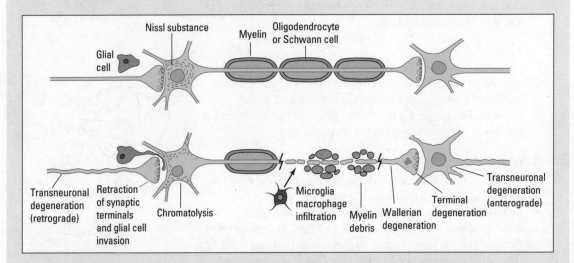

Myelin plays a key role in speeding electrical impulses to the brain for interpretation. The myelin sheath is a lipoprotein complex formed by glial cells. It protects the neuron's long nerve fiber (axon) much like the insulation on an electrical wire. Because of its high electrical resistance and weak ability to store an electrical charge, the myelin sheath permits conduction of nerve impulses from one node of Ranvier to the next.

Effects of injury
Myelin can be injured by hypoxemia, toxic chemicals, vascular insufficiency, or autoimmune responses. When this occurs, the myelin sheath becomes inflamed and the membrane layers break down into smaller components. These components become well-circumscribed plaques filled with microglial elements, macroglia, and lymphocytes. This process is called *demyelination*.

The damaged myelin sheath impairs normal conduction, causing partial loss or dispersion of the action potential and consequent neurologic dysfunction.

(diplopia), weakness of extremities, chronic fatigue, lack of coordination and loss of balance (due to involvement of the cerebellum), and Lhermitte phenomenon (an abnormal electric-shock-like sensation down the spine or limbs on neck flexion) are characteristic of MS.

Other signs and symptoms may include:
- poorly articulated speech (caused by cerebellar involvement)
- muscle weakness and spasticity (caused by lesions in the cortico-spinal tracts)

- hyperreflexia
- urinary problems
- intention tremor
- gait ataxia
- bowel problems
- cognitive dysfunction
- fatigue
- paralysis, ranging from monoplegia to quadriplegia
- vision problems, such as scotoma (an area of lost vision in the visual field), optic neuritis, and ophthalmoplegia (paralysis of the eye muscles)

Getting complicated

Complications include injuries from falls, urinary tract infections, constipation, joint contractures, pressure ulcers, rectal distention, and pneumonia. (See *Treating MS*.)

Battling illness

Treating MS

Treatment for MS aims to shorten exacerbations and, if possible, relieve neurologic deficits so the patient can resume a near-normal lifestyle.

Drug options

There is no cure for MS; treatment is aimed at the disease process and symptomatic relief. Because MS may have allergic and inflammatory causes, corticotropin, prednisone, or dexamethasone may be used to reduce edema of the myelin sheath during exacerbations, relieving symptoms and hastening remissions. However, these drugs don't prevent future exacerbations.

Current treatment helps to manage MS and increase comfort and quality of life. Progressive and relapsing forms of MS medications include IV interferon beta-1a or IV interferon beta-1b, oral teriflunomide and fingolimod, and infused alemtuzumab and mitoxantrone. High doses of intravenous corticosteroids may help to reduce inflammation and end relapse quicker.

Other useful medications to control symptoms include medications for bladder problems: dantrolene to relieve spasticity; bethanechol or oxybutynin to relieve urine retention and minimize urinary frequency and urgency; Cipro to manage infection; venlafaxine and paroxetine for depression; meclizine for dizziness and vertigo; and modafinil for fatigue.

Supportive measures

During acute exacerbations, supportive measures include bed rest, massage, prevention of fatigue and pressure ulcers, bowel and bladder training, treatment of bladder infections with antibiotics, physical therapy, and counseling.

What tests tell you

Diagnosing MS can be difficult due to periods of remission. These tests help diagnose the disease:

- MRI is the most sensitive method of detecting lesions and is also used to evaluate disease progression.
- CSF analysis reveals elevated immunoglobulin G levels but normal total protein levels. This elevation is significant only when serum gamma globulin levels are normal, and it reflects hyperactivity of the immune system due to chronic demyelination. The WBC count may be slightly increased.
- Evoked potential tests measure electrical activity of the brain and may detect slowing of electrical conduction caused by damage.

Myasthenia gravis

Myasthenia gravis is an autoimmune disease, which produces sporadic, progressive weakness and abnormal fatigue of voluntary skeletal muscles. These weaknesses increase with muscle use, and effects are exacerbated by exercise and repeated movement.

A menace to muscles

Myasthenia gravis usually affects muscles in the face, lips, tongue, neck, and throat, which are innervated by the cranial nerves—however, it can affect any muscle group. Eventually, muscle fibers may degenerate, and weakness (especially of the head, neck, trunk, and limb muscles) may become irreversible. When the disease involves the respiratory system, it may be life-threatening.

Myasthenia gravis affects 14 to 20 people per 100,000 and occurs at any age. The average age of onset is 28 years in females and 42 years in males. More females than males are affected, although in older adults, the disease affects females and males equally.

The ups and downs

The disease follows an unpredictable course with periodic exacerbations and remissions. Spontaneous remissions occur in about 25% of patients. No cure exists, but, thanks to drug therapy, patients may lead relatively normal lives except during exacerbations.

How it happens

The cause of myasthenia gravis is unknown. It commonly accompanies autoimmune disorders and disorders of the thymus. In fact, 10% of patients with myasthenia gravis have thymic tumors.

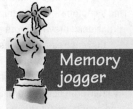

Memory jogger

Remember that myasthenia **gravis** means **grave** muscular weakness.

We interrupt this transmission…

For some reason, the patient's blood cells and thymus gland produce antibodies that block, destroy, or weaken the acetylcholine neuroreceptors that transmit nerve impulses, causing a failure in transmission of nerve impulses at the neuromuscular junction. (See *What happens in myasthenia gravis*, page 219.)

Now I get it!

What happens in myasthenia gravis

During normal neuromuscular transmission, a motor nerve impulse travels to a motor nerve terminal, stimulating the release of a chemical neurotransmitter called *acetylcholine.* When acetylcholine diffuses across the synapse, receptor sites in the motor end plate react and depolarize the muscle fiber. The depolarization spreads through the muscle fiber, causing muscle contraction.

Those darn antibodies

In myasthenia gravis, antibodies attach to the acetylcholine receptor sites. They block, destroy, and weaken these sites, leaving them insensitive to acetylcholine, thereby blocking neuromuscular transmission.

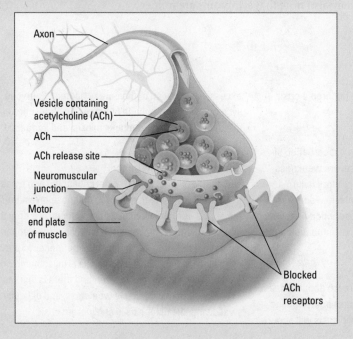

What to look for

Signs and symptoms of myasthenia gravis vary, depending on the muscles involved and the severity of the disease. However, in all cases, muscle weakness is progressive, and eventually some muscles may lose function entirely.

Common signs and symptoms include:
- extreme muscle weakness
- fatigue
- ptosis
- diplopia
- difficulty chewing and swallowing
- sleepy, masklike expression
- drooping jaw
- bobbing head
- arm or hand muscle weakness
(See Two types of crisis, page 220.)

Listen to your patient

The patient may report tilting their head back to see properly. Ptosis and dysfunction of the ocular muscles are common initial signs of myasthenia gravis, sometimes called ocular myasthenia. Ptosis (drooping of eyelids) and ocular muscle weakness cause visual impairment. The patient may also note that symptoms are milder

Two types of crisis

A patient with myasthenia gravis can undergo a crisis in one of two ways.

Myasthenic crisis
Myasthenic crisis is a life-threatening exacerbation of the disease that is characterized by severe weakness affecting the diaphragm muscle. Respiratory failure and severe bulbar (oropharyngeal) muscle weakness often occur, causing upper airway obstruction or severe dysphagia with aspiration. Endotracheal intubation and mechanical ventilation are necessary.

Cholinergic crisis
A cholinergic crisis is caused by too much anticholinesterase medication, which causes excess acetylcholine stimulation. The patient in a cholinergic crisis will show excessive activation of the parasympathetic nervous system. Symptoms include hypotension, bradycardia, diarrhea, abdominal cramping, miosis, and increased respiratory secretions.

How to know the difference
The diagnostic test used to differentiate the two types of crises is the same test used to diagnose myasthenia gravis: the edrophonium test. Edrophonium is a drug that prevents the breakdown of acetylcholine. After administration of this drug, if the patient experiences improvement in the symptoms, the diagnosis is myasthenic crisis. If the patient's symptoms worsen and there is increased salivation, increased muscle weakness, and difficulty swallowing, the diagnosis is cholinergic crisis.

on awakening and worsen as the day progresses and that short rest periods temporarily restore muscle function. Patients also report that symptoms become more intense during menses and after emotional stress, prolonged exposure to sunlight or cold, or infections.

If respiratory muscles are involved

Auscultation may reveal hypoventilation if the respiratory muscles are involved. This may lead to decreased tidal volume, making breathing difficult and predisposing the patient to pneumonia and other respiratory tract infections. Progressive weakness of the diaphragm and the intercostal muscles may eventually lead to myasthenic crisis (an acute exacerbation that causes severe respiratory distress). (See *Treating myasthenia gravis*, page 221.)

Battling illness

Treating myasthenia gravis

The main treatment for myasthenia gravis is anticholinesterase drugs such as pyridostigmine. Acetylcholinesterase is the enzyme the breaks down acetylcholine. Pyridostigmine counteracts acetylcholinesterase and allows the neurotransmitter acetylcholine to remain in neuro-muscle synapses longer. This drug counteracts fatigue and muscle weakness, and certain muscles get stronger. Corticosteroids may also help to relieve symptoms; more than 75% of patients treated with prednisone report improvement of symptoms. However, corticosteroids cannot be used long term due to side effects. Plasma exchange to improve strength and intravenous immune globulin (IVIG) are alternative treatment options.

Options and alternatives

If medications aren't effective, some patients undergo plasmapheresis to remove acetylcholine receptor antibodies and temporarily lessen the severity of symptoms. Thymectomy (removal of the thymus) is often recommended. Young people early in the disease have the best response to a thymectomy. A new drug, efgartigimod, counteracts the antibodies that are attacking the acetylcholine receptors.

Yikes! It's an emergency!

Myasthenic crisis necessitates immediate hospitalization. Endotracheal intubation and mechanical ventilation, combined with vigorous suctioning to remove secretions, usually bring improvement in a few days. Because anticholinesterase drugs aren't effective in myasthenic crisis, they're discontinued until respiratory function improves.

What tests tell you

These tests are used to diagnose myasthenia gravis:

- Edrophonium test confirms diagnosis by temporarily improving muscle function after an IV injection of edrophonium or, occasionally, neostigmine. However, long-standing ocular muscle dysfunction may not respond. This test also differentiates a myasthenic crisis from a cholinergic crisis.
- Electromyography measures the electrical potential of muscle cells and helps differentiate nerve disorders from muscle disorders. In myasthenia gravis, the amplitude of motor unit potential falls off with continued use. Muscle contractions decrease with each test, reflecting fatigue.
- Nerve conduction studies measure the speed at which electrical impulses travel along a nerve and also help distinguish nerve disorders from muscle disorders.
- Chest x-ray or CT scan may identify a thymoma.

Parkinson disease

Parkinson disease (PD) produces progressive muscle rigidity, loss of muscle movement (*akinesia*), and involuntary tremors. The patient's condition may deteriorate over the course of many years. PD is more prevalent in males and usually begins after the age of 40 years, with incidence increasing after the age of 60 years; approximately 90,000 new cases are diagnosed in the United States each year. This number is expected to rise to 1.2 million by 2030. PD is the second-most common neurodegenerative disease after AD.

How it happens

In most cases, the cause of PD is unknown. Genetic and environmental factors should be considered and evaluated. Some cases result from exposure to toxins, such as manganese dust and carbon monoxide, that destroy cells in the substantia nigra of the brain.

A defect in the dopamine pathway...

PD affects the extrapyramidal system, which influences the initiation, modulation, and completion of movement. The extrapyramidal system includes the corpus striatum, globus pallidus, and substantia nigra, all of which are within the basal ganglia.

In PD, a dopamine deficiency occurs in the basal ganglia, the dopamine-releasing pathway that connects the substantia nigra to the corpus striatum.

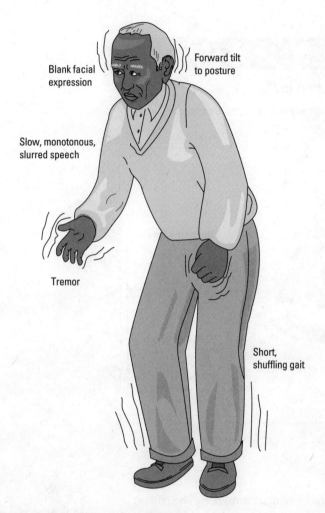

Blank facial expression

Forward tilt to posture

Slow, monotonous, slurred speech

Tremor

Short, shuffling gait

...causes an imbalance of neurotransmitters

Reduction of dopamine in the corpus striatum upsets the normal balance between the inhibitory dopamine and excitatory acetylcholine neurotransmitters. This prevents affected brain cells from performing their normal inhibitory function within the CNS and causes most parkinsonian symptoms.

(See *Neurotransmitter action in PD*, page 224.)

Important signs of PD include:

- Muscle rigidity results in resistance to passive muscle stretching, which may be uniform (lead-pipe rigidity) or jerky (cogwheel rigidity).

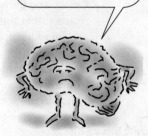

A deficiency of dopamine isn't good news...

Now I get it!

Neurotransmitter action in PD

Degeneration of the dopaminergic neurons and loss of available dopamine lead to rigidity, tremors, and bradykinesia.

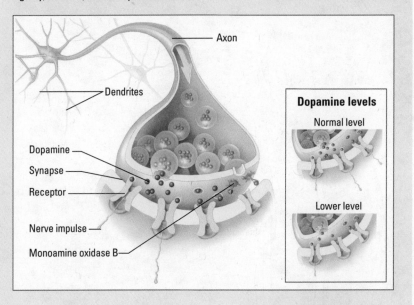

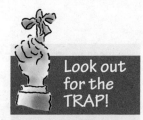

Look out for the TRAP!

Use **TRAP** to remember the classic symptoms of PD:

Tremor

Rigidity

Akinesia

Postural instability

- Akinesia causes gait and movement disturbances. The patient walks with their body bent forward, takes a long time initiating movement when performing a purposeful action, pivots with difficulty, and easily loses their balance. Gait is often described as shuffling, and decreased arm swing may be evident. Akinesia may also cause other signs, which include:
  - masklike facial expression
  - blepharospasm, in which the eyelids stay closed
- "Pill-roll" tremor is insidious. It begins in the fingers, increases during stress or anxiety, and decreases with purposeful movement and sleep. (See *Treating PD*, page 225.)

And there's more

Other signs and symptoms of PD include:
- a high-pitched, monotone voice
- drooling

Treating PD

Treatment for PD aims to relieve symptoms and keep the patient functional as long as possible. It consists of drugs, physical therapy, and stereotactic neurosurgery in extreme cases.

Looking at levodopa and other drugs

Levodopa, dopamine agonists, monoamine oxidase-B (MAO-B) inhibitors, and catechol-o-methyltransferase (COMT) inhibitors are the pharmacological therapies used in PD. Levodopa and dopamine agonists are used to replace the dopamine that is insufficient in the brain. Levodopa is combined with an agent called carbidopa. Carbidopa delays conversion of levodopa into dopamine in peripheral nerves so that more will remain in the CNS. Dopamine agonists include ropinirole and pramipexole; these agents mimic dopamine action. MAO-B inhibitors and COMT inhibitors block the enzyme that breaks down dopamine so that more will remain in the neuron synapses. A variety of medications is necessary in PD because over time, individuals commonly require more frequent levodopa doses (e.g., every 2-3 hours), in addition to higher doses, until it is ineffective.

Anticholinergics may control tremor and rigidity and may also be used in combination with levodopa. Other medications include antihistamines, which may help decrease tremors because of their central anticholinergic and sedative effects, and amantadine, an antiviral agent, is used early in treatment to reduce rigidity, tremors, and akinesia (Parkinson's disease, 2017).

Deep brain stimulation

In the past, pallidotomy and thalamotomy were the only available surgical options. However, deep brain stimulation is now the preferred surgical option. With deep brain stimulation, electrodes are implanted into the targeted brain area. These electrodes are connected to wires attached to an impulse generator that's implanted under the collarbone. The electrodes control symptoms on the opposite side of the body by sending electrical impulses to the brain.

Physical therapy

Physical therapy helps maintain the patient's normal muscle tone and function. It includes both active and passive range-of-motion exercises, routine daily activities, walking, and baths and massage to help relax muscles.

- dysarthria (impaired speech due to a disturbance in muscle control)
- dysphagia (difficulty swallowing)
- fatigue
- muscle cramps in the legs, neck, and trunk
- oily skin
- increased perspiration
- insomnia
- mood changes

Getting complicated

Common complications of PD include injury from falls, food aspiration due to impaired swallowing, urinary tract infections, and skin breakdown due to increased immobility.

What tests tell you

Diagnosis of PD is based on the patient's age, history, and signs and symptoms, so laboratory tests are generally of little value. However, urinalysis may reveal decreased dopamine levels, and CT scan or MRI may rule out other disorders such as intracranial tumors.

Stroke

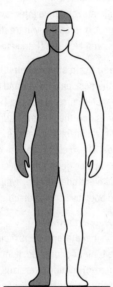

Right-brain damage
(stroke on right side of the brain)

- Paralyzed left side: hemiplegia
- Left-sided neglect
- Spatial-perceptual deficits
- Tends to deny or minimize problems
- Rapid performance, short attention span
- Impulsive, safety problems
- Impaired judgment
- Impaired concept of time

Left-brain damage
(stroke on left side of the brain)

- Paralyzed right side: hemiplegia
- Impaired speech/language aphasias
- Impaired right/left discrimination
- Slow performance, cautious
- Aware of deficits: depression, anxiety
- Impaired comprehension related to language, math

Previously known as *cerebrovascular accident (CVA)*, stroke or cerebral infarct is a sudden impairment of cerebral circulation in one or more of the blood vessels supplying the brain. It interrupts or diminishes oxygen supply, causing serious damage or necrosis in brain tissues. A stroke can be due to either of two processes:

- **Ischemic stroke:** A thrombus or clot lodges in a cerebral artery and causes cerebral ischemia, which becomes cerebral infarction (brain cell death). This is the more common type of stroke; it occurs in 87% of persons experiencing stroke.
- **Hemorrhagic stroke:** A cerebral arterial vessel ruptures, causing a cerebral hemorrhage. This type of stroke is less common, occurring in 13% of persons experiencing stroke. Brain cell death is due to the lack of circulation because of the discontinuous arterial flow, the large mass created by the hemorrhage, and the toxic damage caused to surrounding cells by the hemorrhagic blood.

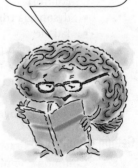

Oh, no! Says here that in stroke, circulation is impaired in the vessels that supply me with blood.

The sooner, the better

Stroke is the leading cause of long-term disability. The sooner circulation returns to normal after a stroke, the better chances are for complete recovery. Quick treatment is critical, and symptoms require emergency care.

Statistically speaking

The CDC reports that in 2020, 1 in 6 deaths from cardiovascular disease was due to stroke. Every 40 seconds, someone in the United States has a stroke. Every 3.5 minutes, someone dies of stroke. Every year, more than 795,000 people in the United States have a stroke. About 610,000 of these are first or new strokes. Although strokes mostly affect older adults, they can strike people of any age. Black adults are more likely to die from stroke than other than other population groups.

Transient ischemic attacks

A transient ischemic attack (TIA) is caused by a temporary interruption of blood flow, usually in the carotid and vertebrobasilar arteries. Although this is similar to ischemic stroke, with TIA the patient recovers circulation and has no neurological deficit. (See *Understanding TIA*.)

Act FAST!

Remember to act FAST when you see signs of a stroke:

Face drooping

Arm weakness

Speech difficulty

Time to call 911

Now I get it!

Understanding TIA

A transient ischemic attack (TIA) is a recurrent episode of neurologic deficit, lasting from seconds to hours, that clears within 12 to 24 hours. This is usually considered a warning sign of an impending thrombotic stroke. In fact, more than a third of people who have a TIA do not seek treatment, and as many as 10% to 15% will have a major stroke within 3 months of a TIA.

Interrupting blood flow
In TIA, microemboli released from a thrombus may temporarily interrupt blood flow, especially in the small distal branches of the brain's arterial tree. Small spasms in those arterioles may precede TIA and also impair blood flow.

A transient experience
The most distinctive characteristics of TIAs are the transient duration of neurologic deficits and the complete return of normal function. The signs and symptoms of TIA correlate with the location of the affected artery. They include double vision, unilateral blindness, staggering or uncoordinated gait, unilateral weakness or numbness, falling because of weakness in the legs, dizziness, and speech deficits, such as slurring or thickness.

Preventing a complete stroke
During an active TIA, treatment aims to prevent a completed stroke and consists of aspirin (or other antiplatelet medications) or anticoagulants to minimize the risk of thrombosis. After or between attacks, preventive treatment includes carotid endarterectomy or cerebral microvascular bypass.

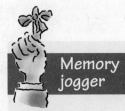

Memory jogger

Here are some key points to remember about **TIAs**:

Temporary episode that clears within 12 to 24 hours

Impending stroke in near future (TIA is considered a warning sign for this possibility)

Aspirin and Anticoagulant given during a TIA may minimize the risk of thrombosis

How it happens

Factors that increase the risk of stroke include:

- history of TIA
- atherosclerosis
- hypertension
- arrhythmias, especially atrial fibrillation
- carotid artery stenosis (arteriosclerosis of the carotid artery)
- rheumatic heart disease
- diabetes mellitus
- orthostatic hypotension
- cardiac enlargement
- high serum triglyceride levels
- lack of exercise
- hormonal contraceptive use
- drug misuse
- smoking
- family history of cerebrovascular disease
- sickle cell disease

Ranking stroke causes

The top three causes of stroke are:

1. thrombosis (clot): The majority of strokes (87%) are ischemic and happen when blood flow to the brain is blocked by a clot that lodges in a cerebral artery, most commonly the middle cerebral artery. The risk increases with obesity, arteriosclerosis, diabetes, atrial fibrillation, carotid stenosis, smoking, hormonal contraceptive use, and sedentary lifestyle.
2. embolism (traveling clot): Similar to thrombotic ischemic strokes, an embolism is caused by a thrombus. However, the thrombus is traveling in the bloodstream from another site and lodges in the middle cerebral artery. This type of stroke can occur at any age, especially in patients with a history of rheumatic heart disease, endocarditis, valvular disease, carotid stenosis, atrial fibrillation, or other cardiac arrhythmias. It can also occur after open-heart surgery. Embolism usually develops rapidly—in 10 to 20 seconds—and without warning. (See *Ischemic stroke*, page 229.)
3. hemorrhage (ruptured cerebral artery): May also occur suddenly at any age. It arises from chronic hypertension or aneurysms, which cause a sudden rupture of a cerebral artery. Increasing cocaine use by younger people has also increased the number of hemorrhagic strokes because of the severe hypertension caused by this drug. Other causes include trauma, brain tumors, and coagulation disorders.

Now I get it!

Ischemic stroke

The illustrations below show common sites of cardiac thrombosis and the resulting sites of embolism and infarction.

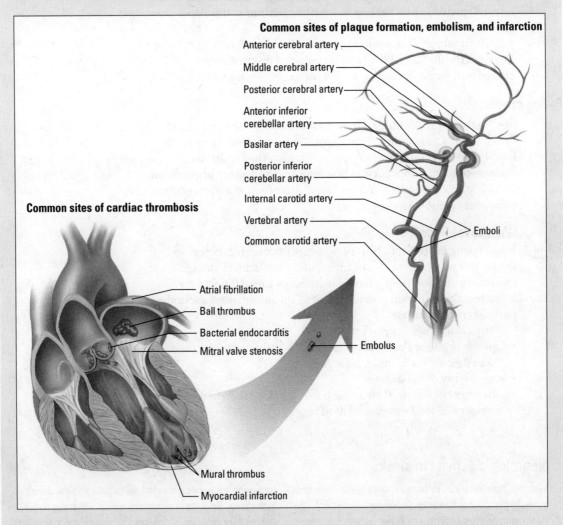

Common sites of plaque formation, embolism, and infarction

Anterior cerebral artery

Middle cerebral artery

Posterior cerebral artery

Anterior inferior cerebellar artery

Basilar artery

Posterior inferior cerebellar artery

Internal carotid artery

Vertebral artery

Common carotid artery

Emboli

Embolus

Common sites of cardiac thrombosis

Atrial fibrillation

Ball thrombus

Bacterial endocarditis

Mitral valve stenosis

Mural thrombus

Myocardial infarction

Damage report

Thrombosis, embolus, and hemorrhage affect the body in different ways.

Thrombosis causes congestion and edema in the affected vessel as well as ischemia in the brain tissue supplied by the vessel. Ischemia can progress to cerebral infarction, which is death of brain tissue.

An embolus is a traveling thrombus that cuts off circulation in the cerebral vasculature by lodging in a narrow portion of the artery, causing ischemia and edema.

In hemorrhage, a brain artery bursts, diminishing blood supply to the area served by the artery. Blood also accumulates deep within the brain, causing even greater damage by further compromising neural tissue.

Getting complicated

Among the many possible complications of stroke are neurological deficit (loss of motor and sensory function in extremities), unstable blood pressure from loss of vasomotor control, fluid imbalances, malnutrition, infections such as pneumonia, and sensory impairment, including vision problems. Altered LOC, aspiration, contractures, and pulmonary emboli may also occur.

What to look for

When taking the patient's history, you may uncover risk factors for stroke. You may observe loss of consciousness, dizziness, or seizures. Obtain information from a family member or friend if necessary. Neurologic examination provides most of the information about the physical effects of stroke.

Physical findings depend on:
- the artery affected and the portion of the brain it supplies (See *Neurologic deficits in stroke*, page 230.)
- the severity of the damage
- the extent of collateral circulation that develops to help the brain compensate for a decreased blood supply

Neurologic deficits in stroke

In stroke, functional loss reflects damage to the brain area normally perfused by the occluded or ruptured artery. The most common artery affected by either ischemic or hemorrhagic stroke is the middle cerebral artery. In stroke, the affected parts of the body are on the opposite side (also called contralateral side) of where the stroke occurs in the brain. A left cerebral hemisphere stroke causes right-sided neurological deficit in the body. A right cerebral hemisphere stroke causes left-sided neurological deficit in the body. Severity of symptoms varies. Whereas one patient may experience only mild hand weakness, another may develop hemiparesis (weakness) or hemiplegia (paralysis). Hypoxia and ischemia may produce edema that affects surrounding areas of the brain, causing further neurologic deficits. The signs and symptoms that accompany stroke at different sites are described below.

Neurologic deficits in stroke *(continued)*

Site	Signs and symptoms
Middle cerebral artery (most common site of stroke)	• Aphasia (speech difficulty; most commonly if stroke occurs in left hemisphere) • Facial droop • Dysphagia (lack of swallow and gag reflex) • Visual field cuts • Hemiparesis or hemiplegia (paralysis) on the contralateral side of the body; often arm is affected worse than leg • Sensory loss on the contralateral side of the body (face, arm, and leg)
Internal carotid artery	• Headaches • Weakness • Paralysis • Numbness • Sensory changes • Monocular visual disturbance or loss • Altered level of consciousness • Bruits over the carotid artery • Aphasia • Dysphasia • Ptosis
Anterior cerebral artery	• Confusion • Weakness • Numbness on the affected side (especially in the arm) • Paralysis of the contralateral foot and leg with accompanying foot drop • Incontinence • Poor coordination • Impaired motor and sensory functions • Personality changes, such as flat affect and distractibility
Vertebral or basilar artery	• Mouth and lip numbness • Dizziness • Weakness on the affected side • Vision deficits, such as color blindness, lack of depth perception, and diplopia • Poor coordination • Dysphagia • Slurred speech • Amnesia • Ataxia
Posterior cerebral artery	• Visual field cuts • Sensory impairment • Dyslexia • Coma • Blindness from ischemia in the occipital area

Reflecting on reflexes

Assessment of motor function and muscle strength commonly shows a loss of voluntary muscle control and hemiparesis or hemiplegia on one side of the body. In the initial phase, flaccid paralysis with decreased deep tendon reflexes may occur. These reflexes return to normal after the initial phase, accompanied by an increase in muscle tone and, in some cases, muscle spasticity on the affected side.

Sensory impairment: Slight to severe

Vision testing usually reveals reduced vision or blindness on the affected side of the body and, in patients with left-sided hemiplegia, problems with visual-spatial relations. Sensory assessment may reveal sensory losses, ranging from slight impairment of touch to the inability to perceive the position and motion of body parts. The patient also may have difficulty interpreting visual, tactile, and auditory stimuli.

Whose side are you on, anyway?

If the stroke occurs in the brain's left hemisphere, it produces signs and symptoms on the right side of the body. If it occurs in the right hemisphere, signs and symptoms appear on the left side. In the majority of individuals, speech is controlled by the left cerebral hemisphere; therefore stroke affecting the left side of the brain commonly causes aphasia (speech difficulty). (See *Treating stroke*, page 232.)

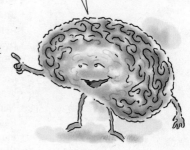

Remember that my right hemisphere controls the left side of the body and my left hemisphere controls the right side of the body.

What tests tell you

These tests are used to diagnose stroke:

- A CT scan is the imaging test that should be done as soon as possible after a patient demonstrates symptoms of stroke. It can differentiate between an ischemic stroke and hemorrhagic stroke, and it can detect structural abnormalities, edema, and lesions, infarction, and aneurysms. It differentiates stroke from other disorders, such as primary metastatic tumor and subdural, intracerebral, or epidural hematoma. Patients with TIA commonly have a normal CT scan.
- Cerebral angiography details disruption or displacement of the cerebral circulation by occlusion or hemorrhage. It's the test of choice for examining the entire cerebral circulation.
- Digital subtraction angiography evaluates the patency of the cerebral vessels and identifies their position in the head and neck. It also detects and evaluates lesions and vascular abnormalities.

Battling illness

Treating stroke

Medical treatment for stroke commonly includes physical rehabilitation, dietary and drug regimens to help decrease risk factors, and measures to help the patient adapt to specific deficits, such as speech impairment and paralysis.

Drug therapy
Drugs commonly used for stroke therapy include:
• thrombolytic therapy such as recombinant tissue plasminogen activator given within the first 3 hours of an ischemic stroke to dissolve the thrombus, restore circulation of the affected brain tissue, and limit the extent of brain injury
• anticonvulsants such as phenytoin (Dilantin) to treat or prevent seizures
• stool softeners to avoid straining, which increases intracranial pressure
• corticosteroids such as dexamethasone to minimize cerebral edema
• anticoagulants, such as heparin, warfarin (Coumadin), and ticlopidine, to reduce the risk of development of clots
• analgesics such as codeine to relieve headache that may follow hemorrhagic stroke

Surgery
Depending on the stroke's cause and extent, the patient may also undergo surgery. A craniotomy may be done to remove a hematoma, an endarterectomy to remove atherosclerotic plaque from the inner arterial wall, or extracranial-intracranial bypass to circumvent an artery that's blocked by occlusion or stenosis. Ventricular shunts may be necessary to drain cerebrospinal fluid if hydrocephalus occurs.

• A PET scan provides data on cerebral metabolism and cerebral blood flow changes, especially in ischemic stroke.
• Single-photon emission computed tomography identifies cerebral blood flow and helps diagnose cerebral infarction.
• MRI and magnetic resonance angiography evaluate the lesion's location and size. MRI doesn't distinguish hemorrhage, tumor, or infarction as well as a CT scan, but it provides superior images of the cerebellum and brain stem.
• Transcranial Doppler studies evaluate the velocity of blood flow through major intracranial vessels, which can indicate the vessels' diameter.
• Cerebral blood flow studies measure blood flow to the brain and help detect abnormalities.
• Ophthalmoscopy may show signs of hypertension and atherosclerotic changes in the retinal arteries.
• EEG may detect reduced electrical activity in an area of cortical infarction and is especially useful when CT scan results are inconclusive. It can also differentiate seizure activity from stroke.

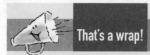
That's a wrap!

Neurologic system review

Understanding the neurologic system
The neurologic system is the body's communication network. It coordinates and organizes the functions of all other body systems. There are two divisions of this network:
• The CNS, made up of the brain and spinal cord, is the body's control center.
• The PNS, containing cranial and spinal nerves, provides communication between the CNS and remote body parts.

CNS
• Protects the brain and spinal cord by the skull and vertebrae, cerebrospinal fluid, and three membranes—the dura mater, the arachnoid mater, and the pia mater
• Houses the nerve center, called the *cerebrum*, that controls sensory and motor activities and intelligence
• Transmits impulses to and from the cerebrum by the thalamus and maintains connections to the brain, spinal cord, autonomic nervous system, and pituitary gland by the hypothalamus
• Coordinates muscle movements, controls posture, and maintains equilibrium by the cerebellum and the brain stem
• Relays sensations that are needed for voluntary or reflex motor activity through the spinal cord

PNS
• Originates in 31 pairs of spinal nerves arranged in segments and attached to the spinal cord
• Divided into the somatic nervous system, which regulates voluntary motor control, and the autonomic nervous

system, which helps to regulate the body's internal environment through involuntary control of the organ systems

Neurologic disorders
• *Alzheimer disease (AD)*—progressive degenerative disorder of the cerebral cortex
• *Amyotrophic lateral sclerosis (ALS)*—most common of the motor neurodegenerative diseases; causes progressive muscular weakness and atrophy
• *Bell palsy*—a disorder characterized by impairment of the facial nerve (cranial nerve VII) on one side and in the absence of any other condition such as stroke
• *Epilepsy*—brain condition characterized by recurrent seizures
• *Guillain-Barré syndrome (GBS)*—acute, rapidly progressive, potentially fatal syndrome that's associated with segmented demyelination of the peripheral nerves
• *Multiple sclerosis (MS)*—results from progressive demyelination of the white matter of the brain and spinal cord, leading to widespread neurologic dysfunction
• *Meningitis*—condition that causes inflammation of the brain and spinal cord meninges
• *Migraine*—a recurring unilateral headache with throbbing pain, with or without aura
• *Myasthenia gravis*—condition that produces sporadic, progressive weakness and abnormal fatigue of the voluntary skeletal muscles
• *Parkinson disease (PD)*—produces progressive muscle rigidity, loss of muscle movement, and involuntary tremors
• *Stroke*—sudden impairment of cerebral circulation in one or more of the blood vessels supplying the brain

Quick quiz

1. What physiologic changes cause the symptoms associated with multiple sclerosis (MS)?
   A. Decreased dopamine in the central nervous system (CNS)
   B. Demyelination of nerve fibers in the CNS
   C. The development of neurofibril webs in the CNS
   D. Reduced amounts of acetylcholine at the neuromuscular junction

Answer: B. Symptoms are dependent on the extent and site of demyelination of the nerve fibers.

2. A patient has left-sided weakness of the upper and lower extremities. Symptoms lasted less than an hour and resolved. The patient most likely experienced a(n):
   A. hemorrhagic stroke.
   B. transient ischemic attack.
   C. episode of hypertension.
   D. stroke caused by an embolism.

Answer: B. A transient ischemic attach (TIA) is often short in duration and patients may not experience any residual effects.

3. Brudzinski sign and Kernig sign are two tests that help diagnose which neurologic disorder?
   A. Stroke
   B. Meningitis
   C. Epilepsy
   D. ALS

Answer: B. A positive response to one or both tests indicates meningeal irritation seen with meningitis.

4. MS is characterized by:
   A. progressive demyelination of the white matter of the CNS.
   B. impairment of cerebral circulation.
   C. deficiency of the neurotransmitter dopamine.
   D. beta-amyloid plaques.

Answer: A. Patches of demyelination cause widespread neurologic dysfunction.

Scoring

☆☆☆   If you answered all four items correctly, unbelievable! Your dedication to dendrites and dopamine is downright unnerving.

☆☆   If you answered four items correctly, congratulations! We are honored to extend congratulations not only to you but to both lobes of your cerebrum.

☆   If you answered fewer than four items correctly, stay cool. We'll just chalk it up to one of those "lapses in the synapses."

Suggested references

Aguilar-Shea A. L., Membrilla Md J. A., & Diaz-de-Teran J. (2022). Migraine review for general practice. *Aten Primaria, 54*(2), 102208. https://doi.org/10.1016/j.aprim.2021.102208

Alzheimer's Association. (2023). *Alzheimer's disease facts and figures.* https://www.alz.org/alzheimers-dementia/facts-figures

American Association of Neurological Surgeons. (2023). *Epilepsy.* (Accessed on October 6, 2023). https://www.aans.org/en/Patients/Neurosurgical-Conditions-and-Treatments/Epilepsy

American Heart Association. (2023). *Age-adjusted total stroke mortality rates by race/ethnicity.* https://www.heart.org/en/about-us/2024-health-equity-impact-goal/age-adjusted-total-stroke-mortality-rates-by-raceethnicity

Amyotrophic Lateral Sclerosis (ALS). (Accessed on October 6, 2023). https://www.ninds.nih.gov/health-information/disorders/amyotrophic-lateral-sclerosis-als

Andrews J.A., Jackson C. E., Heiman-Patterson T. D., Bettica P., Brooks B. R., & Pioro E. P. (2020). Real-world evidence of riluzole effectiveness in treating amyotrophic lateral sclerosis. *Amyotroph Lateral Scler Frontotemporal Degener, 21*(7–8), 509–518. https://doi.org/10.1080/21678421.2020.1771734

Armstrong M. J., & Okun M. S. (2020). Diagnosis and treatment of Parkinson disease: A review. *JAMA, 323*(6), 548–560. https://doi.org/10.1001/jama.2019.22360

Breijyeh Z., & Karaman R. (2020). Comprehensive review on Alzheimer's disease: Causes and treatment. *Molecules (Basel, Switzerland), 25*(24), 5789. https://doi.org/10.3390/molecules25245789

Centers for Disease Control and Prevention. (2022). *Alzheimer's disease.* https://www.cdc.gov/dotw/alzheimers/index.html

Centers for Disease Control and Prevention (CDC). (2020). *Epilepsy.* https://www.cdc.gov/epilepsy/data/index.html

Centers for Disease Control and Prevention (CDC). (2021). *Meningococcal vaccination.* https://www.cdc.gov/vaccines/vpd/mening/index.html

Centers for Disease Control and Prevention (CDC). (2022a). *Meningitis.* (Accessed on October 6, 2023). https://www.cdc.gov/meningitis/index.html

Centers for Disease Control and Prevention (CDC). (2022b). *National amyotrophic lateral sclerosis registry.* https://www.cdc.gov/als/researchpublications/2022/Publication_PrevalenceMet2017.html

Centers for Disease Control and Prevention (CDC). (2022c). *Amyotrophic lateral sclerosis*. https://www.cdc.gov/als/WhatisALS.html

Centers for Disease Control and Prevention (CDC). (2022d). *Stroke facts*. https://www.cdc.gov/stroke/facts.htm

Dresser L., Wlodarski R., Rezania K., & Soliven B. (2021). Myasthenia gravis: Epidemiology, pathophysiology and clinical manifestations. *Journal of Clinical Medicine, 10*(11), 2235. https://doi.org/10.3390/jcm10112235

van Dyck C. H., Swanson C. J., Aisen P., Bateman R. J., Chen C., Gee M., Kanekiyo M., Li D., Reyderman L., Cohen S., Froelich L., Katayama S., Sabbagh M., Vellas B., Watson D., Dhadda S., Irizarry M., Kramer L. D., & Iwatsubo T. (2023). Lecanemab in early Alzheimer's disease. *The New England Journal of Medicine, 388*(1), 9–21. https://doi.org/10.1056/NEJMoa2212948

Feldman E. L., Goutman S. A., Petri S., Mazzini L., Savelieff M. G., Shaw P. J., & Sobue G. (2022). Amyotrophic lateral sclerosis. *Lancet (London, England), 400*(10360), 1363–1380. https://doi.org/10.1016/S0140-6736(22)01272-7

Ferrari M. D., Goadsby P. J., Burstein R., Kurth T., Ayata C., Charles A., Ashina M., van den Maagdenberg A. M. J. M., & Dodick D. W. (2022). Migraine. *Nature Reviews Disease Primers, 8*(1), 2. https://doi.org/10.1038/s41572-021-00328-4

Florian I. A., Lupan I., Sur L., Samasca G., & Timiş T. L. (2021). To be, or not to be… Guillain-Barré Syndrome. *Autoimmunity Reviews, 20*(12), 102983. https://doi.org/10.1016/j.autrev.2021.102983

Goutman S. A., Hardiman O., Al-Chalabi A., Chió A., Savelieff M. G., Kiernan M. C., & Feldman E. L. (2022). Recent advances in the diagnosis and prognosis of amyotrophic lateral sclerosis. *The Lancet Neurology, 21*(5), 480–493. https://doi.org/10.1016/S1474-4422(21)00465-8

Guez-Barber D., Swami S. K., Harrison J. B., & McGuire J. L. (2022). Differentiating Bell's palsy from Lyme-related facial palsy. *Pediatrics, 149*(6), e2021053992. https://doi.org/10.1542/peds.2021-053992

Herpich F., & Rincon F. (2020). Management of acute ischemic stroke. *Critical Care Medicine, 48*(11), 1654–1663. https://doi.org/10.1097/CCM.0000000000004597

Kline L. B., Kates M. M., & Tavakoli M. (2021). Bell palsy. *Journal of the American Medical Association, 326*(19), 1983. https://doi.org/10.1001/jama.2021.18504

Kohil A., Jemmieh S., Smatti M. K., & Yassine H. M. (2021). Viral meningitis: An overview. *Archives of Virology, 166*(2), 335–345. https://doi.org/10.1007/s00705-020-04891-1

Lei P., Ayton S., & Bush A. I. (2021). The essential elements of Alzheimer's disease. *Journal of Biological Chemistry, 296*, 100105. https://doi.org/10.1074/jbc.REV120.008207

Leone M., Iqbal A., Hugo Bonatti J. R., Anwar S., & Feaga C. (2022). A patient with SIADH, urinary retention, constipation, and Bell's palsy following a tick bite. *Case Reports in Nephrology, 2022*, 5937131. https://doi.org/10.1155/2022/5937131

Mayo clinic health system. (2021). *What are the stages of migraine headache?* https://www.mayoclinichealthsystem.org/hometown-health/speaking-of-health/what-are-the-stages-of-a-migraine

Montaño A., Hanley D. F., & Hemphill J. C. III. (2021). Hemorrhagic stroke. *Handbook of Clinical Neurology, 176*, 229–248. https://doi.org/10.1016/B978-0-444-64034-5.00019-5

Morren J. A., & Li Y. (2023). Myasthenia gravis: Frequently asked questions. *Cleve Clin J Med, 90*(2), 103–113. https://doi.org/10.3949/ccjm.90a.22017

National Institutes of Health (NIH). National institute of neurological disorders and stroke. (2023). *Migraine.* (Accessed on October 6, 2023). https://www.ninds.nih.gov/health-information/disorders/migraine

National Institutes of Health (NIH). National Institute of Neurological Disorders and Stroke. (2021). Amyotrophic lateral sclerosis (ALS) fact sheet. https://www.ninds.nih.gov/amyotrophic-lateral-sclerosis-als-fact-sheet

National Institutes of Health (NIH). National Institute of Neurological Disorders and Stroke. (2023a). *Myasthenia gravis.* (Accessed October 6, 2023). https://www.ninds.nih.gov/health-information/disorders/myasthenia-gravis

National Institutes of Health (NIH). National Institute of Neurological Disorders and Stroke. (2023b). *Multiple sclerosis.* (Accessed October 6, 2023). https://www.ninds.nih.gov/health-information/disorders/multiple-sclerosis

Norris T. (2025). *Porth's pathophysiology: Concepts of altered health states* (11th ed.). Wolters Kluwer.

Pacheco A., Rutler O., Valenzuela I., Feldman D., Eskin B., & Allegra J. R. (2020). Positive tests for Lyme disease and emergency department visits for Bell's palsy patients. *J Emerg Med, 59*(6), 820–827. https://doi.org/10.1016/j.jemermed.2020.07.038

Parkinson's Foundation. (2023). *Parkinson's disease statistics.* https://www.parkinson.org/understanding-pakinsons/statistics

Patrick L., & Halabi C. (2022). Inpatient management of acute stroke and transient ischemic attack. *Neurologic Clinics, 40*(1), 33–43. https://doi.org/10.1016/j.ncl.2021.08.003

Quinn C., & Elman L. (2020). Amyotrophic lateral sclerosis and other motor neuron diseases. *Continuum (Minneapolis, Minn.), 26*(5), 1323–1347. https://doi.org/10.1212/CON.0000000000000911

Scheltens P., De Strooper B., Kivipelto M., Holstege H., Chételat G., Teunissen C. E., Cummings J., & van der Flier W. M. (2021). Alzheimer's disease. *Lancet (London, England), 397*(10284), 1577–1590. https://doi.org/10.1016/S0140-6736(20)32205-4

Sever B., Ciftci H., DeMirci H., Sever H., Ocak F., Yulug B., Tateishi H., Tateishi T., Otsuka M., Fujita M., & Başak A. N. (2022). Comprehensive research on past and future therapeutic strategies devoted to treatment of amyotrophic lateral sclerosis. *International Journal of Molecular Sciences, 23*(5), 2400. https://doi.org/10.3390/ijms23052400

Silva M. V. F., Loures C. d. M. G., Alves L. C. V., de Souza L. C., Borges K. B. G., & Carvalho M. D. G. (2019). Alzheimer's disease: Risk factors and potentially protective measures. *Journal of Biomedical Science, 26*(1), 33. https://doi.org/10.1186/s12929-019-0524-y

Simon D. K., Tanner C. M., & Brundin P. (2020). Parkinson disease epidemiology, pathology, genetics, and pathophysiology. *Clinics in Geriatric Medicine, 36*(1), 1–12. https://doi.org/10.1016/j.cger.2019.08.002

Strayer D. Saffitz J., & Rubin E. (2020). *Rubin's pathology: Mechanisms of human disease* (8th ed.). Wolters Kluwer.

Thijs R. D., Surges R., O'Brien T. J., & Sander J. W. (2019). Epilepsy in adults. *Lancet (London, England)*, *393*(10172), 689–701. https://doi.org/10.1016/S0140-6736(18)32596-0

Tolosa E., Garrido A., Scholz S. W., & Poewe W. (2021). Challenges in the diagnosis of Parkinson's disease. *Neurology*, *20*(5), 385–397. https://doi.org/10.1016/S1474-4422(21)00030-2

Wall E. C., Chan J. M., Gil E., & Heyderman R. S. (2021). Acute bacterial meningitis. *Current Opinion in Neurology*, *34*(3), 386–395. https://doi.org/10.1097/WCO.0000000000000934

Witzel S., Maier A., Steinbach R., Grosskreutz J., Koch J. C., Sarikidi A., Petri S., Günther R., Wolf J., Hermann A., Prudlo J., Cordts I., Lingor P., Löscher W. N., Kohl Z., Hagenacker T., Ruckes C., Koch B., Spittel S., for the German Motor Neuron Disease Network (MND-NET). Safety and effectiveness of long-term intravenous administration of edaravone for treatment of patients with amyotrophic lateral sclerosis. *JAMA Neurology*, 2022;79(2):121–130. https://doi.org/10.1001/jamaneurol.2021.4893

Yang Q., Tong X., Schieb L., Coronado F., & Merritt R. (2023). Stroke mortality among black and white adults aged ≥35 Years before and during the COVID-19 pandemic—United States, 2015–2021. *MMWR Morbidity and Mortality Weekly Report*, *72*(16), 431–436.

Chapter 7

Gastrointestinal system*

Just the facts

In this chapter, you'll learn:

♦ the structures of the gastrointestinal system and related organs

♦ how the gastrointestinal system functions

♦ pathophysiology, signs and symptoms, diagnostic tests, and treatments for common gastrointestinal disorders.

Understanding the gastrointestinal system

The gastrointestinal (GI) system is the body's food processing complex. It performs the critical task of supplying essential nutrients to fuel the other organs and body systems.

The GI system has two major components. They include:

1. the GI tract, or alimentary canal
2. the accessory glands and organs

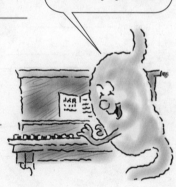

I'm a key player in the GI system, where food is processed into fuel for other organs and body systems.

A GI-ant sphere of influence

A malfunction along the GI tract or in one of the accessory glands or organs can produce far-reaching metabolic effects, which may become life-threatening. (See *A close look at the GI system.*)

GI tract

The GI tract is basically a hollow, muscular tube, approximately 30 feet (9 m) long, that extends from the mouth to the anus. It includes the:

• mouth
• esophagus
• stomach
• small intestine

---

*Note: In this chapter, the term "male" refers to a person assigned male at birth, and the term "female" refers to a person assigned female at birth.

A close look at the GI system

This illustration shows the organs of the GI tract and several accessory organs. The GI tract also includes the mouth and epiglottis.

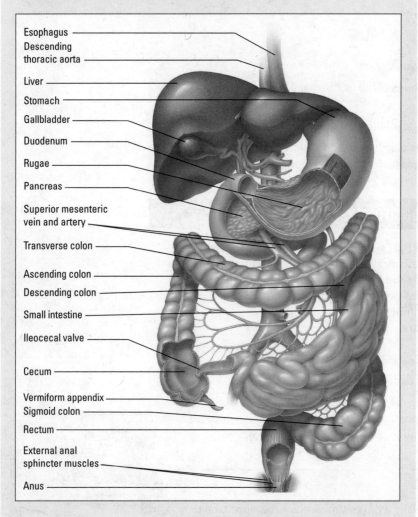

Esophagus
Descending thoracic aorta
Liver
Stomach
Gallbladder
Duodenum
Rugae
Pancreas
Superior mesenteric vein and artery
Transverse colon
Ascending colon
Descending colon
Small intestine
Ileocecal valve
Cecum
Vermiform appendix
Sigmoid colon
Rectum
External anal sphincter muscles
Anus

- large intestine
- anus

Mouth and esophagus

When a person smells, tastes, chews, or merely thinks of food, the digestive system gets ready to go to work.

It begins with the first bite

The digestive process begins in the mouth. Chewing and salivation soften food, making it easy to swallow. An enzyme in saliva called *ptyalin* begins to convert starches to sugars even before food is swallowed.

Riding the peristaltic wave

When a person swallows, the upper esophageal sphincter relaxes, allowing food to enter the esophagus. In the esophagus, peristaltic waves activated by the glossopharyngeal nerve propel food toward the stomach.

Stomach

Digestion occurs in two phases:
1. cephalic phase
2. gastric phase

Phase 1: Break it down

By the time food is traveling through the esophagus on its way to the stomach, the cephalic phase of digestion has begun. In this phase, the stomach secretes hydrochloric acid and pepsin, digestive juices that help break down food.

Phase 2: Set the stomach on start

The gastric phase of digestion begins when food passes the cardiac sphincter, which is a circle of muscle at the end of the esophagus. The food exits the esophagus and enters the stomach, causing the stomach wall to distend. This stimulates the mucosal lining of the stomach to release the hormone gastrin. Gastrin serves two purposes:
• stimulation of gastric juice secretion
• stimulation of the stomach's motor functions

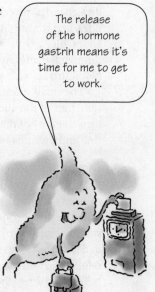

The release of the hormone gastrin means it's time for me to get to work.

Gastric juice, a perfect complement to every meal

Gastric juice secretions are highly acidic, with a pH of about 2. In addition to hydrochloric acid and pepsin, the gastric juices contain intrinsic factor (which helps the body absorb vitamin B_{12}) and proteolytic enzymes (which help the body use protein). The gastric juices mix with the food, which becomes a thick, gruel-like material called *chyme*.

Hold it, mix it, and empty it out

The stomach has three major motor functions:
• holding food
• mixing food by peristaltic contractions with gastric juices
• slowly emptying chyme into the small intestine for further digestion and absorption

Small intestine

Nearly all digestion takes place in the small intestine, which is about 20 feet (6 m) long. Chyme passes through the small intestine and is propelled by peristaltic contractions.

The small intestine has three major sections:
1. the duodenum
2. the jejunum
3. the ileum

Dedicated to the duodenum

The duodenum is a 10-in (25.4-cm) long, C-shaped curve of the small intestine that extends from the stomach. Food passes from the stomach to the duodenum through a narrow opening called the *pylorus*.

The duodenum also has an opening through which bile and pancreatic enzymes enter the intestine to neutralize the acidic chyme and aid digestion. This opening is called the *sphincter of Oddi*.

Just a jejunum? It's the longest part!

The jejunum extends from the duodenum and forms the longest portion of the small intestine. The jejunum leads to the ileum, the narrowest portion of the small intestine.

Let's move these nutrients (and nonnutrients) along

In the ileum, carbohydrates are broken down into monosaccharides and disaccharides, proteins are degraded further into amino acids and peptides, and fats are emulsified and reduced to fatty acids and monoglycerides. Along with water and electrolytes, these nutrients are absorbed through the intestinal mucosa into the bloodstream for use by the body. Nonnutrients such as vegetable fibers are carried through the intestine.

The small intestine ends at the ileocecal valve, located in the lower right part of the abdomen. The ileocecal valve is a sphincter that controls the flow of digested material from the ileum into the large intestine and prevents reflux into the small intestine.

Large intestine

After chyme passes through the small intestine, it enters the ascending colon at the cecum, the pouchlike beginning of the large intestine. By this time, the chyme consists of mostly indigestible material. Off the cecum is small fingerlike projection called the *appendix*. The appendix is not used in digestion but can fill with some of the indigestible material (such as cellulose). From the ascending colon, chyme passes through the transverse colon, then down through the descending colon to the sigmoid colon, and then to the rectum and anal canal, where it's finally expelled.

Superabsorbent

The large intestine produces no hormones or digestive enzymes. Rather, it's where absorption takes place. The large intestine absorbs nearly all of the water remaining in the chyme plus large amounts of sodium and chloride.

The large intestine also harbors the bacteria *Escherichia coli*, *Enterobacter aerogenes*, *Clostridium welchii*, and *Lactobacillus bifidus*, which help produce vitamin K and break down cellulose into usable carbohydrates. These bacteria are part of the normal flora of the body (also called the *microbiome*) and are extremely important.

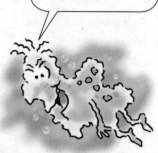

Yeah, it's true. I'm a useful bacterium that hangs out in the large intestine.

Joining a mass movement

In the lower part of the descending colon, long, relatively sluggish contractions cause propulsive waves known as *mass movements*. These movements propel the intestinal contents into the rectum and produce the urge to defecate.

Accessory glands and organs

The liver, gallbladder, and pancreas contribute several substances (such as enzymes, bile, and hormones) that are vital to the digestion of chyme. These structures deliver their secretions to the duodenum through the ampulla of Vater. (See *Accessory GI organs and vessels*.)

Liver

A large, highly vascular organ, the liver is enclosed in a fibrous capsule in the upper right area of the abdomen (often referred to as the right upper quadrant [RUQ] of the abdomen).

No problem with multitasking

The liver performs many complex and important functions, many of which are related to digestion and nutrition:
- It filters and detoxifies blood, removing foreign substances, such as drugs, alcohol, and other toxins.
- It removes naturally occurring ammonia from body fluids, converting it to urea for excretion in urine.
- It produces plasma proteins such as albumin, nonessential amino acids, and vitamin A.
- It synthesizes cholesterol using a key enzyme (HMG-CoA reductase) and has low-density lipoprotein cholesterol (LDL-C) receptors that process LDL cholesterol.
- It stores essential nutrients, such as iron and vitamins K, D, and B_{12}.
- It produces bile to aid digestion.
- It converts glucose to glycogen and stores it as fuel for the muscles.
- It stores fats and converts excess sugars to fats for storage in other parts of the body.

Gallbladder

The gallbladder is a small, pear-shaped organ nestled under the liver and joined to the larger organ by the cystic duct. The gallbladder's job is to store and concentrate bile produced by the liver. Bile is a clear

Accessory GI organs and vessels

Accessory GI organs include the liver, gallbladder, and pancreas, as well as their blood vessels.

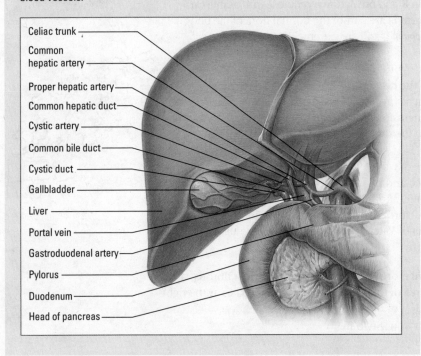

Celiac trunk
Common hepatic artery
Proper hepatic artery
Common hepatic duct
Cystic artery
Common bile duct
Cystic duct
Gallbladder
Liver
Portal vein
Gastroduodenal artery
Pylorus
Duodenum
Head of pancreas

yellowish liquid that helps break down fats and neutralize gastric secretions in the chyme.

You have a delivery

Secretion of the hormone cholecystokinin (CCK) causes the gallbladder to contract and the ampulla of Vater to relax. This allows the release of bile into the common bile duct for delivery to the duodenum. When the ampulla of Vater closes, bile shunts to the gallbladder for storage. Bile accumulates in the gall bladder; it can become static and allow cholesterol to precipitate out of solution to create cholesterol gallstones.

Pancreas

The pancreas lies behind the stomach, with its head and neck extending into the curve of the duodenum and its tail lying against the spleen.

The pancreas is made up of two types of tissue:
- exocrine tissue, from which enzymes are secreted through ducts to the digestive system. Pancreatic exocrine enzymes include proteases (which break down proteins), amylase (which breaks down carbohydrates), and lipase (which breaks down fats). Bicarbonate

is also secreted by the pancreas (which is an alkaline substance that neutralizes acid).
- endocrine tissue, from which hormones are secreted into the blood. Pancreatic endocrine hormones include insulin (which allows glucose to enter cells) and glucagon (which stimulates the liver to break down stored sugar, termed *glycogen*).

An expert analysis…

The pancreas's exocrine function involves acinar cells, which are divided into spherical lobules. These specialized cells are the delivery system for enzymes and alkaline fluids (e.g., bicarbonate), which aid in digestion. These lobules of enzyme-producing cells release their secretions into small ducts that merge to form the pancreatic duct. The pancreatic duct runs the length of the pancreas and joins the bile duct from the gallbladder before entering the duodenum. Vagus nerve stimulation and the release of two intestinal hormones (secretin and CCK) control the rate and amount of pancreatic secretion.

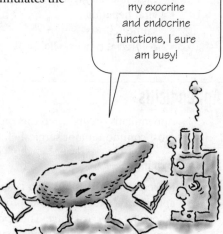

Between my exocrine and endocrine functions, I sure am busy!

…along with an enlightened look

The endocrine function of the pancreas involves the islets of Langerhans, specific groups of cells scattered throughout the pancreas. Over 1 million islets house two major cell types:
- Alpha cells secrete glucagon, a hormone that stimulates glucose breakdown in the liver. Glucagon is released in response to hypoglycemia (low blood sugar).
- Beta cells secrete insulin to promote carbohydrate metabolism. Insulin is released when the body senses a rise in blood glucose (hyperglycemia).

    Both hormones flow directly into the blood; their release is mediated by blood glucose levels.

GI disorders

The disorders discussed in this section include:
- appendicitis
- cholecystitis
- cirrhosis
- esophageal and gastric varices
- Crohn disease
- celiac disease
- diverticular disease
- gastroesophageal reflux disease (GERD)
- hiatal hernia

- irritable bowel syndrome (IBS)
- pancreatitis
- peptic ulcer
- ulcerative colitis
- *Clostridium difficile* infection
- viral hepatitis
- salmonellosis
- colorectal cancer (CRC)

Appendicitis

Appendicitis occurs when the appendix becomes inflamed. It's the most common major surgical emergency.

Let's get specific

More precisely, this disorder is an inflammation of the vermiform appendix, a small, fingerlike projection attached to the cecum just below the ileocecal valve. The appendix is referred to as a vestigial organ; this means it no longer has a function in the body. However, it can become obstructed with resulting inflammation.

Appendicitis is the most common abdominal surgical emergency. The reported lifetime risk of appendicitis in the United States is 8.6% in males and 6.7% in females, with an annual incidence of 90 to 100 cases per 100,000 adults.

How it happens

Appendicitis can result from an obstruction—for instance, from a fecal mass or indigestible material such as cellulose. It can also develop when an infection from bacteria, viruses, fungi, or parasites causes the tissues of the appendix wall to swell.

Apprehending appendicitis

After infection occurs, appendicitis progresses this way:
- Inflammation accompanies the infection and temporarily obstructs the appendix.
- Obstruction, if present, is usually caused by stool accumulation around vegetable fibers (cellulose) (*fecalith* is a fancy name for this). (See *Appendix obstruction and inflammation*.)
- Mucus outflow is blocked, which distends the organ.
- Pressure within the appendix increases, and the appendix contracts.
- Bacteria multiply and inflammation and pressure continue to increase, affecting blood flow to the organ and causing severe abdominal pain.

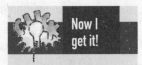

Appendix obstruction and inflammation

This illustration shows a fecal obstruction in the lumen of the appendix with resulting inflammation.

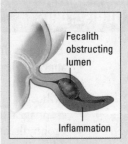

Fecalith obstructing lumen

Inflammation

Getting complicated

Inflammation can lead to infection, clotting, tissue decay, and perforation of the appendix. If the appendix ruptures or perforates, the infected contents spill into the abdominal cavity, causing peritonitis, the most common and dangerous complication.

What to look for

The history and sequence of pain are important in diagnosing appendicitis. The first symptom is almost always vague epigastric pain, sometimes described as a cramping sensation. Over the next 24 hours, the pain becomes more localized and moves to the right lower abdominal area toward the right hip. This is termed *right lower quadrant* (RLQ) pain, and the region of pain is called *McBurney point*. If the appendix is in back of the cecum or in the pelvis, the patient may have flank tenderness instead of abdominal tenderness.

Other signs and symptoms include:

- anorexia
- nausea or vomiting
- low-grade fever
- rebound tenderness on palpation
- lack of appetite

The patient usually wants to remain as still as possible, because any sudden movement causes abdominal pain due to irritation of the peritoneal membrane. Clinical signs of acute appendicitis include:

- Psoas sign is discomfort felt by the patient by hyperextension of the leg.
- Obturator sign is discomfort felt by the patient on the slow internal movement of the hip joint, while the right knee is flexed.

These are physical assessment signs that indicate an inflamed pelvic appendix that is in contact with the obturator and psoas muscle.

Rupture!

In cases of rupture, spasm will occur, sometimes followed by a brief cessation of abdominal pain. Untreated appendicitis is invariably fatal. In recent times, the use of antibiotics has reduced the incidence of death from appendicitis. (See *Treating appendicitis*.)

What tests tell you

These tests are sometimes helpful in diagnosis, but normal findings for these don't rule out appendicitis:

- White blood cell (WBC) count is moderately high with an increased number of immature cells, although levels can be normal in some patients with appendicitis
- Ultrasound of abdomen and pelvis
- Computed tomography (CT) scan of abdomen and pelvis

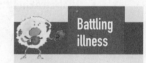

Battling illness

Treating appendicitis

Appendectomy (surgical removal of the inflamed appendix) or antibiotic treatment can be used as an effective treatment for appendicitis. If peritonitis develops, appendectomy, parenteral replacement of fluids and electrolytes, and antibiotic administration are necessary.

Cholecystitis

In cholecystitis, the gallbladder becomes inflamed. Usually, a gallstone becomes lodged in the cystic duct, causing painful gallbladder distention.

In the United States, gallbladder disease affects approximately 20 million people, and acute cholecystitis is diagnosed in approximately 200,000 people each year. Gallstone-associated cystic duct obstruction is responsible for 90% to 95% of the cases of acute cholecystitis.

How it happens

Cholecystitis is caused by the formation of calculi called *gallstones*. Gallstones are deposits—small stones that form from bile, a fluid that helps digestion. There are two major types of gallstones: *pigment stones*, which contain an excess of unconjugated pigments in the bile, and *cholesterol stones* (the more common form), which result from bile supersaturated with cholesterol.

Galling risks

Risk factors that predispose a person to gallstones include:
- obesity and a high-calorie, high-cholesterol diet
- increased estrogen levels from hormonal contraceptives, hormone therapy, or pregnancy
- use of clofibrate, an antilipemic drug
- diabetes mellitus, ileal disease, blood disorders, liver disease, or pancreatitis.

The foundation stone

In acute cholecystitis, inflammation of the gallbladder wall usually develops after a gallstone lodges in the cystic duct. To get to the intestine, bile flows into the cystic duct and then into the common bile duct. When bile flow is blocked, pressure backs up, and the gallbladder becomes inflamed and distended. This causes RUQ abdominal pain. Tenderness over the RUQ is felt by the patient when the abdomen is palpated. The pain in the RUQ is called *Murphy sign*. Bacterial growth, usually *E. coli*, may contribute to the inflammation. (See *Understanding gallstone formation.*)

Then this sequence of events takes place:
- Edema of the gallbladder or cystic duct occurs.
- Edema obstructs bile flow, which chemically irritates the gallbladder.
- Cells in the gallbladder wall may become oxygen starved and die as the distended organ presses on vessels and impairs blood flow.
- Dead cells slough off.
- An exudate covers ulcerated areas, causing the gallbladder to adhere to surrounding structures.

Now I get it!

Understanding gallstone formation

Abnormal metabolism of cholesterol and bile salts plays an important role in gallstone formation. Bile is made continuously by the liver and is concentrated and stored in the gallbladder until the duodenum needs it to help digest fat. Changes in the composition of bile may allow gallstones to form. Changes to the absorptive ability of the gallbladder lining may also contribute to gallstone formation.

Too much cholesterol
Certain conditions, such as age, obesity, and estrogen imbalance, cause the liver to secrete bile that's abnormally high in cholesterol or lacking the proper concentration of bile salts.

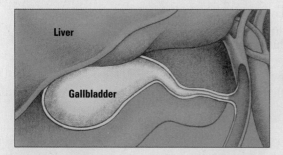

Inside the gallbladder
When the gallbladder concentrates this bile, inflammation may occur. Excessive water and bile salts are reabsorbed, making the bile less soluble. Cholesterol, calcium, and bilirubin precipitate into gallstones. Cholesterol stones are the most common type of gallstones.

Fat entering the duodenum causes the intestinal mucosa to secrete the hormone CCK, which stimulates the gallbladder to contract and empty. If a stone lodges in the cystic duct, the gallbladder contracts but can't empty.

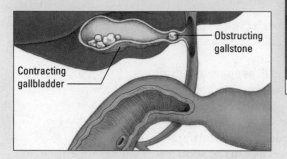

Jaundice, irritation, inflammation
If a stone lodges in the common bile duct, the bile flow into the duodenum becomes obstructed. Bilirubin is absorbed into the blood, causing jaundice.

Biliary narrowing and swelling of the tissue around the stone can also cause irritation and inflammation of the common bile duct.

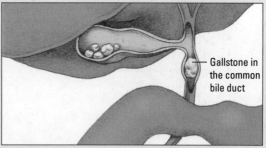

Up the biliary tree
Inflammation can progress up the biliary tree and cause cholangitis, which is inflammation of the common bile duct.

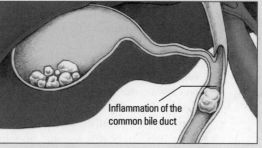

Getting complicated

Cholecystitis may lead to complications:

- Pus may accumulate in the gallbladder.
- Fluid may accumulate in the gallbladder (hydrops).
- The gallbladder may become distended with mucus secretions (mucocele).
- Gangrene may occur, leading to perforation, peritonitis, abnormal passages in the tissues (fistulas), and pancreatitis.
- Chronic cholecystitis may develop.
- Cholangitis (bile duct inflammation) may develop.

What to look for

Signs and symptoms of acute cholecystitis usually strike after meals that are rich in fats and may occur at night, suddenly awakening the patient. They include:

- acute abdominal pain in the RUQ that may radiate to the back, between the shoulders, or to the front of the chest
- colic (spasmodic pain of the abdomen) due to passage of gallstones along the bile duct (biliary colic)
- pain that worsens during deep inspiration
- pain that lasts more than 6 hours, particularly after meals
- belching
- flatulence
- indigestion
- nausea
- vomiting
- low-grade fever
- jaundice (caused by bile in the blood) and clay-colored stools, if a stone obstructs the common bile duct

Older adults with cholecystitis may not have fever or pain. Their only symptom may be a tender area in the abdomen.

With treatment, the prognosis of cholecystitis and surgical cholecystectomy is good. (See *Treating cholecystitis*.)

What tests tell you

These tests are used to diagnose cholecystitis:

- X-rays reveal gallstones if they contain enough calcium to be radiopaque and also help disclose porcelain gallbladder, limy bile, and gallstone ileus.
- Ultrasonography confirms gallstones as small as 2 mm and distinguishes between obstructive and nonobstructive jaundice.
- Oral cholecystography confirms the presence of gallstones, although this test is gradually being replaced by ultrasonography.
- Technetium-labeled scan indicates cystic duct obstruction and acute or chronic cholecystitis if the gallbladder can't be seen.

Treating cholecystitis

Treatment of cholecystitis is mainly determined by the severity of the inflammation. Common surgical approaches include:
• gallbladder removal (cholecystectomy), most commonly by laparotomy

Alternatives to surgery
Other invasive procedures include:
• insertion of a flexible catheter through a sinus tract into the common bile duct and removal of stones using a basket-shaped tool guided by fluoroscopy
• endoscopic retrograde cholangiopancreatography, which removes stones with a balloon or basket-shaped tool passed through an endoscope
• lithotripsy, which breaks up gallstones with ultrasonic waves (contraindicated in patients with pacemakers or implantable defibrillators)

Diet, drugs, and more
Other treatments include:
• a low-fat diet with replacement of vitamins A, D, E, and K and administration of bile salts to facilitate digestion and vitamin absorption
• opioids to relieve pain during an acute attack
• antispasmodic and anticholinergic agents to relax smooth muscles and decrease ductal tone and spasm
• antiemetics to reduce nausea and vomiting
• cholestyramine if the patient has obstructive jaundice with severe itching from accumulation of bile salts in the skin

• Percutaneous transhepatic cholangiography, performed with fluoroscopy, supports the diagnosis of obstructive jaundice and reveals calculi in the ducts.
• Blood studies may reveal high levels of serum alkaline phosphatase, lactate dehydrogenase, aspartate aminotransferase, and total bilirubin. The icteric index, a measure of bilirubin in the blood, is elevated. Bilirubin is a yellow substance that stains skin and sclera (whites of the eyes); this condition is called *jaundice* or *icterus*.
• WBC count is slightly elevated during a cholecystitis attack.

Cirrhosis

Cirrhosis, a chronic liver disease, is characterized by widespread destruction of hepatic cells, which are replaced by fibrous cells (causing scarring of the liver).

Cirrhosis is currently the ninth leading cause of death in the United States. Approximately 51,000 deaths annually in the United States can be attributed to cirrhosis. The most common causes of cirrhosis are alcohol misuse, viral hepatitis (hepatitis B virus [HBV] and hepatitis C virus [HCV]), and nonalcoholic fatty liver disease (NAFLD).

- **NAFLD:** About 100 million individuals in the United States are estimated to have NAFLD. NAFLD is an underdiagnosed disease; numbers are difficult to estimate. NAFLD has more than doubled in incidence over the last 20 years and is linked to being overweight or obese. A high-fat diet and cellular insulin resistance (in which the cells do not respond to insulin) are both causes of NAFLD.
- **Hepatitis:** Approximately 862,000 people in the United States are living with chronic, long-term HBV, and about 2.4 million people are living with chronic, long-term HCV.

How it happens

There are many types of cirrhosis, each with a different cause. The most common include the following:

- Laënnec cirrhosis, also called *portal*, *nutritional*, or *alcoholic cirrhosis*, stems from chronic alcohol use disorder and malnutrition. It's most prevalent among males who are malnourished and who have alcohol use disorder and accounts for more than one-half of all cirrhosis cases in the United States. Many people who are dependent on alcohol never develop the disease; however, others develop it even with adequate nutrition.
- Postnecrotic cirrhosis is usually a complication of viral hepatitis (inflammation of the liver), but it may also occur after exposure to liver toxins. HBV and HCV are leading causes of chronic liver disease. Both HBV and HCV can cause necrotic cirrhosis and hepatocellular carcinoma. Treatment of HCV has been highly successful with oral antiviral drugs that prevent hepatocellular carcinoma. There is a vaccine to prevent HBV; however, treatment is challenging once the disease is present.
- Biliary cirrhosis results from prolonged bile duct obstruction or inflammation.
- Idiopathic cirrhosis may develop in some patients with no known cause.
- NAFLD develops as a result of fatty deposits in the liver over time; it is often seen in people with diabetes mellitus and obese populations, and it is more prevalent in females.
- Nonalcoholic steatohepatitis (NASH) is caused by excess fat in the liver and poor diet. NASH is much more serious than NAFLD. NASH indicates that the liver has fatty changes and has undergone inflammation.

In Laënnec cirrhosis, malnutrition, lack of protein, and misuse of alcohol cause me harm.

No turning back

Cirrhosis is characterized by irreversible chronic injury of the liver, extensive fibrosis, and nodular tissue growth. These changes result from:
- liver cell death (hepatocyte necrosis)
- collapse of the liver's supporting structure (the reticulin network)
- distortion of the vascular bed (blood vessels throughout the liver)
- nodular regeneration of remaining liver tissue (See *Cirrhotic changes in the liver.*)

Getting complicated

When the liver begins to malfunction, blood clotting disorders (coagulopathies), jaundice, edema, and various metabolic problems develop.

Fibrosis and the distortion of blood vessels may impede blood flow in the capillary branches of the portal vein and hepatic artery, leading to portal hypertension (elevated pressure in the portal vein). Increased pressure may lead to the development of esophageal and gastric varices.

Now I get it!

Cirrhotic changes in the liver

The illustration below shows the nodular changes that occur in cirrhosis.

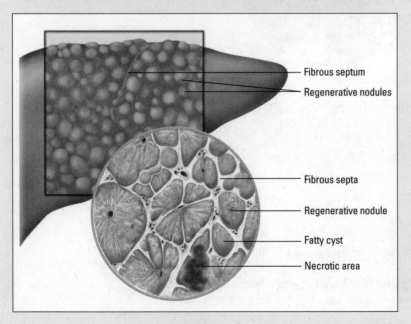

- Fibrous septum
- Regenerative nodules
- Fibrous septa
- Regenerative nodule
- Fatty cyst
- Necrotic area

Esophageal and gastric varices: The engorging truth

Esophageal varices are enlarged, tortuous veins in the lower part of the esophagus. Esophageal varices may easily rupture and leak large amounts of blood into the upper GI tract. They can also bleed slowly over time, with a clinical presentation of coffee-ground emesis, or melena. Gastric varices occur at the top of the stomach, near the esophagus. Approximately 50% of patients with cirrhosis develop esophageal varices, and high-risk varices, which are more likely to rupture and cause GI bleeding, occur in 9% to 36% of patients. The process starts when portal hypertension (high pressure in the portal vein of the liver) develops. With this increase in pressure, varicose veins (varices) can develop in the esophagus and sometimes in the stomach. When pressures become too high, there is an increase in blood flow to these large, engorged veins, and rupture can occur, creating a medical emergency. See *Treating cirrhosis* for treatment of esophageal varices.

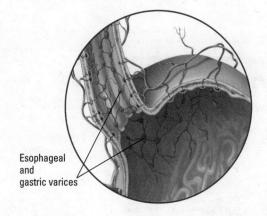

Esophageal
and
gastric varices

What to look for

Early signs and symptoms of cirrhosis are vague but usually include the following:

- loss of appetite
- indigestion
- nausea
- vomiting
- diarrhea
- dull abdominal ache
- jaundice
- bruising easily (because the liver is not producing adequate coagulation factors)
- bilirubin backs up into the blood because it is not being processed (this yellow substance causes jaundice, staining the skin and sclera yellow)

Later signs and symptoms of cirrhosis include the following:

- Hepatomegaly (enlarged liver) due to venous congestion because of portal vein hypertension
- Esophageal varices due to portal vein hypertension can cause GI bleeding and hematemesis (vomiting of blood)
- Accumulation of ammonia in the bloodstream that can cause mental changes such as confusion, lethargy, and stupor; it can also cause sweat and saliva to have an odor
- Ascites, which is fluid in the peritoneal cavity, that can cause swelling of the abdomen
- Bile acids that accumulate and cause pruritus of the skin
- Hormones such as estrogen are not metabolized adequately, causing (in females) amenorrhea and (in males) infertility, gynecomastia, and testicular atrophy
- Renal failure can occur

The final act

Late-stage signs and symptoms affect several body systems and include:

- respiratory effects—fluid in the lungs and weak chest expansion, leading to hypoxia
- central nervous system effects—lethargy, mental changes, slurred speech, asterixis (a motor disturbance marked by intermittent lapses in posture), and peripheral nerve damage
- hematologic effects—nosebleeds, easy bruising, bleeding gums
- endocrine effects—testicular atrophy, menstrual irregularities, gynecomastia, and loss of chest and axillary hair
- skin effects—severe itching and dryness, poor tissue turgor, abnormal pigmentation, and spider veins
- hepatic effects—jaundice, enlarged liver (hepatomegaly), fluid in the abdomen (ascites), and edema
- renal effects—insufficiency that may progress to failure
- miscellaneous effects—musty breath, enlarged superficial abdominal veins, muscle atrophy, pain in the upper right abdominal quadrant that worsens when the patient sits up or leans forward, palpable liver or spleen, temperature of 101° to 103°F (38.3° to 39.4°C), and bleeding from esophageal varices. (See *Treating cirrhosis.*)

What tests tell you

These tests help confirm cirrhosis:

- Liver biopsy, the definitive test, reveals tissue destruction (necrosis) and fibrosis.
- Abdominal x-ray shows liver size, cysts or gas within the biliary tract or liver, liver calcification, and massive fluid accumulation (ascites).

Treating cirrhosis

Therapy for cirrhosis aims to remove or alleviate the underlying cause, prevent further liver damage, and prevent or treat complications.

Drug therapy

Drug therapy requires special caution because the cirrhotic liver can't detoxify harmful substances efficiently. These drugs include:
• vitamins and nutritional supplements to help heal damaged liver cells and improve nutritional status (thiamine is especially important)
• antacids to reduce gastric distress and decrease the potential for GI bleeding
• diuretics such as furosemide to reduce fluid accumulation
• beta-blockers to treat portal hypertension and reduce pressure on esophageal varices.

Noninvasive procedures

To control bleeding from esophageal varices or other GI hemorrhage, two measures are attempted first:
• In gastric intubation, the stomach is lavaged until the contents are clear. Antacids and histamine antagonists are then administered if the bleeding is caused by a gastric ulcer.
• In esophageal balloon tamponade, bleeding vessels are compressed to stop blood loss from esophageal varices.

Esophagogastroduodenoscopy

• Variceal band ligation can be performed during an esophagogastroduodenoscopy (EGD) prophylactically or during acute bleeding to tie off the vessels to stop the bleeding. During this procedure, a scope is passed into the esophagus and a rubber band is used to cut off circulation to the vessel causing the varix to fall off. This creates a banding ulcer, which heals creating scars, and no new varices can form through the scar tissue. Banding an acutely bleeding varix can cut off the blood supply, which stops the bleeding.

Surgery

In patients with ascites, paracentesis may be used to relieve abdominal pressure. A shunt may be inserted to divert ascites into venous circulation. This treatment causes weight loss, decreased abdominal girth, increased sodium excretion from the kidneys, and improved urine output.

Sclerotherapy

If conservative treatment fails to stop GI hemorrhaging from esophageal varices, a sclerosing agent is injected into the oozing vessels to cause clotting and sclerosis. If bleeding from the varices doesn't stop in 2 to 5 minutes, a second injection is given below the bleeding site. Sclerotherapy also may be performed on nonbleeding varices to prevent hemorrhaging.

Radiologic intervention

A radiologic procedure known as *transjugular intrahepatic portosystemic shunt* may be performed. During this procedure, a shunt is placed between the portal vein and the hepatic vein. The procedure reduces pressure in the varices, preventing them from bleeding.

Last resort

As a last resort, portosystemic shunts may be inserted during surgery to control bleeding from esophageal varices and decrease portal hypertension. These shunts divert a portion of the portal vein blood flow away from the liver. This procedure is seldom performed because it can cause bleeding, infection, and shunt thrombosis. Massive hemorrhage requires blood transfusions to maintain blood pressure.

- CT and liver scans show liver size, abnormal masses, and hepatic blood flow and obstruction.
- EGD reveals bleeding esophageal varices, stomach irritation or ulceration, or duodenal bleeding and irritation.
- Blood studies show elevated liver enzymes, total serum bilirubin, and indirect bilirubin levels. Total serum albumin and protein levels decrease; prothrombin time (PT) is prolonged; hemoglobin, hematocrit, and serum electrolyte levels decrease; and vitamins A, C, and K are deficient. Blood ammonia (NH_3) levels may be elevated.
- Urine studies show increased levels of bilirubin and urobilinogen.
- Fecal studies show decreased fecal urobilinogen levels.

Crohn disease

Crohn disease is one of the two major types of inflammatory bowel disease. It may affect any part of the GI tract. Inflammation extends through all layers of the intestinal wall and may involve lymph nodes and supporting membranes in the area. Ulcers form as the inflammation extends into the peritoneum.

Crohn disease commonly peaks during two age ranges. Crohn disease may occur between the ages of 15 and 30 years, and then later in the lifespan, prevalence increases again in patients aged 60 to 70 years with females more commonly affected during this age range. In the United States, the prevalence is estimated at 100 to 300 per 100,000 people, and incidence is increasing.

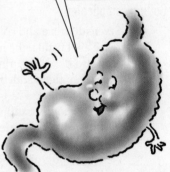

In Crohn disease, severe inflammation can occur in any part of the GI tract.

What's in a name?

When Crohn disease affects only the small bowel, it's known as *regional enteritis*. When it involves the colon or only affects the colon, it's known as *Crohn disease of the colon*. Crohn disease of the colon is sometimes called *granulomatous colitis*; however, not all patients develop granulomas (tumorlike masses of granulation tissue).

How it happens

Current research indicates that Crohn disease is caused by an interplay between genetic susceptibility and environmental factors. A genetic factor that increases risk has been identified (see *NOD2 mutation*). Environmental factors associated with increased risk include smoking, oral contraceptive use, chronic antibiotic use, frequent use of nonsteroidal anti-inflammatory drugs (NSAIDs), and urban environment.

Comprehending Crohn

In Crohn disease, inflammation spreads slowly and progressively. Here's what happens:

- Lymph nodes enlarge and lymph flow in the submucosa is blocked.
- Lymphatic obstruction causes edema, mucosal ulceration, fissures, abscesses, and sometimes granulomas. Mucosal ulcerations are called *skipping lesions* because they aren't continuous as in ulcerative colitis.
- Oval, elevated patches of closely packed lymph follicles—called *Peyer patches*—develop on the lining of the small intestine.
- Fibrosis occurs, thickening the bowel wall and causing stenosis, or narrowing of the lumen. (See *Changes to the bowel in Crohn disease.*)
- Inflammation of the serous membrane (serositis) develops, inflamed bowel loops adhere to other diseased or normal loops, and diseased bowel segments become interspersed with healthy ones.
- Eventually, diseased parts of the bowel become thicker, narrower, and shorter.

The genetic link

NOD2 mutation

Genetic factors may play a major role in Crohn disease. Crohn disease sometimes occurs in identical twins, and 10% to 20% of patients with the disease have one or more affected relatives. People with the *NOD2* gene mutation have a 20- to 40-fold increased risk of developing Crohn disease.

Getting complicated

Severe diarrhea and corrosion of the perineal area by enzymes can cause anal fistula, the most common complication. A perineal abscess may also develop during the active inflammatory state. Fistulas may develop to the bladder, vagina, or even skin in an old scar area. (See *Treating Crohn disease.*)

Other complications include:

- intestinal obstruction
- nutrient deficiencies caused by malabsorption of bile salts and vitamin B_{12} and poor digestion
- fluid imbalances
- rarely, inflammation of abdominal linings (peritonitis)

What to look for

Initially, the patient experiences malaise and diarrhea, usually with pain in the RLQ or generalized abdominal pain and fever.

Chronic diarrhea results from bile salt malabsorption, loss of healthy intestinal surface area, and bacterial growth. Weight loss, nausea, and vomiting also occur. Stools may be bloody.

What tests tell you

These tests and results support a diagnosis of Crohn disease:

- Fecal occult test shows blood in stools.
- Small bowel x-ray shows irregular mucosa, ulceration, and stiffening.

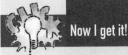

Now I get it!

Changes to the bowel in Crohn disease

As Crohn disease progresses, fibrosis thickens the bowel wall and narrows the lumen. Narrowing—or stenosis—can occur in any part of the intestine and cause varying degrees of intestinal obstruction. At first, the mucosa may appear normal, but as the disease progresses, it takes on a "cobblestone" appearance as shown below.

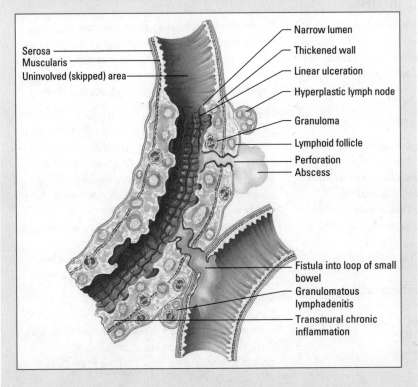

- Barium enema reveals the string sign (segments of stricture separated by normal bowel) and may also show fissures, ulceration, and narrowing of the bowel.
- Sigmoidoscopy and colonoscopy show patchy areas of inflammation, which helps rule out ulcerative colitis. The mucosal surface has a cobblestone appearance. When the colon is involved, ulcers may be seen. Colonoscopy is more accurate than barium enema in assessing the degree of inflammation.
- Biopsy performed during sigmoidoscopy or colonoscopy reveals granulomas in up to one-half of all specimens.

Laboratory tests indicate increased WBC count and erythrocyte sedimentation rate (ESR), both of which suggest infection or inflammation. Other findings include decreased potassium, calcium, magnesium, and hemoglobin levels in the blood.

Battling illness

Treating Crohn disease

Treatment for Crohn disease requires drug therapy, lifestyle changes, and, sometimes, surgery. During acute attacks, maintaining fluid and electrolyte balance is the key. Debilitated patients need total parenteral nutrition to provide adequate calories and nutrition while resting the bowel.

Drug therapy
These drugs combat inflammation and relieve symptoms:
• Corticosteroids such as prednisone reduce diarrhea, pain, and bleeding by decreasing inflammation.
• Immunosuppressants such as azathioprine, methotrexate, and mercaptopurine suppress the body's response to antigens.
• Aminosalicylates such as sulfasalazine and mesalamine reduce inflammation.
• Metronidazole treats perianal complications.
• Antidiarrheals such as diphenoxylate and atropine combat diarrhea but aren't used in patients with significant bowel obstruction.
• Opioids control pain and diarrhea.
• Biologic agents:

— Infliximab, adalimumab, or certolizumab block the inflammatory mediator tumor necrosis factor (TNF) and can be used to treat moderate to severe disease.
— Vedolizumab and ustekinumab inhibit integrins, which are other inflammatory mediators that cause damage.

Lifestyle changes
Stress reduction and reduced physical activity rest the bowel and allow it to heal. Vitamin supplements compensate for the bowel's inability to absorb vitamins. Dietary changes decrease bowel activity while still providing adequate nutrition. The foods usually eliminated include:
• fruits, vegetables, and other high-fiber foods
• dairy products, spicy and fatty foods, and other foods and liquids that irritate the mucosa
• carbonated or caffeinated beverages and other foods or liquids that stimulate excessive intestinal activity

Surgery
Surgery is necessary if bowel perforation, massive hemorrhage, fistulas, or acute intestinal obstruction develop. Colectomy with ileostomy is performed in patients with extensive disease of the large intestine and rectum.

Celiac disease

Celiac disease, also called *gluten-sensitive enteropathy*, is an autoimmune disease caused by antibodies that are stimulated by the ingestion of gluten. Gluten is a protein in wheat, rye, and barley. When gluten is ingested, antibodies attack the intestinal lining, and injury occurs to the epithelial cells of the small intestine. Over time, this leads to the villi in the small intestine flattening out from inflammation, which inhibits their capacity for absorption of nutrients. Celiac disease presently affects approximately one percent of the United States' population, or around three million individuals.

The symptoms

Celiac disease symptoms and severity can vary. One of the determining factors for onset and severity of symptoms is the age at which a patient was first exposed to gluten. Symptoms can be broken into two categories: those occurring in the GI system and those occurring outside of the gut. GI symptoms include:

* diarrhea, abdominal pain and distention, vomiting, anorexia, and constipation
    Extraintestinal symptoms include:
* fatigue, weight loss or failure to grow, delayed puberty, dermatitis herpetiformis, dental enamel hypoplasia, arthritis, osteoporosis, fractures, and neurologic manifestations such as ataxia, neuropathy, and seizures

Making the diagnosis

Celiac disease can be diagnosed through serologic testing. A blood sample is taken and is tested to determine if autoantibodies are present. The sample is tested against tissue transglutaminase IgA, anti-endomysium IgA, and deamidated gliadin peptides. If these studies come back positive, the patient undergoes an EGD to obtain a biopsy of the small intestine. Biopsy confirms the diagnosis and shows the damage within the intestine.

Getting complicated

The major complications of celiac disease relate to vitamin and nutritional deficiencies caused by the malabsorption. Those include hypoprothrombinemia, caused by vitamin K malabsorption, iron and folic acid deficiencies, and vitamin B_{12} deficiency. Patients can also experience loss of bone density. There are three types of cancer associated with celiac disease: enteropathy-associated T-cell lymphoma, non-Hodgkin lymphoma, and adenocarcinoma of the small intestine. It is important to remember, however, that developing cancer due to celiac disease is quite rare.

Let's get treated

Currently, there is only one treatment for celiac disease and that is strict adherence to a gluten-free diet. After approximately 2 years, most patients will have a complete remission of the disease and reversal of damage. Foods that contain gluten include those with wheat, rye, barley, and malt. Those ingredients are also often found in medications, cosmetics, and other products and should be avoided. Patients should be careful when dining out to ensure that food is prepared without gluten, as a small exposure could cause a flare.

Diverticular disease

Diverticular disease is a common problem that affects males and females equally. The risk of disease increases with age. Diverticular disease occurs throughout the world but is more common in developed countries, in which the incidence has increased over time. This suggests that environmental and lifestyle factors may play a role in the development of the disease.

The highs and lows of dietary fiber

One contributing factor may be low intake of dietary fiber. High-fiber diets increase stool bulk, which decreases the wall tension in the colon. High wall tension is thought to increase the risk of developing diverticula.

Diverticula domiciles

In diverticular disease, bulging pouches (diverticula) in the GI wall push the mucosal lining through the surrounding muscle. Although the most common site of diverticula is in the sigmoid colon, they may develop anywhere, from the proximal end of the pharynx to the anus. Other typical sites include the duodenum, near the pancreatic border or the ampulla of Vater, and the jejunum.

Diverticular disease has two clinical forms:

- diverticulosis, in which diverticula are present but don't cause symptoms
- diverticulitis, in which diverticula are inflamed and may cause potentially fatal obstruction, infection, or hemorrhage

How it happens

Diverticula likely result from high intraluminal pressure on an area of weakness in the GI wall, where blood vessels enter. Diet may be a contributing factor because insufficient fiber reduces fecal residue, narrows the bowel lumen, and leads to high intra-abdominal pressure during defecation.

Diverticular sacs under attack

In diverticulitis, retained undigested food and bacteria accumulate in the diverticular sac. This hard mass cuts off the blood supply to the thin walls of the sac, making them more susceptible to attack by colonic bacteria. Inflammation follows and may lead to perforation, abscess, peritonitis, obstruction, or hemorrhage. (See *Diverticulitis of the colon*.)

We can cause lots of trouble if we find some undigested food in a diverticular sac.

Now I get it!

Diverticulitis of the colon

In diverticulitis, retained undigested food and bacteria accumulate in the diverticular sac as shown below.

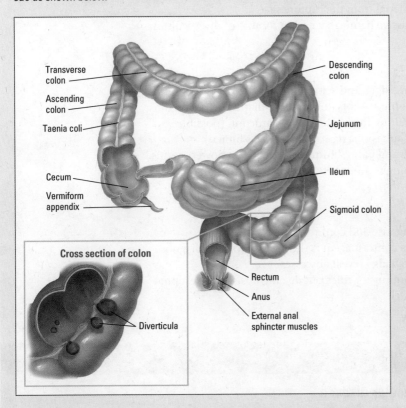

Transverse colon

Descending colon

Ascending colon

Taenia coli

Jejunum

Cecum

Vermiform appendix

Ileum

Sigmoid colon

Cross section of colon

Rectum

Anus

External anal sphincter muscles

Diverticula

What to look for

Typically, the patient with diverticulosis is without symptoms. However, some people may experience crampy pain or discomfort in the lower abdomen, bloating, and constipation.

Mild diverticulitis

In mild diverticulitis, signs and symptoms include:

- moderate left lower quadrant pain secondary to inflammation of diverticula
- low-grade fever and leukocytosis (from infection) due to trapping of bacteria-rich stool in the diverticula

Severe diverticulitis

In severe diverticulitis, signs and symptoms include:

- abdominal rigidity from rupture of the diverticula, abscesses, and peritonitis
- left lower quadrant pain secondary to rupture of the diverticula and subsequent inflammation and infection
- high fever, chills, hypotension from sepsis, and shock from the release of fecal material from the rupture site
- microscopic or massive hemorrhage from rupture of diverticulum near a vessel

Chronic diverticulitis

In chronic diverticulitis, signs and symptoms include:

- constipation, ribbonlike stools, intermittent diarrhea, and abdominal distention resulting from intestinal obstruction (possible when fibrosis and adhesions narrow the bowel's lumen)
- abdominal rigidity and pain, diminishing or absent bowel sounds, nausea, and vomiting secondary to intestinal obstruction (See *Treating diverticular disease.*)

What tests tell you

These tests help to diagnose and confirm diverticular disease:

- CT scanning with a contrast agent is the test of choice to diagnose diverticulitis and can also reveal abscesses.
- Upper GI series confirms or rules out diverticulosis of the esophagus and upper bowel.

Battling illness

Treating diverticular disease

Treatment for diverticular disease may include:
- liquid or bland diet, stool softeners, and occasional doses of mineral oil to relieve symptoms, minimize irritation, and lessen the risk of progression to diverticulitis
- high-residue diet for treatment of diverticulosis after pain has subsided, to help decrease intra-abdominal pressure during defecation, with a switch to a high-fiber, low-fat diet after inflammation subsides
- exercise, to increase the rate of stool passage
- antibiotics, to treat infection of the diverticula

- analgesic agents, such as hydromorphone, to control pain and relax smooth muscle
- antispasmodic agents, to control muscle spasms
- colon resection with removal of involved segment, to correct cases refractory to medical treatment
- temporary colostomy, if necessary, to drain abscesses and rest the colon in diverticulitis accompanied by perforation, peritonitis, obstruction, or fistula
- blood transfusions, if necessary, to treat blood loss from hemorrhage
- fluid replacement as needed

- Barium enema reveals filling of diverticula.
- Biopsy reveals evidence of benign disease, ruling out cancer.
- Blood studies show an elevated ESR and WBC count in diverticulitis.
- Colonoscopy shows the extent of disease and permits biopsy to rule out other disorders.

Gastroesophageal reflux disease

Popularly known as *heartburn*, GERD refers to backflow of gastric or duodenal contents or both into the esophagus and past the lower esophageal sphincter (LES). The backflow occurs when the valve between the stomach and the lower end of the esophagus, the LES, doesn't close tightly enough or relaxes at the wrong time. The reflux of gastric contents causes acute epigastric pain, usually after a meal. The pain may radiate to the chest or arms. Other signs and symptoms include hoarseness, dysphagia, hypersalivation, cough, a feeling of something being stuck in the throat, and nausea.

Heartburn, yet healthy

GERD affects nearly 25% to 40% of adults in the United States to some degree at least once a month, with almost 7% to 10% of adults experiencing GERD weekly or daily. The incidence of GERD increases markedly after age 40. It commonly occurs in people who are pregnant or who have obesity.

How it happens
Various factors can lead to GERD, including:
- weakened LES
- increased abdominal pressure, such as with obesity or pregnancy
- hiatal hernia (the lower esophagus and the top of the stomach are herniated up through an opening in the diaphragm)
- medications, such as morphine, diazepam, calcium channel blockers, meperidine, and anticholinergic agents
- food or alcohol ingestion or cigarette smoking that lowers LES pressure
- nasogastric intubation for more than 4 days (See *How GERD happens.*)

Less LES pressure means more reflux

Normally, the LES maintains enough pressure around the lower end of the esophagus to close it and prevent reflux. Typically, the sphincter relaxes after each swallow to allow food into the stomach. In GERD,

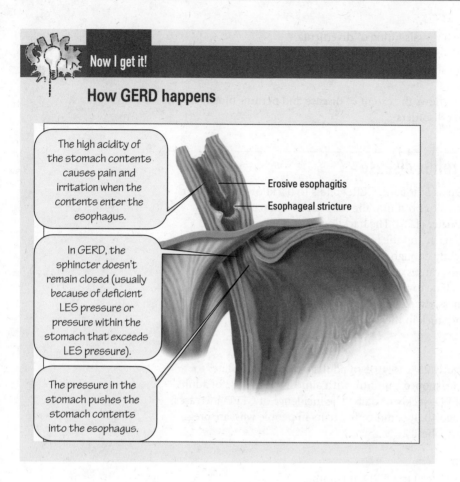

How GERD happens

The high acidity of the stomach contents causes pain and irritation when the contents enter the esophagus.

— Erosive esophagitis

— Esophageal stricture

In GERD, the sphincter doesn't remain closed (usually because of deficient LES pressure or pressure within the stomach that exceeds LES pressure).

The pressure in the stomach pushes the stomach contents into the esophagus.

the sphincter doesn't remain closed (usually because of deficient LES pressure or pressure within the stomach that exceeds LES pressure), and the pressure in the stomach pushes the stomach contents into the esophagus. The high acidity of the stomach contents causes pain and irritation when the contents enter the esophagus.

What to look for

Some patients have GERD without heartburn. However, those with heartburn typically report burning pain in the epigastric area due to the reflux of gastric contents into the esophagus, which causes irritation and esophageal spasm. The pain may radiate to the arms and chest. Pain usually occurs after meals or when the patient lies down because both of these situations cause increased abdominal pressure that leads to reflux.

The patient may also report a feeling of fluid accumulating in the throat; regurgitated contents can cause sore throat. (See *Treating GERD*.)

Potential Complications of GERD

If untreated, chronic GERD can cause lower esophageal epithelial cells to become metaplastic and transform in shape. Although the lower esophageal cells should be squamous cells, they change to look more like columnar stomach cells. This condition, called *Barrett esophagus*, can lead to dysplasia, which is a precancerous change that must be periodically monitored. The dysplasia can lead to adenocarcinoma of the lower esophagus. Symptoms of severe changes in the lower esophagus include dysphagia, odynophagia, melena (blood in stool), hematemesis (blood in vomitus), and abnormal weight loss.

What tests tell you

Diagnostic tests are aimed at determining the underlying cause of GERD:

- Esophageal acidity test (pH monitoring) evaluates the competence of the LES and provides objective measure of reflux.
- Acid perfusion test confirms esophagitis and distinguishes it from cardiac disorders.
- Endoscopy allows visual examination of the lining of the esophagus and stomach to reveal the extent of the disease and to confirm pathologic changes in mucosa.
- Esophageal manometry evaluates the resting pressure of LES and determines sphincter competence.

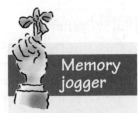

Memory jogger

To recall **GERD**, remember these facts:

Generally known as heartburn.

Epigastric pain and spasm usually follow a meal.

Radiating pain to arms and chest is common.

Diet therapy, raised head of bed for sleep, antacids, histamine-2 receptor antagonists (e.g., famotidine), proton pump inhibitors (e.g., omeprazole), and smoking cessation can help alleviate symptoms.

Battling illness

Treating GERD

Treatment of gastroesophageal reflux disease (GERD) is multifaceted and may include:

- diet therapy with frequent, small meals and avoidance of eating before going to bed, to reduce abdominal pressure and incidence of reflux
- positioning—sitting up during and after meals and sleeping with head of bed elevated—to reduce abdominal pressure and prevent reflux
- increased fluid intake, to wash gastric contents out of the esophagus
- antacids, to neutralize acidic content of the stomach and minimize irritation
- histamine-2 receptor antagonists (e.g., famotidine) to inhibit gastric acid secretion
- proton pump inhibitors (e.g., omeprazole) to reduce gastric acidity
- smoking cessation to improve LES pressure (nicotine lowers LES pressure)
- surgery if hiatal hernia is the cause or patient has refractory symptoms

Hiatal hernia

Hiatal hernia occurs when a defect in the diaphragm permits a portion of the stomach to pass through the diaphragmatic opening (the esophageal hiatus) into the chest cavity. Some people remain without symptoms, whereas others experience reflux, heartburn, and chest pain.

How it happens

Usually, hiatal hernia results from muscle weakening that's common with aging and obesity. It may also be secondary to esophageal cancer, kyphoscoliosis, trauma, and certain surgical procedures. Certain diaphragmatic malformations that cause congenital weakness can also lead to a hiatal hernia. (See *Stomach herniation*.)

Loosening the collar

With a hiatal hernia, the muscular collar around the esophageal and diaphragmatic junction loosens, permitting the lower portion of the esophagus and the stomach to rise into the chest when intra-abdominal pressure increases (possibly causing esophageal reflux). Such increased intra-abdominal pressure may result from ascites, pregnancy, obesity, constrictive clothing, bending, straining, coughing, Valsalva maneuver, or extreme physical exertion.

Two types of hiatal hernia can occur: sliding and paraesophageal. A sliding, or type I, hernia occurs when the upper stomach and gastro-esophageal junction are displaced upward and slide in and out of the thorax. A paraesophageal hernia occurs when all or part of the stomach pushes through the diaphragm beside the esophagus.

What to look for

Typically, a paraesophageal hernia produces no symptoms; it's usually an incidental finding on barium swallow.

A sliding hernia without an incompetent sphincter produces no reflux or symptoms and, consequently, doesn't require treatment. When a sliding hernia does cause symptoms, they're typical of gastric reflux and may include:

- heartburn occurring 1 to 4 hours after eating, aggravated by reclining and belching and may be accompanied by regurgitation or vomiting
- retrosternal or substernal chest pain, occurring usually after meals or at bedtime, aggravated by reclining, belching, and increased intra-abdominal pressure
  Other signs or symptoms that reflect possible complications include:
- dysphagia (difficulty swallowing)
- bleeding due to esophagitis
- severe pain and shock, which occurs when the hernia becomes strangulated (See *Treating hiatal hernia*.)

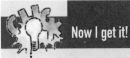

Now I get it!

Stomach herniation

The illustrations in this box show a sliding and paraesophageal hiatal hernia.

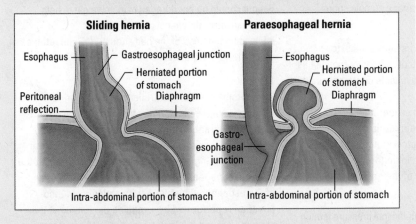

Sliding hernia	Paraesophageal hernia

Esophagus — Gastroesophageal junction — Herniated portion of stomach — Diaphragm — Peritoneal reflection — Intra-abdominal portion of stomach

Esophagus — Herniated portion of stomach — Diaphragm — Gastro-esophageal junction — Intra-abdominal portion of stomach

What tests tell you

A diagnosis of hiatal hernia is based on typical clinical findings as well as the results of these laboratory studies and procedures:

- Chest x-rays occasionally show an air shadow behind the heart with a large hernia and infiltrates in the lower lobes, if the patient has aspirated.
- In a barium study, the hernia may appear as an outpouching that contains barium at the lower end of the esophagus.
- Endoscopy and biopsy differentiate between hiatal hernia, varices, and other small gastroesophageal lesions.
- Esophageal motility studies assess the presence of esophageal motor abnormalities before surgical repair of the hernia.
- pH studies assess for reflux of gastric contents.
- An acid perfusion test indicates that heartburn results from esophageal reflux.

Treating hiatal hernia

The primary goal of treatment for hiatal hernia is to relieve symptoms and to prevent or manage complications.

Drug therapy
• Anticholinergic agents such as bethanechol to strengthen cardiac sphincter tone. Metoclopramide has been used to stimulate smooth muscle contractions and decrease reflux
• Antiemetics, if vomiting is an exacerbating factor; antitussives and antidiarrheals, if appropriate
• Antacids, histamine-2 receptor antagonists (e.g., famotidine), and proton pump inhibitors (e.g., omeprazole), to decrease the acidity of the gastric contents

Noninvasive interventions
• Activity that increases intra-abdominal pressure (coughing, straining, bending) should be restricted. Patient education includes eating small, frequent, bland meals at least 2 hours before lying down; eating slowly; and avoiding spicy foods, fruit juices, alcoholic beverages, and coffee.

• To reduce amount of reflux, the patient who is overweight should be encouraged to lose weight to help decrease intra-abdominal pressure.
• Elevating the head of the bed about 6″ (15 cm) reduces gastric reflux by gravity.

Surgery
If symptoms can't be controlled medically, or complications such as bleeding, stricture, pulmonary aspiration, strangulation, or incarceration (constriction) occur, surgical repair is needed. The procedure involves creating an artificial closing mechanism at the gastroesophageal junction to strengthen the function of the esophageal hiatus. A transabdominal fundoplication is performed by wrapping the fundus of the stomach around the lower esophagus to prevent reflux of stomach contents. Although an abdominal or thoracic approach may be used, hiatal hernia is typically repaired via laparoscopy.

Irritable bowel syndrome

IBS is characterized by chronic symptoms of abdominal pain, alternating constipation and diarrhea, and abdominal distention. IBS is seen in approximately 6% of adults in the United States. Approximately two out of three patients with IBS are female.

Is stress to blame?

IBS is recognized as a multifactorial disorder; causes include GI dysmotility, inflammation, visceral hypersensitivity, and altered intestinal microbiome. Diet and stress exposure have been proposed as contributing factors to this heterogeneous disorder. There is a disturbance in the brain–gut axis. People can have frequent episodes of constipation, diarrhea, or both.

How it happens
Typically, the patient with IBS has a normal-appearing GI tract. However, careful examination of the colon may reveal functional irritability—an abnormality in colonic smooth muscle function marked by excessive peristalsis and spasms, even during remission.

Contract, then relax, contract, then relax…

To understand what happens in IBS, consider how smooth muscle controls bowel function. Normally, segmental muscle contractions mix intestinal contents, while peristalsis propels the contents through the GI tract. Motor activity is most propulsive in the proximal (stomach) and the distal (sigmoid) portions of the intestine. Activity in the rest of the intestines is slower, permitting nutrient and water absorption.

In IBS, the autonomic nervous system, which innervates the large intestine, doesn't cause the alternating contractions and relaxations that propel stools smoothly toward the rectum. The result is constipation or diarrhea, or both. (See *Effects of irritable bowel syndrome*.)

A disturbing pattern

Some patients have spasmodic intestinal contractions that set up a partial obstruction by trapping gas and stools. This causes distention, bloating, gas pain, and constipation.

Other patients have dramatically increased intestinal motility. Usually, eating or cholinergic stimulation triggers the small intestine's contents to rush into the large intestine, dumping watery stools and irritating the mucosa. The result is diarrhea.

If further spasms trap liquid stools, the intestinal mucosa absorbs water from the stools, leaving them dry, hard, and difficult to pass. The result is a pattern of alternating diarrhea and constipation.

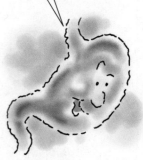

The GI tract may appear normal in a patient with irritable bowel syndrome, but careful examination of the colon may reveal functional irritability.

What to look for

The most commonly reported symptom is intermittent, crampy, lower abdominal pain, usually relieved by defecation or passage of flatus. It usually occurs during the day and intensifies with stress or 1 to 2 hours after meals. The patient may experience constipation alternating with diarrhea, with one being the dominant problem. Abdominal distention and bloating are common. (See *Treating irritable bowel syndrome*.)

What tests tell you

There are no tests that are specific for diagnosing IBS. Other disorders, such as diverticulitis, colon cancer, and lactose intolerance, should be ruled out by these tests:

- Stool samples for ova, parasites, bacteria, and blood rule out infection.
- Lactose intolerance test rules out lactose intolerance.
- Negative fecal calprotectin test rules out inflammatory bowel disease or bowel infection.
- Negative celiac disease serology blood test (elevated levels of specific antibodies) rules out celiac disease.
- Colonoscopy may reveal spastic contractions without evidence of colon cancer or inflammatory bowel disease.

Now I get it!

Effects of irritable bowel syndrome

The illustration below shows partial obstructions in the bowel caused by irritable bowel syndrome (IBS).

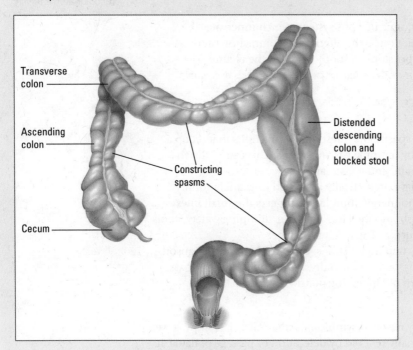

Transverse colon

Ascending colon

Constricting spasms

Cecum

Distended descending colon and blocked stool

Battling illness

Treating irritable bowel syndrome

Treatment for irritable bowel syndrome aims to relieve symptoms.

Medical therapy
Therapy aims to relieve symptoms and includes counseling to help the patient understand the relation between stress and their illness. Dietary restrictions haven't proven to be effective, but the patient is encouraged to be aware of foods that exacerbate symptoms. Rest and heat applied to the abdomen are usually helpful.

In the case of laxative overuse, bowel training is sometimes recommended.

Treating irritable bowel syndrome *(continued)*

Drug therapy

Antispasmodic agents, such as diphenoxylate with atropine, are commonly prescribed. A mild barbiturate such as phenobarbital in judicious doses is sometimes helpful as well. Eluxadoline and rifaximin have been approved to treat IBS with diarrhea, and linaclotide has been approved for IBS with constipation. Eluxadoline works by reducing the spasms in the colon, therefore reducing diarrhea. Rifaximin is an antibiotic therapy that has been shown to change bacteria composition in the colon and is thought to reduce diarrhea that way. Linaclotide works by increasing fluids that the small intestine releases to aid in digestion. This increase in fluid aids in softening and expelling the stool.

Pancreatitis

Pancreatitis is an inflammation of the pancreas. It occurs in acute and chronic forms. In males, the disorder is commonly linked to alcohol use disorder, trauma, or peptic ulcer; in females, to biliary tract disease.

The prognosis is good when pancreatitis follows biliary tract disease but poor when it is a complication of alcohol use disorder. The incidence of acute pancreatitis is estimated at 49 to 35 per 100,000 population, with an estimated more than 300,000 U.S. hospital admissions per year.

Gallstone disease and alcohol misuse are the leading causes of acute pancreatitis. In gallstone disease, the stone obstructs the common bile duct and causes backflow of pancreatic enzymes into the pancreas. Other causes include hypertriglyceridemia (typically >1,000 mg/dL), hypercalcemia, familial pancreatitis (hereditary), and viral infections. Pancreatic tumors can cause obstruction of the pancreatic duct, obstructing the flow of pancreatic enzymes, which may lead to backup of enzymes within the pancreas.

How it happens

The most common causes of pancreatitis are biliary tract disease due to gallstones and alcohol use disorder, but it can also result from:

- abnormal organ structure
- metabolic or endocrine disorders, such as high triglycerides or overactive thyroid
- pancreatic cysts or tumors
- penetrating peptic ulcers
- blunt trauma or surgical trauma
- drugs, such as glucocorticoids, sulfonamides, thiazides, and hormonal contraceptives
- kidney failure or transplantation
- endoscopic retrograde cholangiopancreatography (ERCP); examination of the bile ducts and pancreas can stimulate pancreatitis

In addition, heredity may predispose a patient to pancreatitis. In some patients, emotional or neurogenic factors play a part.

A permanent change for the pancreas

Chronic pancreatitis is a persistent inflammation that produces irreversible changes in the structure and function of the pancreas. It sometimes follows an episode of acute pancreatitis. Here's what probably happens:

- Protein precipitates block the pancreatic duct and eventually harden or calcify.
- Structural changes lead to fibrosis and atrophy of the glands.
- Growths called *pseudocysts*, containing pancreatic enzymes and tissue debris, form.
- An abscess results if these growths become infected.

Acting prematurely

Acute pancreatitis occurs in two forms:

- edematous (interstitial), causing fluid accumulation and swelling
- necrotizing, causing cell death and tissue damage (See *Necrotizing pancreatitis.*)

The inflammation that occurs with both types is caused by premature activation of enzymes, which causes tissue damage. Normally, the cells in the pancreas secrete enzymes in an inactive form.

Two theories explain why enzymes become prematurely activated:

1. A toxic agent, such as alcohol, alters the way the pancreas secretes enzymes. Alcohol probably increases pancreatic secretion, alters

Now I get it!

Necrotizing pancreatitis

Acute pancreatitis can occur as necrotizing pancreatitis when there is cell death and tissue damage.

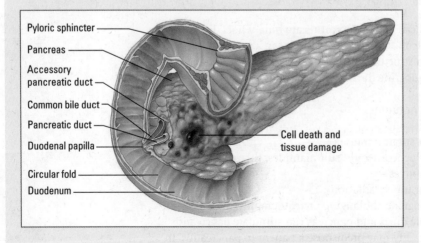

Pyloric sphincter

Pancreas

Accessory pancreatic duct

Common bile duct

Pancreatic duct

Duodenal papilla

Circular fold

Duodenum

Cell death and tissue damage

the metabolism of the acinar cells, and encourages duct obstruction by causing pancreatic secretory proteins to precipitate.

2. A reflux of duodenal contents containing activated enzymes enters the pancreatic duct, activating other enzymes and setting up a cycle of more pancreatic damage.

Pain!!! Why? Why?

Pain can be caused by several factors, including:

- escape of inflammatory exudate and enzymes into the back of the peritoneum
- edema and distention of the pancreatic capsule
- obstruction of the biliary tract

Getting complicated

If pancreatitis damages the islets of Langerhans, diabetes mellitus may result. Sudden, severe pancreatitis causes massive hemorrhage and total destruction of the pancreas. This may lead to diabetic acidosis, shock, or coma.

What to look for

In many patients, the only symptom of mild pancreatitis is steady epigastric pain centered close to the navel and unrelieved by vomiting.

Acute pancreatitis causes severe, persistent, piercing abdominal pain, usually in the midepigastric region, although it may be generalized or occur in the left upper quadrant radiating to the back.

Eat, drink, and be…in pain

The pain usually begins suddenly after eating a large meal or drinking alcohol. It increases when the patient lies on their back and is relieved when they rest on their knees and upper chest. Sitting up or leaning forward can also sometimes decrease the pain. (See *Treating pancreatitis*.)

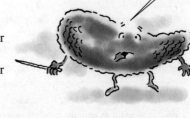

Pancreatitis may start with abdominal pain and progress to swelling, tissue damage, or bleeding.

What tests tell you

These tests are used to diagnose pancreatitis:

- Dramatically elevated serum amylase and lipase levels confirm acute pancreatitis. Dramatically elevated amylase levels are also found in urine, ascites, and pleural fluid.
- Blood and urine glucose tests may reveal transient glucose in urine (glycosuria) and hyperglycemia. In chronic pancreatitis, serum glucose levels may be transiently elevated.
- WBC count is elevated.
- Serum bilirubin levels are elevated in both acute and chronic pancreatitis.
- Blood calcium levels may be decreased.

- Stool analysis shows elevated lipid and trypsin levels in chronic pancreatitis.
- Abdominal and chest x-rays detect pleural effusions and differentiate pancreatitis from diseases that cause similar symptoms.
- CT scan and ultrasonography show an enlarged pancreas and pancreatic cysts and pseudocysts.
- Liver function tests may be elevated, particularly alkaline aminotransferase and alkaline phosphatase, a possible indicator of sudden pancreatitis caused by gallstones.

Battling illness

Treating pancreatitis

The goals of treatment for pancreatitis are to maintain circulation and fluid volume, to relieve pain, and to decrease pancreatic secretions. The patient needs to be counseled to avoid alcohol if they have alcohol use disorder. A cholecystectomy (removal of the gall bladder) may be necessary if there is biliary tract disease due to gall stones.

Acute pancreatitis
For acute cases, treatment includes the following:
- Shock is the most common cause of death in the early stages, so IV replacement of electrolytes and proteins is necessary.
- Metabolic acidosis requires fluid volume replacement.
- Blood transfusions may be needed.
- Food and fluids are withheld to allow the pancreas to rest and to reduce pancreatic enzyme secretion.
- Nasogastric tube suctioning decreases stomach distention and suppresses pancreatic secretions.
- Positioning the patient for comfort in the knee-to-chest position has been helpful in reducing pain.

Drug therapy
Drugs administered for acute pancreatitis include:
- analgesic agents such as hydromorphone or fentanyl can be used to control pain
- antacids to neutralize gastric secretions
- histamine antagonists such as cimetidine, famotidine, or ranitidine to decrease hydrochloric acid production
- antibiotics, such as clindamycin or gentamicin, to fight bacterial infections

- anticholinergics to reduce vagal stimulation, decrease GI motility, and inhibit pancreatic enzyme secretion
- insulin to correct hyperglycemia

Surgery
Surgical drainage is necessary for a pancreatic abscess or a pseudocyst. A laparotomy may be needed if biliary tract obstruction causes acute pancreatitis. Surgical procedures to reduce pain in chronic pancreatitis include removing stones from the pancreas, draining blocked ducts, and destroying certain nerves to reduce pain.

Chronic pancreatitis
Pain control measures are similar to those for acute pancreatitis:
- Intravenous opioids including hydromorphone and fentanyl.
- Some patients require only over-the-counter pain medications.
- Tricyclic antidepressants may be effective in low doses; they suppress the nervous system's reaction to inflammation.

Other treatment depends on the cause. Surgery relieves abdominal pain, restores pancreatic drainage, and reduces the frequency of attacks. Patients with an abscess or pseudocyst, biliary tract disease, or a fibrotic pancreatic sphincter may undergo surgery. Surgery may also help relieve obstruction and allow drainage of pancreatic secretions.

- ERCP shows the anatomy of the pancreas; identifies ductal system abnormalities, such as calcification or strictures; and differentiates pancreatitis from other disorders such as pancreatic cancer.

Peptic ulcer

A peptic ulcer is a circumscribed lesion in the mucosal membrane of the upper GI tract. Peptic ulcers can develop in the lower esophagus, stomach, duodenum, or jejunum. (See *Common ulcer types and sites*.)

Now I get it!

Common ulcer types and sites

This illustration shows common ulcer types and common sites where they can occur. The illustration also shows how an ulcer can penetrate into and through the muscle layers and muscle wall.

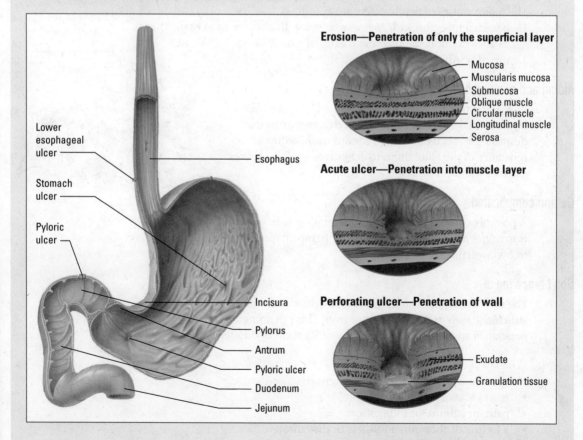

Erosion—Penetration of only the superficial layer
- Mucosa
- Muscularis mucosa
- Submucosa
- Oblique muscle
- Circular muscle
- Longitudinal muscle
- Serosa

Acute ulcer—Penetration into muscle layer

Perforating ulcer—Penetration of wall
- Exudate
- Granulation tissue

Lower esophageal ulcer

Stomach ulcer

Pyloric ulcer

Esophagus

Incisura

Pylorus

Antrum

Pyloric ulcer

Duodenum

Jejunum

How it happens

The two major forms of peptic ulcer are:

- duodenal
- gastric

  Both of these forms of peptic ulcer are chronic conditions.

Upsetting the upper part

Peptic ulcer disease is seen in approximately 4 million individuals every year in the United States

Making the mucosa feel like murder

Gastric ulcers affect the stomach lining (mucosa). They're most common in middle-aged and older adult males, especially males who are undernourished and whose incomes are below the federal poverty threshold. They commonly occur in people who chronically use aspirin or alcohol.

> Chronic use of aspirin or other NSAIDs may cause gastric ulcer.

Peptic promoters

The major causes of peptic ulcers are as follows:

1. bacterial infection with *Helicobacter pylori*; this is seen in as many as 90% of duodenal ulcers and 80% of gastric ulcers
2. use of NSAIDs

Aiding and abetting bacterial infection

In a peptic ulcer due to *H. pylori*, acid adds to the effects of the bacterial infection. *H. pylori* releases a toxin that destroys the mucus coating in the stomach, reduces the resistance of the epithelium to acid digestion, and causes gastritis and ulcer disease.

> Bacteria are a major cause of gastric ulcers.

Getting complicated

A possible complication of severe ulceration is erosion and perforation of the mucosa. This can cause GI hemorrhage, which can progress to hypovolemic shock.

Don't fence me in

The ulcer crater may extend beyond the duodenal wall into nearby structures, such as the pancreas or liver. This phenomenon is called *penetration* and is a fairly common complication of duodenal ulcer.

What to look for

The patient with a gastric ulcer may report:

- recent loss of weight or appetite
- pain, heartburn, or indigestion
- a feeling of abdominal fullness or distention
- pain in the ulcer when fasting or in between meals

The dynamic (if painful) duodenal ulcer

The patient with a duodenal ulcer may describe the pain as sharp, gnawing, burning, boring, aching, or hard to define. The pain may occur several hours after eating when the stomach is empty, and the pain may improve after eating. Because eating usually reduces the pain, the patient may report a recent weight gain. (See *Treating peptic ulcer*.)

What tests tell you

These tests are used to diagnose peptic ulcer:
- Upper GI endoscopy confirms an ulcer and permits cytologic studies and biopsy to rule out *H. pylori* or cancer. Endoscopy is the major diagnostic test for peptic ulcers.
- Upper GI tract x-ray reveals mucosal abnormalities.
- Stool analysis may detect occult blood in stools.
- WBC count is elevated; other blood tests may also disclose clinical signs of infection.
- Serology testing: Test for antibodies to *H. pylori*.
- Gastric secretory studies show excess hydrochloric acid (hyperchlorhydria).
- Carbon-13 urea breath test reflects activity of *H. pylori*.
- Complete blood count may show anemia caused by a bleeding ulcer.

Ulcerative colitis

This inflammatory disease causes ulcerations of the mucosa in the colon and commonly occurs as a chronic condition. Ulcerative colitis is a lifelong inflammatory disease affecting the rectum and colon to a variable extent. In 2023, the prevalence of ulcerative colitis was estimated to be 5 million cases around the world, and the incidence is increasing worldwide.

How it happens

Although the cause of ulcerative colitis is unknown, it may be related to an abnormal immune response in the GI tract, possibly associated with genetic factors. Lymphocytes (T cells) in people with ulcerative colitis may have cytotoxic effects on the epithelial cells of the colon.

Stress doesn't cause the disorder, but it can increase the severity of an attack. Although no specific organism has been linked to ulcerative colitis, infection hasn't been ruled out.

Surveying the damage

Ulcerative colitis damages the large intestine's mucosal and submucosal layers. Here's how it progresses:

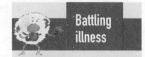

Treating peptic ulcer

Drug therapy
Drug therapy for *Helicobacter pylori* includes 10 to 14 days of bismuth quadruple therapy. This treatment includes a combination of bismuth, proton pump inhibitor (e.g., omeprazole), tetracycline antibiotic, and metronidazole. Other drug options include 10 to 14 days of proton pump inhibitor in combination with clarithromycin, amoxicillin, and metronidazole. The therapy of choice depends on any previous antibiotic treatment, as well as whether or not first-line therapies fail.

More drastic measures
Endoscopy allows visualization of the bleeding site and coagulation by laser or cautery to control bleeding.

Surgery is indicated if the patient doesn't respond to other treatment or has a perforation, a suspected cancer, or other complications.

- Usually, the disease originates in the rectum and lower colon and eventually spreads to the entire colon.
- The mucosa develops diffuse ulceration with hemorrhage, congestion, edema, and exudative inflammation. Unlike Crohn disease, ulcerations are continuous.
- Abscesses formed in the mucosa drain purulent pus, become necrotic, and ulcerate.
- Sloughing occurs, causing bloody, mucus-filled stools.

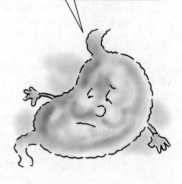

Ulcerative colitis damages the lining of the large intestine.

Looking closer at the colon

As ulcerative colitis progresses, the colon undergoes changes described below:
- Initially, the colon's mucosal surface becomes dark, red, and velvety.
- Abscesses form and coalesce into ulcers.
- Necrosis of the mucosa occurs.
- As abscesses heal, scarring and thickening may appear in the bowel's inner muscle layer.
- As granulation tissue replaces the muscle layer, the colon narrows, shortens, and loses its characteristic pouches (haustral folds). (See *Mucosal changes in ulcerative colitis.*)

Getting complicated

Progression of ulcerative colitis may lead to intestinal obstruction, dehydration, and major fluid and electrolyte imbalances. Malabsorption is common, and chronic anemia may result from loss of blood in the stools.

What to look for

The hallmark of ulcerative colitis is recurrent bloody diarrhea—usually containing pus and mucus—alternating with symptom-free remissions. Accumulation of blood and mucus in the bowel causes cramping abdominal pain, rectal urgency, and diarrhea.

Other symptoms include:
- irritability
- weight loss
- weakness
- anorexia
- anemia
- nausea
- vomiting (See *Treating ulcerative colitis,* below.)

What tests tell you

These tests are used to diagnose ulcerative colitis:
- Sigmoidoscopy confirms rectal involvement by showing mucosal friability (vulnerability to breakdown) and flattening and thick, inflammatory exudate.

Now I get it!

Mucosal changes in ulcerative colitis

In ulcerative colitis, the colon goes through inflammation and ulceration.

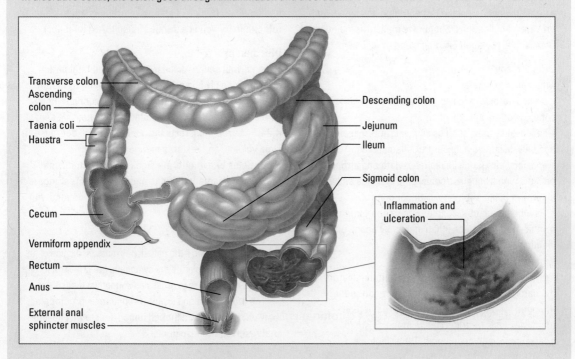

- Transverse colon
- Ascending colon
- Taenia coli
- Haustra
- Cecum
- Vermiform appendix
- Rectum
- Anus
- External anal sphincter muscles

- Descending colon
- Jejunum
- Ileum
- Sigmoid colon

Inflammation and ulceration

- Colonoscopy shows the extent of the disease, strictured areas, and pseudopolyps. It isn't performed when the patient has active signs and symptoms.
- Biopsy during colonoscopy can help confirm the diagnosis.
- Barium enema is used to show the extent of the disease, detect complications, and identify cancer; however, it is not performed in a patient with active signs and symptoms.
- Stool specimen analysis reveals blood, pus, and mucus but no disease-causing organisms.
- Fecal calprotectin test of stool indicates inflammation.
- Stool culture for *C. difficile*.
- Other laboratory tests show decreased serum potassium, magnesium, and albumin levels; decreased WBC count; decreased hemoglobin levels; and prolonged PT. Increase of the ESR correlates with the severity of the attack.

Treating ulcerative colitis

The goals of treatment for ulcerative colitis are to control inflammation, replace lost nutrients and blood, and prevent complications. Supportive measures include bed rest, IV fluid replacement, and blood transfusions.

Drug therapy
Medications include:
- corticosteroids, such as prednisone and hydrocortisone, to control inflammation
- aminosalicylates, such as sulfasalazine, mesalamine, and balsalazide, to help control inflammation
- antidiarrheals, such as diphenoxylate and atropine, for patients with frequent, troublesome diarrhea and whose ulcerative colitis is otherwise under control
- immunomodulators, such as 6-mercaptopurine and azathioprine, to reduce inflammation by acting on the immune system
- iron supplements to correct anemia
- biologic agents that block different inflammatory mediators are the newest agents that can reduce the need for corticosteroids: Drugs that inhibit tumor necrosis factor (TNF) include infliximab, adalimumab, and golimumab. Other biologic drugs include vedolizumab (which is an integrin inhibitor), ustekinumab (which is an anti-interleukin agent), and tofacitinib (which is a Janus kinase [JAK] inhibitor).

Diet therapy
Patients with severe disease usually need total parenteral nutrition (TPN) and are allowed nothing by mouth. TPN is also used for patients awaiting surgery or those who are dehydrated or debilitated from excessive diarrhea. This treatment rests the intestinal tract, decreases stool volume, and restores nitrogen balance.

Patients with moderate signs and symptoms may receive supplemental drinks and elemental feedings. A low-residue diet may be ordered for the patient with mild disease.

Surgery
Surgery is performed if the patient has massive dilation of the colon (toxic megacolon), if the symptoms are unbearable, or if there is no response to drugs and supportive measures.

The most common surgical technique is proctocolectomy with ileostomy, although pouch ileostomy and ileoanal reservoir are also done.

C. difficile infection

C. difficile is a bacterium that causes infection in the colon associated with antibiotic use. The infection causes colitis throughout the large intestine, and the patient experiences diarrhea. Approximately 462,000 patients developed *C. difficile* infection in 2017.

How it happens
C. difficile infection occurs most frequently with overuse of antibiotics. The antibiotics kill off the good, healthy bacteria in the colon, allowing bad bacteria to flourish. The infection is contagious and can be passed via medical equipment, toilet seats, and in the absence of washing hands with soap and water. The *C. difficile* spores invade, proliferate, and cause a pseudomembranous colitis throughout the large intestine. The patient experiences diarrhea, often accompanied by fever, abdominal cramping, and abdominal pain.

What to look for

Anytime a patient experiences three or more liquid stools in a day, for more than 2 days, *C. difficile* is a potential culprit. To obtain a definitive diagnosis, stool samples are collected and tested for the spores in a laboratory. The pseudomembranous colitis can also be visualized during a colonoscopy or flexible sigmoidoscopy. During these tests, a biopsy of tissue can be taken to confirm the suspected diagnosis.

Treatment

The first-line treatment of *C. difficile* infection is oral metronidazole (Flagyl). If that fails, oral vancomycin can be used. Fidaxomicin (Dificid) is a newer treatment, but it is not commonly used at this time due to cost restrictions.

Nonpharmacologic treatment options include fecal bacteriotherapy treatment, which involves transplantation of stool. During this procedure, a donor with healthy flora gives their stool for transplantation into the infected individual. The stool is transplanted into the gut via colonoscopy.

Viral hepatitis

Viral hepatitis is a common infection of the liver. In most patients, damaged liver cells eventually regenerate with little or no permanent damage. Viral hepatitis is reported statistically in accordance with the type.

How it happens

Viral hepatitis is marked by liver cell destruction, tissue death (necrosis), and self-destruction of cells (autolysis). It leads to anorexia, nausea, vomiting, abdominal pain, jaundice, dark-colored urine, clay-colored stools, and hepatomegaly.

The ABCs of viral hepatitis...

Five types of viral hepatitis are recognized, each caused by infection with the virus A, B, C, D, or E. (See *Viral hepatitis from A to E.*)

1. **Hepatitis A virus:** Is transmitted almost exclusively by the fecal–oral route, and outbreaks are common in areas of overcrowding and poor sanitation. Day-care centers and other institutional settings are common sources of outbreaks. It can also be contracted from contaminated food or water. In the United States, hepatitis A outbreaks have been mostly among people experiencing homelessness, men who have sex with men (MSM), and people who use drugs. Hepatitis A is a self-limited disease that does not result in chronic infection. There is a vaccine available to prevent the infection.

Viral hepatitis from A to E

The following chart compares the features of each type of viral hepatitis.

Feature	Hepatitis A	Hepatitis B	Hepatitis C	Hepatitis D	Hepatitis E
Incubation	15–50 days	45–160 days	14–180 days	14–64 days	14–60 days
Onset	Acute	Insidious	Insidious	Acute	Acute
Age group most affected	Children, young adults	Any age	More common in adults	Any age	Ages 20–40
Transmission	Fecal–oral, sexual (especially oral–anal contact), nonpercutaneous (sexual, maternal–neonatal), percutaneous (rare)	Blood-borne; parenteral route, sexual, maternal–neonatal; virus is shed in all body fluids	Blood-borne; parenteral route and sexual transmission	Parenteral route; most people infected with hepatitis D are also infected with hepatitis B	Primarily fecal–oral
Severity	Mild	Usually severe	Moderate	Can be severe and lead to fulminant hepatitis	Highly virulent with common progression to fulminant hepatitis and hepatic failure, especially in pregnant patients
Prognosis	Generally good	Worsens with age and debility	Moderate	Fair; worsens in chronic cases; can lead to chronic hepatitis D and chronic liver disease	Good unless pregnant
Progression to chronicity	None	Occasional	10%–50% of cases	Occasional	None

2. **HBV**: Is seen in approximately 5% of the world's population. During 2021, the United States reported an estimated 13,000 infections. Hepatitis B can be transmitted sexually and can also be contracted via blood, mainly by sharing needles, syringes, or other drug injection equipment or by perinatal transmission from the birthing parent to the fetus during pregnancy or to the baby at birth. It can become a long-term chronic infection that can lead to cirrhosis and liver cancer. A vaccine is commonly given to newborns and is required for healthcare providers and school children.

3. **HCV**: Is transmitted through blood-to-blood contact or through percutaneous exposure to blood. Sexual transmission and perinatal transmission are possible. Intravenous drug use is the most

common risk behavior reported for HCV infection. Sharing of needles and syringes is most strongly associated with hepatitis C. Populations at highest risk for having hepatitis C include HIV-positive MSM, people with a history of incarceration, and people born during 1945–1965 (baby boomer birth cohort). Approximately 75% to 85% of people with acute hepatitis C are not symptomatic; as such, measuring the true burden of disease is difficult. Nearly one-half of people with hepatitis C are unaware of their infection status and can unknowingly transmit the virus to others. Hepatitis C can lead to chronic liver disease and liver cancer. Antiviral treatment has been highly successful to eradicate the infection. Currently, there is no vaccine.

4. **Hepatitis D virus (HDV):** In the United States, is confined to people frequently exposed to blood and blood products, such as people who use IV drugs and people who have hemophilia. Also known as *delta virus*, it requires a concomitant infection with hepatitis B to survive. Hepatitis D can cause severe symptoms and serious illness that can lead to lifelong liver damage and even death. People can become infected with both HBV and HDV at the same time (known as *coinfection*) or get hepatitis D after first being infected with the HBV (known as *superinfection*). Although there is no vaccine to prevent hepatitis D, prevention of hepatitis B with hepatitis B vaccine also protects against future hepatitis D infection.

5. **Hepatitis E virus:** Was formerly grouped with type C under the name non-A, non-B hepatitis. This type mainly occurs in people who live in an endemic area such as India, Africa, Asia, or Central America, or who have visited there. It can be transmitted via the fecal–oral route or vertically from birthing parent to child during childbirth. It is mainly transmitted through contaminated drinking water. The infection is usually self-limited, and treatment is available. No vaccine is available.

> Now you know your ABCs—and also how we cause disease.

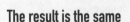

The result is the same

Despite the different causes, changes to the liver are usually similar in each type of viral hepatitis. Varying degrees of liver cell injury and necrosis occur. These changes in the liver are completely reversible when the acute phase of the disease subsides.

Getting complicated

A fairly common complication is chronic persistent hepatitis, which prolongs recovery up to 8 months. Some patients also suffer relapses. A few may develop chronic active hepatitis, which destroys part of the liver and causes cirrhosis. In rare cases, severe and sudden (fulminant) hepatic failure and death may result from massive tissue loss. Primary hepatocellular carcinoma is a late complication that can cause death within 5 years, but it's rare in the United States.

What to look for
Signs and symptoms of viral hepatitis progress in three stages:
1. prodromal
2. clinical
3. recovery

Prodromal stage
In the prodromal stage, the following signs and symptoms may be caused by circulating immune complexes: fatigue, anorexia, mild weight loss, generalized malaise, depression, headache, weakness, joint pain (arthralgia), muscle pain (myalgia), intolerance of light (photophobia), nausea and vomiting, changes in the senses of taste and smell, temperature of 100° to 102°F (37.8° to 38.9°C), RUQ tenderness, and dark-colored urine and clay-colored stools (1 to 5 days before the onset of the clinical jaundice stage).

During this phase, the infection is highly transmissible.

Clinical stage
Also called the *icteric stage*, the clinical stage begins 1 to 2 weeks after the prodromal stage and is the phase of actual illness.

If the patient progresses to this stage, signs and symptoms may include itching, abdominal pain or tenderness, indigestion, appetite loss (in early clinical stage), and jaundice.

Jaundice lasts for 1 to 2 weeks and indicates that the damaged liver can't remove bilirubin from the blood. However, jaundice doesn't indicate disease severity and, occasionally, hepatitis occurs without jaundice.

Recovery stage
Recovery begins with the resolution of jaundice and lasts 2 to 6 weeks in uncomplicated cases. The prognosis is poor if edema and hepatic encephalopathy develop. (See *Treating viral hepatitis*.)

What tests tell you
These tests are used to diagnose viral hepatitis:
- Hepatitis profile establishes the type of hepatitis.
- Liver function studies show disease stage.
- PT is prolonged (coagulation factors are deficient).
- WBC count is elevated.
- Liver biopsy may be performed if chronic hepatitis is suspected.
- FibroScan to determine degree of liver fibrosis, as well as candidacy for treatment.

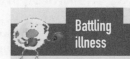
Battling illness

Treating viral hepatitis
Antiviral drugs to treat hepatitis C include boceprevir, telaprevir, simeprevir, sofosbuvir, ledipasvir/sofosbuvir, and sofosbuvir/velpatasvir.

Acute cases
In acute viral hepatitis, hospitalization is usually required only if severe symptoms or complications occur. Parenteral nutrition may be needed if the patient can't eat because of persistent vomiting.

Salmonellosis

Salmonellosis is a bacterial infection caused by *Salmonella* that manifests with diarrhea, fever, and abdominal cramps. One million cases of foodborne *Salmonella* are reported annually. Of those one million cases, approximately 19,000 of those infected require hospitalization, and around 380 cases result in death.

Getting specific

There are two prevalent types of *Salmonella* bacteria in the United States: *Salmonella* serotype *typhimurium* and *Salmonella* serotype *enteritidis*. The most affected age groups are children under 5 years of age and individuals with an underdeveloped or poorly functioning immune system. Complications with *Salmonella* infection are uncommon; however, there are some patients who may experience an extended change to their bowel habits and a small population who may develop reactive arthritis.

Diagnosis

Salmonellosis is diagnosed by taking a sample of blood or stool from the patient. The sample is tested in a laboratory to determine the serotype of *Salmonella*, which is then reported to the CDC.

Treating the bug

Most cases of salmonellosis resolve on their own, requiring only supportive care, such as maintaining good oral hydration. In severe cases, IV hydration may be required. Antibiotics are typically not needed, except in cases where hospitalization is required due to severe diarrhea, bloodstream infection, or high fever or in patients who have a health status that puts them at a higher risk for complications.

Colorectal cancer

CRC is cancer involving the large intestine and rectum. In 2023, approximately 153,020 individuals were diagnosed with CRC, and 52,550 died from the disease, including 19,550 cases and 3,750 deaths in individuals younger than 50 years.

Tumors

CRC can occur anywhere throughout the colon or rectum. Tumors present between the ileocecal valve and the rectum and anus fall into the colorectal category. Tumors most often occur in the rectosigmoid area of the bowel. The most common type of cancer is an adenocarcinoma. (See *Types of colorectal cancer.*)

Tumors often start out as a polyp. There are many types of polyps including hyperplastic polyps (benign) and adenomatous polyps

Now I get it!

Types of colorectal cancer

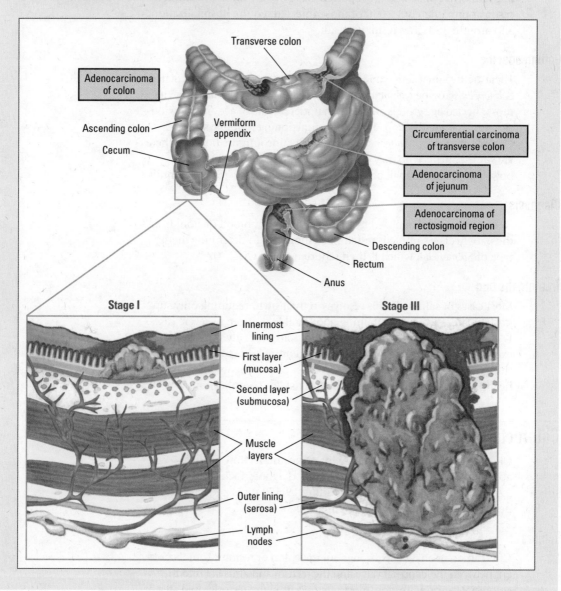

Transverse colon

Adenocarcinoma of colon

Ascending colon

Vermiform appendix

Cecum

Circumferential carcinoma of transverse colon

Adenocarcinoma of jejunum

Adenocarcinoma of rectosigmoid region

Descending colon

Rectum

Anus

Stage I

Stage III

Innermost lining

First layer (mucosa)

Second layer (submucosa)

Muscle layers

Outer lining (serosa)

Lymph nodes

(neoplastic). Adenomatous polyps can be further categorized by their appearance and makeup. They can be tubular, pedunculated (those that have a stalk), or sessile (those that are flat).

Over time, through a series of changes and growth, neoplastic polyps can develop into cancers of the colon and rectum, which is why screening at appropriate intervals is important.

Modifiable and nonmodifiable risk factors

Common risk factors for CRC can be divided into modifiable and nonmodifiable categories. Modifiable risk factors include diet (high fat, low fiber), increased consumption of red meat and other processed meats, large amounts of alcohol intake, cigarette smoking, obesity, and sedentary lifestyle. Nonmodifiable risk factors include age greater than 50 years, genetics, inflammatory bowel diseases such as Crohn disease and ulcerative colitis, and type 2 diabetes mellitus.

The symptoms

Symptoms of CRC can be widely variable, and depending on the location of the tumor or mass, no symptoms may be present. Often, the CRC can be an incidental finding or found during routine screening. When symptoms are present, they are largely related to the location and size of the tumor. Symptoms for tumors on the right side of the colon (ileocecal valve, cecum, ascending colon, and transverse colon) can include pain, palpable mass, anemia, fatigue, and dark red stools. Blood loss from ulcerations in the tumor can also result in anemia. Tumors on the left side of the colon (descending colon, sigmoid, and rectum) can have symptoms including obstruction, narrow ribbonlike stools, abdominal distention and pain, vomiting, constipation, and bright red blood seen on the stool. Due to the wide variance in symptoms and the delay in symptom onset, screening for CRC is integral to prevention and early detection.

Speaking of screening

Screening options for CRC include colonoscopy, flexible sigmoidoscopy, double-contrast barium enema, CT colonography, fecal occult blood testing, fecal immunochemical testing, and stool DNA and RNA testing. The frequency of screening and method of screening are determined by the risk factors, age, and family history. Screening colonoscopy is the most common and effective tool for exams because polyps can be directly visualized with the scope and are often removed the same day. If polyps are found and removed, they are sent to a laboratory for analysis. Once the pathology report is received, the patient is placed on a new screening interval based on the results.

Early detection is key

If not detected early, colon cancer will metastasize to other organs in the body. Colon cancer can take up to 8 to 10 years to progress from a polyp to a tumor, but once a tumor forms and invades the mucosa, metastasis can occur. Common sites for metastasis of CRCs include the liver, the lungs, the prostate in males, the vagina in females, and other systemic sites.

Treatment

Treatment options for CRC predominately include surgical resection of the tumor. Surgery is usually combined with chemotherapy based on the size and stage of the cancer.

Surgery

Surgical options for treatment of CRC include removal of the mass and affected lymph nodes of the surrounding area. Typically, cancers above the rectum can be removed, and depending on the tumor size, the ends of the uninvolved areas can be anastomosed. This prevents an alteration in the way stool is removed. In cases involving the rectum or highly invasive tumors of the rest of the colon, the tumor is removed and a temporary or permanent colostomy is formed. This diverts stool out of the bowel through a stoma created in the abdominal wall. Depending on how much healthy tissue remains, sometimes, the colostomy can be reversed after the bowel has had time to heal.

Chemotherapy

Chemotherapeutic agents are often used prior to and after surgical removal of tumors. Chemotherapy drugs are customized to the type of cells present in the tumor and the degree and location of metastasis. Chemotherapy can be used in conjunction with or separate from radiation prior to surgery, with the goal of shrinking the tumor to make resection easier. Chemotherapy can be used after surgery to prevent growth of new cancer cells. Chemotherapy is often accompanied by side effects, as the drugs cannot differentiate between healthy cells and cancerous cells. These side effects may include diarrhea, mucositis, leukopenia, ulcers in the mouth, and peripheral neuropathy.

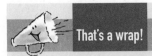

Gastrointestinal system review

Understanding the gastrointestinal system
The body's food processing complex supplies essential nutrients that fuel other organs and body systems. The gastrointestinal system's two major components are the:
- GI tract
- accessory glands and organs

GI tract
Beginning in the mouth and ending at the anus, the GI tract includes the:
- mouth—where chewing and salivation occur to make food soft and easy to swallow
- esophagus—where food enters by peristaltic waves that are activated by the glossopharyngeal nerves
- stomach—where digestion occurs in two phases:
  – cephalic phase
  – gastric phase
- small intestine—where digestion takes place in three major sections:
  – duodenum
  – jejunum
  – ileum
- appendix—a projection off the cecum at the beginning of the ascending colon
- large intestine—ascending, transverse, and descending colon; where absorption takes place and mostly indigestible material passes through the transverse colon and then down through the descending colon to the rectum and is expelled through the anal canal

Accessory glands and organs
Enzymes, bile, and hormones, which are vital to digestion, are produced by the:
- liver—filters and detoxifies blood, removes naturally occurring ammonia from body fluids, produces plasma proteins, stores essential nutrients, produces bile, converts glucose, and stores fat
- gallbladder—stores and concentrates bile
- pancreas—secretes more than 1,000 mL of digestive enzymes daily; houses alpha cells, which stimulate glucose formation in the liver, and beta cells, which secrete insulin to promote carbohydrate metabolism

Digestive disorders
- *Appendicitis*—inflammation of the vermiform appendix
- *Cholecystitis*—inflammation of the gallbladder
- *Cirrhosis*—widespread destruction of hepatic cells in the liver
- *Esophageal and gastric varices*—distended, fragile varicose veins in GI tract
- *Crohn disease*—inflammation of any part of the GI tract
- *Celiac disease*—inflammation in the small intestines caused by ingesting gluten
- *Diverticular disease*—bulging outpouches in the GI wall push the mucosal lining through surrounding muscle
- *Gastroesophageal reflux disease (GERD)*—backflow of gastric or duodenal contents (or both) into the esophagus and past the lower esophageal sphincter
- *Hiatal hernia*—defect in the diaphragm that permits a portion of the stomach to pass through the diaphragmatic opening into the chest cavity
- *Irritable bowel syndrome*—characterized by chronic symptoms of abdominal pain, alternating constipation and diarrhea, and abdominal distention
- *Pancreatitis*—inflammation of the pancreas; two forms:
  – chronic pancreatitis (persistent inflammation)
  – acute pancreatitis (inflammation causes tissue damage)
- *Peptic ulcer*—circumscribed lesion in the mucosal membrane of the upper GI tract
- *Ulcerative colitis*—inflammation of the mucosa in the colon that causes ulcerations
- *Viral hepatitis*—infection of the liver
- *Clostridium difficile* infection—an infection in the colon caused by an imbalance in the normal flora of the gut causing profuse diarrhea
- *Salmonellosis*—a foodborne illness causing nausea, vomiting, diarrhea, and abdominal pain
- *Colorectal cancer*—cancer that occurs anywhere in the large intestine or rectum

Quick quiz

1. What is the most common complication of esophageal varices?
   A. Weight loss
   B. Infection
   C. Diarrhea
   D. Hemorrhage

Answer: D. Hemorrhage occurs as a result of large engorged varices rupturing with increasing portal hypertension. Esophageal varices do not have complications of weight loss, infection, or diarrhea associated with them.

2. What are the two phases of digestion?
   A. Gastric and colonic
   B. Salivation and secretion
   C. Esophageal and abdominal
   D. Cephalic and gastric

Answer: D. The cephalic phase begins when the food is on its way to the stomach. Food entering the stomach initiates the gastric phase.

3. Which of the following is usually the initial event in appendicitis?
   A. Lymph node enlargement
   B. Obstruction of the appendiceal lumen
   C. Ulceration of the mucosa
   D. Perforation of the appendix

Answer: C. Although an obstruction can be identified in some cases, ulceration of the mucosa usually occurs first.

4. In females, pancreatitis is usually associated with:
   A. biliary tract disease (gallstones).
   B. alcohol use disorder.
   C. allergies.
   D. diabetes mellitus.

Answer: A. Biliary tract disease is a leading cause of pancreatitis in females. In males, the leading causes are trauma and peptic ulcer.

Scoring

 If you answered all four items correctly, excellent! When it comes to understanding the GI system, you're on the right "tract."

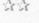 If you answered three items correctly, relax and enjoy! Your performance on this test isn't difficult to digest.

If you answered fewer than three items correctly, don't worry. Take your "chyme," and you'll absorb all the important facts.

Suggested references

Abad, C. L. R., & Safdar, N. (2021). A review of clostridioides difficile infection and antibiotic-associated diarrhea. *Gastroenterol Clinics of North America, 50*(2), 323–340. https://doi.org/10.1016/j.gtc.2021.02.010

Abu-Freha, N., Mathew Jacob, B., Elhoashla, A., Afawi, Z., Abu-Hammad, T., Elsana, F., Paz, S., & Etzion, O. (2022). Chronic hepatitis C: Diagnosis and treatment made easy. *European Journal of General Practice, 28*(1), 102–108. https://doi.org/10.1080/13814788.2022.2056161

American Cancer Society. (2022). Colorectal cancer. Facts and figures 2020-2022. https://www.cancer.org/content/dam/cancer-org/research/cancer-facts-and-statistics/colorectal-cancer-facts-and-figures/colorectal-cancer-facts-and-figures-2020-2022.pdf

American Liver Foundation. (2023). Non-alcoholic fatty liver disease (NAFLD). https://liverfoundation.org/liver-diseases/fatty-liver-disease/nonalcoholic-fatty-liver-disease-nafld/

Baidoun, F., Elshiwy, K., Elkeraie, Y., Merjaneh, Z., Khoudari, G., Sarmini, M. T., Gad, M., Al-Husseini, M., & Saad, A. (2021). Colorectal cancer epidemiology: Recent trends and impact on outcomes. *Current Drug Targets, 22*(9), 998–1009. https://doi.org/10.2174/1389450121999201117115717

Bruner, L. P., White, A. M., & Proksell, S. (2023). Inflammatory bowel disease. *Primary Care: Clinics in Office Practice, 50*(3), 411–427. https://doi.org/10.1016/j.pop.2023.03.009

Catassi, C., Verdu, E. F., Bai, J. C., & Lionetti, E. (2022). Coeliac disease. *Lancet (London, England), 399*(10344), 2413–2426. https://doi.org/10.1016/S0140-6736(22)00794-2

Centers for Disease Control and Prevention (CDC). (2020). *Hepatitis B Surveillance 2020.* https://www.cdc.gov/hepatitis/statistics/2020surveillance/hepatitis-b.htm

Centers for Disease Control and Prevention (CDC). (2021). *Hepatitis C.* https://www.cdc.gov/hepatitis/statistics/2021surveillance/hepatitis-c.htm

Centers for Disease Control and Prevention (CDC). (2023). *Hepatitis C.* https://www.cdc.gov/hepatitis/hcv/index.htm.

Centers for Disease Control and Prevention (CDC). (2024). *Inflammatory bowel disease.* https://www.cdc.gov/dotw/ibd/index.htm

Centers for Disease Control and Prevention (CDC). (2023). *Chronic liver disease and cirrhosis.* https://www.cdc.gov/nchs/fastats/liver-disease.htm

Centers for Disease Control and Prevention (CDC). (2020a). *Clostridioides difficile.* https://www.cdc.gov/cdiff/index.html

Centers for Disease Control and Prevention (CDC). (2020b). *Hepatitis A.* https://www.cdc.gov/hepatitis/hav/index.htm

Centers for Disease Control and Prevention (CDC). (2020c). *Hepatitis D.* https://www.cdc.gov/hepatitis/hdv/index.htm.

Centers for Disease Control and Prevention (CDC). (2021). *Hepatitis B surveillance.* https://www.cdc.gov/hepatitis/statistics/2021surveillance/hepatitis-b.htm

Centers for Disease Control and Prevention (CDC). (2022). *Salmonella*. https://www.cdc.gov/salmonella/index.html

Cohen-Mekelburg, S., & Waljee, A. K. (2021). Inflammatory bowel disease in the older adult. *Clinics in Geriatric Medicine, 37*(1), 185–195. https://doi.org/10.1016/j.cger.2020.08.013

Cushing, K., & Higgins, P. D. R. (2021). Management of Crohn disease: A review. *JAMA, 325*(1), 69–80. https://doi.org/10.1001/jama.2020.18936

Duncanson, K., Tikhe, D., Williams, G. M., & Talley, N. J. (2023). Irritable bowel syndrome—controversies in diagnosis and management. *Expert Review of Gastroenterology & Hepatology, 17*(7), 649–663. https://doi.org/10.1080/17474124.2023.2223975

Eckmann, J. D., & Shaukat, A. (2022). Updates in the understanding and management of diverticular disease. *Current Opinion in Gastroenterology, 38*(1), 48–54. https://doi.org/10.1097/MOG.0000000000000791

Fabregas, J. C., Ramnaraign, B., & George, T. J. (2022). Clinical updates for colon cancer care in 2022. *Clinical Colorectal Cancer, 21*(3), 198–203. https://doi.org/10.1016/j.clcc.2022.05.006

Fichna, J. (2020). Inflammatory bowel disease—from bench to bedside. *Current Drug Targets, 21*(14), 1396. https://doi.org/10.2174/138945012114200925102104

Galica, A. N., Galica, R., & Dumitrașcu, D. L. (2022). Diet, fibers, and probiotics for irritable bowel syndrome. *Journal of Medicine and Life, 15*(2), 174–179. https://doi.org/10.25122/jml-2022-0028

Gallaher, J. R., & Charles, A. (2022). Acute cholecystitis: A review. *JAMA, 327*(10), 965–975. https://doi.org/10.1001/jama.2022.2350

Ginès, P., Krag, A., Abraldes, J. G., Solà, E., Fabrellas, N., & Kamath, P. S. (2021). Liver cirrhosis. *Lancet (London, England), 398*(10308), 1359–1376. https://doi.org/10.1016/S0140-6736(21)01374-X

Guh, A. Y., Mu, Y., Winston, L. G., Johnston, H., Olson, D., Farley, M. M., Wilson, L. E., Holzbauer, S. M., Phipps, E. C., Dumyati, G. K., Beldavs, Z. G., Kainer, M. A., Karlsson, M., Gerding, D. N., McDonald, L. C., & Emerging Infections Program Clostridioides difficile Infection Working Group. (2020). Trends in U.S. Burden of *Clostridioides difficile* infection and outcomes. *New England Journal of Medicne, 382*(14), 1320–1330. https://doi.org/10.1056/NEJMoa1910215

Hart, P. A., & Conwell, D. L. (2020). Chronic pancreatitis: Managing a difficult disease. *American Journal of Gastroenterology, 115*(1), 49–55. https://doi.org/10.14309/ajg.0000000000000421

Hemmer, A., Forest, K., Rath, J., & Bowman, J. (2023). Inflammatory bowel disease: A concise review. *S D Medical Journal, 76*(9), 416–423.

Kaenkumchorn, T., & Wahbeh, G. (2020). Ulcerative colitis: Making the diagnosis. *Gastroenterol Clinics of North America, 49*(4), 655–669. https://doi.org/10.1016/j.gtc.2020.07.001

Kivelä, L., Caminero, A., Leffler, D. A., Pinto-Sanchez, M. I., Tye-Din, J. A., & Lindfors, K. (2021). Current and emerging therapies for coeliac disease. *Nature Reviews Gastroenterology & Hepatology, 18*(3), 181–195. https://doi.org/10.1038/s41575-020-00378-1

Le Berre, C., Honap, S., & Peyrin-Biroulet, L. (2023). Ulcerative colitis. *Lancet (London, England), 402*(10401), 571–584. https://doi.org/10.1016/ S0140-6736(23)00966-2

Li, C. L., Jiang, M., Pan, C. Q., Li, J., & Xu, L. G. (2021). The global, regional, and national burden of acute pancreatitis in 204 countries and territories, 1990-2019. *BMC Gastroenterology, 21*(1), 332. https://doi.org/10.1186/s12876-021-01906-2

Lim, S. C., Knight, D. R., & Riley, T. V. (2020). *Clostridium difficile* and one health. *Clinical Microbiology and Infection, 26*(7), 857–863. https://doi.org/10.1016/j. cmi.2019.10.023

Mederos, M. A., Reber, H. A., & Girgis, M. D. (2021). Acute pancreatitis: A review. *JAMA, 325*(4), 382–390. https://doi.org/10.1001/jama.2020.20317

Moris, D., Paulson, E. K., & Pappas, T. N. (2021). Diagnosis and management of acute appendicitis in adults: A review. *JAMA, 326*(22), 2299–2311. https://doi. org/10.1001/jama.2021.20502

National Institutes of Health (NIH) National Institute of Diabetes, Digestive, and Kidney Disease (NIDDK). Celiac disease. https://www.niddk.nih.gov/ health-information/digestive-diseases/celiac-disease.

National Institutes of Health (NIH) National Institute of Diabetes, Digestive, and Kidney Disease (NIDDK). Non-alcoholic fatty liver disease (NAFLD) and Non-alcoholic steatohepatitis (NASH). https://www.niddk.nih.gov/ health-information/liver-disease/nafld-nash.

Nee, J., & Lembo, A. (2021). Review Article: Current and future treatment approaches for IBS with diarrhoea (IBS-D) and IBS mixed pattern (IBS-M). *Alimentary Pharmacology and Therapeutics, 54*, S63–S74. https://doi.org/10.1111/apt.16625

Nfonsam, V., Wusterbarth, E., Gong, A., & Vij, P. (2022). Early-onset colorectal cancer. *Surgical Oncology Clinics of North America, 31*(2), 143–155. https://doi. org/10.1016/j.soc.2021.11.001

Ouyang, G., Pan, G., Liu, Q., Wu, Y., Liu, Z., Lu, W., Li, S., Zhou, Z., & Wen, Y. (2020). The global, regional, and national burden of pancreatitis in 195 countries and territories, 1990-2017: A systematic analysis for the global burden of disease study 2017. *BMC Medicine, 18*(1), 388. https://doi.org/10.1186/ s12916-020-01859-5

Ozturk, A., Olson, M. C., Samir, A. E., & Venkatesh, S. K. (2022). Liver fibrosis assessment: MR and US elastography. *Abdominal Radiology, 47*(9), 3037–3050. https://doi.org/10.1007/s00261-021-03269-4

Papatheodoridi, M., & Cholongitas, E. (2018). Diagnosis of non-alcoholic fatty liver disease (NAFLD): Current concepts. *Current Pharmaceutical Design, 24*(38), 4574–4586. https://doi.org/10.2174/1381612825666190117102111

Pisano, M., Allievi, N., Gurusamy, K., Borzellino, G., Cimbanassi, S., Boerna, D., Coccolini, F., Tufo, A., Di Martino, M., Leung, J., Sartelli, M., Ceresoli, M., Maier, R. V., Poiasina, E., De Angelis, N., Magnone, S., Fugazzola, P., Paolillo, C., Coimbra, R., … Ansaloni, L. (2020). 2020 World Society of Emergency Surgery updated guidelines for the diagnosis and treatment of acute calculus cholecystitis. *World Journal of Emergency Surgeons, 15*(1), 61. https://doi. org/10.1186/s13017-020-00336-x

Piscopo, N., & Ellul, P. (2020). Diverticular disease: A review on pathophysiology and recent evidence. *The Ulster Medical Journal, 89*(2), 83–88.

Plevris, N., & Lees, C. W. (2022). Disease monitoring in inflammatory bowel disease: Evolving principles and possibilities. *Gastroenterology, 162*(5), 1456–1475.e1. https://doi.org/10.1053/j.gastro.2022.01.024

Pouwels, S., Sakran, N., Graham, Y., Leal, A., Pintar, T., Yang, W., Kassir, R., Singhal, R., Mahawar, K., & Ramnarain, D. (2022). Non-alcoholic fatty liver disease (NAFLD): A review of pathophysiology, clinical management and effects of weight loss. *BMC Endocrine Disorders, 22*(1), 63. https://doi.org/10.1186/s12902-022-00980-1

Raza, S., Rajak, S., Upadhyay, A., Tewari, A., & Anthony Sinha, R. (2021). Current treatment paradigms and emerging therapies for NAFLD/NASH. *Frontiers in Bioscience, 26*(2), 206–237. https://doi.org/10.2741/4892

Roehlen, N., Crouchet, E., & Baumert, T. F. (2020). Liver fibrosis: Mechanistic concepts and therapeutic perspectives. *Cells, 9*(4), 875. https://doi.org/10.3390/cells9040875

Sebastián Domingo, J. J. (2022). Irritable bowel syndrome. *Medicina Clínica, 158*(2), 76–81. https://doi.org/10.1016/j.medcli.2021.04.029

Segal, J. P., LeBlanc, J. F., & Hart, A. L. (2021). Ulcerative colitis: An update. *Clinical Medicine Journal, 21*(2), 135–139. https://doi.org/10.7861/clinmed.2021-0080

Sharma, P., & Yadlapati, R. (2021). Pathophysiology and treatment options for gastroesophageal reflux disease: Looking beyond acid. *Annals of the New York Academy of Sciences, 1486*(1), 3–14. https://doi.org/10.1111/nyas.14501

Siegel, R. L., Wagle, N. S., Cercek, A., Smith, R. A., & Jemal, A. (2023). Colorectal cancer statistics, 2023. *CA A Cancer Journal of Clinicans, 73*(3), 233–254. https://doi.org/10.3322/caac.21772

Tu, T., & Douglas, M. W. (2020). Hepatitis B virus infection: From diagnostics to treatments. *Viruses, 12*(12), 1366. https://doi.org/10.3390/v12121366.

Tuerk, E., Doss, S., & Polsley, K. (2023). Peptic ulcer disease. *Primary Care: Clinics in Office Practice, 50*(3), 351–362. https://doi.org/10.1016/j.pop.2023.03.003

Vege, S. S., & Chari, S. T. (2022). Chronic pancreatitis. *New England Journal of Medicine, 386*(9), 869–878. https://doi.org/10.1056/NEJMcp1809396

Vogel, J. D., Felder, S. I., Bhama, A. R., Hawkins, A. T., Langenfeld, S. J., Shaffer, V. O., Thorsen, A. J., Weiser, M. R., Chang, G. J., Lightner, A. L., Feingold, D. L., & Paquette, I. M. (2022). The American Society of colon and rectal surgeons clinical practice guidelines for the management of colon cancer. *Diseases of the Colon & Rectum, 65*(2), 148–177. https://doi.org/10.1097/DCR.0000000000002323

Walter, K. (2021). Acute appendicitis. *JAMA, 326*(22), 2339. https://doi.org/10.1001/jama.2021.20410

World Health Organization (WHO). (2023). *Hepatitis E.* https://www.who.int/news-room/fact-sheets/detail/hepatitis-e

Young, A., Kumar, M. A., & Thota, P. N. (2020). GERD: A practical approach. *Cleveland Clinic Journal of Medicine, 87*(4), 223–230. https://doi.org/10.3949/ccjm.87a.19114

Zhou, E., Yang, C., & Gao, Y. (2021). Effect of alcohol on the progress of hepatitis B cirrhosis. *Annals of Palliative Medicine, 10*(1), 415–424. https://doi.org/10.21037/apm-20-2353

Chapter 8

Endocrine system*

Just the facts

In this chapter, you'll learn:

◆ the role of the hypothalamus in regulating hormones

◆ the function of the adrenal glands, pancreas, pituitary gland, and thyroid gland

◆ the pathophysiology, signs and symptoms, diagnostic tests, and treatments for several endocrine disorders.

Understanding the endocrine system

The endocrine system consists of glands, specialized cell clusters, and hormones, which are chemical transmitters secreted by the glands in response to stimulation.

Together with the central nervous system (CNS), the endocrine system regulates and integrates the body's metabolic activities and maintains homeostasis.

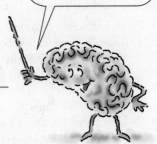

The functions of the endocrine and nervous systems are interrelated.

Hypothalamus: the heart of the system

The hypothalamus is the integrative center for the endocrine and autonomic (involuntary) nervous systems. It helps control some endocrine glands by neural and hormonal pathways.

On the path to the posterior pituitary gland

The posterior pituitary is actually an extension of the hypothalamus, with neural pathways connecting the hypothalamus to the posterior pituitary gland. The effector hormones—antidiuretic hormone (ADH) and oxytocin—are produced in the hypothalamus but are stored in the posterior pituitary. They're released from the posterior pituitary by neural stimulation. When ADH is secreted, the body retains water. Oxytocin stimulates uterine contractions during labor and milk secretion in lactating women.

---

*Note: In this chapter, the term "male" refers to a person assigned male at birth, and the term "female" refers to a person assigned female at birth.

Please release me

The hypothalamus also exerts hormonal control at the anterior pituitary gland by releasing or inhibiting hormones. Hypothalamic hormones stimulate the anterior pituitary gland to release four types of trophic (gland-stimulating) hormones:
1. adrenocorticotropic hormone (ACTH), also called *corticotropin*
2. thyroid-stimulating hormone (TSH)
3. luteinizing hormone (LH)
4. follicle-stimulating hormone (FSH)

The secretion of trophic hormones stimulates their respective target glands, such as the adrenal cortex, the thyroid gland, and the gonads.

Hypothalamic hormones also control the release of effector hormones from the anterior pituitary gland. Examples are growth hormone (GH) and prolactin.

Getting feedback

A negative feedback system regulates the endocrine system by inhibiting hormone overproduction. This system may be simple or complex. (See *The feedback loop*.)

What can cause an endocrine disorder?

Endocrine disorders may be caused by:
*   hypersecretion or hyposecretion of hormones: These phenomena may originate in the hypothalamus, the pituitary gland, or the target endocrine gland. Regardless of origin, however, the result is abnormal hormone concentrations in the blood. Hypersecretion of the target gland hormone leads to elevated blood levels, which feed back to the pituitary to decrease stimulation of the target gland; hyposecretion of target gland hormones leads to deficient blood levels, which feed back to the pituitary to increase stimulation of the target gland.
*   hyporesponsiveness of hormone receptors: The cells of the target organ don't have appropriate receptors for a hormone, so the effects of the hormone aren't detected. Because the receptors don't detect the hormone, there's no feedback mechanism to the pituitary gland to turn off the hormone. Blood levels of the hormone become high, which feed back to the pituitary to shut off stimulation to the target gland. Hyporesponsiveness causes the same clinical symptoms as hyposecretion.
*   inflammation of glands: Inflammation is usually chronic, commonly resulting in glandular secretion of hormones. However, it may be acute or subacute, as in thyroiditis.

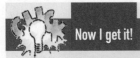

Now I get it!

The feedback loop

This diagram shows the negative feedback mechanism that helps regulate the endocrine system.

From simple …

Simple feedback occurs when the level of one substance regulates secretion of hormones (simple loop). For example, a low serum calcium level stimulates the parathyroid gland to release parathyroid hormone (PTH). PTH, in turn, promotes resorption of calcium from bones. A high serum calcium level inhibits PTH secretion.

… to complex

When the hypothalamus receives feedback from target glands, the mechanism is more complicated (complex loop). Complex feedback occurs through an axis established between the hypothalamus, pituitary gland, and target organ. For example, secretion of the hypothalamic corticotropin–releasing hormone stimulates release of pituitary corticotropin, which in turn stimulates cortisol secretion by the adrenal glands (the target organs). A rise in serum cortisol levels inhibits corticotropin secretion by decreasing corticotropin-releasing hormone.

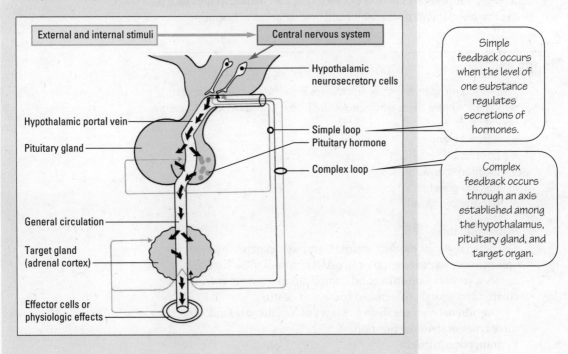

External and internal stimuli → Central nervous system

Hypothalamic neurosecretory cells

Hypothalamic portal vein

Pituitary gland

Simple loop
Pituitary hormone

Complex loop

General circulation

Target gland (adrenal cortex)

Effector cells or physiologic effects

Simple feedback occurs when the level of one substance regulates secretions of hormones.

Complex feedback occurs through an axis established among the hypothalamus, pituitary gland, and target organ.

- gland tumors: Tumors can occur within a gland, such as thyroid carcinoma. Tumors occurring in other areas of the body can cause abnormal hormone production (ectopic hormone production)—for example, certain lung tumors secrete ADH or parathyroid hormone (PTH).

A patient with a possible endocrine disorder needs careful assessment to identify the cause of the dysfunction. Dysfunction may result from defects:

- in the target endocrine gland
- in the release of trophic hormones from the pituitary gland
- in hormone transport or receptors of the target gland
- of the target tissue

Primary versus secondary endocrine disorders

In *primary endocrine disorders*, the endocrine target gland is dysfunctional. In *secondary endocrine disorders,* the pituitary gland that stimulates the endocrine gland is the cause of the dysfunction. For example, in primary hypothyroidism, the thyroid gland itself is not releasing sufficient thyroid hormone (T_3 and T_4), whereas in secondary hypothyroidism, the pituitary gland is not secreting TSH, which in turn causes the thyroid gland to release an insufficient amount of hormone.

Glands

The endocrine glands release hormones into the circulatory system, which distributes them throughout the body. Glands discussed below include the:

- adrenal glands
- pancreas
- pituitary gland
- thyroid gland
- parathyroid glands

Adrenal glands

The adrenal glands produce steroids, amines, epinephrine, and norepinephrine. Hyposecretion or hypersecretion of these substances causes a variety of disorders and complications that range from psychiatric and sexual problems to coma and death.

The adrenal cortex is the outer layer of an adrenal gland. It secretes three types of steroidal hormones:

1. mineralocorticoids
2. glucocorticoids
3. adrenal androgens and estrogens

Aldosterone in action

Aldosterone is a mineralocorticoid. It regulates the reabsorption of sodium and the excretion of potassium by the kidneys. Aldosterone may be involved with other hormones in the development of hypertension.

Cue cortisol

Cortisol, a glucocorticoid, carries out these five important functions:
1. stimulation of gluconeogenesis (formation of glycogen from non-carbohydrate sources), which occurs in the liver in response to low carbohydrate intake or starvation
2. breakdown of increased protein and mobilization of free fatty acid
3. suppression of immune response
4. assistance with stress response
5. assistance with maintenance of blood pressure and cardiovascular function

Androgens (male sex hormones) promote male traits, especially secondary sex characteristics. Examples of such characteristics are facial hair and a low-pitched voice. Estrogens promote female traits. These hormones are also thought to be responsible for sex drive.

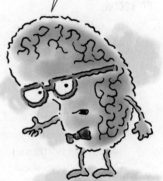

The fight or flight is triggered by the hypothalamus producing a combined response of the sympathetic nervous system and adrenal cortical system.

A gland with a lot of nerve

The adrenal medulla is the inner portion of an adrenal gland. It's an aggregate of nerve tissue that produces the catecholamine hormones epinephrine and norepinephrine that cause vasoconstriction.

Epinephrine causes the response to physical or emotional stress called the *fight or flight response*. This response produces marked dilation of bronchioles and increased blood pressure, blood glucose level, and heart rate.

Pancreas

The pancreas produces glucagon and insulin.

Fasting? You'll need glucose fast . . .

Glucagon is a hormone released when a person is in a fasting state. It stimulates the release of stored glucose from the liver to raise blood glucose levels.

Multiple roles of insulin

Insulin is a hormone released after eating (a time that is also referred to as the postprandial state). This hormone aids glucose transport into the cells and promotes glucose storage. It also stimulates protein synthesis and enhances free fatty acid uptake and storage. Insulin deficiency or cellular resistance to insulin causes diabetes mellitus.

Pituitary gland

The posterior pituitary gland, located at the base of the brain, secretes two hormones:

1. oxytocin, which stimulates uterine contractions during labor and causes the milk letdown reflex in lactating women
2. ADH, which causes reabsorption of water at the collecting duct of the nephrons in the kidney. It raises water content of the blood and counteracts diuresis (loss of water from the body); thus, it is antidiuretic.

> Low blood pressure and low blood volume stimulate the release of ADH.

The ABCs of ADH

ADH secretion depends on plasma osmolality (concentration), which is monitored by hypothalamic neurons. Hypovolemia and hypotension are the most powerful stimulators of ADH release. Other stimulators include pain, stress, trauma, nausea, and the use of morphine, tranquilizers, certain anesthetics, and a positive-pressure breathing apparatus.

It's no secret

In addition to the trophic hormones—ACTH, TSH, LH, and FSH—the anterior pituitary gland secretes prolactin and GH. Prolactin stimulates milk secretion in lactating individuals. GH affects most body tissues. It triggers growth by increasing protein production and fat mobilization and decreasing carbohydrate use.

Thyroid gland

The thyroid gland, located in the anterior neck, secretes the iodine-containing hormones thyroxine (T_4) and triiodothyronine (T_3). Thyroid hormones are necessary for normal growth and development. They also act on many tissues by increasing metabolic activity and protein synthesis.

A good prognosis with treatment

Diseases of the thyroid are caused by thyroid hormone overproduction or deficiency and gland inflammation and enlargement. Most patients have a good prognosis with treatment. Untreated, thyroid disease may progress to an emergency, as in thyroid crisis.

Parathyroid glands

There are four parathyroid glands nestled within the thyroid gland. These glands secrete PTH, which helps regulate blood calcium levels and control bone formation. When hypocalcemia is sensed by the parathyroid glands, they secrete PTH, which stimulates bone to release calcium into the bloodstream.

Disorderly conduct

Disorders of the parathyroid gland involve hyposecretion of PTH, resulting in a reduction of serum calcium (hypocalcemia) that can lead to tetany and seizures, or hypersecretion of PTH, which results in elevated serum calcium levels (hypercalcemia) that can lead to cardiac arrhythmias, muscle and bone weakness, and renal calculi.

Endocrine disorders

The endocrine disorders discussed in this chapter include:
- three adrenal disorders (Addison disease, Cushing syndrome, and pheochromocytoma)
- one pancreatic disorder (diabetes mellitus)
- two pituitary disorders of water metabolism (diabetes insipidus and syndrome of inappropriate ADH)
- three thyroid gland disorders (goiter, hyperthyroidism, and hypothyroidism)

Adrenal disorder: Addison disease

Addison disease, also called *adrenal hypofunction* or *adrenal insufficiency*, occurs in two forms: primary and secondary. It's a disorder that occurs in people of all ages and genders. Either primary or secondary Addison disease can progress into adrenal crisis.

Primary report

The primary form of Addison disease originates within the adrenal glands. It's characterized by decreased secretion by the adrenal glands of mineralocorticoid (aldosterone), glucocorticoid (cortisol), and androgen (testosterone).

Outside influence

The secondary form of Addison disease is caused by a disorder outside the gland, such as a pituitary tumor with corticotropin (ACTH) deficiency. The pituitary is the cause of the disorder because ACTH is not being secreted to stimulate the adrenal glands.

Crisis!

Also called *Addisonian crisis*, adrenal crisis is a critical deficiency of mineralocorticoids (aldosterone) and glucocorticoids (cortisol). It's a medical emergency that requires immediate, vigorous treatment. (See *Understanding adrenal crisis.*)

Now I get it!

Understanding adrenal crisis

Adrenal crisis (acute adrenal insufficiency) is the most serious complication of Addison disease. It may occur gradually or suddenly.

Who's at risk

This potentially lethal condition usually develops in patients who:
- don't respond to hormone therapy
- undergo extreme stress without adequate glucocorticoid replacement
- abruptly stop hormone therapy

- undergo trauma
- undergo bilateral adrenalectomy
- develop adrenal gland thrombosis after a severe infection (Waterhouse–Friderichsen syndrome)

What happens

In adrenal crisis, destruction of the adrenal cortex leads to a rapid decline in the steroid hormones cortisol and aldosterone. This directly affects the liver, stomach, and kidneys. The flowchart below illustrates what happens in adrenal crisis.

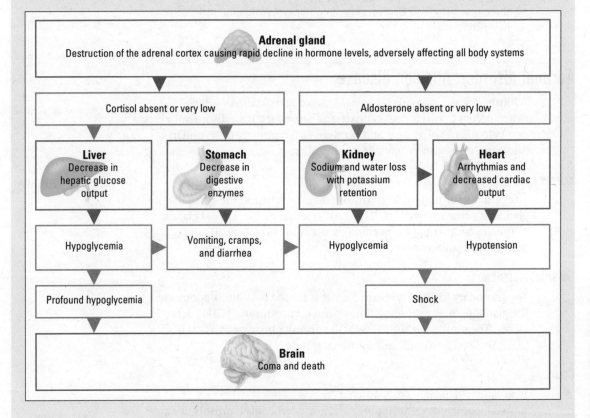

Adrenal gland
Destruction of the adrenal cortex causing rapid decline in hormone levels, adversely affecting all body systems

Cortisol absent or very low

Aldosterone absent or very low

Liver
Decrease in hepatic glucose output

Stomach
Decrease in digestive enzymes

Kidney
Sodium and water loss with potassium retention

Heart
Arrhythmias and decreased cardiac output

Hypoglycemia

Vomiting, cramps, and diarrhea

Hypoglycemia

Hypotension

Profound hypoglycemia

Shock

Brain
Coma and death

How it happens

In primary Addison disease, more than 90% of both adrenal glands are destroyed. In most cases, destruction of the adrenal glands results from an autoimmune process whereby circulating antibodies attack adrenal tissue. Destruction of the gland may also be idiopathic (no known cause). This causes a lack of cortisol secretion by the adrenal glands. Then the pituitary gland, through feedback, senses insufficient cortisol release and secretes excessive ACTH.

Other causes of primary Addison disease include:
* tuberculosis
* removal of both adrenal glands
* hemorrhage into the adrenal glands
* neoplasms
* infections, such as human immunodeficiency virus infection, histoplasmosis, meningococcal pneumonia, and cytomegalovirus (CMV)

The signs and symptoms of primary adrenal insufficiency result from decreased glucocorticoid (cortisol) production. Signs and symptoms may develop slowly and stay unrecognized if production is adequate for the normal demands of life. It may progress to adrenal crisis when trauma, surgery, or other severe physical stress requires greater release of cortisol but the adrenal glands do not have sufficient hormone.

Secondary disease

Secondary Addison disease mainly results from lack of pituitary function:
* hypopituitarism leads to decreased corticotropin (ACTH) secretion, which can occur if patients are on long-term corticosteroid drug treatment. Long-term use of exogenous corticosteroid agents makes the pituitary gland less active; because there is sufficient cortisol coming from a drug, the pituitary gland senses there is sufficient cortisol and stops secreting ACTH. For example, several months of prednisone treatment will diminish the body's natural ability to secrete cortisol. This decrease in the pituitary gland's secretion of ACTH results in adrenal atrophy, which means the patient has lost the natural ability to cope with a stressful situation.

What to look for

These signs and symptoms may indicate Addison disease:
* confusion
* extreme fatigue
* GI disturbances and weight loss
* hyperkalemia

- hyperpigmentation (in primary adrenal insufficiency)
- hypoglycemia
- hyponatremia
- hypotension
- muscle weakness
- low tolerance of any stress to the body

Patient history may reveal synthetic steroid use, adrenal surgery, or recent infection. The patient may complain of fatigue, lightheadedness when rising from a chair or bed (termed *orthostatic hypotension*), cravings for salty food, decreased tolerance for even minor stress, anxiety, irritability, and various GI disturbances, such as nausea, vomiting, anorexia, and chronic diarrhea. The patient may also have reduced urine output and other symptoms of dehydration. Females may have decreased libido from reduced androgen production and amenorrhea. Males also endure low androgen production, which causes erectile dysfunction, decreased libido, and infertility.

Getting physical

During your examination, you may detect poor coordination, dry skin and mucous membranes, and sparse axillary and pubic hair in women. The patient's skin is typically a deep bronze, especially in the creases of the hands and on the knuckles, elbows, and knees. The patient may also have a darkening of scars, areas of vitiligo (an absence of pigmentation), and increased pigmentation of the mucous membranes, especially in the mouth. The darkened pigmentation is caused by the pituitary gland's excessive secretion of ACTH in primary adrenal insufficiency, which occurs when cortisol is low. ACTH stimulates melanocyte-stimulating hormone (MSH), which stimulates melanocytes (skin pigment cells).

Secondary adrenal hypofunction (which is caused by pituitary ACTH deficiency) doesn't cause hyperpigmentation, because ACTH and MSH levels are low.

With early diagnosis and treatment, the prognosis for a patient with either primary or secondary Addison disease is good. (See *Treating Addison disease.*)

What tests tell you

These laboratory tests are used in diagnosing adrenal hypofunction:

- Plasma and urine tests detect decreased corticosteroid concentrations.
- Measurement of corticotropin levels classifies the disease as primary or secondary. A high level indicates the primary disorder, and a low level points to the secondary disorder.
- Rapid corticotropin test (ACTH stimulation test) demonstrates plasma cortisol response to corticotropin. After obtaining

Treating Addison disease

Lifelong corticosteroid replacement is the main treatment for patients with primary or secondary Addison disease. In general, cortisone or hydrocortisone is given because they have a mineralocorticoid effect. Fludrocortisone, a synthetic drug that acts as a mineralocorticoid, may also be given to prevent dehydration and hypotension. Females with muscle weakness and decreased libido may benefit from testosterone injections, but they risk masculinizing effects. Males can also benefit from testosterone administration.

In stressful situations, the patient may need to double or triple the usual corticosteroid dose. These situations include acute illness (because a fever increases the basal metabolic rate), injury, surgery, or psychologically stressful episodes.

Crisis control

Treatment for adrenal crisis is prompt IV bolus administration of 100 mg of hydrocortisone along with 1 L isotonic fluid, followed by hydrocortisone 50 mg every 6 hours (200 mg/d) given IV until the patient's condition stabilizes. An additional 3 to 5 L of IV normal saline solution may be required during the acute stage with caution in older adults, those with heart failure, and those with renal impairment.

With proper treatment, the crisis usually subsides quickly, with blood pressure stabilizing and water and sodium levels returning to normal. Afterward, maintenance doses of hydrocortisone keep the patient's condition stable. Occasionally, mineralocorticoids are required to help provide stabilization, more often in patients who have primary Addison disease. Once glucocorticoid doses have tapered down to 50 mg/d, fludrocortisone may be added at 100 μg/daily to aid in recovery.

Remember to assess the patient for the complications associated with glucocorticoid use while administering medications. Keep alert for hyperglycemia, secondary infections, and peptic ulcers.

---

plasma cortisol samples, an IV infusion of cosyntropin is administered. Plasma samples are taken 30 and 60 minutes later. If the plasma cortisol level doesn't increase, adrenal insufficiency is suspected.

Is it a crisis?

In a patient with typical symptoms of Addison disease, these laboratory findings strongly suggest adrenal crisis:
- reduced serum sodium levels
- increased serum potassium, serum calcium, and blood urea nitrogen levels
- elevated hematocrit and elevated lymphocyte and eosinophil counts
- x-rays showing adrenal calcification, tumor, or adrenal atrophy
- decreased plasma cortisol levels—less than 10 μg/dL in the morning, with lower levels at night

Adrenal disorder: Cushing syndrome

Cushing syndrome is a cluster of physical abnormalities that occur when the adrenal glands secrete excess glucocorticoids (cortisol). It may also cause excessive androgen secretion. When glucocorticoid excess is caused by pituitary-dependent conditions, it's called *Cushing disease (secondary hyperadrenalism)*. However, it is *Cushing syndrome* when caused by the overactivity of the adrenal glands (*primary hyperadrenalism*).

How it happens
Cushing disorders appear in three forms:
- primary, caused by a disease of the adrenal cortex (also called *Cushing syndrome*)
- secondary, caused by hyperfunction of corticotropin-secreting cells of the anterior pituitary gland (also called *Cushing disease*)
- tertiary, caused by hypothalamic dysfunction or injury

Cancel the corticotropin
In about 70% of patients, Cushing disorder results from an excess of corticotropin (ACTH) from the pituitary. This leads to hyperplasia (excessive cell proliferation) of the adrenal cortex. Corticotropin overproduction may stem from:
- pituitary hypersecretion (Cushing disease)
- a corticotropin-producing tumor in another organ (commonly occurs in lung cancer)
- administration of synthetic glucocorticoids (corticosteroid drugs)

In the remaining 30% of patients, Cushing disorder results from a cortisol-secreting adrenal tumor, which is usually benign. This is called *Cushing syndrome*.

Administration of excessive corticosteroid drugs can also lead to Cushing syndrome because it will shut down the pituitary secretion of ACTH and lead to adrenal gland atrophy.

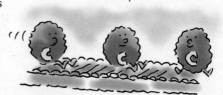

In most patients, Cushing syndrome results from overproduction of the hormone corticotropin.

It's getting complicated
Complications associated with Cushing syndrome are caused by the effects of cortisol, the principal glucocorticoid. These complications may include:
- osteoporosis and pathologic fractures, caused by increased calcium resorption from bone
- peptic ulcer, caused by increased gastric secretions, pepsin production, and decreased gastric mucus
- hyperlipidemia
- high blood glucose (hyperglycemia), a diabetes-like state caused by increased hepatic gluconeogenesis and insulin resistance

- increased risk of venous thromboembolism due to hypercoagulability
- hypertension
- weight gain (round, moon-like facies) and truncal obesity
- hirsutism, skin develops striae
- ruddy complexion
- immunosuppression (white blood cells [WBCs] are suppressed due to high cortisol)
- emotional depression
- mental changes such as concentration difficulty and confusion
- infertility

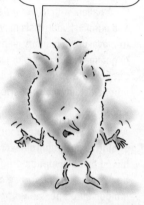

Hypertension is common in Cushing syndrome and can cause ischemic heart disease and heart failure.

Compromised

Frequent infections or slow wound healing due to decreased lymphocyte production, hyperglycemia, and suppressed antibody formation may occur. Suppressed inflammatory response may mask infection.

Taking it to heart

Hypertension due to sodium and water retention is common in Cushing syndrome. It may lead to ischemic heart disease and heart failure.

Sexual and psychological complications

Menstrual disturbances and sexual dysfunction may also occur because of increased adrenal androgen secretion. Decreased ability to handle stress may result in psychiatric problems, ranging from mood swings to psychosis.

What to look for

If your patient has some or all of these signs, Cushing syndrome might be the cause:
- weight gain
- muscle weakness
- fatigue
- buffalo hump
- thinning extremities with muscle wasting and fat mobilization
- thin, fragile skin
- thinning scalp hair
- moon face and ruddy complexion
- hirsutism
- truncal obesity
- broad purple striae
- bruising
- impaired wound healing

The prognosis depends on early diagnosis, identification of the underlying cause, and effective treatment. (See *Treating Cushing syndrome*.)

Battling illness

Treating Cushing syndrome

Restoring hormone balance and reversing Cushing syndrome may require radiation, drug therapy, or surgery. Treatment depends on the cause of the disease.

A patient with pituitary-dependent Cushing disease and adrenal hyperplasia may require hypophysectomy (removal of the pituitary gland) using either traditional or gamma knife surgery or pituitary irradiation. If these treatments are unsuccessful or impractical, bilateral adrenalectomy may be performed.

Diverse drugs

A patient with a nonendocrine corticotropin–producing tumor requires excision of the tumor, followed by combination drug therapy with various agents that can decrease cortisol levels. Such drugs include mitotane, metyrapone, aminoglutethimide, or ketoconazole.

An ounce of prevention

Before surgery, the patient needs to control edema, diabetes, hypertension, and other cardiovascular manifestations and prevent infection. Glucocorticoids given before surgery can help prevent acute adrenal insufficiency during surgery. Cortisol therapy is essential during and after surgery to combat the physiologic stress imposed by the removal of the pituitary or adrenal glands.

If normal cortisol production resumes, steroid therapy may gradually be tapered and eventually discontinued. However, the patient who has a bilateral adrenalectomy or a total hypophysectomy requires lifelong steroid replacement. After surgery, these patients also must be monitored for return to normal sodium, T_4, and prolactin levels. Occasionally, overcorrection can occur, which may require pharmacologic intervention.

What tests tell you

Diagnosis of Cushing syndrome depends on a demonstrated increase in cortisol production and the failure to suppress endogenous cortisol secretion after dexamethasone is given.

These tests may be performed:

- Late night salivary cortisol measured twice. This is performed because it is often the first and most sensitive test to detect elevated cortisol. It is the most widely studied test for Cushing and has an over 93% sensitivity. However, there is a high rate of false positives and a thus a second confirmatory test is required if one scores a positive on this first line test.
- ACTH level determines whether Cushing syndrome is ACTH dependent.
- Low-dose dexamethasone suppression test or 24-hour urine test determines the free cortisol excretion rate. Failure to suppress plasma and urine cortisol levels confirms the diagnosis.
- High-dose dexamethasone suppression test determines whether Cushing syndrome results from pituitary dysfunction. If dexamethasone suppresses plasma cortisol levels, the test result is positive. Failure to suppress plasma cortisol levels indicates an adrenal tumor or a nonendocrine, corticotropin-secreting tumor. This test can produce false-positive results.

- Radiologic evaluation locates a causative tumor in the pituitary or adrenal glands. Tests include ultrasonography, computed tomography (CT) scan, and magnetic resonance imaging (MRI) enhanced with gadolinium.
- WBC count shows levels elevated above 11,000 mm^3.
- Petrosal sinus sampling is the most accurate way to determine whether Cushing syndrome is due to a pituitary tumor or some other cause. ACTH levels higher in the petrosal sinuses than in a forearm vein indicate the presence of a pituitary adenoma. This is done by drawing blood from the veins that drain the pituitary gland, an invasive procedure, in order to obtain ACTH levels.

Adrenal disorder: pheochromocytoma

Pheochromocytoma is a rare adrenal mass that is commonly found incidentally on abdominal CT scans. These tumors, which are sometimes referred to as "incidentalomas," secrete excess catecholamines, norepinephrine, and epinephrine. Hypertension, tachycardia (sensed as palpitations), headaches, diaphoresis, and flushing are common symptoms.

How it happens

Pheochromocytoma tumors can be caused by genetic factors or may arise sporadically. These tumors are often part of other genetic disorders such as multiple endocrine neoplasia, neurofibromatosis, or von Hippel–Lindau disease.

What to look for

Biochemical studies should be performed first followed by imaging. Standard blood tests include glucose, calcium, blood cell count with differential, and 24-hour urine for catecholamines.

Testing is recommended in symptomatic patients, patients with an adrenal incidentaloma, and patients who have a hereditary risk for developing a pheochromocytoma. (See *Treating pheochromocytoma*.)

Complications

In malignancy, the survival rate is less 50%. However, in the benign tumors, the survivor rate is 90% and above. Associated risk includes myocarditis, myocardial infarction, dilated cardiomyopathy, and pulmonary edema.

Common symptoms include:
- extremes in blood pressure (persistently low or high)
- headaches
- palpitations
- abdominal pain
- diaphoresis
- chest pain

Treating pheochromocytoma

Surgery is the treatment of choice. Alternatives to surgery include radiation therapy, chemotherapy, and targeted therapy (substances that destroy cancer cells and not normal cells).

Pancreatic disorder: diabetes mellitus

Diabetes mellitus is a disease in which the body doesn't produce or properly use insulin, leading to hyperglycemia. The disease occurs in two primary forms:

- **Type 1 diabetes mellitus (T1DM)** is caused by insufficient insulin reserves in the pancreas due to autoimmune destruction of beta cells.
- **Type 2 diabetes mellitus (T2DM)** is caused by cellular insulin resistance, meaning that the body cells are insensitive to insulin. This type of diabetes is more prevalent.

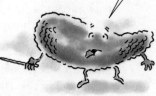

Diabetes mellitus is a pancreatic disorder.

There are also several secondary forms of diabetes mellitus, caused by such conditions as pancreatic disease, pregnancy (gestational diabetes mellitus), hormonal or genetic problems, and certain drugs or chemicals.

Of the estimated 34 million US adults with diabetes, about one in five (21%) is undiagnosed. The Centers for Disease Control and Prevention estimates that 88 million people in the United States have prediabetes and that most of them aren't aware of that fact. The incidence of diabetes increases with age. Diabetes is the seventh leading cause of death in the United States; however, it increases risk of cardiovascular disease, which is the number one cause of death.

How it happens

Normally, insulin allows glucose to enter cells, where it's used for energy and stored as glycogen. Insulin also stimulates protein synthesis and free fatty acid storage in adipose tissue. In T1DM, glucose can't enter body cells because there is a deficiency of pancreatic insulin. In T2DM, body cells' resistance to insulin prevents glucose from entering cells. In both T1DM and T2DM, glucose accumulates in the bloodstream, causing hyperglycemia. Hyperglycemia causes endothelial injury of the lining of all arteries, which enhances development of arteriosclerosis.

Type 1 diabetes

In T1DM, the beta cells in the pancreas are destroyed or suppressed. T1DM is subdivided into idiopathic and immune-mediated types. With the idiopathic type, patients have a permanent insulin deficiency with no evidence of autoimmunity.

In the immune-mediated type, a local or organ-specific deficit may induce an autoimmune attack on beta cells. This attack, in turn, causes an inflammatory response in the pancreas called *insulitis*.

Islet cell antibodies may be present long before symptoms become apparent. These immune markers also precede evidence of beta cell deficiency. Autoantibodies against insulin have also been noted.

By the time the disease becomes apparent, 80% of the beta cells are dysfunctional.

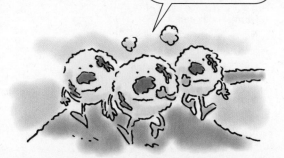

When beta cells stop or slow, it's unlikely that they'll regain function again.

Type 2 diabetes

T2DM is mainly caused by resistance to insulin of target tissues. T2DM often develops as a consequence of obesity. (See *Understanding type 2 diabetes* and *Screening guidelines*.)

Secondary diabetes

Common causes of secondary diabetes are:
- physical or emotional stress, which may cause prolonged elevation in levels of the stress hormones cortisol, epinephrine, glucagon, and GH (this, in turn, raises the blood glucose level and increases demands on the pancreas)
- pregnancy, which causes weight gain and high levels of estrogen and placental hormones
- use of adrenal corticosteroids, hormonal contraceptives, and other drugs that antagonize the effects of insulin
- some viral infections have been implicated, such as CMV, adenovirus, rubella, and mumps

Acute danger

Two acute metabolic complications of diabetes are diabetic ketoacidosis (DKA) and hyperosmolar hyperglycemic nonketotic syndrome (HHNS). These life-threatening conditions require immediate medical intervention. (See *Understanding DKA and HHNS*.)

Chronic complications

Patients with diabetes mellitus also have a higher risk of various chronic complications affecting virtually all body systems. This is

Understanding type 2 diabetes

Normally, in response to blood glucose levels, the pancreatic islet cells release insulin. In type 2 diabetes, problems arise when insufficient insulin is produced or when the body's cells resist insulin.

Normal body cell

Normally, insulin molecules bind to the receptors on the body's cells. When activated by insulin, portals open to allow glucose to enter the cell, where it's converted to energy or stored as glycogen.

Diabetic body cell

In type 2 diabetes, the body's cells develop a resistance to insulin, making it more difficult for glucose to enter the cell. As a result, glucose builds up in the bloodstream, causing hyperglycemia. Hyperglycemia damages endothelial lining of all the arteries throughout the body. This endothelial damage acts as an arteriosclerosis accelerator. People with uncontrolled diabetes develop arteriosclerosis at a greater rate than people without diabetes.

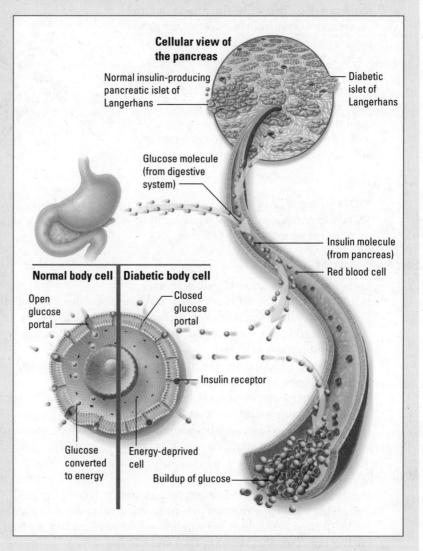

Cellular view of the pancreas

Normal insulin-producing pancreatic islet of Langerhans

Diabetic islet of Langerhans

Glucose molecule (from digestive system)

Insulin molecule (from pancreas)

Red blood cell

| Normal body cell | Diabetic body cell |

Open glucose portal

Closed glucose portal

Insulin receptor

Glucose converted to energy

Energy-deprived cell

Buildup of glucose

Screening guidelines

The guidelines below, from the American Diabetes Association, are also endorsed by the National Institutes of Health.

• Adults should be tested for diabetes every 3 years starting at age 35. Those whose test shows a high glucose reading should have the test repeated on another day.

• People at increased risk may need to be tested earlier or more often. High-risk groups include Native Americans, African Americans, Asians, Pacific Islanders, Alaska Natives, Hispanics, and anyone who is overweight (body mass index > 25) or has high blood pressure or high cholesterol, has a history of gestational diabetes, or has a strong family history of diabetes.

• The cutoff used for a diagnosis of diabetes is a fasting plasma glucose level greater than or equal to 126 mg/dL on at least two occasions or a hemoglobin A1C greater than or equal to 6.5%.

mainly due to the hyperglycemia that damages the endothelial lining of all the arteries in the body, leading to arteriosclerosis. The most common chronic complications are cardiovascular disease, peripheral vascular disease, eye disease (retinopathy), kidney disease (nephropathy), skin disease (diabetic dermopathy), and peripheral and autonomic neuropathy.

Research shows that glucose readings don't have to be as high as previously thought for complications to develop. So meticulous blood glucose control is essential to help prevent acute and chronic complications.

What to look for

Patients with T1DM usually report rapidly developing symptoms, including muscle wasting and loss of subcutaneous fat.

With T2DM, symptoms are generally vague and long-standing and develop gradually. In T2DM, patients generally report a family history of diabetes mellitus, gestational diabetes, delivery of a baby weighing more than 9 lb (4 kg), severe viral infection, another endocrine disease, recent stress or trauma, or use of drugs that increase blood glucose levels. Obesity, especially in the abdominal area, is also common. Patients with a history of hypertension or hyperlipidemia are also at risk.

It takes both types

Patients with T1DM or T2DM may report symptoms related to hyperglycemia and cell starvation, such as:

• excessive urination (polyuria) due to osmotic diuresis
• excessive thirst (polydipsia) due to cellular dehydration

Understanding DKA and HHNS

Diabetic ketoacidosis (DKA) and hyperosmolar hyperglycemic nonketotic syndrome (HHNS) are acute complications of hyperglycemic crisis that may occur with diabetes. If not treated properly, either may result in coma or death.

DKA occurs most often in patients with T1DM or those less than 65 years old. It may be the first evidence of the disease. However, it may also occur in anyone who is experiencing extreme stress such as those undergoing acute trauma, illness, and cardiovascular events. HHNS occurs most often in patients with type 2 diabetes or those older than 65 years, but it also occurs in anyone whose insulin tolerance is stressed and in patients who have undergone certain therapeutic procedures, such as peritoneal dialysis, hemodialysis, tube feedings, or total parenteral nutrition.

Acute insulin deficiency (absolute in DKA; relative in HHNS) precipitates both conditions. Causes include illness, stress, infection, and, in patients with DKA, failure to take insulin.

Buildup of glucose

Inadequate insulin hinders glucose uptake by fat and muscle cells. Because the cells can't take in glucose to convert to energy, glucose accumulates in the blood (hyperglycemia). At the same time, the liver responds to the demands of the energy-starved cells by breaking down glycogen to glucose and releasing glucose into the blood, further increasing the blood glucose level. When this level exceeds the renal threshold, excess glucose is excreted in urine.

As time goes on, insulin-deprived cells can't utilize glucose. The body starts to break down fat and proteins to provide sustenance for the cells. Fatty tissue breaks down, and muscle breaks down to release proteins, which further break down into amino acids. The liver then converts these fatty acids and amino acids into glucose in a process termed *gluconeogenesis*. The liver then releases more and more glucose into the bloodstream.

As a result of these processes, blood glucose levels are grossly elevated. The aftermath is increased serum osmolarity and glycosuria (high amounts of glucose in the urine), leading to osmotic diuresis. Glycosuria is higher in HHNS than in DKA because blood glucose levels are higher in HHNS.

A deadly cycle

The massive fluid loss from osmotic diuresis causes fluid and electrolyte imbalances and dehydration. Dehydration causes excessive thirst; this symptom is termed *polydipsia*. Water loss exceeds glucose and electrolyte loss, contributing to hyperosmolarity. The patient urinates more due to the water loss; this symptom is termed *polyuria*. This leads to a deadly cycle: There is no glucose entry into cells. Glucose accumulates in the bloodstream. Fluid shifts from intracellular space into the extracellular space (bloodstream). Dehydration and excessive urination continue, which can lead to shock, coma, and death.

DKA complication

All of these steps hold true for DKA and HHNS, but DKA involves an additional, simultaneous process that leads to metabolic acidosis. The absolute insulin deficiency causes cells to convert fats into glycerol and fatty acids for energy. The fatty acids can't be metabolized as quickly as they're released, so they accumulate in the liver, where they're converted into ketones (ketoacids). These ketones accumulate in the blood and urine and cause ketoacidosis. Ketoacidosis is a metabolic acidosis that interferes with cellular function and can cause coma and death.

- excessive eating (polyphagia) due to lack of glucose entry into cells
- weight loss due to breakdown of fat and muscle
- fatigue
- weakness
- vision changes

- increased susceptibility to infections; WBCs don't work well in a hyperglycemic environment
- vaginal candidiasis; the accumulation of glucose in vaginal cells can lead to candida (yeast) infection

Patients with either type of diabetes may have poor skin turgor, dry mucous membranes related to dehydration, decreased peripheral pulses, cool skin temperature, and decreased reflexes. Patients in crisis with DKA may have a fruity breath odor, because of ketones in the saliva, as well as deep, rapid respirations (Kussmaul respirations), which develop as an effort to eliminate carbon dioxide and correct acidosis. (See *Treating diabetes mellitus*.)

Battling illness

Treating diabetes mellitus

Effective treatment for diabetes optimizes blood glucose levels and decreases complications. In type 1 diabetes, treatment includes insulin replacement, meal planning, and exercise. Current forms of insulin replacement include single-dose, mixed-dose, split mixed-dose, and multiple-dose regimens. The multiple-dose regimens may use an insulin pump.

Insulin action
Insulin may be rapid acting (Humalog), fast acting (regular), intermediate acting (NPH), or a premixed combination of fast acting and intermediate acting. Purified human insulin is used commonly today. Patients may inject insulin subcutaneously throughout the day or receive insulin through an insulin pump. A common treatment regimen, the basal-bolus insulin regimen, usually consists of 50% of the total daily dose prescribed as basal insulin and 50% prescribed as bolus insulin. Boluses of insulin are commonly administered via insulin pen at or around meal times.

Personalized meal plan
Treatment for both types of diabetes also requires a meal plan to meet nutritional needs, to control blood glucose levels, and to help the patient reach and maintain their ideal body weight. An exercise plan is also needed. A dietitian estimates the total amount of energy a patient needs per day based on their ideal body weight. The dietitian then plans meals with the appropriate carbohydrate, fat, and protein content. For the diet to work, the patient must follow it consistently and eat at regular times.

Weight reduction is a goal for the obese patient with type 2 diabetes.

Other treatments
Exercise is also useful in managing type 2 diabetes because it increases insulin sensitivity, improves glucose tolerance, and promotes weight loss. In addition, patients with type 2 diabetes may need oral antidiabetic drugs to stimulate endogenous insulin production and increase insulin sensitivity at the cellular level. There are now also alternative injectable agents such as GLP-1 agonists that may be used in addition to or in place of oral agents. Oral glucophage (metformin) is a common first-line treatment recommendation for patients with type 2 diabetes. Treatment for long-term complications may include dialysis or kidney transplantation for renal failure, photocoagulation for retinopathy, and vascular surgery for large vessel disease. Pancreas transplantation is also an option.

What tests tell you

In nonpregnant adults, a diagnosis of diabetes mellitus may be confirmed by:

- symptoms of diabetes and a random blood glucose level equal to or above 200 mg/dL
- a fasting plasma glucose level equal to or greater than 126 mg/dL on at least two occasions
- a blood glucose level above 200 mg/dL on the second hour of the glucose tolerance test and on at least one other occasion during a glucose tolerance test

Three other tests may be done:

- An ophthalmologic examination may show diabetic retinopathy.
- Urinalysis shows the presence of ketones and glucose.
- Blood tests for glycosylated hemoglobin (also referred to as hemoglobin A1C) monitor the long-term effectiveness of diabetes therapy. Hemoglobin A1C levels show how well the blood glucose has been controlled over the preceding 3 months. Ideally, the hemoglobin A1C goal is less than 6.5%, although some healthcare providers assert that a hemoglobin A1C less than 7% is adequate.

Pituitary disorder: diabetes insipidus

Diabetes insipidus is a disorder of water metabolism caused by a deficiency of ADH (also called *vasopressin*). The absence of ADH allows filtered water to be excreted in the urine instead of reabsorbed into the bloodstream at the kidney. The disease causes excessive urination and excessive thirst and fluid intake. It may first appear in childhood or early adulthood and is more common in males than in females.

How it happens

Some drugs as well as injury to the posterior pituitary gland can cause abnormalities in ADH secretion. A less common cause is a failure of the kidneys to respond to ADH. Lesions of the hypothalamus, infundibular stem, and posterior pituitary gland can also interfere with ADH synthesis, transport, or release. Lesions may be caused by brain tumor, removal of the pituitary gland (hypophysectomy), aneurysm, thrombus, immunologic disorder, or infection.

When ADH is absent

Normally, ADH is synthesized in the hypothalamus and then stored by the posterior pituitary gland. When it's released into the general circulation, ADH increases the water permeability of the distal and collecting tubules of the kidneys, causing water reabsorption into the bloodstream. If ADH is absent, the filtered water is excreted in the urine instead of being reabsorbed, and the patient excretes large quantities of dilute urine. (See *Understanding ADH.*)

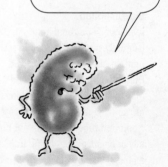

Without ADH, the kidneys are unable to reabsorb fluid, which causes excretion of large quantities of dilute urine and excessive thirst.

Now I get it!

Understanding ADH

In response to increased serum osmolality and reduced circulating volume, the posterior pituitary gland releases antidiuretic hormone (ADH). Circulating ADH alters permeability of the distal renal tubules and collecting ducts in the kidney, resulting in increased reabsorption of water into the bloodstream.

This decreases serum osmolality and increases circulating volume. Through a negative feedback mechanism, decreased osmolality and increased volume halt the release of ADH.

ADH release	Negative feedback halting release of ADH
Hemoconcentration or hypovolemia occurs.	Hemodilution or hypervolemia occurs.
Stimulation of receptors in posterior pituitary releases more ADH.	Stimulation of receptors in posterior pituitary decreases amount of ADH released.
Kidneys become more permeable to water.	Kidneys become less permeable to water.
Water is conserved and reabsorbed.	Water isn't reabsorbed, and diuresis occurs.
Serum osmolality and urine output decrease, and urine osmolality increases.	Serum osmolality and urine output increase, and urine osmolality decreases.

What to look for

The patient's history shows:

- abrupt onset of extreme polyuria (usually 4 to 16 L/d of dilute urine, but sometimes as much as 30 L/d)
- polydipsia (extreme thirst) and consumption of extraordinarily large volumes of fluid

In severe cases, fatigue occurs because sleep is interrupted by the need to void and drink fluids. Children often have enuresis (involuntary urination), sleep disturbances, irritability, anorexia, and decreased weight gain and linear growth.

Additional signs and symptoms may include:

- weight loss
- dizziness
- weakness

- constipation
- dehydration
- increased serum sodium and osmolality

What lies underneath?

The prognosis is good for uncomplicated diabetes insipidus treated with vasopressin; patients usually lead normal lives. However, when the disease is complicated by an underlying disorder such as cancer, a pituitary tumor, or pituitary damage, the prognosis varies. (See *Treating diabetes insipidus*.)

One thing leads to another

Untreated diabetes insipidus can produce hypovolemia, hyperosmolality, circulatory collapse, loss of consciousness, and CNS damage. These complications are most likely to occur if the patient has an impaired or absent thirst mechanism.

A prolonged urine flow may produce chronic complications, such as bladder distention, enlarged calyces, hydroureter (distention of the ureter with fluid), and hydronephrosis (collection of urine in the kidney). Complications may also result from underlying conditions, such as metastatic brain lesions, head trauma, and infections.

What tests tell you

These tests distinguish diabetes insipidus from other disorders causing polyuria:
- Urinalysis reveals almost colorless urine of low osmolality (50 to 200 mOsm/kg of water, less than that of plasma) and low specific gravity (less than 1.005).
- Dehydration test differentiates ADH deficiency from other forms of polyuria by comparing urine osmolality after dehydration and

Battling illness

Treating diabetes insipidus

Until the cause of diabetes insipidus is identified and eliminated, patients are given various forms of vasopressin to control fluid balance and prevent dehydration. The following may be administered:
- Aqueous vasopressin is a replacement agent administered by subcutaneous injection. It's used in the initial management of diabetes insipidus after head trauma or a neurosurgical procedure.

- Desmopressin acetate, a synthetic vasopressin analogue, affects prolonged antidiuretic activity and has no pressor effects. A long-acting drug, desmopressin acetate is administered intranasally, orally, sublingually, subcutaneous, and intravenously.

after ADH administration. Diabetes insipidus is diagnosed if the increase in urine osmolality after ADH administration exceeds 9%. After administration of ADH, patients with pituitary diabetes insipidus have decreased urine output and increased urine specific gravity. This proves the patient has an ADH deficiency due to a pituitary abnormality. People with nephrogenic diabetes insipidus have kidneys that do not respond to ADH, so they show no response to ADH.

- Plasma or urinary ADH evaluation may be performed after fluid restriction or hypertonic saline infusion to determine whether diabetes insipidus originated from damage to the posterior pituitary gland or failure of the kidneys to respond to ADH (nephrogenic). ADH levels are decreased in pituitary-induced diabetes insipidus, but ADH is elevated in the nephrogenic type of diabetes insipidus.

If the patient is critically ill, diagnosis may be based on these laboratory values alone:

- urine osmolality of 200 mOsm/kg (very low osmolality; dilute urine)
- urine specific gravity of 1.005 (very low osmolality; dilute urine)
- serum osmolality of 300 mOsm/kg (high serum osmolality; blood lacks sufficient water)
- serum sodium of 147 mEq/L (hypernatremia due to lack of sufficient water in blood)

Pituitary disorder: syndrome of inappropriate antidiuretic hormone

Syndrome of inappropriate antidiuretic hormone (SIADH) is a disorder of water metabolism caused by an excess of ADH, resulting in serum hypo-osmolality (excessive water in the bloodstream). This syndrome, which is due to excessive ADH, is the opposite of diabetes insipidus (which is a lack of ADH). Excessive water is reabsorbed into the bloodstream due to the excessive ADH effect on the nephron. Dilutional hyponatremia occurs in the setting of fluid overload, creating a hypo-osmolar state.

How it happens

An abundance of water in the bloodstream is the major problem in SIADH, with consequent low serum osmolality and dilutional hyponatremia. Excessive release of ADH can be due to the dysfunction of the pituitary gland or other disorders, such as small cell carcinoma of the lung. Lung cancers often secrete inappropriate hormones such as ADH. Excessive ADH causes excessive reabsorption of water at the collecting ducts in the nephrons; this causes blood to become highly diluted. Dilutional hyponatremia and excessive urination occur.

Causes

The most common causes of SIADH are brain surgery, head trauma, and lung cancer. SIADH can also occur as a side effect of some medications. Any CNS abnormality—including stroke, hemorrhage, infection, and trauma—can enhance ADH release from the pituitary gland, leading to SIADH. Small cell lung cancer (SCLC) is the most common tumor leading to inappropriate ADH secretion. A number of drugs associated with SIADH act by enhancing the release or effect of ADH. The most common drugs include carbamazepine, oxcarbazepine, chlorpropamide, cyclophosphamide, and selective serotonin reuptake inhibitors (SSRIs).

Ecstasy (methylenedioxymethamphetamine), an illicit psychoactive drug that is often misused, is particularly associated with the direct release of ADH.

What to watch for

The earliest clinical manifestations of SIADH occur due to acute dilutional hyponatremia when the serum sodium concentration falls below 125 to 130 mEq/L (normal 135 to 145 mEq/L). These nonspecific, vague symptoms, which may not prompt electrolyte measurement, can include:
- malaise
- nausea
- anorexia

As the dilutional hyponatremia progresses, further symptoms can occur, such as:
- weakness
- irritability
- drowsiness
- confusion

If the serum sodium level falls below 115 to 120 mEq/L, the following can happen:
- seizures
- coma
- respiratory arrest

It's important to remember that a patient with a slow, steady fall in their sodium level will present with more subtle symptoms than a patient with a rapid fall in their sodium level. Additionally, the more severe neurological symptoms do not typically occur with sodium levels at or above 120 mEq/L.

What is the treatment?

In addition to a fluid (water) restriction, a hypertonic saline solution (3% saline) is typically required to correct the hyponatremia. However, the sodium level must be corrected carefully and slowly to avoid cerebral effects.

Diagnostics

SIADH can be difficult to diagnose because it is not a common disorder, and symptoms can be subtle and nonspecific. In slow-developing, chronic hyponatremia, cerebral adaptation occurs, and patients can remain without symptoms despite a serum sodium concentration below 120 mmol/L. Serum hyponatremia (less than 135 mg/dL), normal urine sodium (greater than 40 mEq/L), low serum osmolality (less than 275 mOsmol/kg), and normal urine osmolality (greater than 100 mOsmol/kg) are diagnostic findings in SIADH.

Thyroid disorder: goiter

A goiter is simply an enlargement of the thyroid gland. With a goiter present, the thyroid gland may or may not function normally. In resource-limited countries, a goiter can be related to a diet deficient in iodine. In the United States, the most likely cause of a goiter is that thyroid gland enlargement is causing dysfunctional activity of the gland. The possible dysfunctional gland states are hypothyroidism, hyperthyroidism, and thyroid cancer.

Thyroid disorder: hyperthyroidism

When thyroid hormone is overproduced, it creates a metabolic imbalance called *hyperthyroidism* or *thyrotoxicosis*. Excess thyroid hormone is most often caused by Graves disease. Graves disease occurs when the body's own antibodies overstimulate the thyroid gland; what triggers the antibodies is unknown. Graves disease is considered an autoimmune disease. (See *Types of hyperthyroidism*.)

How grave is Graves disease?

Graves disease is an autoimmune disorder that causes hyperthyroidism, which leads to multiple systemic changes. It occurs mostly in people ages 30 to 60, especially those whose family histories include thyroid abnormalities. Only 5% of patients are younger than age 15.

How it happens

In Graves disease, thyroid-stimulating antibodies bind to and stimulate the TSH receptors of the thyroid gland.

The trigger for this autoimmune response is unclear; it may have several causes. Genetic factors may play a part; the disease tends to occur in identical twins. Immunologic factors may also be a culprit; the disease occasionally coexists with other autoimmune endocrine abnormalities, such as T1DM, thyroiditis, and hyperparathyroidism. Stressful life situations often precede Grave disease; therefore, stress may be a cause.

Graves disease may result from genetic and immunologic influences.

Genetic Information

DNA

Types of hyperthyroidism

In addition to Graves disease, other forms of hyperthyroidism include toxic adenoma, thyrotoxicosis factitia, thyroid carcinoma, TSH-secreting pituitary tumor, and subacute thyroiditis.

Toxic adenoma

The second most common cause of hyperthyroidism, toxic adenoma, is a small benign nodule in the thyroid gland that secretes excessive thyroid hormone. The cause of toxic adenoma is unknown; its incidence is highest in older adults.

Thyrotoxicosis factitia (exogenous thyroid)

Thyrotoxicosis factitia results from chronic overingestion of thyroid hormone, which causes TSH suppression of the pituitary gland. It is most often due to misuse of thyroid hormone by people trying to lose weight.

Thyroid carcinoma

Cancer of the thyroid gland can cause excessive thyroid hormone or deficient thyroid hormone.

TSH-secreting pituitary tumor

This occurs when there is excess production of TSH from the anterior pituitary gland that then overstimulates the thyroid gland to secrete excessive thyroid hormone.

Subacute thyroiditis

A virus-induced granulomatous inflammation of the thyroid, subacute thyroiditis produces transient hyperthyroidism associated with fever, pain, pharyngitis, and tenderness of the thyroid gland.

What to look for

The classic features of Graves disease are:
- an enlarged thyroid gland
- exophthalmos (abnormal protrusion of the eyes)
- nervousness
- heat intolerance
- weight loss despite increased appetite
- excessive sweating
- diarrhea
- tremors
- palpitations (See *Recognizing hyperthyroidism.*)

Because thyroid hormones have widespread effects on almost all body systems, many other signs and symptoms are common with hyperthyroidism:
- CNS (most common in younger patients)—difficulty concentrating, anxiety, excitability or nervousness, fine tremor, shaky handwriting, clumsiness, emotional instability, and mood swings
- cardiovascular system (most common in older adult patients)—arrhythmias, especially atrial fibrillation
- integumentary system—vitiligo and skin hyperpigmentation; warm, moist, flushed skin with a velvety texture; fine, soft hair; premature graying; hair loss; fragile nails; and pretibial myxedema producing raised, thickened skin and plaquelike or nodular lesions

Recognizing hyperthyroidism

The below figure illustrates the common signs of an overactive thyroid.

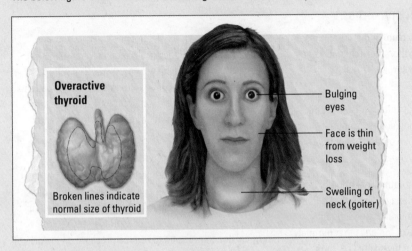

Overactive thyroid

Broken lines indicate normal size of thyroid

Bulging eyes

Face is thin from weight loss

Swelling of neck (goiter)

- respiratory system—dyspnea on exertion and, possibly, at rest and breathlessness when climbing stairs
- GI system—anorexia, nausea, and vomiting
- musculoskeletal system—muscle weakness, generalized or localized muscle atrophy, and osteoporosis
- reproductive system—menstrual abnormalities, impaired fertility, decreased libido, and gynecomastia (abnormal development of mammary glands in males)
- eyes—infrequent blinking, lid lag, reddened conjunctiva and cornea, corneal ulcers, impaired upward gaze, convergence, strabismus (eye deviation), and exophthalmos, which causes the characteristic staring gaze (See *Treating hyperthyroidism.*)

Touch tells you

On palpation, the thyroid gland may feel asymmetrical, lobular, and enlarged to three or four times its normal size. The liver may also be enlarged. Hyperthyroidism may cause tachycardia, commonly accompanied by a full, bounding, palpable pulse. Hyperreflexia is also present.

Listen and learn

Auscultation of the heart may detect an accelerated heart rate, which may prove to be paroxysmal supraventricular tachycardia or atrial fibrillation when verified by electrocardiogram, especially in older

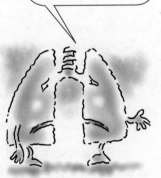

Breathlessness when taking a slow jog or climbing stairs could mean Graves disease is affecting the respiratory system.

Battling illness

Treating hyperthyroidism

In Graves disease, the most common hyperthyroid disorder, treatment consists of drug therapy, including radioactive iodine (^{131}I) therapy, and surgery.

Drug therapy

Antithyroid drugs, such as propylthiouracil and methimazole, are used for children, young adults, pregnant patients, and patients who refuse other treatments.

Radioactive iodine therapy

A single oral dose of ^{131}I is the treatment of choice. During treatment, the thyroid gland picks up the radioactive element as it would regular iodine. Subsequently, the radioactivity destroys some of the cells that normally concentrate iodine and produce thyroxine (T_4), thus decreasing thyroid hormone production and normalizing thyroid size and function.

In most patients, hypermetabolic symptoms diminish within 6 to 8 weeks. However, some patients may require a second dose. This treatment is contraindicated in people who are pregnant or planning to become pregnant; a pregnancy test must be done prior to treatment in those of childbearing age. A patient treated with radioactive iodine also needs to avoid close proximity to pregnant people.

Surgery

Partial or total thyroidectomy is indicated for patients younger than age 40 whose hyperthyroidism relapses after drug therapy, for pregnant patients, and for patients allergic to ^{131}I and other antithyroid drugs. After total thyroidectomy, the patient needs to be on replacement thyroid hormone for life.

Other treatments

Therapy for hyperthyroid ophthalmopathy includes local applications of topical drugs but may require high doses of corticosteroids. A patient with severe exophthalmos that causes pressure on the optic nerve may require surgical decompression to reduce pressure on the orbital contents.

Treatment for thyrotoxic crisis includes giving an antithyroid drug, IV propranolol to block sympathetic effects, a corticosteroid to inhibit the conversion of triiodothyronine to T_4 and replace depleted cortisol, and an iodide to block the release of thyroid hormones. Supportive measures include the administration of nutrients, vitamins, fluids, oxygen, and sedatives.

adult patients. Occasionally, a systolic murmur occurs at the left sternal border. Wide pulse pressures may be audible when blood pressure readings are taken. In Graves disease, an audible bruit over the thyroid gland indicates high blood flow indicative of thyrotoxicity, but, occasionally, it may also be present in other hyperthyroid disorders. With treatment, most patients can lead normal lives.

What tests tell you

These laboratory tests confirm Graves disease:

- Radioimmunoassay shows increased serum T_3 and T_4 concentrations.
- TSH level is low in primary hyperthyroidism, caused by Graves disease.
- Thyroid scan reveals increased uptake of ^{131}I.

Taken by storm

Thyrotoxic crisis, also known as *thyroid storm*, is an acute exacerbation of hyperthyroidism. It's a medical emergency that may lead to life-threatening cardiac, hepatic, or renal failure. Inadequately treated hyperthyroidism and stressful conditions, such as surgery, infection, toxemia of pregnancy, and DKA, can lead to thyrotoxic crisis. (See *Understanding thyroid storm.*)

Now I get it!

Understanding thyroid storm

Thyrotoxic crisis—also known as *thyroid storm*—usually occurs in patients with preexisting, though often unrecognized, thyrotoxicosis.

Pathophysiology
The thyroid gland secretes excessive thyroid hormones triiodothyronine (T_3) and thyroxine (T_4). When T_3 and T_4 are overproduced, systemic adrenergic activity increases. The result is epinephrine overproduction and severe hypermetabolism, leading rapidly to cardiac, GI, and sympathetic nervous system decompensation.

Assessment findings
Initially, the patient may have marked tachycardia, vomiting, and stupor. If left untreated, the patient may experience vascular collapse, hypotension, coma, and death. Other findings may include a combination of irritability and restlessness, visual disturbance (such as diplopia), tremor and weakness, angina, shortness of breath, cough, and swollen extremities. Palpation may disclose warm, moist, flushed skin and a high fever that begins and rises rapidly to a lethal level. Laboratory assessment

will likely reveal low TSH with a high free T_4/T_3. Additionally, hyperglycemia may occur due to increased glycogenolysis and inhibited insulin release by catecholamines. Bone reabsorption and hemoconcentration can result in hypercalcemia. Finally, nonspecific alterations such as abnormal liver function tests, leukocytosis, or leukopenia may occur.

Precipitating factors
Onset is almost always abrupt and evoked by a stressful event, such as trauma, surgery, or infection. Other less common precipitating factors include:
* hypoglycemia or diabetic ketoacidosis
* stroke
* myocardial infarction
* pulmonary embolism
* sudden discontinuation of antithyroid drug therapy
* initiation of radioactive iodine therapy
* preeclampsia
* subtotal thyroidectomy with accompanying excessive intake of synthetic thyroid hormone

Thyroid disorder: hypothyroidism

Hypothyroidism is thyroid hormone deficiency that causes all the body's metabolic processes to slow down because of a deficit in T_3 or T_4, both of which regulate metabolism. The disorder is most prevalent in females and in people with Down syndrome. In the United States, the incidence rate increases by 10% for those older than 65 years of age.

Primary or secondary

Hypothyroidism is classified as primary or secondary. The primary form stems from a disorder of the thyroid gland itself. The secondary form stems from a failure of the pituitary gland to secrete TSH to stimulate normal thyroid function. This form may progress to myxedema coma, a medical emergency. (See *Understanding myxedema coma*, page 332.)

How it happens

Primary hypothyroidism has several possible causes:
- autoimmune destruction of thyroid tissue, termed *Hashimoto thyroiditis*
- thyroidectomy without replacement of thyroid hormone
- inflammation from radiation therapy of neck
  Secondary hypothyroidism, which is uncommon, is caused by a failure of the pituitary gland to stimulate normal thyroid function. The pituitary may fail to produce TSH (thyrotropin), or the hypothalamus may fail to produce thyrotropin-releasing hormone.

Throughout the organization

Because insufficient synthesis of thyroid hormones affects almost every organ system in the body, signs and symptoms vary according to the organs involved as well as the duration and severity of the condition.

What to look for

The signs and symptoms of hypothyroidism may be vague and varied. Early signs include:
- energy loss
- fatigue
- forgetfulness
- sensitivity to cold
- unexplained weight gain
- constipation
  As the disease progresses, the patient may have:
- anorexia
- decreased libido
- menorrhagia (excessive blood loss in menstruation)
- paresthesia (numbness, prickling, or tingling)
- joint stiffness
- muscle cramping
  Other signs and symptoms include:
- CNS—psychiatric disturbances, ataxia (loss of coordination), intention tremor (tremor during voluntary motion), carpal

tunnel syndrome, benign intracranial hypertension, and behavioral changes ranging from slight mental slowing to severe impairment
- integumentary system—dry, flaky, inelastic skin; puffy face, hands, and feet; dry, sparse hair with patchy hair loss and loss of the outer third of the eyebrow; thick, brittle nails with transverse and longitudinal grooves; and a thick, dry tongue, causing hoarseness and slow, slurred speech (See *Recognizing hypothyroidism.*)
- cardiovascular system—hypercholesterolemia (high cholesterol) with associated arteriosclerosis and ischemic heart disease, poor peripheral circulation, heart enlargement, heart failure, and pleural and pericardial effusions
- GI system—achlorhydria (absence of free hydrochloric acid in the stomach), pernicious anemia, and adynamic (weak) colon, resulting in megacolon (extremely dilated colon) and intestinal obstruction
- reproductive system—impaired fertility
- eyes and ears—conductive or sensorineural deafness and nystagmus
- hematologic system—anemia, which may result in bleeding tendencies and iron deficiency anemia

Going to extremes

Severe hypothyroidism, or myxedema, is characterized by thickening of the facial features and induration of the skin. The skin may

Recognizing hypothyroidism

The figure below illustrates common signs of an underactive thyroid.

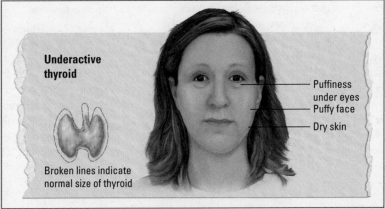

Underactive thyroid

Puffiness under eyes
Puffy face
Dry skin

Broken lines indicate normal size of thyroid

feel rough, doughy, and cool. Other signs and symptoms are weak pulse, bradycardia, muscle weakness, sacral or peripheral edema, and delayed reflex relaxation time (especially in the Achilles tendon). (See *Understanding myxedema coma.*)

Hyponatremia (low blood sodium) may result from impaired water excretion and from poor regulation of ADH secretion. (See *Treating hypothyroidism.*)

What tests tell you
Primary hypothyroidism is confirmed by an elevated TSH level and low serum free T_4 level. Additional tests may be performed:
- Serum TSH levels determine whether the disorder is primary or secondary. An increased serum TSH level is due to thyroid insufficiency; a decreased or normal level is due to hypothalamic or pituitary insufficiency.
- The levels of serum antithyroid antibodies are elevated in Hashimoto thyroiditis, an autoimmune disorder.
- Perchlorate discharge tests identify enzyme deficiency within the thyroid gland. A deficiency will affect the uptake of iodine.
- Radioisotope scanning identifies ectopic thyroid tissue.
- Skull x-ray, CT scan, and MRI locate pituitary or hypothalamic lesions that may cause secondary hypothyroidism.

Now I get it!

Understanding myxedema coma

A medical emergency, myxedema coma commonly has a fatal outcome. Progression is usually gradual but when stress, such as infection, exposure to cold, or trauma, aggravates severe or prolonged hypothyroidism, coma may develop abruptly. Other precipitating factors are thyroid medication withdrawal and the use of sedatives, opioids, or anesthetics.

What happens
Patients in myxedema coma have significantly depressed respirations, so their partial pressure of carbon dioxide in arterial blood may rise. Decreased cardiac output and worsening cerebral hypoxia may also occur. The patient becomes stuporous and hypothermic. Vital signs reflect bradycardia and hypotension. Lifesaving interventions are needed.

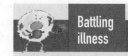

Treating hypothyroidism
Treatment consists of gradual thyroid hormone replacement with the synthetic hormone levothyroxine. Treatment begins slowly, particularly in older adult patients, to avoid adverse cardiovascular effects. The dosage is increased every 2 to 3 weeks until the desired response is obtained.

No time to waste
Rapid treatment is necessary for patients with myxedema coma and those having emergency surgery. These patients need both IV administration of levothyroxine and hydrocortisone therapy.

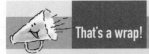

Endocrine system review

Understanding the endocrine system
- Hypothalamus helps control endocrine glands by secreting releasing factors that stimulate the pituitary gland.
- Adrenal cortex secretes mineralocorticoids (aldosterone), glucocorticoids (cortisol), adrenal androgens (testosterone), and estrogen.
- Adrenal medulla produces epinephrine and norepinephrine.
- Pancreas produces glucagon and insulin.
- Anterior pituitary gland produces TSH, ACTH, FSH, LH, and GH.
- Posterior pituitary gland secretes oxytocin and antidiuretic hormone (ADH).
- Thyroid gland secretes thyroxine (T_4) and triiodothyronine (T_3).
- Parathyroid glands secrete parathyroid hormone (PTH).

Major causes of endocrine disorders
- Hypersecretion or hyposecretion of hormones
- Hyporesponsiveness of receptors of hormones
- Inflammation of gland
- Tumor of gland

Endocrine disorders
- *Addison disease*—most commonly caused by autoimmune disease of the adrenal glands, which causes lack of cortisol secretion by the glands
- *Cushing syndrome*—most commonly caused by excess cortisol secretion by the adrenal glands
- Pheochromocytoma—caused by tumor of adrenal that releases catecholamines
- *Diabetes mellitus*—occurs in two primary forms:
  - *Type 1*—beta cells in pancreas are destroyed or suppressed; insulin isn't secreted
  - *Type 2*—cells of the body have insulin resistance, which leads to exhaustion of the pancreas
- *Diabetes insipidus*—caused by deficiency of ADH
- *SIADH*—caused by excess secretion of ADH
- *Goiter*—enlargement of the thyroid gland; may or may not cause a thyroid hormone disorder

Quick quiz

1. A patient with weight loss, orthostatic hypotension, weakness, GI disturbances, dehydration, fatigue, and a craving for salty food may have which disorder?
    A. Cushing syndrome
    B. Addison disease
    C. Hypothyroidism
    D. Diabetes insipidus

Answer: B. Addison disease is due to a lack of secretion of cortisol (glucocorticoid), aldosterone (mineralocorticoid), and adrenal androgens and estrogen. Lack of cortisol causes weakness and hypotension. Lack of aldosterone causes lack of sodium reabsorption into the blood, and therefore hyponatremia and dehydration. Other classic symptoms of Addison disease are anxiety, lightheadedness, and amenorrhea. People will have a poor response to stress due to lack of cortisol and low blood pressure due to lack of aldosterone. Low blood pressure causes fatigue and weakness. Lack of cortisol changes circadian rhythms and impairs digestion, which can lead to changes in bowel habits and weight loss.

2. Cushing syndrome may be caused by which of the following?
    A. Destruction of more than 90% of the adrenal glands
    B. Thyroid hormone overproduction
    C. Glucocorticoid excess
    D. Insufficient antidiuretic hormone production

Answer: C. Cushing syndrome is caused by an excess of cortisol secretion by the adrenal glands. Cushing syndrome is characterized by weight gain, fat redistribution causing truncal obesity, hypertension, hyperglycemia and diabetes-like state, striae, and osteoporosis.

3. Which treatment is commonly indicated for type 2 diabetes mellitus?
    A. High-fiber, low-fat diet
    B. Fluid restriction
    C. Insulin
    D. Oral antidiabetic agent

Answer: D. Oral antidiabetic agents are commonly indicated for treatment of type 2 diabetes mellitus.

4. Hyperthyroidism is more common in:
    A. females.
    B. African Americans.
    C. older adults.
    D. children.

Answer: A. The disorder occurs more commonly in females, often as part of Graves disease, which is an autoimmune disorder. Antibodies produced by the body overstimulate the thyroid gland, causing hyperthyroidism.

Scoring

☆☆☆   If you answered all four items correctly, hooray! You're hyperinformed about hormones.

☆☆   If you answered three items correctly, exceptional! Your endocrine expertise is indeed endearing.

☆   If you answered fewer than three items correctly, just remember—never give up. Let's hope your glands will release test-taking hormones that will stimulate you to stick with it.

Suggested references

American Diabetes Association. (2023). *ADA diabetes standard of care 2023 guideline summary.* https://www.guidelinecentral.com/guideline/14119/#section-anchor-1226404

Barthel, A., Benker, G., Berens, K., Diederich, S., Manfras, B., Gruber, M., Kanczkowski, W., Kline, G., Kamvissi-Lorenz, V., Hahner, S., Beuschlein, F., Brennand, A., Boehm, B. O., Torpy, D. J., & Bornstein, S. R. (2019). An update on Addison's disease. *Experimental and Clinical Endocrinology & Diabetes, 127*(2–03), 165–175. https://doi.org/10.1055/a-0804-2715

Betterle, C., Presotto, F., & Furmaniak, J. (2019). Epidemiology, pathogenesis, and diagnosis of Addison's disease in adults. *Journal of Endocrinological Investigation, 42*(12), 1407–1433. https://doi.org/10.1007/s40618-019-01079-6

Bilic-Curcic, I., Cigrovski Berkovic, M., Bozek, T., Simel, A., Klobucar Majanovic, S., & Canecki-Varzic, S. (2022). Comparative efficacy and safety of two fixed ratio combinations in type 2 diabetes mellitus patients previously poorly controlled on different insulin regimens: A multi-centric observational study. *European Review of Medical and Pharmacological Sciences, 26*(8), 2782–2793. https://doi.org/10.26355/eurrev_202204_28608

Christ-Crain, M., Winzeler, B., & Refardt, J. (2021). Diagnosis and management of diabetes insipidus for the internist: An update. *Journal of Internal Medicine, 290*(1), 73–87. https://doi.org/10.1111/joim.13261

Cloete, L. (2022). Diabetes mellitus: An overview of the types, symptoms, complications and management. *Nursing Standard, 37*(1), 61–66. https://doi.org/10.7748/ns.2021.e11709

Diri, H., & Aycicek, B. (2023). A retrospective comparison between intensive and non-intensive insulin regimens in type 2 diabetes mellitus. *Minerva Endocrinology, 48*(3), 311–317. https://doi.org/10.23736/S2724-6507.20.03323-4

Duan, D., Kengne, A. P., & Echouffo-Tcheugui, J. B. (2021). Screening for diabetes and prediabetes. *Endocrinology and Metabolism Clinics of North America, 50*(3), 369–385. https://doi.org/10.1016/j.ecl.2021.05.002

ElSayed, N. A., Aleppo, G., Aroda, V. R., Bannuru, R. R., Brown, F. M., Bruemmer, D., Collins, B. S., Cusi, K., Das, S. R., Gibbons, C. H., Giurini, J. M., Hilliard, M. E., Isaacs, D., Johnson, E. L., Kahan, S., Khunti, K., Kosiborod, M., Leon, J., Lyons, S. K., … Gabbay, R. S. (2023). Summary of revisions standards of care in diabetes-2023. *Diabetes Care, 46*(Suppl 1), S5–S9. https://doi.org/10.2337/dc23-Srev

Evans, K. (2019). Diabetic ketoacidosis: Update on management. *Clinical Medicine Journal, 19*(5), 396–398. https://doi.org/10.7861/clinmed.2019-0284

Farrugia, F. A., & Charalampopoulos, A. (2019). Pheochromocytoma. *Endocrine Regulations, 53*(3), 191–212. https://doi.org/10.2478/enr-2019-0020

Ferriere, A., & Tabarin, A. (2020). Cushing's syndrome: Treatment and new therapeutic approaches. *Best Practice & Research Clinical Endocrinology & Metabolism, 34*(2), 101381. https://doi.org/10.1016/j.beem.2020.101381

Ferriere, A., & Tabarin, A. (2021). Cushing's disease. *La Presse Médicale, 50*(4), 104091. https://doi.org/10.1016/j.lpm.2021.104091

Healy, A. M., Faherty, M., Khan, Z., Emara, N., Carter, C., Scheidemantel, A., Abu-Jubara, M., & Young, R. (2023). Diabetic ketoacidosis diagnosis in a hospital setting. *Journal of Osteopathic Medicine, 123*(10), 499–503. https://doi.org/10.1515/jom-2023-0019

Libianto, R., Yang, J., & Fuller, P. J. (2021). Adrenal disease: An update. *Australian Journal of General Practice, 50*(1–2), 9–14. https://doi.org/10.31128/AJGP-09-20-5619

Luo, Y., Xia, J., Zhao, Z., Chang, Y., Bee, Y. M., Nguyen, K. T., Lim, S., Yabe, D., McGill, M., Kong, A. P. S., Chan, S. P., Deodat, M., Deerochanawong, C., Suastika, K., Xu, C., Chen, L., Chen, W., Li, X., Zhao, W., … Ji, L. (2023). Effectiveness, safety, initial optimal dose, and optimal maintenance dose range of basal insulin regimens for type 2 diabetes: A systematic review with meta-analysis. *Journal of Diabetes, 15*(5), 419–435. https://doi.org/10.1111/1753-0407.13381

Majety, P., Lozada Orquera, F. A., Edem, D., & Hamdy, O. (2023). Pharmacological approaches to the prevention of type 2 diabetes mellitus. *Frontiers in Endocrinology, 14*, 1118848. https://doi.org/10.3389/fendo.2023.1118848

Norris, T. (2025). *Porth's pathophysiology: Concepts of altered health states* (11th ed.). Wolters Kluwer.

Pasarica, M., St Onge, E., & Lee, E. (2021). Diabetes: Type 1 diabetes. *FP Essentials, 504*, 11–15.

Poch, E., Molina, A., & Piñeiro, G. (2022). Syndrome of inappropriate antidiuretic hormone secretion. *Medicina Clínica, 159*(3), 139–146. https://doi.org/10.1016/j.medcli.2022.02.015

Priya, G., Kalra, S., Bahendeka, S., Jawad, F., Aye, T. T., Shahjada, S., Sehgal, A., Uloko, A., Ruder, S., Somasundaram, N., Naseri, M. W., & Chaudhary, S. (2020). Initiation of basal bolus insulin therapy. *Journal of the Pakistan Medical Association, 70*(8), 1462–1467.

Refardt, J., Winzeler, B., & Christ-Crain, M. (2020). Diabetes insipidus: An update. *Endocrinology and Metabolism Clinics of North America, 49*(3), 517–531. https://doi.org/10.1016/j.ecl.2020.05.012

Tomkins, M., Lawless, S., Martin-Grace, J., Sherlock, M., & Thompson, C. J. (2022). Diagnosis and management of central diabetes insipidus in adults. *The Journal of Clinical Endocrinology & Metabolism, 107*(10), 2701–2715. https://doi.org/10.1210/clinem/dgac381

Vaz de Castro, P. A. S., Bitencourt, L., de Oliveira Campos, J. L., Fischer, B. L., Soares de Brito, S. B. C., Soares, B. S., Drummond, J. B., & Simões E Silva, A. C. (2022). Nephrogenic diabetes insipidus: A comprehensive overview. *Journal of Pediatric Endocrinology and Metabolism, 35*(4), 421–434. https://doi.org/10.1515/jpem-2021-0566

Chapter 9

Renal system*

Just the facts

In this chapter, you'll learn:

♦ the structures of the renal system

♦ how the renal system functions

♦ pathophysiology, signs and symptoms, diagnostic tests, and treatments for several common renal system disorders.

Understanding the renal system

The renal system, which consists of the kidneys, ureters, bladder, and ure-thra, serves as the body's water treatment plant by collecting the body's waste products and expelling them as urine. It also filters electrolytes.

The kidneys are located on each side of the vertebral column in the upper abdomen in the posterior region outside the peritoneal cavity. The kidneys are located at the costovertebral angles of the back, where the ribs meet the vertebrae on both sides. These compact organs contain an amaz-ingly efficient filtration system—they filter about 45 gallons of fluid each day. The by-product of this filtration is urine, which contains water, elec-trolytes, and waste products. (See *A close look at the kidney*, page 338.)

The kidneys can be divided into three primary sections:

* cortex (outer)—contains the glomeruli and their capillaries, most of the proximal tubules and arteries
* medulla (middle)—contains the collecting ducts, pyramids, and most of the blood vessels and distal tubules
* pelvis (inner) section (See *A close look at the kidney*, page 338.)

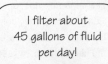

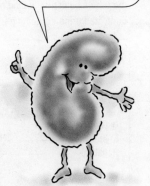

I filter about 45 gallons of fluid per day!

It's all downhill from here

After it is produced by the kidneys, urine passes through the urinary system and is expelled from the body via the urethra. Passing urine

*Note: In this chapter, the term "male" refers to a person assigned male at birth, and the term "female" refers to a person assigned female at birth.

A close look at the kidney

Illustrated below is a kidney along with an enlargement of a nephron, the kidney's functional unit. Major structures of the kidney include:
- cortex—outer layer of the kidney
- medulla—inner portion of the kidney, made up of renal pyramids and tubular structures
- renal artery—supplies blood to the kidney
- renal calyx—channels formed urine from the renal pyramids to the renal pelvis
- renal pelvis—after blood that contains waste products is processed in the kidney, formed urine is channeled to the renal pelvis
- renal vein—about 99% of filtered blood is reabsorbed and circulated through the renal vein back to the general circulation; the remaining 1%, which contains waste products, undergoes further processing in the kidney
- ureters—tubes that move urine from the kidneys to the bladder before excretion

Note the nephron

The nephron is the functional and structural unit of the kidney. Each kidney contains about 1 million nephrons. Its two main actions are reabsorption of water back into the bloodstream and secretion of ions and wastes into the tubule fluid; tubule fluid eventually becomes a concentrated urine containing wastes. The nephron filters the blood to remove fluid, wastes, and electrolytes and regulates acids and bases.

Components of the nephron include:
- glomerulus—a network of twisted capillaries, which acts as a filter for the passage of protein-free and red blood cell–free filtrate to Bowman capsule.
- Bowman capsule—contains the glomerulus and acts as a reservoir for glomerular filtrate.
- proximal convoluted tubule—site of reabsorption of water, glucose, amino acids, metabolites, and electrolytes from filtrate; reabsorbed substances return to circulation.
- loop of Henle—a U-shaped nephron tubule located in the medulla and extending from the proximal convoluted tubule to the distal convoluted tubule; site for further concentration of filtrate through reabsorption of water. Secretion of urea into the nephron tubules also occurs at the loop of Henle. Urea is a conglomeration of nitrogen waste products.
- distal convoluted tubule—site from which filtrate enters the collecting tubule; aldosterone affects the distal tubule by increasing reabsorption of sodium and water into the bloodstream.
- collecting tubule or collecting duct—at this site, ADH affects the tubule fluid by enhancing reabsorption of water into the bloodstream. This then results in a concentrated urine that is released into the renal pelvis.

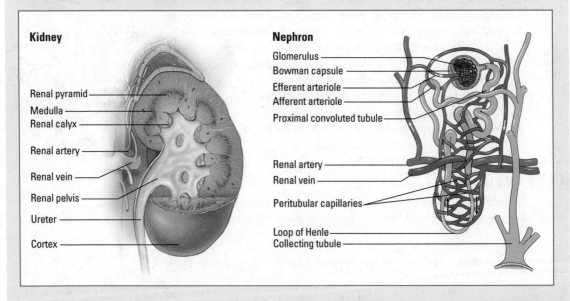

Kidney

Renal pyramid
Medulla
Renal calyx
Renal artery
Renal vein
Renal pelvis
Ureter
Cortex

Nephron

Glomerulus
Bowman capsule
Efferent arteriole
Afferent arteriole
Proximal convoluted tubule

Renal artery
Renal vein
Peritubular capillaries
Loop of Henle
Collecting tubule

from the body is urination (also referred to as micturition). Other structures of the renal system, extending downward from the kidneys, include:

- ureters—16 to 18″ (40.5- to 45.5-cm) muscular tubes that contract rhythmically (peristaltic action) to transport urine from each kidney to the bladder
- urinary bladder—a sac with muscular walls that collects and holds urine (300 to 500 mL) that's expelled from the ureters every few seconds
- urethra—a narrow passageway, surrounded by the prostate gland in males, from the bladder to the outside of the body through which urine is excreted

Renal labor

Vital functions that the kidneys perform include:

- maintaining fluid as well as regulating electrolyte concentration (an important function is water conservation by reabsorption of fluid back into the bloodstream from the nephron tubules)
- detoxifying the blood and eliminating wastes (nitrogen wastes are mainly filtered out of the blood)
- regulating blood pressure by releasing renin in response to low circulation
- regulating acid–base balance (releasing acid or conserving acid and releasing base or conserving base)
- regulation of release of excess potassium from the blood into the urine
- red blood cell (RBC) production (erythropoiesis) (the kidney secretes erythropoietin in response to low oxygen in the bloodstream (hypoxemia); erythropoietin stimulates the bone marrow to manufacture RBCs
- producing a portion of vitamin D (vitamin D enhances reabsorption of calcium from the GI tract into the blood; therefore, calcium balance is controlled by the kidney)

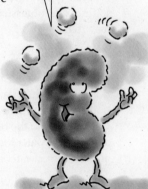

Regulating, balancing, and detoxifying—no wonder the body finds me vital!

Maintaining fluid and acid–base balance

Two important kidney functions are maintaining fluid and acid–base balance.

Fluid balance

The kidneys maintain fluid balance in the body by regulating the amount and makeup of the fluids inside and around the cells.

At the exchange

The kidneys maintain the volume and composition of extracellular and, to a lesser extent, intracellular fluid by continuously exchanging water and solutes, such as hydrogen, sodium, potassium, chloride, bicarbonate, sulfate, and phosphate ions, across their cell membranes.

Hormones…sometimes a help…

Hormones partially control the kidneys' role in fluid balance. This control depends on the response of specialized sensory nerve endings (osmoreceptors) to changes in osmolality (the ionic or solute, concentration of a solution).

The two hormones involved are:
- antidiuretic hormone (ADH), produced by the pituitary gland, which works at the collecting duct of the nephrons
- aldosterone, produced by the adrenal cortex, which works at the distal tubule of the nephrons

…sometimes a hindrance

Problems in hormone concentration may cause fluctuations in sodium and potassium concentrations that, in turn, may lead to hypertension.

The ABCs of ADH

ADH alters the collecting tubules' permeability to water. Antidiuretic hormone performs antidiuresis, meaning it stops water loss from the body. ADH stimulates the collecting duct at the nephron to reabsorb water back into the bloodstream. This then increases blood volume and reduces water lost in the urine. ADH creates a concentrated urine and conserves water in the body.

The renin–angiotensin–aldosterone system

The *renin–angiotensin–aldosterone system (RAAS)* of the body is a key regulator of fluid and blood pressure. Here is how it works:
1. When the kidney senses low perfusion due to hypovolemia (low blood volume), it secretes *renin*.
2. Renin stimulates the liver to secrete a large protein called *angiotensinogen*.
3. Angiotensinogen is broken down in the circulation into *angiotensin I*.
4. An essential enzyme, *angiotensin-converting enzyme (ACE)*, transforms angiotensin I into *angiotensin II*.
5. Angiotensin II stimulates arterial vasoconstriction, which raises BP. Angiotensin II also stimulates the adrenal gland to secrete *aldosterone*.

Aldosterone is produced and released by the adrenal cortex but works in the kidney. Aldosterone causes reabsorption of sodium and water into the bloodstream at the distal tubule of the nephron. This raises blood volume and blood pressure.

Aldosterone also stimulates the secretion of potassium from the bloodstream into the distal tubules. A high aldosterone concentration increases the excretion of potassium into the urine. (See *Understanding hypertension: Constant cycling of the renin–angiotensin–aldosterone system*, page 77.)

Other key hormones

The kidney is also home to several other very important hormones.
- Calcitriol—assists with converting vitamin D to its active form
- Erythropoietin—stimulates RBC production
- Renin—helps regulate blood pressure through the RAAS

Going against the current

The kidneys concentrate urine through the countercurrent exchange system in nephron's loop of Henle. In this system, fluid flows in opposite directions through parallel tubes, up and down parallel sides of the loop of Henle. The loop of Henle is an ingenious apparatus of the nephron that reabsorbs water back into the bloodstream from the tubule fluid and releases waste products (particularly urea) into the tubule fluid. The tubule fluid then contains urea (nitrogenous wastes) and is highly concentrated. The loop of Henle conserves water while concentrating tubule fluid that becomes urine.

Acid–base balance

To regulate acid–base balance, the kidneys:
- secrete hydrogen ions
- reabsorb sodium and bicarbonate ions
- acidify phosphate salts
- produce ammonia (chemically, this is NH_3)

Earning a PhD in pH balance

All of these regulating activities keep the blood at its normal pH of 7.35 to 7.45. Acidosis occurs when the pH falls below 7.35, and alkalosis occurs when the pH rises above 7.45. (For more information on acid–base balance, see Chapter 4.)

Waste collection

The kidneys collect and eliminate wastes from the body via a three-step process:
1. *Glomerular filtration*—The *glomeruli*, a collection of nephron capillaries, filter blood flowing through them to form filtrate.

2. *Tubular reabsorption*—Next, the tubules (tiny canals that make up the nephron) reabsorb the filtered fluid into the surrounding blood vessels.

3. *Tubular secretion*—The filtered substance, known as *glomerular filtrate*, passes through the tubules to the collecting tubules and ducts and eventually becomes urine.

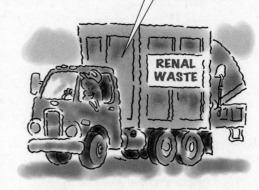

How do I go about waste collection? Easy. First, I get to work by filtering the blood.

Clear the way

Clearance is the complete removal of a substance from the blood—commonly described in terms of the amount of blood that can be cleared in a specific amount of time. Creatinine is a muscle breakdown product that needs to be almost completely cleared from the blood and excreted into the urine. Therefore, the amount of creatinine in the bloodstream is a good gauge of how well the kidneys are functioning. Serum creatinine is used as a measure of how well the kidneys are clearing creatinine from the bloodstream. For example, creatinine clearance is the volume of blood in milliliters that the kidneys can clear of creatinine in 1 minute.

Some substances are filtered out of the blood by the glomeruli. Dissolved substances that remain in the tubule fluid may be reabsorbed back into the bloodstream. (See *Understanding the glomerular filtration rate*, page 343.)

Too little, too late

In a patient whose kidneys have shrunk from disease, healthy nephrons (the filtering units of the kidney) enlarge to compensate. However, as nephron damage progresses, the enlargement can no longer adequately compensate, and the GFR slows.

Don't saturate the system

The amount of a substance that's reabsorbed or secreted depends on the substance's maximum tubular transport capacity—the maximum amount of a substance that can be reabsorbed or secreted in 1 minute without saturating the renal system.

For example, in diabetes mellitus, excess glucose in the blood overwhelms the renal tubules and causes glucose to appear in the urine (glycosuria). In other cases, when glomeruli are damaged, protein appears in the urine (proteinuria) because the large protein molecules pass into the urine by a damaged glomerulus. Damaged glomeruli allow large proteins to pass into the tubule fluid; these proteins then become urine-containing protein (proteinuria).

Understanding the glomerular filtration rate

The glomerular filtration rate (GFR) is the rate at which the glomeruli filter blood. The normal GFR is between 107 and 139 mL/minute for males and 87 and 107 mL/minute for females. GFR depends on:
- permeability of capillary walls
- vascular pressure
- filtration pressure

GFR and clearance

Clearance is the complete removal of a substance from the blood. The most accurate measure of glomerular filtration is *creatinine clearance*, because creatinine is filtered by the glomeruli but not reabsorbed by the tubules. Creatinine is a breakdown product of skeletal muscle that should be completely excreted by the kidney; it should not accumulate in the bloodstream.

Equal to, greater than, or less than

Here's more about how the GFR affects clearance measurements for a substance in the blood:
- If the tubules neither reabsorb nor secrete the substance—as happens with creatinine—creatinine clearance equals the GFR. Creatinine is an ideal substance to use to gauge how well the kidneys are functioning. This is why *serum creatinine* is used as a measure of kidney function and that *creatinine clearance* is another measure of how well the kidneys are functioning.

Blood pressure regulation and the RAAS

The kidneys help regulate blood pressure by producing and secreting the enzyme renin in response to decreased perfusion of the kidney, most commonly due to hypovolemia. Renin, in turn, stimulates formation of angiotensin I, which is converted to angiotensin II by a key enzyme, *ACE*.

Angiotensin II raises low arterial blood pressure levels by:
- increasing peripheral vasoconstriction
- stimulating aldosterone secretion by the adrenal gland

Aldosterone then acts at the distal tubule of the nephrons to promote the reabsorption of sodium and water into the bloodstream. Remember that two essential functions of aldosterone are:
- sodium and water reabsorption into the bloodstream raises blood volume and blood pressure
- aldosterone enhances excretion of potassium at the distal tubule of the nephron

Hypertension: a serious threat

Hypertension can stem from a fluid and electrolyte imbalance as well as RAAS hyperactivity. High blood pressure can damage blood vessels and cause hardening of the kidneys (nephrosclerosis), one of the leading causes of chronic renal failure.

RBC production

Erythropoietin is a hormone that prompts the bone marrow to increase RBC production.

"Eryth"-ing you need to know about erythropoietin

The kidneys secrete erythropoietin when the oxygen supply in blood circulating through the tissues drops (hypoxia). Loss of renal function causes loss of erythropoietin response, which results in lack of stimulus to the bone marrow to manufacture RBCs. This leads to chronic anemia.

Vitamin D regulation and calcium formation

The kidneys help convert vitamin D to its active form. Active vitamin D helps regulate calcium and phosphorus balance and bone metabolism. When the kidneys fail, vitamin D is not produced, which causes lack of calcium (Ca^{++}) absorption from the GI tract. This results in hypocalcemia. Calcium (Ca^{++}) and phosphate (PO_4^-) have an inverse relationship in the blood. They are both contained in bone and can be released by bone. When calcium decreases in the bloodstream, phosphate increases in the bloodstream. Therefore, with hypocalcemia comes hyperphosphatemia. When kidneys fail, calcium decreases in the blood, and phosphate accumulates in the blood.

However, that's not the end of the story...

When calcium decreases in the blood (hypocalcemia), the parathyroid glands are stimulated to release parathyroid hormone (PTH), and hyperparathyroidism (overactivity of the parathyroid glands) can occur. PTH specifically activates bone to release calcium. The result is that bone density decreases, and osteoporosis can occur. This type of osteoporosis is called *renal osteodystrophy*.

Renal disorders

The renal disorders discussed in this chapter include:
- acute kidney injury (AKI)
- acute tubular necrosis

- glomerulonephritis
- hydronephrosis
- kidney disease, chronic (chronic renal failure)
- renal calculi (kidney stones; also called *nephrolithiasis*)
- urinary tract infection (UTI), pyelonephritis (kidney infection), and urosepsis

Acute kidney injury

AKI, previously known as *acute renal failure*, is the sudden interruption of renal function. It can be caused by obstruction, poor circulation, or kidney disease. It's potentially reversible; however, if left untreated, permanent damage can lead to chronic renal failure.

How it happens

AKI may be classified as prerenal, intrarenal, or postrenal. Each type has separate causes. (See *Causes of acute renal injury*, below.)
- Prerenal failure results from conditions that diminish blood flow to the kidneys (hypoperfusion). Examples include hypovolemia, hypotension, hemorrhage causing low blood volume, or inadequate cardiac output. Prerenal failure can also be termed *prerenal azotemia*, which means excessive nitrogenous wastes in the blood (increased blood urea nitrogen [BUN]). When there is

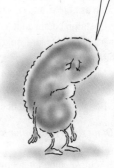

Tubule trouble can be traumatic—75% of all renal failure is caused by the destruction of my tubules.

Causes of acute kidney injury

Acute kidney injury is classified as prerenal, intrarenal, or postrenal. All conditions that lead to prerenal failure impair blood flow to the kidneys (renal hypoperfusion), resulting in decreased glomerular filtration rate. Intrarenal failure results from damage to the kidneys themselves, postrenal failure, from obstructed urine flow. The causes of each type of acute kidney injury are listed below.

Prerenal failure
Cardiovascular disorders
- Arrhythmias
- Cardiac tamponade
- Cardiogenic shock
- Heart failure
- Myocardial infarction

Hypovolemia
- Burns
- Dehydration
- Diuretic overuse
- Hemorrhage
- Hypovolemic shock
- Trauma

Peripheral vasodilation
- Antihypertensive drugs
- Sepsis

Renovascular obstruction
- Arterial or pulmonary embolism
- Arterial or venous thrombosis
- Tumor

(Continued)

Causes of acute kidney injury *(continued)*

Severe vasoconstriction
- Disseminated intravascular coagulation
- Eclampsia
- Malignant hypertension
- Vasculitis

Intrarenal failure
Acute tubular necrosis
- Ischemic damage to renal tissue
- Nephrotoxins including NSAIDS such as ibuprofen, aminoglycosides such as tobramycin, and heavy metals such as lead, radiographic contrast media, illicit drugs such as heroin, and organic solvents
- Obstetric complications such as eclampsia, post-partum renal failure, septic abortion, and uterine hemorrhage
- Myoglobin release from crush injury, myopathy, or rhabdomyolysis
- Renal ischemia that occurs during surgery

Other renal tissue disorders that lead to intrarenal failure
- Acute glomerulonephritis
- Acute interstitial nephritis
- Acute pyelonephritis
- Bilateral renal vein thrombosis
- Hemolytic uremic syndrome (pediatric)
- Malignant nephrosclerosis
- Papillary necrosis

- Periarteritis nodosa (inflammatory disease of the arteries)
- Renal cancer
- Sickle cell disease
- Systemic lupus erythematosus
- Vasculitis

Postrenal failure
Bladder obstruction
- Anticholinergic drugs
- Autonomic nerve dysfunction
- Infection
- Trauma
- Tumor

Ureteral obstruction
- Blood clots
- Calculi (commonly calcium, uric acid, or struvite crystals)
- Edema or inflammation
- Necrotic renal papillae
- Retroperitoneal fibrosis or hemorrhage
- Surgery (accidental ligation)
- Tumor

Urethral obstruction
- Prostatic hyperplasia or prostate cancer
- Urethral strictures
- Urethral valve malformation or blockage
- Ureteropelvic junction obstruction

inadequate circulation in the body, prerenal azotemia occurs due to renal hypoperfusion (the kidneys are not getting enough circulation). Usually, this condition can be rapidly reversed by restoring renal blood flow and glomerular filtration with increasing fluid administration.
- Intrarenal failure, also called *intrinsic renal failure*, results from damage to the filtering structures of the kidneys, usually from acute tubular necrosis, a disorder that causes nephron cell death, kidney infection, autoimmune disease that affects the kidney, or from nephrotoxic substances such as certain antibiotics.

- Postrenal failure results from obstruction of urine outflow, as occurs in nephrolithiasis (kidney stone), prostatic hyperplasia, prostate cancer, or bladder outlet obstruction due to bladder tumor.

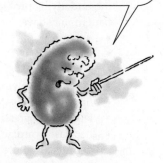

Postrenal failure is caused by any condition that blocks urine flow from both kidneys.

Going through phases

With treatment, each type of AKI passes through three distinct phases:
1. oliguric (decreased urine output)
2. diuretic (increased urine output)
3. recovery (glomerular filtration rate normalizes)

On the decrease…

The oliguric phase lasts from 2 weeks to several months. Oliguria is a decreased urine output (less than 400 mL/24 hours). Prerenal oliguria results from decreased blood flow to the kidney. Before damage occurs, the kidney responds to decreased blood flow by conserving sodium and water. After damage occurs, the kidney's ability to conserve sodium is impaired. Untreated prerenal oliguria may lead to acute tubular necrosis.

During this phase, BUN and creatinine levels rise, and the ratio of BUN to creatinine falls from 20:1 (normal) to 10:1. Hypervolemia occurs, causing edema, weight gain, and elevated blood pressure.

On the increase…

The diuretic phase may last from 1 to 2 weeks, but possibly longer, and is marked by urine output that can range from normal (1 to 2 L/day) to as high as 4 to 5 L/day. High urine volume has two causes:
- the kidney's inability to conserve sodium and water
- osmotic diuresis produced by high BUN levels

During this phase, BUN and creatinine slowly rise, and hypovolemia and weight loss result. These conditions can lead to deficits of potassium, sodium, and water that can be deadly if left untreated. If the cause of the diuresis is corrected, azotemia gradually disappears and the patient improves greatly—leading to the recovery stage.

The recovery phase is reached when BUN and creatinine levels have returned to normal and urine output is between 1 and 2 L/day.

Getting complicated

Primary damage to the renal tubules or blood vessels results in kidney failure (intrarenal failure). The causes of intrarenal failure are classified as nephrotoxic, inflammatory, or ischemic.

When the damage is caused by nephrotoxicity or inflammation, the delicate layer under the epithelium (basement membrane) becomes irreparably damaged, commonly proceeding to chronic renal failure. Severe or prolonged lack of blood flow (ischemia) may lead to renal damage (ischemic parenchymal injury) and excess nitrogen in the blood (intrinsic renal azotemia).

What to look for

The signs and symptoms of prerenal failure depend on the cause. If the underlying problem is a change in blood pressure and volume, the patient may have:

- oliguria
- tachycardia
- hypotension
- dry mucous membranes
- flat neck veins
- lethargy progressing to coma
- decreased cardiac output and cool, clammy skin in a patient with heart failure

As renal failure progresses, the patient may show signs and symptoms of uremia, including:

- confusion
- GI complaints
- fluid in the lungs
- infection

About 5% of all hospitalized patients develop AKI. The condition is usually reversible with treatment, but if it isn't treated, it may progress to end-stage renal disease, excess urea in the blood (prerenal azotemia or uremia), and death. (See *Treating acute kidney injury*, page 348.)

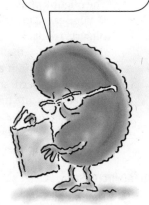

Hmm... It says here that acute kidney injury is usually reversible with medical treatment but can be fatal without it.

 Battling illness

Treating acute kidney injury

Supportive measures for acute kidney injury include:
- a high-calorie diet, low in protein, sodium, and potassium
- fluid and electrolyte balance
- monitoring signs and symptoms of uremia
- fluid restriction
- diuretic therapy during the oliguric phase
- prevention of infection
- renal dose dopamine (Intropin) to improve renal perfusion
- corticosteroids

Halting hyperkalemia

Meticulous electrolyte monitoring is needed to detect excess potassium in the blood (hyperkalemia). If symptoms occur, hypertonic glucose, insulin, and sodium bicarbonate are given IV, and sodium polystyrene sulfonate (Kayexalate) is given by mouth or enema.

If these measures fail to control uremia, the patient may need hemodialysis or continuous renal replacement therapy.

What tests tell you

These tests are used to diagnose AKI:

- Blood studies reveal elevated BUN, serum creatinine, and potassium levels and decreased blood pH, bicarbonate, hematocrit (HCT), and hemoglobin levels.
- Urine specimens show casts, cellular debris, decreased specific gravity, and, in glomerular diseases, proteinuria and urine osmolality close to serum osmolality. Urine sodium level is less than 20 mEq/L if oliguria results from decreased perfusion and more than 40 mEq/L if it results from an intrarenal problem.
- Creatinine clearance test measures GFR and is used to estimate the number of remaining functioning nephrons.
- Electrocardiogram (ECG) shows tall, peaked T waves, a widening QRS complex, and disappearing P waves if increased serum potassium (hyperkalemia) level is present.
- Other studies that help determine the cause of renal failure include kidney ultrasonography; plain films of the abdomen; kidney, ureter, and bladder (KUB) radiography; excretory urography; renal scan; retrograde pyelography; computed tomography scan; and nephrotomography.

Acute tubular necrosis

Acute tubular necrosis is responsible for the majority of cases of AKI. Also called *acute tubulointerstitial nephritis*, this disorder destroys the tubular segment of the nephron, causing uremia (the excess accumulation of nitrogen by-products of protein metabolism in the blood) and renal failure.

How it happens

Acute tubular necrosis may follow two types of kidney injury:

1. ischemic injury, the most common cause
2. nephrotoxic injury, commonly due to drugs

Disruption!

In ischemic injury, blood flow to the kidneys is disrupted. The longer the blood flow is interrupted, the worse the kidney damage. Blood flow to the kidneys may be disrupted by:

- circulatory collapse
- severe hypotension
- trauma
- hemorrhage

- dehydration
- cardiogenic or septic shock
- surgery
- anesthetics
- transfusion reactions

Warning! Toxic materials

Nephrotoxic injury can result from:

- ingesting or inhaling toxic chemicals, such as carbon tetrachloride, heavy metals, or excessive nonsteroidal anti-inflammatory drug–type medications or other nephrotoxic drugs
- a hypersensitivity reaction of the kidneys to substances as antibiotics and radiographic contrast agents

Let's get specific

Some specific causes of acute tubular necrosis and their effects include:

- diseased tubular epithelium that allows glomerular filtrate (that should be excreted) to leak through the membranes and be reabsorbed into the blood
- obstructed urine flow from the collection of damaged cells, casts, RBCs, and other cellular debris within the tubular walls
- ischemic injury to glomerular epithelial cells, causing cellular collapse and poor glomerular capillary permeability
- ischemic injury to the vascular endothelium, eventually causing cellular swelling, and tubular obstruction

A lesson on lesions

Deep or shallow lesions may occur in acute tubular necrosis. With ischemic injury, necrosis creates deep lesions, destroying the tubular epithelium and basement membrane (the delicate layer underlying the epithelium). Ischemic injury causes patches of necrosis in the tubules. Ischemia can also cause lesions in the connective tissue of the kidney.

With nephrotoxic injury, necrosis occurs only in the epithelium of the tubules, leaving the basement membrane of the nephrons intact. This type of damage may be reversible. (See *A close look at acute tubular necrosis*, page 351.)

Taking its toll

Toxicity takes a toll. Nephrotoxic agents can injure tubular cells by:

- direct cellular toxic effects
- coagulation and destruction (lysis) of RBCs
- disruption of normal function causing decreased perfusion
- oxygen deprivation (hypoxia)
- crystal formation of solutes

Now I get it!

A close look at acute tubular necrosis

In acute tubular necrosis caused by ischemia, patches of necrosis occur, usually in the straight portion of the proximal tubules as shown below. In areas without lesions, tubules are usually dilated.

In acute tubular necrosis caused by nephrotoxicity, the tubules have a more uniform appearance, as shown in the second illustration.

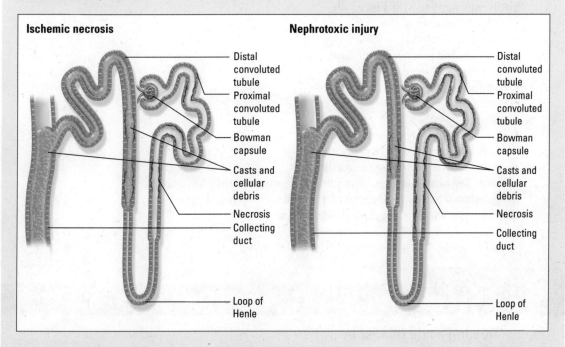

Getting complicated

There are several common complications of acute tubular necrosis:
- Infections (typically septicemia) are the leading cause of death.
- GI hemorrhage, fluid and electrolyte imbalance, and cardiovascular dysfunction may occur during the acute phase or the recovery phase.
- Neurologic complications are common in older adult patients and occur occasionally in younger patients.
- Excess blood calcium (hypercalcemia) may occur during the recovery phase.

What to look for

Early-stage acute tubular necrosis may be hard to spot because the patient's primary disease may obscure the signs and symptoms. The first recognizable sign may be decreased urine output (termed *oliguria*), usually less than 400 mL/24 hours.

Oliguria is an important term to understand; it means an inadequate amount of urine for waste elimination. The kidney needs a certain amount of water (urine volume) in order to excrete wastes.

Other signs and symptoms depend on the severity of systemic involvement and may include:
- bleeding abnormalities
- vomiting of blood
- dry skin and mucous membranes
- lethargy
- confusion
- agitation
- edema
- fluid and electrolyte imbalances
- muscle weakness with hyperkalemia
- tachycardia and an irregular rhythm

Mortality can be as high, depending on complications from underlying diseases. Nonoliguric forms of acute tubular necrosis have a better prognosis. (See *Treating acute tubular necrosis*.)

Battling illness

Treating acute tubular necrosis

Acute tubular necrosis requires vigorous supportive measures during the acute phase until normal kidney function is restored.
- Initially, diuretics are given and fluids are infused to flush tubules of cellular casts and debris and replace lost fluids.
- Projected and calculated fluid losses require daily replacement.
- Transfusion of packed red blood cells is administered for anemia.

- Nonnephrotoxic antibiotics are given for infection.
- Hyperkalemia requires an emergency IV infusion of 50% glucose and regular insulin.
- Sodium bicarbonate may be needed to combat metabolic acidosis.
- Sodium polystyrene sulfonate is given by mouth or by enema to reduce potassium levels.
- Hemodialysis or peritoneal dialysis is used to prevent severe fluid and electrolyte imbalance and uremia.

What tests tell you

Acute tubular necrosis is hard to diagnose except in advanced stages.
These tests are commonly performed:
- Urinalysis shows dilute urine, low osmolality, high sodium levels,
  and urine sediment containing RBCs and casts.
- Blood studies reveal high BUN and serum creatinine levels, low
  serum protein levels, anemia, platelet adherence defects, metabolic
  acidosis, and hyperkalemia.
- ECG may show arrhythmias from electrolyte imbalances and, with
  hyperkalemia, a widening QRS complex, disappearing P waves,
  and tall, peaked T waves.

Glomerulonephritis

Glomerulonephritis is a bilateral inflammation of the glomeruli,
commonly following a streptococcal infection.

In acute situations

Acute glomerulonephritis is most common in males between 5 and
15 years old, but it can occur at any age and in any gender. Although
many patients recover fully, others, especially older adult patients,
may progress to chronic renal failure within months.

This is all happening too quickly

Rapidly progressive glomerulonephritis most commonly occurs
between ages 50 and 60. It may be idiopathic or associated with a
proliferative glomerular disease such as *poststreptococcal glomerulonephritis*. After strep pharyngitis (strep throat), the kidney can be affected
by antibodies that have developed against the strep organism, group
A beta-hemolytic streptococci. The antibodies against the strep organism mistakenly also attack the nephrons.

This is an immunological reaction against the kidney. The trigger
of the antibodies is the strep infection.

Another immunological disease that involves the kidney is
Goodpasture disease, also called *antiglomerular basement membrane* disease. This disorder is a rare type of rapidly progressive glomerulonephritis. It most often occurs in males younger than 30 years old and
females who are older than 50. In this autoimmune disease, antibodies destroy the glomerulus. The trigger of the antibodies is unknown.

Chronic cases

Chronic glomerulonephritis is a slowly progressive disease characterized by inflammation, sclerosis, scarring, and eventual renal failure.
It usually remains undetected until the progressive phase, which is
irreversible.

How it happens

In nearly all types of glomerulonephritis, the glomerular membrane is disturbed. A damaged glomerulus is highly permeable and filters out water and proteins from the blood. A healthy glomerulus retains the proteins in the bloodstream and filters out the water into the nephron tubules. A key sign of glomerulonephritis is protein in the urine (termed *proteinuria*) and low protein in the bloodstream (termed *hypoalbuminemia*). The low protein in the blood causes low oncotic pressure in the bloodstream, which leads to fluid shifts, resulting in pulmonary edema and periorbital edema.

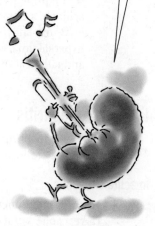

If this glomerulonephritis isn't detected, I'll soon be playing the blues!

Unwelcome lodger

Acute poststreptococcal glomerulonephritis results from an immune response that occurs in the glomerulus. The antigen, group A beta-hemolytic streptococci, stimulates antibody formation. As an antigen–antibody complex forms, it becomes lodged in the glomerular capillaries, causing an inflammatory response.

Glomerular injury occurs as a result of the inflammatory process when complexes initiate the release of immunologic substances that break down cells and increase membrane permeability. The severity of glomerular damage and renal insufficiency is related to the size, number, location, duration of exposure, and type of antigen–antibody complexes. (See *Immune complex deposits on the glomerulus.*)

What's so "good" about Goodpasture disease?

In Goodpasture disease (antiglomerular membrane disease), antibodies are produced against the pulmonary capillaries and glomerular basement membrane. Goodpasture disease is a disorder of both the lungs and the kidney. Glomerular filtration rate becomes reduced, and renal failure occurs within weeks or months.

What to look for

Possible signs and symptoms of glomerulonephritis include:
- decreased urination or oliguria (oliguria = less than 400 mL urine/day)
- coffee-colored urine (blood in urine)
- proteins in urine (proteinuria)
- shortness of breath due to pulmonary edema
- orthopnea due to pulmonary edema
- periorbital edema
- mild to severe hypertension (kidney damage commonly causes high renin release)
- bibasilar crackles on lung auscultation due to pulmonary edema
- nausea
- malaise
- weight loss
- arthralgia (See *Treating chronic glomerulonephritis.*)

Immune complex deposits on the glomerulus

The illustrations below show where the immune complex deposits appear in the glomerulus in glomerulonephritis.

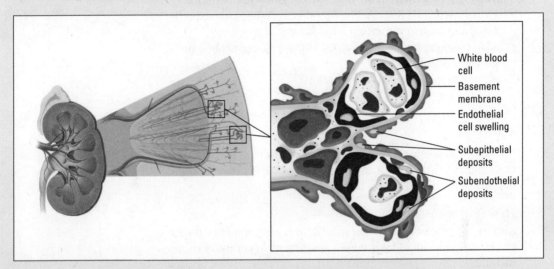

- White blood cell
- Basement membrane
- Endothelial cell swelling
- Subepithelial deposits
- Subendothelial deposits

What tests tell you

These blood study results aid in the diagnosis of glomerulonephritis:

- BUN and creatinine levels are elevated.
- Serum protein levels are decreased.
- Urine protein is high (proteinuria).
- Hemoglobin levels may be decreased in chronic glomerulonephritis.

Battling illness

Treating chronic glomerulonephritis

Treatment focuses on the underlying disease.

Drug therapy

Drugs used to treat chronic glomerulonephritis include:

- antibiotics (7 to 10 days) to treat infections contributing to ongoing antigen–antibody response
- diuretics such as furosemide to reduce fluid overload
- vasodilators such as hydralazine to control hypertension
- corticosteroids to decrease antibody synthesis and suppress inflammation

Other interventions

In rapidly progressive glomerulonephritis, the patient may require plasmapheresis to suppress rebound antibody production. Plasmapheresis is a procedure that removes antibodies from the bloodstream. This procedure may be combined with corticosteroids and cyclophosphamide.

Dialysis or kidney transplantation may be necessary.

- Antistreptolysin O titers are elevated in many patients.
- Serum phosphorous levels are increased.
- Serum calcium levels are decreased.
  These tests also help in the diagnosis of glomerulonephritis:
- Urinalysis reveals RBCs, white blood cells (WBCs), mixed cell casts, and protein indicating renal failure.
- KUB radiography reveals bilateral kidney enlargement (acute glomerulonephritis).
  A renal biopsy confirms the diagnosis.

Hydronephrosis

An abnormal dilation of the renal pelvis and the calyces of one or both kidneys, hydronephrosis is caused by an obstruction of urine outflow in the genitourinary tract.

How it happens

Almost any type of disease that results from obstruction of the urinary tract can result in hydronephrosis. The most common causes include:
- benign prostatic hyperplasia
- urethral strictures
- stenosis of the ureter or bladder outlet
  Less common causes include:
- congenital abnormalities
- abdominal tumors
- neurogenic bladder
- tumors of the ureter and bladder

Instruction on obstruction

If the obstruction is in the urethra or bladder, hydronephrosis usually affects both kidneys; if the obstruction is in a ureter, it usually affects one kidney. Obstructions distal to the bladder cause the bladder to dilate and act as a buffer zone, delaying hydronephrosis. Total obstruction of urine flow with dilation of the collecting system ultimately causes complete atrophy of the cortex (the outer portion of the kidney) and cessation of glomerular filtration. (See *Renal damage in hydronephrosis*.)

From bad to worse

Untreated hydronephrosis can result in infection, or pyelonephritis, due to stasis that exacerbates renal damage and may create a life-threatening crisis.

Now I get it!

Renal damage in hydronephrosis

In hydronephrosis, the ureters dilate, the renal pelvis dilates, and the parenchyma and papilla atrophy.

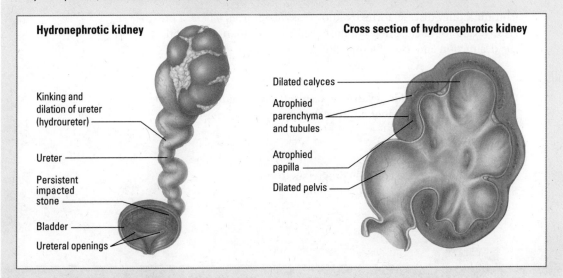

Hydronephrotic kidney

Kinking and dilation of ureter (hydroureter)

Ureter

Persistent impacted stone

Bladder

Ureteral openings

Cross section of hydronephrotic kidney

Dilated calyces

Atrophied parenchyma and tubules

Atrophied papilla

Dilated pelvis

What to look for

Signs and symptoms depend on the cause of the obstruction. In mild cases, hydronephrosis produces either no symptoms or mild pain and slightly decreased urine flow. In more severe cases, it may produce severe, colicky renal pain or dull flank pain that may radiate to the groin and gross urinary abnormalities, such as hematuria, pyuria, dysuria, alternating polyuria and oliguria, and complete anuria.

Generally speaking

Other symptoms of hydronephrosis are generalized and include:
• nausea and vomiting
• abdominal fullness
• dribbling of urine
• urinary hesitancy

What tests tell you

These tests are essential to the diagnosis of hydronephrosis:
• Excretory urography confirms hydronephrosis.
• Retrograde pyelography reveals hydronephrosis.

- Renal ultrasonography reveals an obstruction and confirms hydronephrosis.
- Renal function studies demonstrate hydronephrosis.

Kidney disease, chronic (chronic renal failure)

Chronic kidney disease, formerly known as *chronic renal failure*, a progressive and irreversible deterioration, is the end result of gradual tissue destruction and loss of kidney function.

Blitz!

Occasionally, chronic kidney disease results from a rapidly progressing disease of sudden onset that destroys the nephrons and causes irreversible kidney damage.

How it happens

Chronic kidney disease typically progresses through five stages. (See *Stages of chronic kidney disease.*)

Now I get it!

Stages of chronic kidney disease

Stages	GFR	Nursing interventions
Stage 1—Patient is "at risk" due to structural abnormalities, genetic concerns, or urine findings, although kidney function is normal.	GFR > 90 mL/minute	Screen for risk factors and provide education to reduce risks of conditions such as diabetes and hypertension.
Stage 2—Mild chronic kidney disease; renal function has begun to be impaired; diagnostic testing indicates kidney disease.	GFR 60–89 mL/minute	Continue to reduce risk factors.
Stage 3—Moderate chronic kidney disease; renal function shows impairment.	GFR 30–59 mL/minute	Provide interventions to slow the development of the disease process.
Stage 4—Severe chronic kidney disease; renal function is severely impaired.	GFR 15–29 mL/minute	Focus on management of complications; educate about options available when in stage 5.
Stage 5—End-stage renal disease (ESRD); kidneys cannot maintain homeostasis; waste elimination is severely impaired as urea and creatinine build up in the blood.	GFR < 15 mL/minute	Educate patient about options and prepare for dialysis, kidney transplant, or withdrawal from therapy based on patient's wishes.

It may result from

- chronic glomerular disease, such as glomerulonephritis, which affects the capillaries in the glomeruli
- chronic infections, such as chronic pyelonephritis and tuberculosis
- congenital anomalies such as polycystic kidney disease
- vascular diseases, such as hypertension and nephrosclerosis, which causes hardening of the kidneys
- obstructions such as renal calculi
- collagen diseases such as systemic lupus erythematosus
- nephrotoxic agents such as long-term aminoglycoside therapy
- endocrine diseases such as diabetic nephropathy

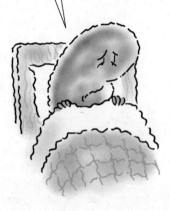

Healthy nephrons work hard to keep me going, but eventually they're overwhelmed.

Fight to the finish

Nephron damage is progressive. Damaged nephrons can no longer function. Healthy nephrons compensate for destroyed nephrons by enlarging and increasing their clearance capacity. The kidneys can maintain relatively normal function until about 75% of the nephrons are nonfunctional.

Eventually, when the healthy glomeruli are so overburdened, they become sclerotic and stiff, leading to their destruction. If this condition continues unchecked, toxins accumulate and produce potentially fatal changes in all major organ systems.

Getting complicated

Even if the patient can tolerate life-sustaining maintenance dialysis or a kidney transplant, conditions such as anemia, nervous system effects (peripheral neuropathy), cardiopulmonary and GI complications, sexual dysfunction, and skeletal defects may develop.

What to look for

Symptoms may not develop until more than 75% of glomerular filtration is lost. Then, the remaining normal tissue deteriorates progressively. Symptoms worsen as kidney function decreases. Because the kidneys perform so many processes in the body, the profound changes that characterize chronic kidney disease affect all body systems. Major findings include:

- hypervolemia (abnormal increase in plasma volume) (the kidney is not adequately filtering the blood and is not excreting water)
- peripheral edema (the excess water in the body causes edema)
- hyperphosphatemia
- hyperkalemia (the kidney is not excreting K^+)
- hypocalcemia (the kidney is not synthesizing vitamin D)
- azotemia (high amount of nitrogen wastes in the blood [high BUN])

- metabolic acidosis (the kidney is not excreting H^+ from the bloodstream)
- anemia (the kidney is not secreting erythropoietin)
- peripheral neuropathy (nitrogen waste accumulation irritates nerve endings)
- encephalopathy (confusion, lethargy, disorientation, possible stupor, coma) (the nitrogen waste accumulation affects the brain)

Body count
Other signs and symptoms, by body system, include:
- *renal*—dry mouth, fatigue, nausea, hypotension, loss of skin turgor, and listlessness that may progress to somnolence and confusion, decreased or dilute urine, irregular pulses, and edema
- *cardiovascular*—hypertension, irregular pulse, life-threatening arrhythmias, and heart failure
- *respiratory*—infection, crackles, and pleuritic pain
- *GI*—gum sores and bleeding, hiccups, metallic taste, anorexia, nausea, vomiting, ammonia smell to the breath, and abdominal pain on palpation
- *skin*—pallid, yellowish-bronze color; dry, scaly skin; thin, brittle nails; dry, brittle hair that may change color and fall out easily; severe itching; and white, flaky urea deposits (uremic frost) in critically ill patients
- *neurologic*—altered level of consciousness, muscle cramps and twitching, and pain, burning, and itching in legs and feet (restless leg syndrome)
- *endocrine*—growth retardation in children, infertility, decreased libido, amenorrhea, and impotence
- *hematologic*—GI bleeding and hemorrhage from body orifices and easy bruising
- *musculoskeletal*—fractures, bone and muscle pain, abnormal gait, and impaired bone growth and bowed legs in children

The progression of chronic renal failure can sometimes be slowed, but it's ultimately irreversible, culminating in end-stage renal disease. Although it's fatal without treatment, dialysis or a kidney transplant can sustain life. (See *Treating chronic kidney disease*.)

What tests tell you
These tests are used to diagnose chronic kidney disease:
- Blood studies show decreased arterial pH and bicarbonate levels, low HCT and low hemoglobin levels, and elevated BUN, serum creatinine, sodium, and potassium levels.
- Arterial blood gas analysis reveals metabolic acidosis.
- Urine specific gravity becomes fixed at 1.010; urinalysis may show proteinuria, glycosuria, RBCs, leukocytes, casts, or crystals, depending on the cause.

Treating chronic kidney disease

Treatment for chronic kidney disease may consist of one or more of these treatments, depending on the stage of failure.

Conservative measures

Conservative treatment includes:
- a low-protein diet to reduce end products of protein metabolism that the kidneys can't excrete
- a high-protein diet for patients on continuous dialysis
- a high-calorie diet to prevent ketoacidosis (the accumulation of ketones, in the blood) and tissue atrophy
- sodium and potassium restrictions
- phosphorus restriction
- fluid restrictions to maintain fluid balance
- fat restrictions for patients with hyperlipidemia

Drug therapy

Drugs used to treat chronic kidney disease include:
- loop diuretics such as furosemide, if some renal function remains, to maintain fluid balance
- antihypertensive medications to control blood pressure and edema
- antiemetic drugs to relieve nausea and vomiting
- histamine-2 receptor antagonists such as famotidine to decrease gastric irritation
- stool softeners to prevent constipation
- iron and folate supplements or red blood cell (RBC) infusion for anemia
- synthetic erythropoietin to stimulate the bone marrow to produce RBCs
- antipruritic drugs, such as trimeprazine or diphenhydramine to relieve itching
- aluminum hydroxide gel to lower serum phosphate levels
- supplementary vitamins, particularly B and D, and essential amino acids

Dialysis

When the kidneys fail, kidney transplantation or dialysis may be the patient's only chance for survival. Dialysis options include:
- hemodialysis, which filters blood through a dialysis machine. During hemodialysis, a dialysis machine and a special filter called an *artificial kidney*, or a dialyzer, are used to clear blood of excess waste products and fluid. This procedure requires surgical insertion of a fistula implanted in the forearm for access to the dialysis machine.
- peritoneal dialysis, in which a catheter is placed in the peritoneal cavity for instillation of dialysate. This procedure is a renal replacement therapy based on infusing a sterile solution into the peritoneal cavity through a catheter; it provides for the removal of solutes and water using the peritoneal membrane as the exchange surface.

Emergency measures

Potassium levels in the blood must be monitored to detect hyperkalemia. Hyperkalemia is an emergency due its potential to cause cardiac arrest. Emergency treatment includes dialysis therapy, oral or rectal administration of cation exchange resins, such as sodium polystyrene sulfonate (Kayexalate), and IV administration of calcium gluconate, sodium bicarbonate, 50% hypertonic glucose, and regular insulin.

- X-ray studies, including KUB radiography, excretory urography, nephrotomography, renal scan, and renal arteriography, show reduced kidney size.
- Renal biopsy is used to identify underlying disease.
- EEG shows changes that indicate brain disease (metabolic encephalopathy).

Renal calculi (kidney stones; also called *nephrolithiasis*)

Renal calculi, or *kidney stones,* may form anywhere in the urinary tract, but they usually develop in the renal pelvis or calices. Calculi form when crystalline substances that normally dissolve in the urine precipitate. The most common calculi are made of calcium oxalate. Calculi vary in size, shape, and number. (See *A close look at renal calculi.*)

Lifetime prevalence of kidney stones for Americans is approximately 12% for males and 7% for females. They're more common in males, with a higher incidence in the White population, and they are more prevalent in specific geographic areas such as the South and Southwestern United States. Geographic areas with hot weather have a higher incidence of kidney stones because of the higher risk of dehydration.

How it happens

Although their exact cause is unknown, there are several predisposing factors to the development of renal calculi:

* *Dehydration*—decreased water and urine excretion concentrates calculus-forming substances.

Now I get it!

A close look at renal calculi

Renal calculi vary in size and type. Small calculi may remain in the renal pelvis or pass down the ureter as shown below left. A staghorn calculus, shown below right, is a cast of the innermost part of the kidney—the calyx and renal pelvis. A staghorn calculus may develop from a calculus that stays in the kidney.

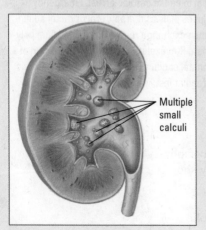

Multiple small calculi

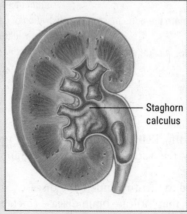

Staghorn calculus

- *Infection*—infected, scarred tissue provides a site for calculus development. Calculi may become infected if bacteria are the nucleus in calculi formation. Calculi that result from *Proteus* infections may lead to destruction of kidney tissue.
- *Changes in urine pH*—consistently acidic or alkaline urine provides a favorable medium for calculus formation. An alkaline pH favors the crystallization of calcium- and phosphate-containing stones, whereas an acidic urine pH promotes uric acid or cystine stones.
- *Obstruction*—urinary stasis allows calculus constituents to collect and adhere, forming calculi. Obstruction also encourages infection, which compounds the obstruction.
- *Immobilization*—immobility allows calcium to be released into the circulation and, eventually, to be filtered by the kidneys.
- *Diet*—increased intake of calcium or oxalate-rich foods encourages calculi formation.
- *Metabolic factors*—hyperparathyroidism, renal tubular acidosis, elevated uric acid (usually with gout), defective oxalate metabolism, a genetic defect in cystine metabolism, and excessive intake of vitamin D or dietary calcium may predispose a person to renal calculi.

A delicate balance

Renal calculi usually arise because the delicate excretory balance breaks down.

Here's how it happens:
- Urine becomes concentrated with insoluble materials.
- Crystals form from these materials and then consolidate, forming calculi. These calculi contain an organic mucoprotein framework and crystalloids, such as calcium, oxalate, phosphate, urate, uric acid, struvite, cystine, and xanthine.
- Calculi remain in the renal pelvis and damage or destroy kidney tissue, or they enter the ureter.
- Large calculi in the kidneys may cause tissue damage (pressure necrosis).
- In certain locations, calculi obstruct urine, which collects in the renal pelvis (hydronephrosis). These calculi also tend to recur. Intractable pain and serious bleeding can result. The pain of kidney stones is usually flank pain or costovertebral angle pain (back) into the groin.
- Initially, hydrostatic pressure increases in the collection system near the obstruction, forcing nearby renal structures to dilate as well. The farther the obstruction is from the kidney, the less serious the dilation because the pressure is diffused over a larger surface area.
- With a complete obstruction, pressure in the renal pelvis and tubules increases, the GFR falls, and a disruption occurs in the junctional complexes between tubular cells. If left untreated, tubular atrophy and destruction of the medulla leave connective tissue in place of the glomeruli, causing irreversible damage.

What to look for

The key symptom of renal calculi is severe flank pain (costovertebral angle), which usually occurs when large calculi obstruct the opening of the ureter and increase the frequency and force of peristaltic contractions. Pain may travel from the lower back to the sides and then to the groin region and external genitalia. Pain intensity fluctuates and may be excruciating at its peak.

The patient with calculi in the renal pelvis and calices may complain of more constant, dull pain. They may report back pain from an obstruction within a kidney and severe abdominal pain from calculi traveling down a ureter. Severe pain is typically accompanied by nausea, vomiting, and, possibly, fever and chills. (See *Treating renal calculi*.)

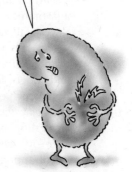

The pain from renal stones can be excruciating!

It's more than just a pain

Other signs and symptoms include:
- hematuria (when stones abrade a ureter)
- abdominal distention

Battling illness

Treating renal calculi

Renal calculi that are smaller than 4 mm in diameter have an 80% chance of passing naturally with vigorous hydration (more than 3 L/day). Drinking large amounts of water can flush out the calculus, and straining the urine to capture the calculus for analysis. Other treatments may include drug therapy for infection or other effects of illness and measures to prevent recurrence of calculi. If calculi are too large for natural passage, they may be removed by surgery or first broken down with the use of ultrasonic lithotripsy. Lithotripsy uses sound waves to break up the stone into smaller particles, which can more easily pass through the urinary tract.

Drug therapy

Drugs used to treat renal calculi include:
- antimicrobial agents for infection (varying with the cultured organism)
- analgesic agents, such as hydromorphone (Dilaudid) and morphine (Duramorph) for pain
- diuretics to prevent urinary stasis and further calculi formation
- thiazides to decrease calcium excretion into the urine

- methenamine to suppress calculi formation when infection is present

Preventive measures

Measures to prevent recurrence of renal calculi include:
- a low-calcium oxalate diet
- oxalate-binding cholestyramine for absorptive hypercalciuria
- parathyroidectomy for hyperparathyroidism
- allopurinol for uric acid calculi
- daily oral doses of ascorbic acid (vitamin C) to acidify the urine
- adequate hydration

Removing calculi

Calculi lodged in the ureter may be removed by inserting a cystoscope through the urethra and then manipulating the calculi with catheters or retrieval instruments. A flank or lower abdominal approach may be needed to extract calculi from other areas, such as the kidney calyx or renal pelvis. Percutaneous ultrasonic lithotripsy and extracorporeal shock wave lithotripsy shatter the calculi into fragments for removal by suction or natural passage.

- oliguria (from an obstruction in urine flow)
- dysuria
- frequency of urination
- nausea and vomiting
  Most small calculi can be flushed out of a person's system by drinking lots of fluids.

What tests tell you

Diagnosis is based on clinical signs and symptoms, and these tests:
- KUB radiography reveals most renal calculi.
- Excretory urography helps confirm the diagnosis and shows the size and location of calculi.
- Kidney ultrasonography is easy to perform, noninvasive, and nontoxic and detects obstructions not seen on the KUB radiography.
- Urinalysis may indicate pus in the urine (pyuria), a sign of UTI.
- 24-hour urine collection reveals calcium oxalate, phosphorus, and uric acid levels. Three separate collections, along with blood samples, are needed for accurate testing.
- Calculus analysis shows mineral content.
  These tests may identify the cause of calculus formation:
- Blood calcium and phosphorus levels detect hyperparathyroidism and show an increased calcium level in proportion to normal serum protein levels.
- Blood protein levels determine the level of free calcium unbound to protein.
- Differential diagnosis rules out appendicitis, cholecystitis, peptic ulcer, and pancreatitis as sources of pain.

Urinary tract infection, pyelonephritis (kidney infection), and urosepsis

A UTI is an infection anywhere in the urinary tract. This includes the two kidneys and ureters, the bladder, and the urethra. The bladder and urethra are referred to as the lower urinary tract.

Who gets it: gender bias

Not fair! Unfortunately, females are four times more likely than males to get a UTI. For females, this is mostly due to a much shorter urethra, 1.5″, compared to the male, nearly 8″ urethra. Another cause is the proximity of the urethral and anal openings in females. In females, bacteria from the bowel (such as *Escherichia coli*) can easily travel into the urethra; because the bacteria have a much shorter distance to travel, the body has less of an opportunity to fight against the attacking pathogen. When a male gets a UTI, it is usually structurally related and associated with impaired flow of the urine.

Raising the risk

Although a UTI can happen to anyone, certain populations are more vulnerable. Patients with diabetes are at higher risk of developing a UTI due to reduced circulation, reduced bladder emptying, reduced WBC function, and increased glucose in the urine.

Germs feed on sugar! Other special populations at risk include those who have a urinary catheter inserted to eliminate urine from the body.

How it happens: getting specific

UTIs are usually caused by bacteria, but they may also be related to a virus, yeast, or fungi growth.

- The most common bacteria to cause UTIs are *Escherichia coli*.
- The next most common bacteria to cause UTIs are *Klebsiella pneumoniae*.
- The third most common bacteria to cause UTIs vary widely and are often dependent on the location and the season of the year; these can include *Staphylococcus epidermidis*, *Pseudomonas aeruginosa*, *Enterococcus*, and various strains of *Streptococcus*.
- Sometimes *Candida albicans*, a yeast, can cause a UTI.

What is the main malfunction?

The urinary tract system is made to prevent infection by having built-in one-way valves and a natural flushing action that occurs with urination. UTIs can be caused by the failure of one of more natural defenses of anatomy, immunity, or action of the WBCs. The pathogens can gain entry to the urinary tract due to poor hygiene in the perineal region or introduction of foreign objects like a catheter. A lack of adequate flushing action allows for further entry of the pathogen and continued growth. Inadequate emptying of the bladder, low immunity, and high glucose levels can stimulate growth of foreign pathogens in the urinary tract.

Will it stay or will it go?

Most UTIs are acute, meaning they begin fast and are not serious in nature. However, some people have chronic or recurrent UTIs. Characteristics of chronic UTIs include:

- having 3 or more UTIs in 12 months
- bacterial persistence after 2 weeks of treatment
- infection with new bacteria, or
- a sterile intervening culture

A sterile intervening culture means that a sterile, or bacteria-free, urine sample was collected following treatment of a UTI; however, another UTI developed following collection of this sample.

Recurrent or chronic UTIs tend to happen to certain people. These people include:

- postmenopausal females, which is hormone related
- those who insert birth control devices or medications into the vagina
- males with prostate enlargement (benign prostatic hyperplasia)
- those with diseases that cause delayed or incomplete bladder emptying
- those with genetic predisposition, and
- those with structural abnormalities of the urologic system

Getting complicated

An untreated lower UTI can lead to:

- pyelonephritis (upper UTI, which is more serious than lower UTI)
- permanent kidney damage
- kidney failure
- risk of low birth weight or premature birth for those who are pregnant
- urethral narrowing (stricture) in men
- recurrent UTIs
- urosepsis (See *Pyelonephritis and urosepsis.*)

What to look for

- Initially, a urinary tract infection is suspected based on signs and symptoms, which are usually subjective until further testing can be completed. Your patient may report:
  - urination that is painful, frequent, urgent, or occurring at night
  - urine that is dark, red, milky, or cloudy or has a foul odor

---

Pyelonephritis and urosepsis

Complications of lower UTI can include:

• **Pyelonephritis:** A serious urinary tract infection that involves the kidney, it causes fever, chills, abdominal pain, and costovertebral angle tenderness, and it requires high doses of antibiotic treatment.

• **Urosepsis:** A body-wide infection that can also be called *septicemia* (bloodstream infection), it can lead to multiple organ dysfunction. This serious infection can also lead to septic shock and can be fatal. It is a common cause of sepsis in adults ages 65 and older with unrecognized urinary tract infection. Up to 25% of all cases of sepsis are urosepsis, meaning they began in the urinary tract. Signs and symptoms of urosepsis include:

- fever, chills (often older adults do not have fever)
- pain on the lower sides of the back, where the kidneys are located
- anorexia, nausea
- extreme fatigue
- decreased urine output
- dark urine
- confusion, disorientation
- difficulty breathing
- abnormal heart function

Sepsis requires high doses of antibiotics, IV therapy, supportive care, and hospitalization.

- pain in the back or tenderness in the costovertebral region
- pressure in the abdomen area
- fever, fatigue, altered mental status, or shakiness/chills
- confusion in older adults
- the return of incontinence in a child who has already accomplished toilet training
- urethral discharge, scrotal mass, or scrotal or prostatic tenderness in males

What tests tell you

Most healthcare providers will begin with obtaining a urinalysis. An initial urinalysis will come back quickly, but a culture and susceptibility will take between 1 and 3 days and usually at least 48 hours.

- Mid-stream or clean catch urinalysis with culture and susceptibility (sensitivity) and gram staining. The following are indicators of infection:
  - two or more WBCs and two or more RBCs
  - 15 or more bacteria in a high-powered field
  - >100,000 colony-forming units of one bacteria
  - positive for nitrites and leukocyte esterase
  - 2 g or more of protein is an indicator of infection

Let's take a look

Imaging is generally not used to diagnose a UTI unless the condition is expected to be complicated in nature; however, it can be helpful in identifying functional impairment. Methods of imaging include:

- CT urogram with and without contrast
- Abdominopelvic ultrasound
- X-ray, which is sometimes ordered in conjunction with an ultrasound
- MRI

Proceed to procedures

At times, additional procedures may need to be performed to gain a full understanding of what is causing the malfunction. These include:

- Cystoscopy to identify structural abnormalities
- Postvoid residual to identify retention
- Uroflowmetry or urodynamic to determine function and flow

Treating urinary tract infections

Drug therapy
Medications used to treat a simple UTI include trimethoprim/
sulfamethoxazole, fosfomycin, nitrofurantoin, or cephalexin.
More complicated UTIs may require treatment with a fluoro-
quinolone, such as ciprofloxacin or levofloxacin.

Self-care
A patient can do certain things to help prevent a urinary
tract infection or assist with eliminating the infection.
These things include:
• Practicing good perineal hygiene: wiping from front
to back, showering instead of bathing, and washing the
perianal and pubic area with soap
• Avoidance of sprays, creams, or birth prevention
devices in the genital area
• Frequent urination, especially after intercourse
• Drinking plenty of water—six to eight glasses daily
• Avoidance of tight-fitting and nonbreathable pants and
underclothes
• If a person has diabetes, keeping blood glucose within
normal limits

Cancer: a few words about that
Cancer can occur anywhere in the renal system but
is most common in the kidneys and then the bladder.
The most common is renal cell cancer in adults and
Wilms tumor in children, also called *nephroblastoma*.
Risk factors associated with renal cancer include
certain inherited disorders (such as polycystic kidney
disease), obesity, smoking, long-term pain medication use, and exposure to arsenic, aniline dyes, or
trichloroethylene.
    The signs and symptoms of renal-related cancers
often come late, with no signs in early stages. Late stage
symptoms may include:
• hematuria
• dull flank pain
• anemia
• weight loss
• anorexia
• fatigue
• sometimes an intermittent recurrent fever

Renal system review

Understanding the renal system
The renal system collects the body's
waste products and expels them as
urine. The renal system includes:
• kidneys
• ureters
• urinary bladder
• prostate gland (in males)
• urethra

Kidneys
• Located on each side of the vertebral column in the upper abdomen
outside the peritoneal cavity (the
region where kidneys are located
is the costovertebral angle on both
sides of the back)

• Work with the urinary system to
collect the body's waste products
and expel them as urine
• Filter about 45 gallons of fluid each day

Ureters
• Muscular tubes that contract
rhythmically to transport urine from
each kidney to the bladder

(Continued)

Renal system review *(continued)*

Urinary bladder
• A sac with muscular walls that collects and holds urine that's expelled from the ureters every few seconds

Prostate gland (in males)
• A gland that sits under the bladder only in males
• Manufactures fluid for sperm
• Enlarges as a male ages (usually beginning at age 70); benign prostatic hyperplasia (BPH) is a common cause of urinary outflow obstruction

Urethra
• A narrow passageway from the bladder to the outside of the body through which urine is excreted

How the kidneys perform
• Maintain fluid balance (the kidney reabsorbs water back into the bloodstream if water is needed or eliminates excess water from the bloodstream)
• Detoxify the blood and eliminate wastes, particularly nitrogen waste products (urea)
• Regulate blood pressure by secretion of renin in response to renal hypoperfusion
• Aid RBC production by secretion of erythropoietin, which is triggered by hypoxia sensed by the kidney
• Regulate vitamin D; the kidney is necessary to make a portion of vitamin D (vitamin D then enhances reabsorption of calcium from the GI tract)

Controlling fluid balance
• Antidiuretic hormone (ADH), produced by the pituitary gland, causes reabsorption of water back into the bloodstream at the collecting duct of the nephron, which creates a concentrated urine
• Aldosterone, produced by the adrenal cortex, causes reabsorption of sodium and water into the bloodstream at the distal tubules

Regulating acid–base balance
The kidneys:
• excrete hydrogen ions into the urine if blood is acidotic
• reabsorb bicarbonate ions (HCO_3^-), which are basic substances, to neutralize acidosis
• acidify phosphate salts: add hydrogen to PO_4^- and excrete HPO_4^-
• produce ammonia (NH_3): combine nitrogen and H^+, which becomes ammonia and is excreted in urine

Collecting and eliminating waste
The kidneys:
• filter blood flowing through the glomeruli; tubule fluid eventually becomes urine
• reabsorb water filtered at the glomerulus back into the bloodstream
• release the filtered substance from the tubules as urine

Regulating blood pressure
The kidneys:
• produce and secrete renin in response to a decline in blood volume and blood pressure that causes low perfusion of the kidney.

Low circulation sensed by the kidney triggers the renin–angiotensin–aldosterone system (RAAS).

Producing RBCs
The kidneys:
• secrete erythropoietin (a hormone that prompts increased RBC production) when the oxygen supply in tissue blood drops.

Regulating vitamin D and calcium formation
• The kidneys help convert vitamin D to its active form.
• Active vitamin D helps regulate calcium and phosphorus.

Renal disorders
• *Acute kidney injury*—sudden interruption of renal function caused by obstruction, poor circulation, or kidney disease; is usually reversible
• *Acute tubular necrosis*—destruction of the tubular segments of the nephron, causing renal failure and uremia; is most commonly due to renal ischemia or nephrotoxic injury of the kidney
• *Chronic kidney disease*—irreversible deterioration of tissue and eventual loss of kidney function leading to end-stage renal disease; hemodialysis or renal transplant is necessary
• *Glomerulonephritis*—bilateral inflammation of the glomeruli, commonly following a streptococcal infection
• *Goodpasture syndrome (antiglomerular basement membrane disease)*: autoimmune disease of the kidney in which antibodies are stimulated to destroy glomeruli

(Continued)

Renal system review *(continued)*

• *Hydronephrosis*—abnormal dilation of the renal pelvis and the calyces of one or both kidneys due to obstruction of urine outflow
• *Renal calculi (nephrolithiasis)*—substances that normally dissolve in the urine precipitate to form "kidney stones"; most commonly calcium oxalate stones
• *Lower urinary tract infection*—an infection located in the bladder and urethra
• *Pyelonephritis*—upper urinary tract infection; infection that has ascended from the lower urinary tract into the kidney
• *Urosepsis*—body-wide infection that began as a urinary tract infection and can lead to shock and multiple organ failure

Quick quiz

1. Which hormone helps control the secretion of potassium by the distal tubules?
    A. Antidiuretic hormone
    B. Renin
    C. Aldosterone
    D. Calcitriol

Answer: C. Aldosterone, along with ADH, is one of the two hormones that partially effects the kidney's ability to maintain fluid balance. Aldosterone, which is secreted by the adrenal gland, enhances potassium excretion at the distal tubule.

2. One potential cause of intrarenal failure is:
    A. arterial embolism.
    B. acute tubular necrosis.
    C. venous thrombosis.
    D. cardiogenic shock.

Answer: B. This can be caused by nephrotoxins, such as aminoglycosides. The other potential causes are associated with prerenal failure.

3. Which is the main complication of glomerulonephritis?
    A. Bilateral inflammation of the glomeruli
    B. Sudden interruption of renal function
    C. Destruction of the tubular segment of the nephron
    D. An infection in the urinary tract

Answer: A. This often follows a streptococcal infection and is most common in young males between the ages of 3 and 7.

4. The kidneys secrete renin in response to:
    A. hypoxia in the bloodstream.
    B. high sodium content in the bloodstream.
    C. low potassium content in the bloodstream.
    D. hypovolemia, which causes low circulation and low perfusion of the kidney.

Answer: D. Hypovolemia causes low circulation, which leads to low perfusion of the kidney. Low circulation sensed by the kidney will cause it to secrete renin, which then triggers the renin–angiotensin–aldosterone system (RAAS). This will raise blood volume.

5. Which is a way that the kidneys help maintain acid–base balance?
    A. Excrete sodium and bicarbonate
    B. Excrete hydrogen ions
    C. Regulate vitamin D
    D. Secrete erythropoietin

Answer: B. The kidneys maintain acid–base balance of the bloodstream by excreting H^+ if the blood becomes acidotic. The kidneys also conserve HCO_3^- (bicarbonate) in acidosis.

Scoring

☆☆☆ If you answered all five items correctly, wow! Your ability to concentrate, absorb, and secrete data about the kidneys is amazing!

☆☆ If you answered four items correctly, fantastic! Your knowledge of things renal isn't venal.

☆ If you answered fewer than four items correctly, don't worry. We recommend reading the chapter once more. After all, that's what reabsorption is all about.

Suggested references

Abou Heidar, N. F., Degheili, J. A., Yacoubian, A. A., & Khauli, R. B. (2019). Management of urinary tract infection in women: A practical approach for everyday practice. *Urology Annals*, *11*(4), 339–346. https://doi.org/10.4103/UA.UA_104_19

Acute kidney injury. (2021). Nature reviews. *Disease Primers*, *7*(1), 51. https://doi.org/10.1038/s41572-021-00291-0

Akhtar, M., Taha, N. M., & Asim, M. (2021). Anti-glomerular basement membrane disease: What have we learned? *Advances in Anatomic Pathology*, *28*(1), 59–65. https://doi.org/10.1097/PAP.0000000000000280

American Association for Cancer Research. (2023). Renal cancer treatment PDQ. https://www.aacr.org/patients-caregivers/cancer/kidney-cancer/renal-cell-cancer-treatment-pdq/

American Cancer Society. (2022). What is kidney cancer? https://www.cancer.org/cancer/kidney-cancer/about/what-is-kidney-cancer.html

Basile, C., Davenport, A., Mitra, S., Pal, A., Stamatialis, D., Chrysochou, C., & Kirmizis, D. (2021). Frontiers in hemodialysis: Innovations and technological advances. *Artificial Organs*, *45*(2), 175–182. https://doi.org/10.1111/aor.13798

Centers for Disease Control and Prevention (CDC). 2022. Post-streptococcal glomerulonephritis. https://www.cdc.gov/groupastrep/diseases-public/post-streptococcal.html

Centers for Disease Control and Prevention (CDC). (2022). Kidney disease. https://www.cdc.gov/nchs/fastats/kidney-disease.htm

Centers for Disease Control and Prevention (CDC). 2022. Kidney cancer. https://www.cdc.gov/cancer/kidney/index.htm

Centers for Disease Control and Prevention (CDC). 2022. Urinary tract infection. https://www.cdc.gov/antibiotic-use/uti.html

Charles, C., & Ferris, A. H. (2020). Chronic kidney disease. *Journal of Primary Care*, *47*(4), 585–595. https://doi.org/10.1016/j.pop.2020.08.001

Chenoweth, C. E. (2021). Urinary tract infections: 2021 update. *Infectious Disease Clinics of North America*, *35*(4), 857–870. https://doi.org/10.1016/j.idc.2021.08.003

Coffman, T. J., Boothe, A., & Watson, J. (2022). Rising prevalence of renal calculi: Treatments and considerations. *Nursing*, *52*(4), 19–24. https://doi.org/10.1097/01.NURSE.0000823264.55591.8c

Devlin, C. M., Simms, M. S., & Maitland, N. J. (2021). Benign prostatic hyperplasia—What do we know? *BJU International*, *127*(4), 389–399. https://doi.org/10.1111/bju.15229

Dowsett, T., & Oni, L. (2022). Anti-glomerular basement membrane disease in children: A brief overview. *Pediatr Nephrology*, *37*(8), 1713–1719. https://doi.org/10.1007/s00467-021-05333-z

Flagg, A. J. (2018). Chronic renal therapy. *Nursing Clinics of North America*, *53*(4), 511–519. https://doi.org/10.1016/j.cnur.2018.07.002

Guliciuc, M., Maier, A. C., Maier, I. M., Kraft, A., Cucuruzac, R. R., Marinescu, M., Şerban, C., Rebegea, L., Constantin, G. B., & Firescu, D. (2021). The urosepsis—A literature review. *Medicina (Kaunas, Lithuania)*, *57*(9), 872. https://doi.org/10.3390/medicina57090872

Herness, J., Buttolph, A., & Hammer, N. C. (2020). Acute pyelonephritis in adults: Rapid evidence review. *American Family Physician*, *102*(3), 173–180.

Kamijo, Y., Fujimoto, S., & Ishibashi, Y. (2018). Total renal care approach for patients with end-stage renal disease. *Contributions to Nephrology*, *196*, 78–82. https://doi.org/10.1159/000485703

Konwar, M., Gogtay, N. J., Ravi, R., Thatte, U. M., & Bose, D. (2022). Evaluation of efficacy and safety of fosfomycin versus nitrofurantoin for the treatment of uncomplicated lower urinary tract infection (UTI) in women—A systematic review and meta-analysis. *Journal of Chemotheraphy*, *34*(3), 139–148.

Laquerre, J. (2020). Hydronephrosis: Diagnosis, grading, and treatment. *Radiologic Technology*, *92*(2), 135–151.

Manrique-Caballero, C. L., Del Rio-Pertuz, G., & Gomez, H. (2021). Sepsis-associated acute kidney injury. *Critical Care Clinics*, *37*(2), 279–301. https://doi.org/10.1016/j.ccc.2020.11.010

Matuszkiewicz-Rowińska, J., & Małyszko, J. (2020). Acute kidney injury, its definition, and treatment in adults: Guidelines and reality. *Polish Archives of Internal Medicine, 130*(12), 1074–1080. https://doi.org/10.20452/pamw.15373

Mayans, L. (2019). Nephrolithiasis. *Journal of Primary Care, 46*(2), 203–212. https://doi.org/10.1016/j.pop.2019.02.001

Menon, S., Symons, J. M., & Selewski, D. T. (2023). Acute kidney injury. *Pediatrics Review, 44*(5), 265–279. https://doi.org/10.1542/pir.2021-005438

Mody, H., Ramakrishnan, V., Chaar, M., Lezeau, J., Rump, A., Taha, K., Lesko, L., & Ait-Oudhia, S. (2020). A review on drug-induced nephrotoxicity: Pathophysiological mechanisms, drug classes, clinical management, and recent advances in mathematical modeling and simulation approaches. *Clinical Pharmacology in Drug Development, 9*(8), 896–909. https://doi.org/10.1002/cpdd.879

Mohammad, D., & Baracco, R. (2020). Postinfectious glomerulonephritis. *Pediatrics Annals, 49*(6), e273–e277. https://doi.org/10.3928/19382359-20200519-01

National Kidney Foundation. (2022a). Kidney stones. https://www.kidney.org/atoz/kidneystones

National Kidney Foundation. (2022b). Goodpasture's syndrome. https://www.kidney.org/atoz/content/goodpasture

National Kidney Foundation. (2022c). What is glomerulonephritis? https://www.kidney.org/atoz/content/glomerulonephritis

Neyra, J. A., & Chawla, L. S. (2021). Acute kidney disease to chronic kidney disease. *Critical Care Clinics, 37*(2), 453–474. https://doi.org/10.1016/j.ccc.2020.11.013

Norris, T. L. (2025). *Porth's pathophysiology: Concepts of altered health states* (11th ed.). Wolters Kluwer.

Patel, K., & Batura, D. (2020). An overview of hydronephrosis in adults. *British Journal of Hospital Medicine, 81*(1), 1–8. https://doi.org/10.12968/hmed.2019.0274

Patel, S., Rauf, A., Khan, H., & Abu-Izneid, T. (2017). Renin-angiotensin-aldosterone (RAAS): The ubiquitous system for homeostasis and pathologies. *Biomedicine & Pharmacotherapy, 94*, 317–325. https://doi.org/10.1016/j.biopha.2017.07.091

Peck, J., & Shepherd, J. P. (2021). Recurrent urinary tract infections: Diagnosis, treatment, and prevention. *Obstetrics and Gynecology Clinics of North America, 48*(3), 501–513. https://doi.org/10.1016/j.ogc.2021.05.005

Peerapornratana, S., Manrique-Caballero, C. L., Gómez, H., & Kellum, J. A. (2019). Acute kidney injury from sepsis: Current concepts, epidemiology, pathophysiology, prevention and treatment. *Kidney International, 96*(5), 1083–1099. https://doi.org/10.1016/j.kint.2019.05.026

Ponticelli, C., Calatroni, M., & Moroni, G. (2023). Anti-glomerular basement membrane vasculitis. *Autoimmunity Review, 22*(1), 103212. https://doi.org/10.1016/j.autrev.2022.103212

Porat, A., Bhutta, B. S., & Kesler, S. (2023). *Urosepsis*. In *StatPearls*. StatPearls Publishing.

Reggiani, F., L'Imperio, V., Calatroni, M., Pagni, F., & Sinico, R. A. (2023). Goodpasture syndrome and anti-glomerular basement membrane disease. *Clinical and Experimental Rheumatology, 41*(4), 964–974. https://doi.org/10.55563/clinexprheumatol/tep3k5

Rivera, S. (2022). Principles for the prevention of medication-induced nephrotoxicity. *Critical Care Nursing Clinics of North America, 34*(4), 361–371. https://doi.org/10.1016/j.cnc.2022.08.005

Satoskar, A. A., Parikh, S. V., & Nadasdy, T. (2020). Epidemiology, pathogenesis, treatment and outcomes of infection-associated glomerulonephritis. *Nature Reviews Nephrology, 16*(1), 32–50. https://doi.org/10.1038/s41581-019-0178-8

Sepsis Alliance. (2023). *Sepsis and Urinary Tract Infections.* https://www.sepsis.org/sepsisand/urinary-tract-infections/

Strayer, D., Saffitz, J., Rubin, E. (2020). *Rubin's pathology: Mechanisms of disease* (8th ed.). Wolters Kluwer.

Tolani, M. A., Suleiman, A., Awaisu, M., Abdulaziz, M. M., Lawal, A. T., & Bello, A. (2020). Acute urinary tract infection in patients with underlying benign prostatic hyperplasia and prostate cancer. *The Pan African Medical Journal, 36,* 169. https://doi.org/10.11604/pamj.2020.36.169.21038

Tyagi, A., & Aeddula, N. R. (2023). *Azotemia.* In *StatPearls.* StatPearls Publishing.

Vargas Vargas, R. A., Varela Millán, J. M., & Fajardo Bonilla, E. (2022). Renin-angiotensin system: Basic and clinical aspects—A general perspective. *Endocrinology, Diabetes and Nutrition, 69*(1), 52–62. https://doi.org/10.1016/j.endien.2022.01.005

Yang, J., Sun, B. G., Min, H. J., Son, Y. B., Kim, T. B., Lee, J., Oh, S. W., Kim, M. G., Cho, W. Y., Ahn, S. Y., Ko, G. J., Kwon, Y. J., Cha, J. J., Kang, Y. S., Cha, D. R., & Jo, S. K. (2021). Impact of acute kidney injury on long-term adverse outcomes in obstructive uropathy. *Scientific Reports, 11*(1), 23639. https://doi.org/10.1038/s41598-021-03033-0

Yang, T., & Xu, C. (2017). Physiology and pathophysiology of the intrarenal renin-angiotensin system: An update. *Journal of the American Society of Nephrology, 28*(4), 1040–1049. https://doi.org/10.1681/ASN.2016070734

Yoon, S. Y., Kim, J. S., Jeong, K. H., & Kim, S. K. (2022). Acute kidney injury: Biomarker-guided diagnosis and management. *Medicina (Kaunas, Lithuania), 58*(3), 340. https://doi.org/10.3390/medicina58030340

Zare, M., Vehreschild, M. J. G. T., & Wagenlehner, F. (2022). Management of uncomplicated recurrent urinary tract infections. *BJU International, 129*(6), 668–678. https://doi.org/10.1111/bju.15630

Immune system*

Understanding the immune system

The body protects itself from infectious organisms and other harmful invaders through an elaborate network of safeguards called the *host defense system*. This system has three lines of defense:

1. physical and chemical barriers to infection
2. the inflammatory response
3. the immune response

Physical barriers, such as the skin and mucous membranes, prevent most organisms from invading the body. Organisms that penetrate this first barrier simultaneously trigger the inflammatory and immune responses. Both responses involve white blood cells (WBCs). Inflammation commonly involves macrophages, neutrophils, eosinophils, and basophils. The immune system involves T and B lymphocytes, called T and B cells.

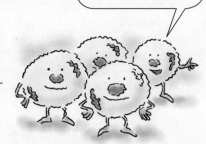

We cells have a lot to do with the immune system.

Structures of the immune system

These five structures in the body make up the immune system:

- bone marrow
- lymph nodes
- thymus
- spleen
- tonsils and other lymphoid tissue in the body

*Note: In this chapter, the term "male" refers to a person assigned male at birth, and the term "female" refers to a person assigned female at birth.

Bone marrow
B cells and T cells are produced and develop in the bone marrow and then migrate to the lymph nodes.

Lymph nodes
Lymph nodes are distributed along lymphatic vessels throughout the body. They filter lymphatic fluid, which drains from body tissues and later returns to the blood as plasma. Lymph nodes are also the place where lymphocytes mature after they are released from the bone marrow. Lymph nodes that are actively secreting lymphocytes enlarge.

Double agents?
The lymph nodes also remove bacteria and toxins from the circulatory system. This means that, on occasion, infectious agents can be spread by the lymphatic system.

Thymus
The thymus, located in the mediastinal area (between the lungs), secretes a group of hormones that enable lymphocytes to develop into mature T cells. The thymus gland naturally degenerates as a person ages.

"T" stands for "tough"
T cells originate in the bone marrow and mature in the thymus. They attack foreign or abnormal cells and regulate cell-mediated immunity.

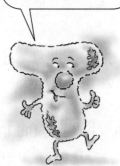

My job is to attack foreign cells and regulate cell-mediated immunity. And I can do that job to a T!

Spleen
The largest lymphatic organ, the spleen functions as the "graveyard for dead red blood cells" and serves as a place where B lymphocytes mature and are released. Cells in the splenic tissue, called *macrophages*, clear cellular debris and process hemoglobin.

Tonsils
The tonsils consist of lymphoid tissue and also produce lymphocytes. These are visible on both sides of the pharynx.

Guarding against air raids
The location of the tonsils allows them to guard the body against airborne and ingested pathogens. Tonsils often enlarge when they are actively releasing lymphocytes for fighting upper respiratory infection.

Types of immunity
Certain cells have the ability to distinguish between foreign matter and what belongs to the body—a skill known as *immunocompetence*. When foreign substances invade the body, two types of immune responses are possible: cell-mediated immunity and humoral immunity.

Cell-mediated immunity

In cell-mediated immunity, T cells respond directly to *antigens* (foreign substances, such as bacteria or toxins). This response involves destruction of target cells—such as virus-infected cells and cancer cells—through the secretion of lymphokines (lymph proteins). Examples of cell-mediated immunity are rejection of transplanted organs and delayed allergic reactions.

Approximately one-third of WBCs are T cells. They are thought to originate from stem cells in the bone marrow; the thymus gland controls their maturity. In the process, a large number of antigen-specific cells are produced.

A license to kill, help, or suppress

T cells can be killer, helper, or suppressor T cells.
- Killer cells bind to the surface of the invading cell, disrupt the membrane, and destroy it by altering its internal environment.
- Helper cells stimulate B cells to mature into plasma cells, which begin to synthesize and secrete *immunoglobulins* (proteins with known antibody activity). Immunoglobulins are also termed antibodies.
- Suppressor cells reduce the humoral response.

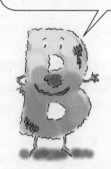

My job is to produce antibodies that, in turn, will attack an antigen.

Humoral immunity

B cells act in a different way than T cells to recognize and destroy antigens. B cells are responsible for humoral or immunoglobulin-mediated immunity. B cells originate in the bone marrow and mature into plasma cells that produce *antibodies* (immunoglobulins that interact with a specific antigen). Antibodies destroy bacteria and viruses, thereby preventing them from entering host cells.

Get to know your immunoglobulin

Five major classes of immunoglobulin exist; IgG and IgA have subclasses, as well. For purposes of this reference, focus is placed on the five major classes:
1. Immunoglobulin G (IgG) makes up about 80% to 85% of plasma antibodies. It is primarily responsible for protective factors against infection.
2. Immunoglobulin M (IgM) is the largest immunoglobulin and the first produced during an immune response.
3. Immunoglobulin A (IgA) is found mainly in body secretions, such as saliva, sweat, tears, mucus, bile, and colostrum. It defends against pathogens on body surfaces, especially those that enter through secretions.
4. Immunoglobulin D (IgD) is present in plasma and is easily broken down. It's the predominant antibody on the surface of early B cells and is mainly an antigen receptor.

5. Immunoglobulin E (IgE) is the antibody involved in immediate hypersensitivity reactions, or allergic reactions that develop within minutes of exposure to an antigen. IgE stimulates the release of mast cell granules, which contain histamine and heparin.

Thanks for the complement

Part of humoral immunity, the complement system is a major mediator of the inflammatory response. The complement system assists both T and B lymphocytes to attack antigens.

The system causes inflammation by increasing:
- vascular permeability
- chemotaxis (movement of additional WBCs to an area of inflammation)
- phagocytosis (engulfing and disposing of foreign particles by cells called *macrophages* or *phagocytes*)
- lysis of the antigen

In most cases, an antigen–antibody reaction is necessary for the complement system to activate, a process called the *complement cascade.*

Immune disorders

Common immune disorders include:
- allergic rhinitis (AR)
- anaphylaxis
- human immunodeficiency virus (HIV)
- systemic lupus erythematosus (SLE)
- rheumatoid arthritis

What's the response?

Disorders of the immune response are of three main types:
- immunodeficiency disorders
- hypersensitivity disorders
- autoimmune disorders

Absent or depressed

Immunodeficiency disorders result from an absent or depressed immune system. These deficiencies can be primary or acquired. Some examples include HIV disease, DiGeorge syndrome, chronic fatigue syndrome, Wiskott–Aldrich syndrome, and severe combined immunodeficiency.

An allergen is the culprit

When an allergen (a substance the person is allergic to) enters the body, a hypersensitivity reaction occurs. It may be immediate or delayed. Hypersensitivity reactions are classified as follows.

Type	Onset	Immunoglobulin	Example
Type I	Immediate	Mediated by IgE, mast cells, or basophils	Allergic reactions; mediated by humoral immunity; immunoglobulins
Type II	Delayed	Usually caused by IgG	Mediated cell destruction; tissue-specific
Type III	Delayed	Caused by IgG	Immune complex deposition and complement activation
Type IV	Delayed	T cell mediated	Cell-mediated; subcategories include type IVa, IVb, IVc, and IVd

A body divided against itself

With autoimmune disorders, the body launches an immunologic response against itself. This leads to a sequence of tissue reactions and damage that may produce diffuse systemic signs and symptoms.

Examples of autoimmune disorders include rheumatoid arthritis, SLE, scleroderma, sarcoidosis, Goodpasture syndrome, dermatomyositis, and vasculitis.

Allergic rhinitis

Inhaled, airborne allergens may trigger an immune response in the upper airway. This causes two problems:
- rhinitis, or inflammation of the nasal mucous membrane
- conjunctivitis, or inflammation of the membrane lining the eyelids and covering the eyeball

Hey, is this just hay fever?

When AR occurs seasonally, some people call this *hay fever,* even though hay doesn't cause it and no fever occurs. When it occurs year-round, it's called *perennial allergic rhinitis.*

It is estimated that between 10% and 30% of the world's population has AR, making it the most common allergic reaction. Although it can affect anyone at any age, it's most common in young children and adolescents.

How it happens

AR is a type I, IgE-mediated hypersensitivity response to an environmental allergen in a genetically susceptible patient.

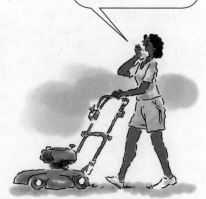

Ah-choo! Seasonal allergic rhinitis ("hay fever") is usually caused by airborne pollens from trees, grass, and weeds, as well as by mold spores.

Hay fever occurs in the spring, summer, and fall and is usually induced by airborne pollens from trees, grass, and weeds. In the summer and fall, mold spores also cause it.

Major perennial allergens and irritants include house dust and dust mites, feathers, molds, fungi, tobacco smoke, processed materials or industrial chemicals, and animal dander.

Swelling of the nasal and mucous membranes may trigger secondary sinus infections and middle ear infections, especially in perennial AR. Nasal polyps caused by edema and infection may increase nasal obstruction. Bronchitis and pneumonia are possible complications.

What to look for

In hay fever, the patient will report sneezing attacks, rhinorrhea (profuse, watery nasal discharge), nasal obstruction or congestion, itching nose and eyes, and headache or sinus pain. An itchy throat and malaise also may occur, along with cough, irritability, and fatigue.

Perennial AR causes chronic, extensive nasal obstruction or stuffiness, which can obstruct the eustachian tube, particularly in children. Conjunctivitis or other extranasal signs and symptoms can occur but are rare. (See *Types of rhinitis*.)

Would you look at that shiner!

Both conditions can cause dark circles under the eyes, known commonly as "allergic shiners," from venous congestion in the maxillary sinuses. The severity of signs and symptoms may vary from year to year. (See *Treating allergic rhinitis*.)

What tests tell you

IgE levels are commonly elevated in allergic disorders. Microscopic examination of sputum and nasal secretions shows a high number of eosinophils (granular leukocytes).

Types of rhinitis

Characteristics of the three common disorders of the nasal mucosa are listed below.

Chronic vasomotor rhinitis
- Eyes aren't affected.
- Nasal discharge contains mucus.
- There's no seasonal variation.

Infectious rhinitis (common cold)
- Nasal mucosa is beet red.
- Nasal secretions contain exudate.
- Fever and sore throat occur.

Rhinitis medicamentosa
- The disorder is caused by excessive use of nasal sprays or drops.
- Nasal drainage and mucosal redness and swelling subside when the medication is discontinued.

Treating allergic rhinitis

Treatment of allergic rhinitis involves controlling signs and symptoms and preventing infection. Treatment may include removing the environmental allergen. Drug therapy and immunotherapy may be used to treat perennial allergic rhinitis. Seasonal allergic rhinitis treatment includes combining an intranasal corticosteroid with an oral H1 antihistamine or an intranasal corticosteroid. Perennial treatment includes an intranasal corticosteroid.

Annoying aftereffects

Antihistamines, such as chlorpheniramine, diphenhydramine, and promethazine, are effective in stopping a runny nose and watery eyes, but they usually produce sedation, dry mouth, nausea, dizziness, blurred vision, and nervousness. Nonsedating antihistamines, such as loratadine, desloratadine, fexofenadine, and cetirizine, produce fewer side effects and are the treatment of choice.

Try these treatments, too

Topical intranasal corticosteroids may reduce local inflammation with minimal systemic adverse effects.

Long-term management may include immunotherapy or desensitization with injections of allergen extracts administered preseasonally, seasonally, or throughout the entire year.

Anaphylaxis

Anaphylaxis, an acute type I allergic reaction, causes sudden, rapidly progressive urticaria (hives) and respiratory distress. A severe reaction may lead to vascular collapse, systemic shock, and even death.

How it happens

Anaphylactic reactions can result from exposure to sensitizing drugs or other antigens in people with genetic predisposition to allergy, including:

- serums such as vaccines
- allergen extracts such as pollen
- enzymes such as L-asparaginase
- hormones
- penicillin and other antibiotics
- local anesthetics
- salicylates
- latex (found in gloves, catheters, tubing, or balloons)
- polysaccharides such as iron dextran
- diagnostic chemicals such as radiographic contrast media
- foods, such as nuts and seafood
- sulfite-containing food additives

- insect venom, such as that from honeybees, wasps, and certain spiders

Penicillin and other antibiotics, bee stings, seafood, peanuts, and tree nuts are the most common anaphylaxis-causing antigens.

Reenacting the reaction

Here's how an anaphylactic reaction occurs:

- After initial exposure to an antigen, the immune system responds by producing IgE antibodies in the lymph nodes. Helper T cells enhance the process.
- Antibodies bind to membrane receptors located on mast cells in connective tissues and on basophils, which are a type of leukocyte. Mast cells are stimulated to secrete histamine.
- On reexposure, the antigen binds to adjacent IgE antibodies or cross-linked IgE receptors, activating inflammatory reactions such as the release of histamine.

Untreated anaphylaxis causes respiratory obstruction, systemic vascular collapse, and death—minutes to hours after the first symptoms occur. However, a delayed or persistent reaction may last up to 24 hours. (See *Treating anaphylaxis* and *Understanding anaphylaxis*.)

What to look for

Immediately after exposure, the patient may report a feeling of impending doom or fright, progressing to a fear of impending death, weakness, sweating, sneezing, dyspnea, pruritus, and urticaria.

Battling illness

Treating anaphylaxis

Anaphylaxis is always a medical emergency. It requires an immediate treatment with epinephrine, delivered intramuscularly or subcutaneously. IV diphenhydramine is used to counteract the histamine release, and IV corticosteroids are used to counteract the inflammation.

Emphasis on epinephrine

In the early stages of anaphylaxis, when the patient remains conscious and normotensive, epinephrine IM or subQ is most likely to be ordered. Massage the injection site to speed the drug into the circulation. In severe reactions, when the patient is unconscious and hypotensive, give the drug intravenously as ordered. IV therapy is necessary to prevent vascular collapse after a severe reaction is treated.

Be certain to establish and maintain a patent airway. Watch for early signs of laryngeal edema, such as stridor, hoarseness, and dyspnea. If these occur, oxygen therapy along with endotracheal tube insertion or a tracheotomy is required.

Now I get it!

Understanding anaphylaxis

The illustrations below teach the development of anaphylaxis.

1. Response to antigen
Immunoglobulins (Ig) M and G recognize and bind the antigen.

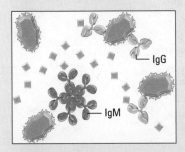

2. Release of chemical mediators
Activated IgE on basophils promotes the release of mediators: histamine, serotonin, and leukotrienes.

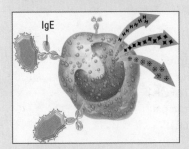

3. Intensified response
Mast cells release more histamine and eosinophil chemotactic factor of anaphylaxis (ECF-A). Vasodilation occurs.

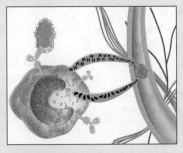

4. Respiratory distress
In the lungs, histamine causes endothelial cell destruction and fluid to leak into alveoli.

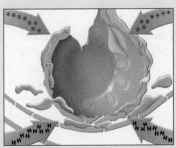

5. Deterioration
Meanwhile, mediators increase vascular permeability, causing fluid to leak from the vessels.

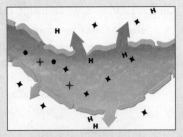

6. Failure of compensatory mechanisms
Endothelial cell damage causes basophils and mast cells to release heparin and mediator-neutralizing substances. However, anaphylaxis is now irreversible.

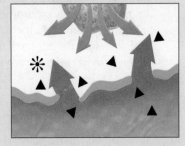

Key		
Complement cascade ■	Serotonin ✦	ECF-A ◗
Histamine **H**	Leukotrienes ✳	Bradykinin ●
	Prostaglandins +	Heparin ▲

The skinny on skin effects

The skin may look cyanotic and pallid. Well-circumscribed, discrete, cutaneous wheals with red, raised wavy or indented borders and blanched centers usually appear and may merge to form giant hives.

That's just swell...

Angioedema may cause the patient to report difficulty breathing; swelling of the tongue and larynx also occur. You may hear hoarseness, stridor, or wheezing. Chest tightness signals bronchial obstruction. These are all early signs of potentially fatal respiratory failure.

GI, cardiovascular, and neurologic effects

The patient may report severe stomach cramps, nausea, diarrhea, urinary urgency, and urinary incontinence.

Cardiovascular effects include hypotension, shock, and cardiac arrhythmias, which may precipitate vascular collapse if untreated.

Neurologic signs and symptoms may include dizziness, drowsiness, headache, restlessness, and seizures.

What tests tell you

The patient's history and signs and symptoms, such as increased heart and respiratory rate and decreased blood pressure, will help the healthcare provider to diagnose anaphylaxis.

Human immunodeficiency virus

HIV is the infectious agent responsible for HIV infection and acquired immunodeficiency syndrome (AIDS). Characterized by progressive immune system impairment, HIV destroys T cells (also called CD4 cells) and, therefore, the cell-mediated response. The CD4 cells also participate in the humoral immune response (B-cell immunity). In addition, HIV

Facts about HIV infection and AIDS

Acquired immunodeficiency syndrome (AIDS) was first described by the Centers for Disease Control and Prevention (CDC) in 1981. In 2021, the CDC estimated that approximately 1.2 million people aged 13 and older were living with human immunodeficiency virus (HIV). However, the incidence of AIDS has been gradually decreasing in the United States due to effective antiretroviral treatment and newer HIV prophylactic medications. In the United States, HIV infection and AIDS is highest in MSM (men who have sex with men) and people who use illicit IV drugs.

attacks macrophages, which are integral to innate immunity. In these ways, HIV causes a gradual deactivation of all levels of natural immunity in the individual, resulting in severe immunosuppression. This immunodeficiency makes the patient more susceptible to infections and unusual cancers. (See *Facts about HIV infection and AIDS.*)

The Centers for Disease Control and Prevention (CDC) established laboratory testing criteria for making a diagnosis of HIV disease. The course of HIV disease can vary. Many people, with appropriate and early treatment, can live long and mostly normal lives. Others, especially those who do not seek or do not have access to medical care, may die from opportunistic infections. The average onset of symptoms associated with AIDS, in the absence of treatment, is 10 years after becoming infected with HIV (University of California, San Francisco, 2018). (See *HIV infection classification.*)

How it happens

HIV is an RNA-based retrovirus that requires a human host to replicate. HIV infection has three stages:
1. stage 1: acute HIV infection
2. stage 2: latent or chronic HIV infection
3. stage 3: AIDS

The average time between acute HIV infection and the development of AIDS is 10 years. Note that because of effective treatments, most people never enter stage 3.

HIV destroys CD4$^+$ cells—also known as *helper T cells*—that regulate the normal immune response. In addition, HIV enters macrophages (key WBCs) in the first line of defense. Afterward, the virus mainly replicates within the CD4$^+$ cell, killing the CD4$^+$ cell, and gradually causing depletion of the patient's CD4$^+$ cells. This can take many years.

Modes of transmission

HIV is transmitted in three ways:
1. through contact with infected blood or blood products, or by sharing a contaminated needle
2. through contact with infected body fluids, such as semen and vaginal fluids, during unprotected sex (anal intercourse is especially dangerous because it causes mucosal trauma)
3. across the placental barrier from an infected pregnant person to a fetus or from birthing parent to an infant either through cervical or blood contact at delivery or through breast milk

Blood, semen, vaginal secretions, and breast milk are the body fluids that most readily transmit HIV.

HIV infection classification

The Clinical Staging and Disease Classification System developed by the World Health Organization and the Centers for Disease Control and Prevention is an important tool to track the HIV epidemic. It also gives healthcare providers and patients important information about HIV staging and associated clinical management.

Two main measures—the viral load and the CD4 cell count—are used in this classification system. The viral load indicates the amount of viral replication, and the CD4 cell count predicts the progress of the disease and the effectiveness of treatment. CD4 cell counts are monitored throughout disease; when CD4 cell count is less than or equal to 200, the individual is susceptible to AIDS.

What to look for

After initial exposure, the infected person may have no signs or symptoms, or they may have a flu-like illness (acute HIV infection [stage 1]) and then remain with no symptoms with latent HIV infection (stage 2) for many years. As the syndrome progresses and CD4$^+$ cells become depleted, the patient may develop an opportunistic infection, such as *Pneumocystis jirovecii* pneumonia, tuberculosis, *Candida* infection, toxoplasmosis, cryptococcosis, cytomegalovirus, or cancer, particularly Kaposi sarcoma or lymphoma. Eventually, repeated opportunistic infections can overwhelm the patient's weakened immune defenses, invading every body system. AIDS (stage 3) is diagnosed when the patient's CD4$^+$ count is less than or equal to 200 and there is evidence of an opportunistic infection (See *Opportunistic diseases associated with AIDS.*)

Opportunistic diseases associated with AIDS

This chart describes some common diseases associated with acquired immunodeficiency syndrome (AIDS), their characteristic signs and symptoms, and their treatments.

Disease	Signs and symptoms	Treatment
Bacterial infections		
Tuberculosis A disease caused by *Mycobacterium tuberculosis*, an aerobic, acid-fast bacillus spread through inhalation of droplet nuclei that are aerosolized by coughing, sneezing, or talking	Fever, weight loss, night sweats, cough, and fatigue, followed by dyspnea, chills, hemoptysis, and chest pain	Isoniazid, rifampin, pyrazinamide, and ethambutol are given during the first 2 months of therapy, followed by rifampin and isoniazid for a minimum of 9 months and for at least 6 months after culture is negative for bacteria.
Mycobacterium avium A primary infection acquired by oral ingestion or inhalation; can infect the bone marrow, liver, spleen, GI tract, lymph nodes, lungs, skin, brain, adrenal glands, and kidneys; is chronic and may be localized and disseminated in its course of infection; incidence is decreasing because of changes in treatment of human immunodeficiency virus (HIV)	Multiple, nonspecific symptoms consistent with systemic illness: fever, fatigue, weight loss, anorexia, night sweats, abdominal pain, and chronic diarrhea; *physical assessment findings:* emaciation, generalized lymphadenopathy, diffuse tenderness, jaundice, and hepatosplenomegaly; *laboratory findings:* anemia, leukopenia, and thrombocytopenia	Treatment includes clarithromycin or azithromycin and ethambutol. These drugs are given with one or more of the following: amikacin, ciprofloxacin, rifabutin, or rifampin.

Opportunistic diseases associated with AIDS *(continued)*

Disease	Signs and symptoms	Treatment
Fungal infections		
Coccidioidomycosis An infectious disease caused by the fungus *Coccidioides immitis*, which grows in soil in arid regions in the Southwestern United States, Mexico, Central America, and South America	Flu-like illness (malaise, fever, backache, headache, cough, arthralgia), periarticular swelling in knees and ankles, meningitis, bony lesions, difficulty breathing, skin findings, and pulmonary or genitourinary involvement	Fluconazole, itraconazole, or amphotericin B is given.
Candidiasis A disease caused by the fungus *Candida albicans* that exists on teeth, gingivae, and skin and in the oropharynx, vagina, and large intestine; majority of infections are endogenous and related to interruption of normal defense mechanisms; possible human-to-human transmission, including congenital transmission in neonates, in whom thrush develops after vaginal delivery	*Thrush* (the most common form in HIV-infected individuals): creamy, curdlike, white patches, surrounded by an erythematous base, found on any oral mucosal surface; *nail infection:* inflammation and tenderness of tissue surrounding the nails or the nail itself; *vaginitis:* intense pruritus of the vulva and curdlike vaginal discharge	Nystatin suspension and clotrimazole troches are administered for thrush; nystatin suspension or pastilles, clotrimazole troches, fluconazole, or itraconazole for esophagitis; topical clotrimazole, miconazole, or ketoconazole for cutaneous candidiasis; topical imidazole or oral fluconazole, ketoconazole, or both for candidiasis of nails; and topical clotrimazole, miconazole, or oral fluconazole for vaginitis.
Cryptococcosis An infectious disease caused by the fungus *Cryptococcus neoformans;* can be found in nature (particularly in bird droppings); can be aerosolized and inhaled; settles in the lungs, where it can remain dormant or spread to other parts of the body, particularly the central nervous system (CNS); responsible for three forms of infection: pulmonary, CNS, and disseminated; most pulmonary cases found serendipitously	*Pulmonary cryptococcosis:* fever, cough, dyspnea, and pleuritic chest pain; *CNS cryptococcosis:* fever, malaise, headaches, stiff neck, nausea and vomiting, and altered mentation; *disseminated cryptococcosis:* lymphadenopathy, multifocal cutaneous lesions; *other symptoms:* macules, papules, skin lesions, oral lesions, placental infection, myocarditis, prostatic infection, optic neuropathy, rectal abscess, and lymph node infection	Primary therapy for initial infection is amphotericin B, administered IV for 6 to 8 weeks; sometimes amphotericin B and flucytosine are used in combination. Fluconazole and itraconazole are also used. After initial treatment, the patient is typically maintained on lifelong fluconazole therapy.
Histoplasmosis A disease caused by the fungus *Histoplasma capsulatum* that exists in nature, is readily airborne, and can reach the bronchioles and alveoli when inhaled	*Most common:* fever, weight loss, hepatomegaly, splenomegaly, and pancytopenia; *less common:* diarrhea, cerebritis, chorioretinitis, meningitis, oral and cutaneous lesions, and GI mucosal lesions causing bleeding	Drug of choice is amphotericin B for acute treatment of illness and then for lifelong suppressive therapy. Itraconazole is also used.

(Continued)

Opportunistic diseases associated with AIDS *(continued)*

Disease	Signs and symptoms	Treatment
Protozoan infections		
Pneumocystis jirovecii pneumonia Pneumonia caused by *P. jirovecii;* also has properties of fungal infection, exists in human lungs, and is transmitted by airborne exposure; the most common life-threatening opportunistic infection in individuals with AIDS	Fever, fatigue, and weight loss for several weeks to months before respiratory symptoms develop; *respiratory symptoms:* dyspnea, usually noted initially on exertion and later at rest, and cough, usually starting out dry and nonproductive and later becoming productive	Co-trimoxazole may be given orally or IV, although about 20% of AIDS patients are hypersensitive to sulfa drugs. IV pentamidine isethionate may be given but can cause many adverse effects, including permanent diabetes mellitus. Dapsone with trimethoprim, clindamycin, primaquine, atovaquone, or corticosteroids is also used. Prophylaxis for disease prevention and following treatment includes co-trimoxazole, atovaquone, or dapsone.
Cryptosporidiosis An intestinal infection by the protozoan *Cryptosporidium;* transmitted by person-to-person contact, water, food contaminants, and airborne exposure; most common site: small intestine	Abdominal cramping, flatulence, weight loss, anorexia, malaise, fever, nausea, vomiting, myalgia, and profuse, watery diarrhea	Most medical therapy is palliative and directed toward symptom control, focusing on fluid replacement, total parenteral nutrition (TPN), correction of electrolyte imbalances, and analgesic, antidiarrheal, and antiperistaltic agents. Paromomycin and octreotides are used.
Toxoplasmosis A disease caused by *Toxoplasma gondii;* major means of transmission through ingestion of undercooked meats and vegetables containing oocysts; can also be transmitted through handling cat feces, because this organism can grow in litter boxes; causes focal or diffuse meningoencephalitis with cellular necrosis and progresses unchecked to the lungs, heart, and skeletal muscle	Localized neurologic deficits, fever, headache, altered mental status, and seizures	Sulfadiazine may be given, or clindamycin with pyrimethamine can be given for patients who are hypersensitive to sulfa drugs. Folinic acid may be given to prevent marrow suppression. Patients must receive maintenance combination drug therapy in lower doses to prevent relapse.
Viral infections		
Herpes simplex virus Chronic infection caused by a herpes virus; often a reactivation of an earlier herpes infection	Red, blister-like lesions occurring in oral, anal, and genital areas; also found on the esophageal and tracheobronchial mucosa; pain, bleeding, and discharge	Acyclovir, famciclovir, or valacyclovir is given IV or PO. Lower maintenance doses may be given to prevent recurrence of symptoms.

Opportunistic diseases associated with AIDS *(continued)*

Disease	Signs and symptoms	Treatment
Cytomegalovirus (CMV) A viral infection of the herpes virus that may result in serious, widespread infection; most common sites: lungs, adrenal glands, eyes, CNS, GI tract, male GU tract, and blood	Unexplained fever, malaise, GI ulcers, diarrhea, weight loss, swollen lymph nodes, hepatomegaly, splenomegaly, blurred vision, floaters, dyspnea (especially on exertion), dry nonproductive cough, and vision changes leading to blindness in patients with ocular infection	Ganciclovir is used to treat CMV. Ganciclovir has shown some anti-HIV properties. Intraocular ganciclovir implants may be used to treat CMV retinitis.
Progressive multifocal leukoencephalopathy (PML) Progressive demyelinating disorder caused by hyperactivation of a papovavirus that leads to gradual brain degeneration	Progressive dementia, memory loss, headache, confusion, weakness, and other possible neurologic complications such as seizures	No form of therapy for PML has been effective, but attempted therapies include prednisone and acyclovir administered both IV and intrathecally.
Herpes zoster A disease also known as *acute posterior ganglionitis, shingles, zona,* and *zoster;* acute infection caused by reactivation of the chickenpox virus	Small clusters of painful, reddened papules that follow the route of inflamed nerves; may be disseminated, involving two or more dermatomes	Herpes zoster is most often treated with oral acyclovir capsules until healed. Treatment may have to continue at lower doses indefinitely to prevent recurrence. IV acyclovir is effective in disseminated varicella zoster lesions in some patients. Medications, such as capsaicin, may relieve pain associated with the infection and postherpetic neuropathies. Famciclovir and valacyclovir can also be used.

No bones about it! These infections can affect all my body systems.

(Continued)

Opportunistic diseases associated with AIDS *(continued)*

Disease	Signs and symptoms	Treatment
Neoplasms		
Kaposi sarcoma A generalized disease with characteristic lesions involving all skin surfaces, including the face (tip of the nose, eyelids), head, upper and lower limbs, soles of the feet, palms of the hands, conjunctivae, sclerae, pharynx, larynx, trachea, hard palate, stomach, liver, small and large intestines, and glans penis	Manifested cutaneously and subcutaneously; usually painless, nonpruritic tumor nodules that are pigmented and violaceous (red to blue), nonblanching and palpable; patchy lesions appearing early and possibly mistaken for bruises, purpura, or diffuse cutaneous hemorrhages	Treatment is focused on palliation and prevention of spread. Systemic chemotherapy or radiation therapy may be used. Intralesional therapy with vinblastine may be given for cosmetic purposes to treat small cutaneous lesions, and laser therapy and cryotherapy may be used to treat small isolated lesions. Interferon alfa-2a may also be used.
Malignant lymphomas Immune system cancer in which lymph tissue cells begin growing abnormally and spread to other organs; incidence in people with AIDS: diagnosed in HIV-infected individuals as widespread disease involving extranodal sites, most commonly in the GI tract, CNS, bone marrow, and liver	Unexplained fever, night sweats, or weight loss greater than 10% of patient's total body weight; signs and symptoms commonly confined to one body system: CNS (confusion, lethargy, and memory loss) or GI tract (pain, obstruction, changes in bowel habits, bleeding, and fever)	Individualized therapy may include a modified combination of methotrexate, bleomycin, doxorubicin, cyclophosphamide, vincristine, and dexamethasone. Radiation therapy is used to treat primary CNS lymphoma.
Cervical cancer Females who are HIV-positive are at increased risk for cervical neoplasm associated with human papillomavirus (HPV) infections	*Possible indicators of early invasive disease:* abnormal vaginal bleeding, persistent vaginal discharge, or postcoital pain and bleeding; *possible indicators of advanced disease:* pelvic pain, vaginal leakage of urine and feces from a fistula, anorexia, weight loss, and fatigue	Treatment is tailored to the disease stage. Preinvasive lesions may require total excisional biopsy, cryosurgery, laser destruction, conization (and frequent Papanicolaou test follow-up), and possibly hysterectomy. Invasive squamous cell carcinoma may require radical hysterectomy and radiation therapy.

Child watch

In children, the incubation period for HIV infection averages only 18 months. Signs and symptoms resemble those for adults, except that children are more likely to have a history of bacterial infections, such as otitis media and lymphoid interstitial pneumonia, as well as types of pneumonia not caused by *P. jirovecii*, sepsis, and chronic salivary gland enlargement.

What tests tell you

Tests that detect HIV have a "window period," the time between exposure to HIV and when the test can detect antibodies. Antibodies to HIV require 2 weeks to 6 months to develop in the bloodstream.

Therefore, the antibody test detects HIV infection after the virus has had time to invade and kill many CD4 cells. Nucleic acid tests can detect HIV between 10 and 33 days postexposure; antigen/antibody tests can detect HIV between 18 and 45 days after exposure; antibody tests can take between 23 and 90 days to obtain a confirmed result. Antibody tests in neonates may also be unreliable because transferred maternal antibodies persist for up to 18 months, causing a false-positive result.

If a person tests negative via an antigen/antibody test after a known exposure to HIV, the CDC advise getting retested 45 days after the most recent exposure. For other tests, the CDC states that a patient should be tested again at least 90 days after the most recent exposure to gain a definitive result.

Many opportunistic infections in AIDS patients are reactivations of previous infections. Therefore, patients may also be tested for syphilis, hepatitis B, tuberculosis, toxoplasmosis, and histoplasmosis. (See *Treating HIV disease*.)

 Battling illness

Treating HIV disease

There is no cure for human immunodeficiency virus (HIV) disease; however, several types of drugs are used to treat the disease and prolong life.

Antiretrovirals
Antiretroviral drugs are used to control the reproduction of the virus and to slow the progression of HIV-related disease. Antiretroviral therapy, commonly referred to as ART, is the recommended treatment for HIV infection. ART combines medications from six major drug classes.
• Nonnucleoside reverse transcriptase inhibitors (NNRTI)—bind to and disable reverse transcriptase, a protein that HIV needs to make more copies of itself.
• Nucleoside reverse transcriptase inhibitors (NRTI)—are faulty versions of building blocks that HIV requires to make more copies of itself. When HIV uses one of these drugs instead of a normal building block, reproduction of the virus is halted.
• Protease inhibitors (PI)—disable protease, a protein that HIV needs to make more copies of itself.

• Fusion inhibitors (FI)—block HIV entry into cells. These are only used for patients with multidrug-resistant virus.
• Integrase strand inhibitors—inhibit the insertion of HIV DNA into human DNA via the integrase enzyme.
• CCR antagonist—blocks the CCR5 coreceptor on an immune cell's surface, preventing HIV from entering the cell.

Preexposure Prophylaxis
A regimen of antiretroviral agents combined in one pill or injection can be given to people with high risk of exposure to HIV infection to prevent infection.

Postexposure Prophylaxis
A regimen of antiretroviral agents combined in one pill or injection can be given to people who have known exposure to HIV infection to prevent infection.

Anti-infectives and antineoplastics
In addition to antiretroviral drugs, anti-infective drugs are prescribed to treat opportunistic infections. Antineoplastic drugs are used to treat associated cancers.

Systemic lupus erythematosus

A chronic, inflammatory, autoimmune disorder affecting the connective tissues, SLE is classified as cutaneous, drug-induced, neonatal, or systemic. The first type affects only the skin; the second type is caused by high doses of certain medications; the third type is a rare neonatal condition in which the pregnant person's antibodies affect the fetus (and the condition later resolves); the fourth affects multiple organs and can be fatal.

Cutaneous lupus causes superficial lesions—typically over the cheeks and bridge of the nose—that leave scars after healing. SLE is characterized by recurrent remissions and exacerbations.

About 16,000 new cases of SLE are diagnosed each year. Lupus erythematosus strikes females more often than males and often occurs during the childbearing years. It is two to three times more prevalent among females of color.

Get to it early

Although there's no cure for lupus, the prognosis improves with early detection and treatment. Prognosis remains poor for patients who develop cardiovascular, renal, or neurologic complications or severe bacterial infections. The goal of treatment is to control symptoms. (See *Treating SLE*.)

Battling illness

Treating SLE

Drugs are the mainstay of treatment for systemic lupus erythematosus (SLE). In patients who have mild disease, nonsteroidal anti-inflammatory drugs such as ibuprofen usually control arthritis and arthralgia. Skin lesions require sun protection and topical corticosteroid creams, such as triamcinolone and hydrocortisone.

Fluorinated steroids may control acute or discoid lesions. Stubborn lesions may respond to intralesional or systemic corticosteroids or antimalarials, such as hydroxychloroquine, chloroquine, and dapsone. Because hydroxychloroquine and chloroquine can cause retinal damage, patients receiving them should have an ophthalmologic examination every 6 months.

Corticosteroids are the treatment of choice for systemic symptoms, acute generalized exacerbations, and injury to vital organs from pleuritis, pericarditis, nephritis, vasculitis, and central nervous system involvement. With initial prednisone doses of 60 mg or more, the patient's condition usually improves noticeably within 48 hours. After symptoms are under control, the drug dosage is gradually tapered and then discontinued. In patients whose kidneys or central nervous system is affected by SLE, immunosuppressive drugs, such as cyclophosphamide and mycophenolate, may be used. Methotrexate is sometimes effective in controlling the disease. Corticosteroids and immunosuppressive drugs can induce many adverse reactions such as infection, opportunistic infections, and metabolic abnormalities.

There is an array of different biological agents that specifically attack the cytokines or enzymes involved in the inflammation reaction in SLE. These drugs include belimumab, ustekinumab, and baricitinib.

How it happens

The exact cause of lupus erythematosus remains a mystery, but auto-immunity is thought to be the primary cause, along with environmental, hormonal, genetic, and, possibly, viral factors. (See *The lowdown on lupus.*)

In autoimmunity, the body produces antibodies against its own cells. The formed antigen–antibody complexes can suppress the body's normal immunity and damage tissues. A significant feature of patients with SLE is their ability to produce antibodies against many different tissue components, such as red blood cells, neutrophils, platelets, lymphocytes, or almost any organ or tissue in the body.

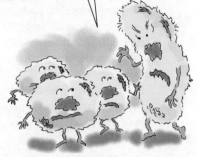

We didn't do anything wrong! Why are you attacking your own cells?!

SLE susceptibility

Most people with SLE have a genetic predisposition. Other predisposing factors include stress, streptococcal or viral infections, exposure to sunlight or ultraviolet light, immunization, pregnancy, and abnormal estrogen metabolism. Drugs may also trigger or aggravate the disease. (See *Drugs that spark SLE.*)

The genetic link

The lowdown on lupus

Apoptosis

Researchers have identified that a genetic defect in a cellular process called *apoptosis* appears to be present in people with lupus. Apoptosis allows the body to eliminate cells that have fulfilled their function and need to be replaced. If a problem with apoptosis occurs, harmful cells may linger, causing damage to the body's own tissue.

Complement

Researchers continue to study how *complement,* a series of proteins in the blood, factor into SLE.

Complement acts as a backup for antibodies, helping them destroy foreign substances that invade the body. A decrease in the amount of complement makes the body less able to fight or destroy foreign substances. If these substances aren't removed from the body, the immune system may become overactive and make autoantibodies. Research updates have focused on mutations in complement receptors 2 and 3 and complement inhibitors.

Drugs that spark SLE

Many drugs can cause symptoms that resemble those of systemic lupus erythematosus (SLE). Other drugs may actually trigger SLE or activate it. These drugs include (National Resource Center on Lupus, 2018):

- procainamide
- hydralazine
- quinidine

What to look for

The onset of SLE may be acute or insidious, but the disease has no characteristic clinical pattern. Patients may report fever, anorexia, weight loss, malaise, fatigue, abdominal pain, nausea, vomiting, diarrhea, constipation, rashes, and polyarthralgia (multiple joint pain).

Blood disorders, such as anemia, leukopenia, lymphopenia, thrombocytopenia, and an elevated erythrocyte sedimentation rate (ESR), occur because of circulating antibodies. Females may report irregular menstruation or amenorrhea, particularly during exacerbations.

Most patients have joint involvement that resembles rheumatoid arthritis. Many have Raynaud phenomenon—intermittent, severe pallor of the fingers, toes, ears, or nose.

Shedding light on lupus

The skin eruption characteristic of SLE is a rash on areas exposed to light. The rash varies in severity from red areas to disc-shaped plaque. The classic "butterfly" rash occurs after sun exposure. Patchy alopecia is a lesser common symptom associated with SLE.

Cardiopulmonary effects

Cardiopulmonary signs and symptoms include pericarditis, endocarditis, myocarditis, and coronary artery disease.

Neurologic effects

Neurological signs and symptoms occur in patients with SLE and often include seizure disorders, aseptic meningitis, cognitive dysfunction, organic brain syndromes, delirium, psychosis, migraine, and mood disorder.

Urinary system effects

Renal damage is the most common cause of death in patients with SLE. Most patients with SLE develop glomerular disease. Other renal concerns include acute or chronic renal failure, nephrotic syndrome, and lupus nephritis.

What tests tell you

These tests are used to diagnose lupus erythematosus:
- Complete blood count with differential may show anemia and a reduced WBC count.

- Serum electrophoresis may show hypergammaglobulinemia.
- Other blood tests may show a decreased platelet count and an elevated ESR. Active disease is diagnosed by decreased serum complement levels, leukopenia, mild thrombocytopenia, and anemia.
- Chest x-rays may reveal pleurisy or lupus pneumonitis.
- Antinuclear antibodies are elevated.

Rheumatoid arthritis

A chronic, systemic, inflammatory disease, rheumatoid arthritis usually attacks peripheral joints, particularly the hands, the cervical spine, and surrounding muscles, tendons, ligaments, and blood vessels. Spontaneous remissions and unpredictable exacerbations mark the course of this potentially crippling disease.

Rheumatoid arthritis affects between 1.28 and 1.36 million Americans, with more females affected than males. The peak onset is highest in people in their 60s.

Lifelong treatment

Rheumatoid arthritis usually requires lifelong treatment and sometimes surgery. In most patients, the disease is intermittent, allowing for in-between periods of normal activity. However, some patients suffer total disability from severe joint deformity, associated symptoms, or both. The prognosis worsens with the development of nodules, vasculitis (inflammation of a blood or lymph vessel), and high titers of rheumatoid factor.

How it happens

The cause of rheumatoid arthritis isn't known, but infections, genetics, and endocrine factors may play a part.

When exposed to an antigen, a person susceptible to rheumatoid arthritis may develop abnormal or altered IgG antibodies. The body doesn't recognize these antibodies as "self," so it forms an antibody known as *rheumatoid factor* against them. By aggregating into complexes, rheumatoid factor causes inflammation.

Eventually, inflammation causes cartilage damage. Immune responses continue, including complement system activation. Complement system activation attracts leukocytes and stimulates the release of inflammatory mediators, which then exacerbate joint destruction. (See *Treating rheumatoid arthritis*.)

Battling illness

Treating rheumatoid arthritis

Treatment measures are used to reduce pain and inflammation and preserve the patient's functional capacity and quality of life.

Drug therapy

Nonsteroidal anti-inflammatory drugs (NSAIDs), systemic and intra-articular glucocorticoids, and nonbiologic and biologic disease-modifying antirheumatic drugs (DMARDs) are the treatments of choice. A wide array of biologic agents have been developed for treatment of RA and are proving effective.

These drugs target the inflammatory mediators (cytokines) involved in the joint disease. These include etanercept, infliximab, adalimumab, abatacept, and tofacitinib.

Physical and other therapies

Joint function can be preserved through range-of-motion exercises and a carefully individualized physical and occupational therapy program. Surgery is available for joints that are damaged or painful.

The genetic link

HLA susceptibility genes

The human leukocyte antigen (*HLA*)-*DRB1* gene is the major center for susceptibility for rheumatoid arthritis.

Four-alarm inflammation

If unarrested, joint inflammation occurs in four stages:

1. Initial inflammation in the joint capsule is accompanied by swelling of the synovial tissue. The patient begins feeling joint pain, swelling, and stiffness.
2. Formation of pannus (thickened layers of granulation tissue) marks the onset of the second stage. Pannus covers and invades cartilage and eventually destroys the joint capsule and bone.
3. The third stage is characterized by fibrous ankylosis (fibrous invasion of the pannus and scar formation that occludes the joint space). Bone atrophy and misalignment cause visible deformities and restrict movement, causing muscle atrophy, imbalance, and, possibly, partial dislocations.
4. In the fourth stage, fibrous tissue calcifies, resulting in bony ankylosis (fixation of a joint) and total immobility. Pain associated with movement may restrict active joint use and cause fibrous or bony ankylosis, soft-tissue contractures, and joint deformities. (See *The effects of rheumatoid arthritis on certain joints.*)

Now I get it!

The effects of rheumatoid arthritis on certain joints

Many joints can be affected by RA, including the knee, the hip, the wrist, and the joints in the hand.

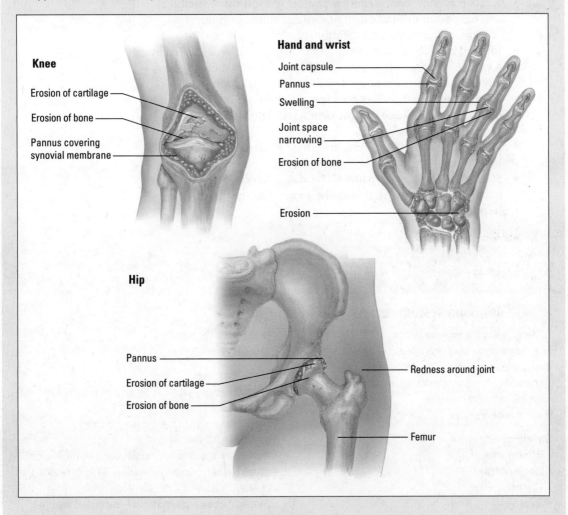

Knee

Erosion of cartilage

Erosion of bone

Pannus covering synovial membrane

Hand and wrist

Joint capsule

Pannus

Swelling

Joint space narrowing

Erosion of bone

Erosion

Hip

Pannus

Erosion of cartilage

Erosion of bone

Redness around joint

Femur

What to look for

At first, the patient may complain of nonspecific symptoms, including fatigue, malaise, anorexia, persistent low-grade fever, weight loss, and vague articular symptoms. As inflammation progresses through the four stages, specific symptoms develop, frequently in the fingers. They usually occur bilaterally and symmetrically and may extend to the wrists, elbows, knees, and ankles.

What tests tell you

Although no test can be used to definitively diagnose rheumatoid arthritis, these tests are useful:

- X-rays may show bone demineralization and soft-tissue swelling and help determine the extent of cartilage and bone destruction, erosion, subluxations, and deformities.
- Rheumatoid factor test is positive in many patients, as indicated by a value of less than 60 units/mL. Antinuclear antibodies are generally elevated above the normal finding of 1:40 dilution.
- Synovial fluid analysis shows increased volume and turbidity but decreased viscosity and complement levels. The WBC count often exceeds 10,000/mm³.
- Serum protein electrophoresis may show elevated serum globulin levels.
- ESR is elevated in many patients. Because an elevated rate often parallels disease activity, this test helps monitor the patient's response to therapy.

That's a wrap!

Immune system review

Understanding the immune system

The body protects itself from infectious organisms through the host defense system. Three lines of defense include:
- physical and chemical barriers to infection
- the inflammatory response
- the immune response

Structures
- Bone marrow
- Lymph nodes
- Thymus
- Spleen
- Tonsils

Types of immunity
- Cell-mediated immunity—T cells respond to antigen.
- Humoral immunity—B cells respond to antigen.

Types of disorders
- Immunodeficiency disorders
- Hypersensitivity disorders
- Autoimmune disorders

Immune disorders
- *Allergic rhinitis*—type I, IgE-mediated response to allergen.
- *Anaphylaxis*—type I allergic reaction from systemic exposure to antigen.
- *Human immunodeficiency virus disease*—ribonucleic acid retrovirus replicates within the CD4⁺ cell, resulting in cell death.
- *Systemic lupus erythematosus*—antibodies are produced against body's own cells; normal immunity suppressed by formed antigen–antibody complex that results in tissue damage.
- *Rheumatoid arthritis*—exposure to an antigen causes altered IgG antibodies to develop; the body doesn't recognize these antibodies, and an antibody known as *rheumatoid factor* forms against them.

Quick quiz

1. Which is the most concerning symptom of anaphylactic shock?
   A. Hives (urticaria)
   B. Respiratory distress
   C. Allergic shiners
   D. Fever

Answer: B. Respiratory distress is the most dangerous symptom of anaphylactic shock. Hives comes on suddenly and often accompanies severe respiratory distress, followed by stridor and possible vascular collapse.

2. What is the most common assessment finding in a patient with systemic lupus erythematosus?
   A. Joint pain
   B. Nausea and vomiting
   C. Itchy skin
   D. Insomnia

Answer: A. Joint pain. Most patients with lupus report to have joint pain, which resembles that of rheumatoid arthritis.

3. What is the most common life-threatening opportunistic disease associated with acquired immunodeficiency syndrome (AIDS)?
   A. *Candida* infection
   B. Tuberculosis
   C. *Pneumocystis jirovecii* pneumonia
   D. Toxoplasmosis

Answer: C. *Pneumocystis jirovecii* pneumonia is the most common life-threatening protozoal infection in human lungs, transmitted by airborne exposure.

4. Systemic lupus erythematosus is characterized by:
   A. ulnar rotation of the hand.
   B. butterfly rash.
   C. flu-like syndrome.
   D. dark circles under the eyes.

Answer: B. About 30% of patients get the characteristic butterfly rash over their noses and cheeks.

5. Common concerns associated with rheumatoid arthritis include:
   A. painful joints, weak muscles, and peripheral neuropathy.
   B. dizziness, dyspnea, and tachycardia.
   C. anemia, Raynaud phenomenon, and amenorrhea.
   D. headache, emotional lability, and patchy alopecia.

Answer: A. These symptoms typically develop in the fingers and extend bilaterally to the wrists, elbows, knees, and ankles.

Scoring

☆☆☆ If you answered all five items correctly, bravo! Your performance is immune to criticism.

☆☆ If you answered four items correctly, congratulations! Clearly, the quick quiz provided a stimulus that evoked an effective and appropriate response.

☆ If you answered fewer than four items correctly, that's okay. We still have plenty of body systems to cover, so now is no time to become hypersensitive.

Suggested references

Akhouri, S., & House, S. A. (2023 January). *Allergic rhinitis*. [Updated 2023, July 16]. In: *StatPearls* [Internet]. StatPearls Publishing; Available from https://www.ncbi.nlm.nih.gov/books/NBK538186/

Ambrosioni, J., Petit, E., Liegeon, G., Laguno, M., & Miró, J. M. (2021). Primary HIV-1 infection in users of pre-exposure prophylaxis. *The Lancet HIV, 8*(3), e166–e174. https://doi.org/10.1016/S2352-3018(20)30271-X

American Academy of Allergy Asthma and Immunology. (2023). Allergy facts. https://acaai.org/allergies/allergies-101/facts-stats/

Barbaud, A., & Romano, A. (2022). Skin testing approaches for immediate and delayed hypersensitivity reactions. *Immunology and Allergy Clinics of North America, 42*(2), 307–322. https://doi.org/10.1016/j.iac.2022.01.003

Centers for Disease Control and Prevention. (2019). Understanding the HIV care continuum. https://www.cdc.gov/hiv/pdf/library/factsheets/cdc-hiv-care-continuum.pdf

Centers for Disease Control and Prevention. (2021). Recognizing and responding to anaphylaxis. https://www.cdc.gov/vaccines/covid-19/downloads/recognizing-responding-to-anaphylaxis-508.pdf

Centers for Disease Control and Prevention. (2022). Preventing and managing adverse reactions. https://www.cdc.gov/vaccines/hcp/acip-recs/general-recs/adverse-reactions.html

Centers for Disease Control and Prevention. (2022a). HIV statistics overview. https://www.cdc.gov/hiv/statistics/overview/index.html

Centers for Disease Control and Prevention. (2022b). HIV basics. https://www.cdc.gov/hiv/basics/index.html

Centers for Disease Control and Prevention. (2022c). HIV risk and prevention. https://www.cdc.gov/hiv/risk/index.html

Centers for Disease Control and Prevention. (2022d). HIV treatment. https://www.cdc.gov/hiv/basics/livingwithhiv/treatment.html

Centers for Disease Control and Prevention. (2022e). Systemic lupus erythematosus. https://www.cdc.gov/lupus/facts/detailed.html

Centers for Disease Control and Prevention. (2023). Diagnosed allergic conditions in adults: United States, 2021. https://www.cdc.gov/nchs/products/databriefs/db460.htm

Dispenza, M. C. (2019). Classification of hypersensitivity reactions. *Allergy and Asthma Proceedings, 40*(6), 470–473. https://doi.org/10.2500/aap.2019.40.4274

Elkon, K. (2023). Apoptosis and autoimmune disease. Retrieved from www.Uptodate .com

Goodsell, D. S. (2015). Illustrations of the HIV life cycle. *Current Topics in Microbiology and Immunology, 389*, 243–252. https://doi.org/10.1007/82_2015_437

HIVinfo NIH.gov. (2021). *HIV overview*. HIV Life Cycle. https://hivinfo.nih.gov/ understanding-hiv/fact-sheets/hiv-life-cycle

Huang, J., Fu, X., Chen, X., Li, Z., Huang, Y., & Liang, C. (2021). Promising therapeutic targets for treatment of rheumatoid arthritis. *Frontiers in Immunology, 12*, 686155. https://doi.org/10.3389/fimmu.2021.686155

Huynh, K., & Kahwaji, C. I. (2022). *HIV testing*. In *StatPearls*. StatPearls Publishing.

Kiriakidou, M., & Ching, C. L. (2020). Systemic lupus erythematosus. *Annals of Internal Medicine, 172*(11), ITC81–ITC96. https://doi.org/10.7326/ AITC202006020

Motosue, M. S., Li, J. T., & Campbell, R. L. (2022). Anaphylaxis: Epidemiology and differential diagnosis. *Immunology and Allergy Clinics of North America, 42*(1), 13–25. https://doi.org/10.1016/j.iac.2021.09.010

Muraro, A., Worm, M., Alviani, C., Cardona, V., DunnGalvin, A., Garvey, L. H., Riggioni, C., de Silva, D., Angier, E., Arasi, S., Bellou, A., Beyer, K., Bijlhout, D., Bilò, M. B., Bindslev-Jensen, C., Brockow, K., Fernandez-Rivas, M., Halken, S., Jensen, B., … European Academy of Allergy and Clinical Immunology, Food Allergy, Anaphylaxis Guidelines Group. (2022). EAACI guidelines: Anaphylaxis (2021 update). *Allergy, 77*(2), 357–377. https://doi.org/10.1111/ all.15032

National Institutes of Health (NIH). National Institute of Arthritis and Musculoskeletal and Skin Diseases. (2022a). *Systemic lupus erythematosus*. https://www.niams. nih.gov/health-topics/lupus

National Institutes of Health (NIH). National Institute of Arthritis and Musculoskeletal and Skin Diseases. (2022b). *Rheumatoid arthritis*. https://www.niams.nih.gov/ health-topics/rheumatoid-arthritis

Norris, T. (2025). *Porth's pathophysiology: Concepts of altered health states* (11th ed.). Wolters Kluwer.

Peters, R. L., Krawiec, M., Koplin, J. J., & Santos, A. F. (2021). Update on food allergy. *Pediatric Allergy and Immunology: Official Publication of the European Society of Pediatric Allergy and Immunology, 32*(4), 647–657. https://doi.org/10.1111/ pai.13443

Phanuphak, N., & Gulick, R. M. (2020). HIV treatment and prevention 2019: Current standards of care. *Current Opinion in HIV and AIDS, 15*(1), 4–12. https://doi. org/10.1097/COH.0000000000000588

Radu, A. F., & Bungau, S. G. (2021). Management of rheumatoid arthritis: An overview. *Cells, 10*(11), 2857. https://doi.org/10.3390/cells10112857

Schuler Iv, C. F., & Montejo, J. M. (2021). Allergic rhinitis in children and adolescents. *Immunology and Allergy Clinics of North America, 41*(4), 613–625. https://doi. org/10.1016/j.iac.2021.07.010

Smith, M. H., & Berman, J. R. (2022). What is rheumatoid arthritis? *JAMA, 327*(12), 1194. https://doi.org/10.1001/jama.2022.0786

Tedner, S. G., Asarnoj, A., Thulin, H., Westman, M., Konradsen, J. R., & Nilsson, C. (2022). Food allergy and hypersensitivity reactions in children and adults-A review. *Journal of Internal Medicine, 291*(3), 283–302. https://doi.org/10.1111/joim.13422

Tsoi, B. W., Fine, S. M., McGowan, J. P., Vail, R., Merrick, S. T., Radix, A., Gonzalez, C. J., & Hoffmann, C. J. (2022). *HIV testing.* Johns Hopkins University.

Tumarkin, E., Siedner, M. J., & Bogoch, I. I. (2019). HIV pre-exposure prophylaxis (PrEP). *BMJ (Clinical Research ed.), 364,* k4681. https://doi.org/10.1136/bmj.k4681

Zhang, Y., Lan, F., & Zhang, L. (2021). Advances and highlights in allergic rhinitis. *Allergy, 76*(11), 3383–3389. https://doi.org/10.1111/all.15044

Chapter 11

Integumentary system

Just the facts

In this chapter, you'll learn:

 ◆ structures of the skin

 ◆ functions of the skin

 ◆ how the integumentary system works

 ◆ pathophysiology, diagnostic tests, and treatments for several skin disorders.

Understanding the integumentary system

The skin is the body's largest organ whose main function is to protect the body. Weighing in at approximately 20% of the body's weight, the average adult has two square yards of skin. Each inch of skin contains millions of cells and many special nerve endings for sensing heat, cold, and pain.

The average thickness of the skin is one-tenth of an inch, but it ranges from the thinnest of coverage on the eyelids to much thicker on the soles of the feet. Skin keeps harmful microbes out and helps prevent infections. It holds body fluids in, preventing dehydration, and keeps the body temperature even while allowing the individual to still feel things like heat, cold, and pain. Skin activates vitamin D in cooperation with sunlight.

Layer upon layer

The epidermis, dermis, and hypodermis form the layers of the skin that house hair follicles, sweat glands, fat, connective tissue, and blood vessels.

The **epidermis**, the outermost layer of the skin, provides a defensive and waterproof barrier for the body. The superficial layer, the *stratum corneum*, perpetually renews through the process of shedding. New cells called *keratinocytes* originate in the stratum basale. As they move upward and differentiate, the stratum spinosum is formed. Together, the *stratum basal* and *stratum spinosum* form the *stratum germinativum*.

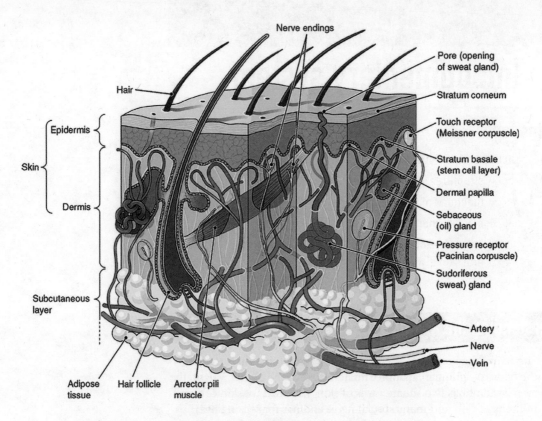

Hair

Nerve endings

Epidermis

Skin

Dermis

Subcutaneous layer

Pore (opening of sweat gland)

Stratum corneum

Touch receptor (Meissner corpuscle)

Stratum basale (stem cell layer)

Dermal papilla

Sebaceous (oil) gland

Pressure receptor (Pacinian corpuscle)

Sudoriferous (sweat) gland

Artery

Nerve

Vein

Adipose tissue

Hair follicle

Arrector pili muscle

Melanocytes, *Langerhans cells*, and *Merkel cells* live in the epidermis. Melanocytes are responsible for synthesis and secretion of the pigment melanin when exposed to UV light that responds to melanocyte-stimulating hormone. Within the epidermis, melanin shields the skin against UV radiation and is responsible for skin color.

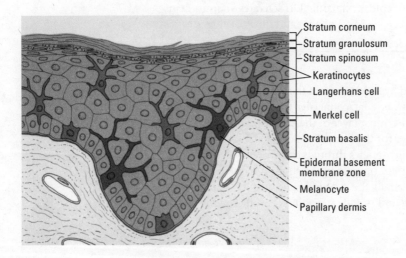

Stratum corneum

Stratum granulosum

Stratum spinosum

Keratinocytes

Langerhans cell

Merkel cell

Stratum basalis

Epidermal basement membrane zone

Melanocyte

Papillary dermis

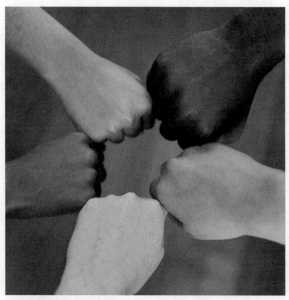

(Shutterstock/Meeko Media.)

Langerhans cells, a type of dendritic cell, move to the epidermis from the bone marrow; in cooperation with dermal dendritic cells, they start an immune response, which acts as a defense against environmental allergies. *Merkel cells* are responsible for the sensation and are situated in areas of high-touch reception, such as in the fingertips.

The **dermis** is 1 to 4 mm thick and contains collagen, elastin and reticulin, and a gel-like ground substance. This combination provides mobility and stretch of the skin in response of bodily movement. Nerves, lymphatic and blood vessels, sweat glands, sebaceous glands, and hair follicles live within the dermis. Dermal cells include fibroblasts, mast cells, and macrophages.

The **subcutaneous** layer of the skin, containing fat cells and subcutaneous tissue, also houses the nails, hair, sebaceous glands, and sweat glands.

Health promotion first!

Maintaining healthy skin and prevention of infection and other skin problems is important to a patient's overall state of health. Teach patients to:
- keep skin clean
- protect skin from direct sunlight and to avoid tanning beds
- participate in regular physical activity
- consume a healthy diet (fruits, vegetables, whole grains, proteins, and low-fat dairy products)
- maintain a healthy weight
- get enough sleep—adults need at least 7 to 9 hours of sleep nightly; teens need 9 hours of sleep; infants and children need even more!

Types of skin lesions

Skin lesions can be classified as primary or secondary.

Primary lesions

Primary lesions are directly connected to the immediate health problem.

Type	Description	Examples	Image
Bulla	• A vesicle that is 1 cm or larger, filled with serous fluid	• Blister	Bulla
Cyst	• Located in the dermis or subcutaneous layer of the skin • Elevated, circumscribed, and encapsulated • Filled with an expressible liquid or semisolid material	• Sebaceous cyst	Cyst
Macule and patch	• A flat, nonpalpable area; macules are up to 1 cm, and patches are greater than 1 cm • Represents a change in normal color of the skin	Macule: • Freckle • Birthmark Patch: • Vitiligo • Port-wine stain	Macule and Patch
Nodule	• An elevated, firm, circumscribed, palpable lesion, 1–2 cm in diameter • Deeper and firmer than a papule	• Lipoma	Nodule

(Continued)

Primary lesions *(continued)*

Type	Description	Examples	Image
Papule	• An elevated, palpable, firm, circumscribed lesion less than 1 cm in diameter	• Wart • Insect bite	 Papule
Plaque	• An elevated, flat-topped, firm, rough, super-ficial lesion greater than 1 cm in diameter	• Psoriasis • Seborrheic keratoses • Actinic keratoses	 Plaque
Pustule	• An elevated and superficial lesion, similar to a vesicle but filled with purulent fluid	• Impetigo • Acne	 Pustule
Tumor	• An elevated, solid mass, greater than 2 cm in diameter • Originated deeper in the dermis than other lesions	• Neoplasm • Neurofibroma	 Tumor

(Continued)

Primary lesions *(continued)*

Type	Description	Examples	Image
Vesicle	• An elevated, circumscribed, superficial lesion filled with serous fluid, less than 1 cm in diameter	• Varicella zoster • Herpes zoster • Herpes simplex	 Vesicle
Wheal	• Transient, elevated, irregularly shaped area of localized skin edema	• Urticaria	 Wheal

Image credit: *Tumor:* Reprinted with permission from Weber, J. R., & Kelley, J. H. (2022). *Health assessment in nursing* (7th ed., unnumbered figure in Table 14-3). Wolters Kluwer.

Secondary lesions

Secondary lesions result from the primary lesion or develop as the result of a different health problem.

Type	Description	Examples	Image
Scar	• Thin to thick fibrous tissue that replaces normal tissue after injury or laceration	• Health wound • Surgical incision	
Atrophy	• Thinning of the skin surface; loss of skin markings	• Aging skin	

(Continued)

Secondary lesions *(continued)*

Type	Description	Examples	Image
Scale	• Heaps of keratinized cells; irregularly shaped flakes	• Dry skin • Dandruff	
Crust	• Dried residue of skin exudates such as serum, pus, or blood	• Dried drainage that originated from varicella vesicles	
Lichenification	• Rough thickening of the epidermis • Often caused by persistent rubbing or scratching	• Chronic dermatitis	
Excoriation	• Epidermal loss represented by linear, hollowed-out areas	• Scabies	

Images reprinted with permission from the following sources: *Scar:* Krakowski, A. C., & Shumaker, P. R. (2017). *The* scar book. Wolters Kluwer; *Atrophy:* Carter, P. Lippincott textbook for nursing assistants (4th ed., Fig. 28-4). Wolters Kluwer; *Scale:* Hall, J. C., & Hall, B. J. (2017). *Sauer's manual of skin diseases* (11th ed., Fig. 16-1). Wolters Kluwer; *Crust:* Edwards, L., & Lynch, P. (2017). *Genital dermatology atlas and manual* (3rd ed., Fig. 10-41). Wolters Kluwer; *Lichenification:* Goodheart, H., & Gonzalez, M. (2015). *Goodheart's photoguide to common pediatric and adult skin disorders* (4th ed., Fig. 13-19). Wolters Kluwer; *Excoriation:* Krajbich, J. I., Pinzur, M. S., Potter, B. K., & Stevens, P. M. Atlas of amputations and limb deficiencies (5th ed., Fig. 52-6). Wolters Kluwer.

"Seeing" the skin

Assessment of the skin can reveal actual integumentary disorders or clues about other health conditions that are not immediately visible to the eye. A thorough skin assessment and associated documentation includes:

Assessment	Common findings	Things to document
Color	Color will be consistent with ethnicity, injury, stage of healing, and/or health condition	Color of patient's normal skin, area of injury, and/or lesion(s)
Temperature	Warmth or coolness	Warmth or coolness of area of injury and/or lesion(s), and surrounding skin; warmth or coolness of overall body temperature via thermometer
Texture	Roughness or smoothness	Characteristics of texture
Moisture	Moistness or dryness	Characteristics of moisture or degree of dryness
Turgor	Elasticity	Presence or absence of elasticity and location of assessment
Edema	Absence or presence of swelling	Area(s) of edema Quality of edema—pitting vs. nonpitting
Lesions (see *Types of Skin Lesions*)	Primary or secondary	Type Location Distribution Size (measure!) Shape Color Texture Characteristics of surface Presence of tenderness Type of exudate (color, consistency, odor, amount)

Skin disorders

The skin disorders discussed in this chapter include:
- basal cell carcinoma (BCC)
- bedbugs
- burns
- cellulitis
- herpes simplex
- herpes zoster
- malignant melanoma
- pediculosis
- pressure injury
- scabies
- tinea infections
- trauma

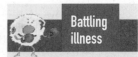

Battling illness

Treating basal cell carcinoma

Treatment measures for BCC include:
- surgical excision
- cryotherapy
- radiotherapy
- photodynamic therapy
- topical application of imiquimod or 5-fluorouracil

Basal cell carcinoma

An epithelial tumor of the skin, BCCs are the most common kind of skin cancer in White individuals. They can grow upward or downward, usually have depressed centers, and borders that are rolled.

How it happens

BCCs are thought to be caused by exposure to UV radiation, arsenic from groundwater wells, or a mutation in the TP53 tumor suppressor gene.

What to look for

BCCs may not be visible in their earliest stages. As they progress, look for nodules greater than 5 mm that are ivory or pearl with small surface blood vessels. They are often found around the nose, ear, or eyelid.

Bedbugs (*Cimex lectularius*)

Bedbugs are nocturnal parasites found in cracks of floors, walls, furniture, and bedding. These creatures are 3 to 5 mm long and feed for 5 to 15 minutes at a time.

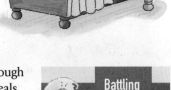

How it happens

Bedbugs attach themselves to a host and suck blood.

What to look for

Reddened, pruritic papules result from the saliva of bedbugs, although sensitized individuals may also develop papules, vesicles, and wheals. Areas that remain uncovered during sleep (for example, face, hands) are often involved. Symptoms may last up to 2 weeks.

Burns

Burns are thermal, chemical, or electrical injuries of the skin. Ranging in severity from extremely mild to life threatening, burns can cause local or systemic injury dependent upon the intensity of the energy experienced, the duration of exposure, and the type of tissue injury. Burns are classified by burn wound depth, which is assessed by noticing the physical appearance of the wound and observing the associated symptoms.

How it happens

Common causes of burns include fire, chemical exposure, electrical exposure, frostbite, and radiation.

What to look for

Superficial (formerly known as first-degree) burns are localized to the epidermis and do not involve the dermis or subcutaneous tissue. The skin still has water vapor and can function as a bacterial barrier. The patient may experience discomfort localized to the site after exposure. Mild sunburns are a good example of a superficial

---

Battling illness

Treating bedbugs

Treatment of bedbugs involves administration of antihistamine and corticosteroids. Bedding, mattresses, furniture, and other contaminated items should be discarded or cleaned by a professional using appropriate insecticides.

burn. Superficial burns usually heal after 3 to 5 days and do not cause scarring to the skin.

Partial-thickness (formerly known as second-degree) burns are deeper than superficial burns. These affect the epidermis and extend to the dermis. Partial-thickness injuries involve fluid-filled blisters that arise quickly after injury and pain. Deeper partial-thickness burns often appear waxy white and look much like full-thickness burns, although healing processes are notable after 7 to 10 days following the injury. Partial-thickness burns take weeks to heal depending again on the extent of injury.

Full-thickness (formerly known as third-degree) burns involve destruction of the epidermis and dermis and extend into the subcutaneous tissue and below. Muscle or bone may be affected, and nerve endings are destroyed, making these burns painless. Full-thickness burns have no elasticity and may appear white, dry, and leathery.

See the below figure for images of each type of burn.

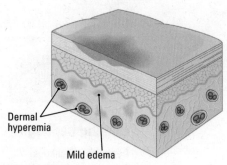

A. Superficial burn

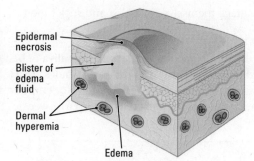

B. Partial-thickness burn

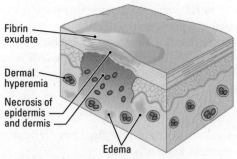

C. Full-thickness burn

The "rule of nines" can be used to determine the total body surface area (TBSA) affected. (See *Rule of nines*.) Another method of determining the TBSA is to use a Lund and Browder chart.

Now I get it!

Rule of nines

The rule of nines is a method that divides the body's surface area into percentages (multiples of nine) so you can quickly estimate the extent of burns. The nurse records on the diagram areas of partial-thickness and full-thickness burns.

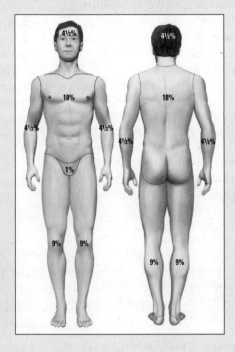

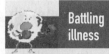

Battling illness

Treating burns

Treatment measures for burns includes:
• Superficial burns: comfort measures, over-the-counter pain relievers, frequent application of water-soluble lotion
• Partial-thickness burns: various pharmacologic ointments and possible antibiotics, wound dressings, surgical removal of the burn followed by grafting is a possible treatment for deep partial-thickness burns
• Full-thickness burns: prevention of, or treatment for, burn shock; IV resuscitation; escharotomy (cutting through burned skin to relieve pressure)

Cellulitis

Cellulitis is a skin infection, usually caused by *Staphylococcus*, methicillin-resistant *Staphylococcus aureus* (MRSA), or group B streptococci, affecting the dermis and subcutaneous tissue.

How it happens

Cellulitis usually occurs as an extension of an ulcer, furuncle, carbuncle, or other skin wound.

What to look for

Areas affected by cellulitis are often red and warm to the touch, swollen, and painful.

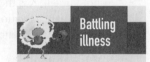

Battling illness

Treating cellulitis

Treatment measures for cellulitis include:
• antibiotics
• corticosteroids (as adjuvant therapy)

Herpes simplex virus

The herpes simplex virus (HSV) is responsible for blistering infections. HSV-1, called *oral herpes*, causes "cold sores" and fever blisters around the mouth and on the face; it can sometimes cause genital herpes, although HSV-2, which is more virulent, is usually the main causative agent.

How it happens

Both serotypes of HSV can be transmitted by genital skin or mucosal contact with an infected individual who is shedding the virus. After introduction of the virus, replication takes place in the dermis and epidermis. The virus spreads through cells and intra-axonally to the dorsal root where is can stay dormant until reactivation.

What to look for

During primary infection, some patients may report generalized flu-like symptoms including fever, malaise, lymphadenopathy, and muscle pain. Recurrent symptoms involve wet lesions that are often unilateral and crust over after 4 to 5 days. Recovery occurs in about 10 days, and then the virus may again lay dormant until reactivation, which occurs on average between five and eight times annually.

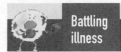
Battling illness

Treating herpes simplex virus

Treatment measures for HSV include:
• Oral lesions: supportive care, refraining from oral or genital contact when virus is active, antiviral therapy may be initiated
• Genital lesions: refraining from oral or genital contact when virus is active; antiviral therapy; educate that exposure, even with no symptoms, is possible

Herpes zoster

Herpes zoster—also known as shingles—is caused by the varicella zoster virus (VZV), the same virus that causes chickenpox (varicella). After initial exposure to the virus, shingles arise years later from viral reactivation.

How it happens

After initial exposure, the VZV lies dormant in the trigeminal and dorsal root ganglia. Although the specific cause of viral reactivation is not known, it is thought that stress or immunosuppression may play a part in reactivation. There is a vaccine available to prevent shingles, usually recommended for adults aged 60 and older.

What to look for

Unilateral lesions are present, often accompanied by pain and paresthesias around the affected dermatome (the area of skin innervated by a single spinal nerve).

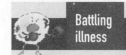
Battling illness

Treating herpes zoster

Treatment measures for herpes zoster include:
• vaccination (preventative)
• compresses to the localized area affected, antiviral drugs, topical lidocaine patch, tricycle antidepressants (for pain control), and topical capsaicin

Malignant melanoma

Malignant melanoma originates from malignant degeneration of melanocytes. Often associated with moles (nevi), healthcare providers often use the ABCDE rule to evaluate changes in Asymmetry, Border irregularity, Color variation, Diameter (larger than 6 mm), and Evolving of these lesions.

How it happens
Malignant degeneration of melanocytes either along the basal layer of the epidermis or in a benign melanocytic nevus is the causative agent of malignant melanoma.

What to look for

Look for changes in symmetry, border, color, diameter, and evolution of any known lesions. New lesions should be evaluated by the same criteria. Because this condition is often found in individuals with light skin and fair hair, patients should consider a total body skin examination to locate lesions that may not be readily visible.

Pediculosis

Pediculosis is a lice infestation that can take up residence on the head (*Pediculus capitis*), in the body (*Pediculus corporis*), or in the groin ("crabs") (*Phthirus pubis*). These blood-sucking parasites reproduce every 2 weeks and are very difficult to treat because of the hundreds of new lice hatch so quickly. Head and body lice are transmitted by personal contact and sharing of combs and clothing; pubic lice are spread by body contact with an infected individual.

How it happens
As lice pierce the skin to suck blood, they secrete a toxic saliva, which results in pruritic dermatitis.

What to look for

Patients with lice report itching. Some types of lice may be visible on hairs or eyebrows. Other types must be visualized under a Wood lamp, a type of ultraviolet light, or via a microscope.

Pressure injury

Formerly known as "decubitus ulcers," pressure injuries are ischemic ulcers caused by pressure, shearing, friction, and moisture.

How it happens
Interruption to arterial and venous blood flow to the skin and tissues because of pressure is the main cause of pressure injuries.

What to look for

Pressure injuries are classified by stages (National Pressure Injury Advisory Panel, n.d.). Please see https://npiap.com/page/PressureInjuryStages for descriptions and images of each of these stages.

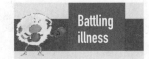

Treating malignant melanoma
Treatment measures for malignant melanoma are based upon thickness of lesion, mitotic index, ulceration, metastasis, and other immunohistochemical assessment measures. Treatments may include:
- surgical excision
- immunotherapy

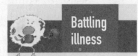

Treating pediculosis
Treatment for pediculosis involves:
- topical ivermectin
- washing and drying of clothing, towels, bedding, combs, and brushes in extremely hot or boiling water

Treating pressure injury

The best treatment for pressure injury is prevention. Other treatments include:
- frequent skin inspection
- frequent repositioning to reduce pressure
- use of special equipment (for example, pressure-reducing mattresses, padding devices)
- use of special wound care products (for example, dressings, gels, cleansers, foams)

- frequent and thorough skin care, especially following urination or bowel movements
- maintenance of a dry skin environment
- barrier creams or ointments
- adequate nutrition
- use of specialized wound pharmaceutical treatments
- negative-pressure wound healing

Scabies

Scabies, a common skin infection, is caused by *Sarcoptes scabiei*, the itch mite, which colonizes in the epidermis. It frequently affects children and people living in areas of overcrowding or poor sanitation and is transmitted by personal contact, infected clothing, and bedding.

How it happens

Infestation begins with a female mite that burrows into the stratum corneum, where she lays eggs that hatch 3 weeks later. Symptoms appear 3 to 5 weeks later when papules and vesicular lesions appear, accompanied by intense itching, especially at night.

What to look for

Finger webs, axillae, arm and wrist creases, waistline, and genitalia and buttocks are often most affected in children and adults; infants may have scabies on their palms, soles, head, back, neck, and face. Areas of infestation appear red and bumpy and may have crusting or secondary infection due to scratching.

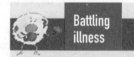

Treating scabies

Treatment of scabies includes:
- Topical permethrin cream
- Oral ivermectin (for generalized scabies)
- Washing of clothing and linens in hot water

Tinea infections

Tinea infections are fungal in nature. They are classified by their location on the skin and are also known as "ringworm"; however, they aren't caused by a worm.

How it happens
Dermatophytes, the fungi that cause superficial skin infections, thrive on keratin found in the nails, hair, and stratum corneum.

What to look for
Specific areas affected will have unique symptoms. These include:
- tinea capitis (scalp)—scaly, pruritic scalp; bald patches; hair that breaks easily
- tinea corporis (body, except for the scalp, face, hands, feet, and groin)—circular, circumscribed reddened scaly patches; some are dry and macular while others are moist and vesicular
- tinea cruris (groin; also known as "jock itch")—small, scaling, reddened vesicular patches over the inner and upper thigh surfaces; increase with heat and high humidity
- tinea pedis (foot; also known as "athlete's foot")—scaling, macerated, and sometimes painful skin between the toes; may spread over the soles of the feet
- tinea manus (hand)—dry, scaly, reddened lesions that originate with itchy, clear vesicles; often accompanies tinea pedis
- tinea unguium (nails; also known as "onychomycosis")—superficial or deep inflammation of the nails; yellow or brown accumulation of brittle keratin all over the nail

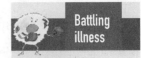

Battling illness

Treating tinea infections

Treatment of tinea infections is dependent upon the type of fungi, diagnosed by cultures, and includes topical and systemic antifungal medication.

That's a wrap!

Integumentary system review

Understanding the integumentary system
The major function of the integumentary system is protection.

Components consist of the epidermis, dermis, and subcutaneous tissue.

Primary lesions are specific to the current health condition and are distinguished as one of the following:
- Bullae
- Cyst
- Macule
- Nodule
- Papule
- Patch
- Plaque
- Pustule
- Tumor
- Vesicle
- Wheal

Secondary lesions arise from primary lesions or arise as the result of a different health problem and are distinguished as one of the following:
- Scar
- Atrophy
- Scale
- Crust
- Lichenification
- Excoriation

Assessment and documentation
Assessment and documentation of integumentary information should include skin color, temperature, texture, moisture level, turgor, and presence of edema or lesions.

Integumentary system review *(continued)*

Integumentary disorders
- Basal cell carcinoma—the most common form of skin cancer in White individuals
- Bedbugs—blood-sucking nocturnal parasite found in bedding, floors, walls, and furniture
- Burns—thermal, chemical, or electrical injuries to the skin
- Cellulitis—a skin infection, usually caused by *Staphylococcus*, MRSA, or group B streptococci, affecting the dermis and subcutaneous tissue
- Herpes simplex—causes blistering ulcerations around the mouth and face, or on the genitals
- Herpes zoster—"shingles," caused by the varicella zoster virus
- Malignant melanoma—lesion arising from malignant degeneration of melanocytes
- Pediculosis—lice infestation
- Pressure injury—ischemic ulcers caused by pressure, shearing, friction, and moisture
- Scabies—a common skin infection caused by *Sarcoptes scabiei*, the itch mite
- Tinea infection—fungal infections of the skin

Quick quiz

1. The nurse palpates an elevated, firm, circumscribed, encapsulated 2-cm lesion on a patient's shoulder. How will the nurse document this finding?
   A. Papule
   B. Macule
   C. Nodule
   D. Excoriation

Answer: C. Lesions that are elevated, firm, circumscribed, and encapsulated and are 1 to 2 cm in diameter are described as nodules.

2. Which is responsible for skin color?
   A. Melanin
   B. Keratinocytes
   C. Langerhans cells
   D. Fibroblasts

Answer: A. Melanin shields the skin against UV radiation and is responsible for skin color.

3. Which is the priority intervention within the first 24 hours of third-degree burn exposure?
   A. Prevention of scarring
   B. Administration of IV fluids
   C. Planning for exercise and therapy
   D. Initiation of high-calorie, high-protein diet

Answer: B. IV fluids must be initiated within the first 24 hours to preserve systemic function.

4. Which is fungal infection of the scalp?
    A. Tinea pedis
    B. Tinea capitis
    C. Tinea corporis
    D. Tinea unguium

Answer: B. Tinea capitis refers to a fungal infection of the scalp.

5. Which skin condition is caused by the same virus that causes chicken pox?
    A. Cellulitis
    B. Scabies
    C. Tinea barbae
    D. Shingles

Answer: D. Shingles (herpes zoster) is a reactivation of the same virus that causes chicken pox (varicella zoster).

Scoring

☆☆☆ If you answered all five items correctly, excellent! When it comes to understanding the integumentary system, you have smooth understanding!

☆☆ If you answered four items correctly, well done! Keep up the good work!

☆ If you answered fewer than four items correctly, keep reviewing! It's just a temporary rough patch!

Suggested references

Ahmed, B., Qadir, M. I., & Ghafoor, S. (2020). Malignant melanoma: Skin cancer-diagnosis, prevention, and treatment. *Critical Reviews in Eukaryotic Gene Expression, 30*(4), 291–297. https://doi.org/10.1615/CritRevEukaryotGeneExpr.2020028454

Alshahrani, B., Sim, J., & Middleton, R. (2021). Nursing interventions for pressure injury prevention among critically ill patients: A systematic review. *Journal of Clinical Nursing, 30*(15–16), 2151–2168. https://doi.org/10.1111/jocn.15709

American Academy of Dermatology Association. (2022). Scabies diagnosis and treatment. https://www.aad.org/public/diseases/a-z/scabies-treatment

American Cancer Society. (2023). Melanoma skin cancer. https://www.cancer.org/cancer/melanoma-skin-cancer.html

Basset-Seguin, N., & Herms, F. (2020). Update in the management of basal cell carcinoma. *Acta Dermato-Venereologica, 100*(11), adv00140. https://doi.org/10.2340/00015555-3495

Boettler, M. A., Kaffenberger, B. H, Chung, C. G. (2022, March). Cellulitis: A review of current practice guidelines and differentiation from Pseudocellulitis. *American Journal of Clinical Dermatology, 23*(2), 153–165. https://doi.org/10.1007/s40257-021-00659-8

Centers for Disease Control and Prevention (CDC). (2021). About ringworm. https://www.cdc.gov/fungal/diseases/ringworm/definition.html.

Centers for Disease Control and Prevention (CDC). (2023). Pediculosis. https://www.cdc.gov/dpdx/pediculosis/index.html

Chung, M. L., Widdel, M., Kirchhoff, J., Sellin, J., Jelali, M., Geiser, F., Mücke, M., & Conrad, R. (2022, January 11). Risk factors for pressure injuries in adult patients: A narrative synthesis. *International Journal of Environmental Research and Public Health, 19*(2), 761. https://doi.org/10.3390/ijerph19020761

Cole, S. (2020). Herpes simplex virus: Epidemiology, diagnosis, and treatment. *Nursing Clinics of North America, 55*(3), 337–345. https://doi.org/10.1016/j.cnur.2020.05.004

Jeschke, M. G., van Baar, M. E., Choudhry, M. A., Chung, K. K., Gibran, N. S., & Logsetty, S. (2020). Burn injury. *Nature Review Disease Primers, 6*(1), 11. https://doi.org/10.1038/s41572-020-0145-5

National Cancer Institute. (2022). Melanoma treatment. https://www.cancer.gov/types/skin/patient/melanoma-treatment-pdq

National Pressure Injury Advisory Panel. (n.d.). Pressure injury stages. Retrieved from https://npiap.com/page/PressureInjuryStages

Norris, T. (2025). *Porth's pathophysiology: Concepts of altered health states* (11th ed.). Wolters Kluwer.

Rosamilia, L. L. (2020, February). Herpes zoster presentation, management, and prevention: A modern case-based review. *American Journal of Clinical Dermatology, 21*(1), 97–107. https://doi.org/10.1007/s40257-019-00483-1

Strayer, D., Saffitz, J., & Rubin, E. (2020). *Rubin's pathology: Mechanisms of human disease* (8th ed.). Wolters Kluwer.

U.S. Environmental Protection Agency (EPA).(2022). How to find bedbugs. https://www.epa.gov/bedbugs/how-find-bed-bugs

Warby, R., & Maani, C. (2022). *Burn classification*. Stat Pearls [Internet]. https://www.ncbi.nlm.nih.gov/books/NBK539773/

Weber, J. R., & Kelley, J. H. (2022). *Health assessment in nursing* (7th ed.). Wolters Kluwer.

Chapter 12

Sensory system*

Just the facts

In this chapter, you'll learn:

♦ visual and auditory functions and their components

♦ risk factors for visual and auditory abnormalities

♦ causes, pathophysiology, diagnostic tests, and treatments for common visual and auditory disorders.

Understanding the eye

The human eye is one of the most fascinating and complex parts of the body, ranking second only to the brain in complexity. Eyes are composed of over 200 million working parts with 107 million light-sensitive cells. Eyes contain 7 million cones to help see color and detail and 100 million rods to assist with night vision. A human can see 500 shades of gray, blinks an average of 4,200,000 times a year, and can process 36,000 pieces of information in an hour. Often, the eye is compared to a camera as it gathers light and transforms it into a picture. The eye is made up of both external and internal structures, which work in harmony to protect the eye and produce continuous images which are transmitted to the brain.

---

*Note: In this chapter, the term "male" refers to a person assigned male at birth, and the term "female" refers to a person assigned female at birth.

The eye

The following illustrations will help you visualize the structures and processes of the eye.

The anatomy of the eye

This figure shows external and internal structures of the eye.

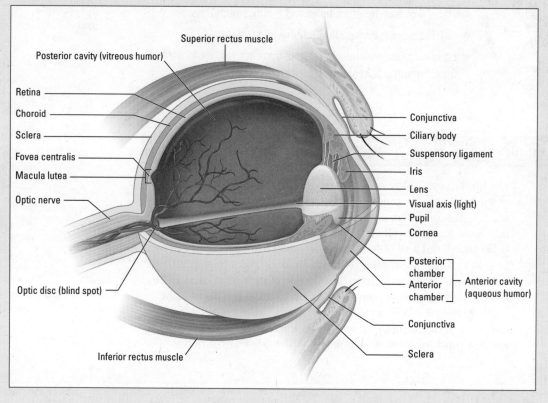

(Continued)

The eye *(continued)*

Normal flow and drainage of the aqueous humor

The aqueous humor flows through the anterior chamber and into the canal of Schlemm.

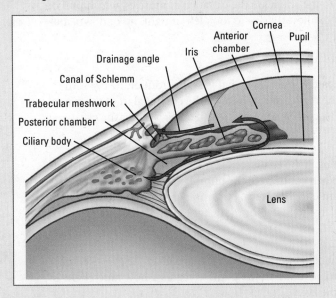

The external structures of the eye

Each structure of the eye plays an important role in the transmission of images to the brain.

Eyelids and eyelashes

- The eyelids are thin folds of skin that cover and protect the cornea and conjunctiva from injury, excessive light, dust, dirt, and other foreign matter. Blinking allows for the eyelids to help spread tears over the eye's surface to keep the eye from getting dry.
- The eyelashes are short, stiff hairs, which help to filter out dust and debris from entering the eye.

Conjunctiva

- The bulbar conjunctiva is a thin, transparent layer of tissues which cover the front of the eye. The palpebral conjunctiva is the pink lining under the eye. It also serves to keep foreign material and bacteria from getting behind the eye. The conjunctiva also contains visible blood vessels, which can be seen against the white background of the sclera.

Sclera

- The sclera is often referred to as the "white part of the eye." This leather-like tissue surrounds the eye to give it its shape and protects the inner structures of the eye.
- Attached to the sclera are the extraocular muscles, which pull on the sclera to allow the eye to look left or right, up or down, and diagonally.

Cornea

- The transparent, clear layer that is at the front of the eye is the cornea. The cornea sits in front of the colored part of the eye called the iris. The cornea helps to focus light as it enters the eye.

Pupil

- The opening at the center of the iris, which permits light to enter the eye. When contracted, the pupil becomes small and restricts the amount of light entering the inner eye. When dilated, the pupil becomes large to allow for more light to enter the inner eye.

Iris

- This pigmented layer of muscular tissue gives the eye its color and controls the size of the pupil to regulate how much light is entering the eye.
- Circular and radial involuntary muscles are located within the iris to control the diameter of the pupil. They contract and relax in an opposing manner to regulate the size of the pupil.

The internal structures of the eye

Choroid

- The choroid is the middle layer between the sclera and the retina. It is the black-pigmented layer under the sclera, which prevents the internal reflection of light rays. Its rich blood vessels bring oxygen and nutrients to nourish the eye. It is modified to form the ciliary body at the front of the eye.

Ciliary body

- The ciliary body is a circular band of tissue at the front of the choroid, which supports the lens. It contains ciliary muscles, which adjust the curvature of the lens.

Lens

- The lens is a transparent, round, and biconvex structure whose elasticity allows the curvature to change to adjust its focusing power. The lens is responsible for fine-tuning the light onto the retina.

Macula

- The macula is located near the central portion of the retina. The macula enables the eye to view detailed central vision that is sharp, and to perceive colors and assist with reading and other tasks, which require central vision.

Retina

- The retina is the innermost, light-sensitive layer of the eyeball, where images are formed. The retina contains neurons called photoreceptors (light-sensitive cells called cones or rods), which convert light waves into nerve impulses.
- Cones enable the eye to see colors in bright lights, and rods enable the eye to see in black and white when the light is dim.

Aqueous humor

- The aqueous humor is a clear, watery fluid, which is produced in the ciliary body, that fills the area between the lens and cornea. It supplies the cornea and lens with nutrients, maintains the convex shape of the cornea, and refracts light rays into the pupil.

Vitreous humor

- This transparent, gel-like substance forms the main bulk of the eyeball. It maintains the shape of the eye and refracts light onto the retina.

Optic nerve

The optic nerve is located at the back of the eye and transmits nerve impulses from the photoreceptors to the brain.

How the eye works

1. The cornea is the transparent front surface of the eye, which is responsible for focusing light.
2. The iris of the eye controls the amount of light reaching the back of the eye by adjusting the size of the pupil, much like the diaphragm of a camera.
3. Like the automatic focus camera lens, the eye's lens sits directly behind the pupil, and pupil automatically focuses the light.
4. The light, which the cornea and lens focuses, reaches the retina. The retina, acting as an electronic sensor of a camera, converts images into electronic signals. The optic nerve takes over and transmits these electronic signals to the visual cortex area of the brain, which controls our sense of sight.

Common disorders of the eye

In this section, you'll find information on some common eye disorders:

- Blindness
- Cataracts
- Conjunctivitis (pinkeye)
- Glaucoma
- Hordeolum (stye)
- Macular degeneration
- Ocular trauma
- Refractive errors
- Retinal detachment and retinal tears
- Strabismus (crossed eyes)
- Retinoblastoma

Blindness

The state of blindness is the inability to see anything including shapes, objects, or light. Complete blindness means that the individual is in a state of total darkness. Legal blindness refers to vision that is highly reduced. In legal blindness, vision is 20/200 or less, or the field of vision is less than 20°.

What to look for

Individuals with eye diseases such as macular degeneration and glaucoma are at an increased risk of developing blindness. Those with diabetes or have had a stroke are at an increased risk for blindness. People who have had eye surgery or work near sharp objects or toxic chemicals are at risk of becoming blind. Lastly, premature babies are at an increased risk for blindness.

What tests tell you

In infants, visual system development begins in the womb and is not fully formed until 2 years old. At 6 to 8 weeks, babies should be able to fix their gaze on an object and follow movement. At 4 months, a baby's eyes should be properly aligned and not turned inward or outward. In young children with eye disorders, caregivers often report symptoms of light sensitivity, poor focusing, chronic eye redness, white or black pupil, poor visual tracking and trouble following an object, and abnormal eye alignment or movement after 6 months of age.

Battling illness

Treating vision loss or blindness

The goal of treating blindness is to assist with restoring vision to the highest functioning state possible. The following are common assistive devices or modifications, which can aid those experiencing vision loss or blindness.

- Eyeglasses
- Contact lenses
- Surgery
- Medication
- Reading Braille
- Use of a service dog/animal
- Organize home so the patient can find things easily
- Remove obstacles in the home environment that can cause a fall (e.g., throw rugs, toys)
- Demonstrate how to use a white mobility cane for the person's safe ambulation

Cataracts

Cataracts are the clouding of the normally translucent lens of the eye. Cataracts are most often associated with aging. As the lens ages, its weight and thickness increases. With each additional cortical layer being added to the lens, the central nucleus of the lens is compressed. As the central nucleus is compressed, it also begins to harden in a process called nuclear sclerosis. The once clear lens begins to lose epithelium cell density, which leads to the reduction in which water and other water-soluble low-molecular-weight metabolites enter the cells of the lens nucleus via the epithelium and cortex. The result is a decrease in the transport rate of water, nutrients, and antioxidants. Another result of the aging process is the progressive oxidative damage to the lens leading to cataract development.

Cataracts progress through four stages. In the early stage, some light is transmitted through the lens, allowing for useful vision. Vision significantly decreases in the second stage of cataract development. The cataract appears completely opaque during the second stage. In the third stage of cataract development, the lens absorbs water and increases in size. The result is an increase in intraocular pressure (IOP). During the final stage of cataract progression, it becomes very difficult for the patient to see clearly. Vision is reported as cloudy during the day, and a noticeable white spot on the lens with milky or yellowish pupils appears. This stage also may cause IOP to increase as the cataract may start leaking protein as the lens breaks down. This increase in protein fluid may block the trabecular meshwork, which causes pain and decreased vision.

What to look for

Cataracts are the largest cause of blindness in the world. Those working in bright sunlight for long periods of time and those who live at higher altitudes have an increased risk of developing cataracts younger in life.

Cataracts are also prevalent in those who have experienced ocular trauma, lacerations, foreign bodies, radiation, exposure to infrared light, have a history of retinal detachment, inflammation of the retina, and chronic use of glucocorticosteroid drugs. A genetic predisposition is also found in patients who have systemic disorders such as diabetes mellitus or Down syndrome.

What tests tell you

Cataracts are painless and cause a decrease in visual acuity. They are often associated with blurred vision and increased sensitivity to bright lights (photophobia) or glares. In some patients, color perception decreases with the development of the cataract. Using an ophthalmoscope to examine the lens, the red reflex normally observed is absent and the lens appears cloudy.

Battling illness

Treating cataracts

The goal of cataract treatment is to restore visual acuity and reduce discomfort.
• Surgical removal is the most common and successful intervention.
• The use of ultraviolet-protective glasses in sunny climates may slow the progression and reduce the discomfort of the cataract.
• Following surgery, pain is minimal. Acute pain indicates IOP and should be reported immediately.
• Document visual acuity in both eyes.
• Following surgery, advise the patient to leave the eye patch in place, use eye drops as prescribed, and avoid rubbing the eye.
• Instruct patient to sleep on the opposite side of the surgical eye.
• Avoid lifting anything over 5 lb.
• Avoid bearing down.
• Avoid aspirin to reduce the chance of bleeding.
• Acetaminophen for discomfort should be encouraged.

Conjunctivitis (pinkeye)

Infections and inflammatory responses of the eye are the most common conditions affecting the external structures of the eye. Both are caused by the body's response to microorganisms, usually bacteria or virus, which have entered the body and begin damaging cells. The same bacteria and viruses that result in colds, ear infections, and sinus infections also can cause an infection or inflammatory response in the eye.

Conjunctivitis is an inflammation and redness of the transparent, mucous membrane (conjunctiva) covering the white part of the eye (sclera). There are several different causes for conjunctivitis. Infectious causes of conjunctivitis include bacteria, viruses, and fungi. Noninfectious causes include allergies, foreign bodies, and chemicals. When the term "pinkeye" is used to refer to conjunctivitis, it is because the redness of the conjunctiva is the most noticeable symptom. The three most common types of conjunctivitis are bacterial, viral, and allergic conjunctivitis.

Bacterial conjunctivitis

Bacteria such as *Staphylococcus aureus, Haemophilus influenzae, Streptococcus pneumoniae,* and *Pseudomonas aeruginosa* are the most common types of bacteria that cause conjunctivitis. The thick eye discharge that causes difficulty opening the eye upon waking in the morning usually indicates that the cause is bacterial conjunctivitis. Antibiotics are required to eliminate the bacteria. Antibiotics typically prescribed are topical eye drops or eye ointments. The treatment time depends on the severity of the infection but is usually between 7 and 14 days.

Viral conjunctivitis

Viral conjunctivitis often accompanies a viral upper respiratory infection, the common cold or influenza. Discharge associated with this highly contagious viral conjunctivitis is watery. Both eyes may be affected by viral conjunctivitis. Antibiotics will not work against viral conjunctivitis. Supportive therapies such as eye drops to reduce itching and swelling can help to reduce the symptoms.

Allergic conjunctivitis

Pollen, animal dander, and dust mites can trigger eye allergies. Such allergens may cause allergic conjunctivitis. Itchy eyes are usually the predominant symptoms of allergic conjunctivitis and can be relieved with over-the-counter or prescription eye drops containing antihistamines and corticosteroids.

Keratoconjunctivitis sicca (dry eye disease)

Keratoconjunctivitis sicca, also called dry eye disease, is frequently associated with Sjögren syndrome and other autoimmune diseases. Dry eye is a dysfunction of the nasolacrimal glands, corneal surface, and eyelids that results in insufficient tears. Patients experience ocular irritation often described as a burning, gritty sensation or dryness. The mechanism of disease is unclear, but the condition is thought to stem from antibodies that attack the tear-producing glands.

 Battling illness

Preventing and treating conjunctivitis

• Proper hygiene and frequent hand washing is encouraged.
• Avoid touching or rubbing the eye(s).
• Avoid sharing personal cloths with others and always use a clean towel and wash cloth.
• Change pillow cases frequently and wash in hot water.
• Replace eye makeup (especially mascara) every 6 months, and never share with others.
• Avoid contacts and eye makeup with conjunctivitis symptoms.
• Apply warm compresses over eye, and wipe discharge with a clean tissue. Dispose of tissue in a trash receptacle.
• Avoid work or school as directed by the provider to prevent spreading to others.
• Keratoconjunctivitis sicca (dry eye disease) can be treated with artificial tears and medications. Agents used to provide relief include tear secretion stimulators, such as cyclosporine A, cevimeline, and pilocarpine.

Glaucoma

Glaucoma is characterized by an increase in IOP within the anterior chamber of the eye. Aqueous humor fills the anterior chamber of the eye and nourishes the cornea and lens by providing oxygen and nutrients. The trabecular meshwork, an area located around the base of the cornea, is responsible for draining the aqueous humor from the eye. The shape of the eye is also a direct result of the necessary pressure which the aqueous humor provides. Normal pressure within the anterior chamber does not exceed 2 to 3 mm Hg. As the aqueous fluid increases, the pressure within the anterior chamber increases. The increased pressure interferes with the blood supply to the optic nerve and the retina and can cause permanent damage to the optic nerve.

Glaucoma is characterized as either acute or chronic. Open-angle glaucoma is chronic, which results from degenerative changes. Open-angle glaucoma is commonly linked to genetic predisposition. It is generally slow to develop and occurs bilaterally, and it is difficult to determine the onset. The angle between the cornea and the iris is wide in open-angle glaucoma; however, the trabecular meshwork impaired causing a buildup of aqueous humor. In acute angle-closure glaucoma, also known as closed-angle glaucoma, the angle between the cornea and the iris is narrow, and obstruction to the outflow of the aqueous humor is present. Acute-angle glaucoma is noted by the elevated IOP.

What to look for

Glaucoma is five times more prevalent in Black individuals between the ages of 45 and 65 years than in White individuals in the same age category. Ninety percent of glaucoma occurs in individuals who have open angles. Acute-angle glaucoma is more prevalent in those individuals who have a narrow anterior chamber angle. Risk factors for glaucoma include hypertension, cardiovascular disease, obesity, and diabetes mellitus. Smoking, caffeine, alcohol, and the use of illicit drugs may also cause elevations of IOP.

What tests tell you

In open-angle glaucoma, central vision remains intact until late in the progression of the disease. Over time, the patient experiences a slow, progressive vision loss. IOP is normal until later stages of the disease. Closed-angle glaucoma is usually unilateral, has a sudden onset, and is accompanied by severe pain and blurry vision. Patients often report a rainbow halo around lights, and some will also experience nausea and vomiting. To diagnose glaucoma, a physician will use a gonio-scope, a lens with a simple microscope called a slit lamp, to look into the eye. A beam of light checks the angle between the iris and cornea to see how the aqueous humor is draining. Next, a tonometer is used to measure the pressure in the eye. Patients with at least three of the following signs are considered to be experiencing an acute-angle glaucoma: IOP exceeding 21 mm Hg, corneal epithelial edema, mid-dilated nonreactive pupil, and a shallow anterior chamber with a noted occlusion.

Treating glaucoma

The goal of open-angle glaucoma is to reduce the pressure before it causes progressive loss of vision. Treatment is usually lifelong.
• Prostaglandins: Increase the outflow of aqueous humor and reduce pressure.
• Beta-blockers: Reduce the production of fluid in the eye.
• Alpha-adrenergic agonists: Reduce the production of aqueous humor and increase outflow of the fluid in the eye.
• Miotic or cholinergic agents: Increase the outflow of fluid from the eye.
The goal of treatment for acute angle-closure glaucoma consists of IOP reduction, suppression of inflammation, and the reversal of angle closure.
• Treatment should not be delayed, or eyesight can be permanently damaged.
• Treatment will require both medication and a surgical procedure.
• Medication to constrict the pupil and reduce aqueous humor production will be used.
• Surgical procedure: Laser iridotomy to make a small opening in the iris. This allows for the fluid to flow freely.
• Instruct patient to sleep on the opposite side of the surgical eye.
• Avoid lifting anything over 5 lb.
• Avoid bearing down.
• Avoid aspirin to reduce the chance of bleeding.

Hordeolum (stye)

A common infection of the external structure of the eye is called a hordeolum or stye. Debris becomes blocked in the sebaceous gland of the eyelid and a small, painful, pus-filled lump on the underside or outside of the eyelid begins to form. A stye is usually caused from a *Staphylococcus* bacterial infection. Usually, external styes begin as a small spot next to an eyelash, which turns into a red, painful and swollen area and can last for several days. Once it bursts, it will begin to heal. A stye can also occur on the underside of the eyelid. This internal stye is less common but more severe. It will also cause a red, painful lump, but because of where it is located, a white head will never form.

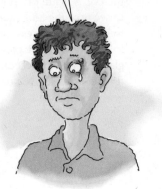

I guess I should have washed my hands after petting that pig...I now have a stye!

Preventing and treating styes

- Wash hands prior to touching the eye to reduce dirt and bacteria from entering the eye.
- Discourage rubbing the eye as this can increase irritation and bacteria.
- Protect eyes from foreign debris by wearing protective glasses when working outside.
- Replace eye makeup every 6 months as bacteria can grow in makeup.
- For frequent styes, wash eyelids regularly with baby shampoo mixed in warm water.
- Promptly treat any inflammation or infection of the eyelid.
- Warm, wet compresses for 5 to 10 minutes, three to six times a day.
- Do not squeeze or open the stye.
- Avoid contact lenses or wearing eye makeup with a stye.
- Antibiotic eye ointment or drops may be prescribed for difficult styes.
- The physician may lance a large stye to allow for drainage and healing.

Macular degeneration

Macular degeneration is the breakdown of cells in the macula; a portion of the retina, and surrounding tissues of the eye. Most of the time, macular degeneration begins appearing between the ages of 50 and 60 years. Age-related macular degeneration is known as the leading cause of vision loss in persons over the age of 65 years. There are two stages of macular degeneration, which affect different structures within the eye. The first stage is known as the "dry" stage. During this stage, the eye tissues will begin to degenerate.

The pigmented epithelial cells produce yellowish-white spots, which are deposited on the retina. These deposits eventually calcify, enlarge, and multiply. The second stage of macular degeneration is known as the exudative or "wet" stage. This stage affects the choroid, which is the layer immediately beneath the epithelial cells of the retina. A serous fluid leak containing choroidal blood vessels occurs and as a result, central vision is lost.

What to look for

Those who spend large amounts of time outdoors in the sunlight without wearing sunglasses are at an increased risk for developing macular degeneration. Several other risk factors for developing macular degeneration include hypertension, diets low in nutrients, a blue or light-colored iris, and hyperopia.

Battling illness

Treating macular degeneration

• Patients should be encouraged to eat a diet rich in vitamins A, E, C, zinc, and beta-carotene.
• Eating a diet rich in dark-green leafy vegetables may reduce the chances of developing the exudative "wet" stage of macular degeneration.
• Encourage the patient to use low-vision aids such as large-print books and magnifying screens, which can assist with the immediate vision loss.

What tests tell you

The loss of central vision is the primary sign of macular degeneration. Often patients will experience blurred vision due to the leaking of the serous fluid from the choroid. A physician may note yellowish round spots on the retina and macula or a dome-shaped deposit of retinal pigment epithelium by using an ophthalmoscope.

Ocular trauma

Trauma to the eye is a very common presenting problem in emergency departments. A total of 10% to 20% of ocular traumas result in temporary or permanent vision loss. The most common types of ocular injuries are foreign bodies, open wounds and contusions, and burns. Most ocular injuries could be prevented by wearing protective eyewear.

The Ocular Trauma Score (OTS) is a tool for predicting visual outcomes in trauma. The OTS has six variables, which provide the clinician with an understanding of the extent of the injury. The six variables are:

• initial vision (initial visual acuity)
• globe rupture
• endophthalmitis
• perforating injury
• retinal detachment
• relative afferent pupillary defect.

Common ocular injuries

- **Ruptured Globe:** Any full-thickness injury to the cornea, sclera, or both is considered an open-globe injury. Globe rupture occurs when the integrity of the outer membranes of the eye is disrupted by blunt or penetrating trauma. It may be accompanied by low visual clarity, visual impairment, or complete loss of vision.
- **Posttraumatic Endophthalmitis:** An intraocular infection involving the anterior and posterior segment of the eye after a traumatic open globe injury.
- **Hyphema:** A hemorrhage at the bottom of the anterior chamber of the eye.
- **Orbital Hematoma:** A true ocular emergency. Can cause vision loss within 90 minutes. The optic nerve is compressed by a hematoma.

- **Foreign Bodies:** Common foreign objects in the eye are eyelashes, sawdust, dirt, sand, cosmetics, contact lenses, metal particles.
- Young males are the most commonly affected population.
- **Chemical Injuries:** The most concerning chemical injuries are alkali injuries; alkali-containing agents (for example, bleach, commercial cleaners, fertilizers) cause the rapid disruption of the cell membranes and penetrate deep inside tissues.
- **Lens Dislocation/Detachment:** Most common cause is a direct blow to the eye or blunt trauma to the head or orbit. Retinal detachment is one of the most serious complications of a dislocated/displaced lens.

Treating ocular injuries

Foreign body in the eye
- Instruct the patient to not rub eyes.
- Blink repeatedly.
- If the particle is still in the eye, rinse with water or saline.

Direct blow to the eye
- Apply a cold compress without putting pressure on the eye.
- Over-the-counter pain medication like acetaminophen or ibuprofen can be used for pain.

Chemical exposure
- Instruct the patient to not rub eyes.

- Immediately flush out the eye with water for at least 15 minutes.
- Do not bandage the eye.

Ocular trauma
- Remove patient's glasses or contact lenses.
- Anesthetic eye drops should be instilled.
- Treat pain according to pain score.
- Attempt to irrigate nonpenetrating foreign body with 1 L of 0.9% saline.
- Use fluorescein drops to stain the eye to assess for minor corneal or subconjunctival abrasions.

Refractive errors

Common refractive errors include hyperopia (farsightedness) and myopia (nearsightedness).

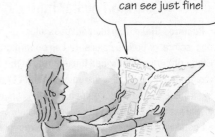

Wonder why the doctor thinks I need reading glasses. I can see just fine!

Hyperopia: farsightedness

Hyperopia is a visual problem associated with difficulty seeing objects that are near. Distance vision is not affected by hyperopia. Hyperopia is known as farsightedness and is the result of a shortened eyeball and a misshaped lens, which appears less round. When light enters the eye, the focus is behind the retina instead of directly to the retina in hyperopia patients.

What to look for

Individuals over 40 years of age are most commonly affected by hyperopia. Due to the aging process, the lens is less able to accommodate light, resulting in blurred vision. As a person ages, the lens naturally develops extra layers of tissue, which results in less lens flexibility. Age-related hyperopia is termed *presbyopia*. Presbyopia usually can be corrected using reading glasses.

A child diagnosed with hyperopia may outgrow the vision problem due to the ability to accommodate refractive error; however, in individuals over the age of 40, the ability to accommodate refractive errors is less likely, resulting in blurred vision.

Hyperopia is linked to genetics. If one or both biological parents have hyperopia, their children may experience the same vision problem. Diseases or disorders such as an eye tumor and retinopathy may also cause hyperopia.

What tests tell you

Individuals often report eyestrain after reading for long periods of time. Blurred vision, frequent headaches, and difficulty seeing at night are common symptoms of hyperopia. In children, frequent headaches, strabismus, rubbing, itching or blinking the eyes often, and reports of reading difficulties are common symptoms of hyperopia.

Treatment

Hyperopia may be corrected with prescription corrective eyeglasses or contact lenses. The prescription is based on the eye examination. Refractive procedures such as laser-assisted in situ keratomileusis (LASIK) can assist in reducing the refractive error. LASIK is a surgical procedure that permanently changes the shape of the cornea which, in turn, changes the refraction of light rays and can improve vision.

Myopia: nearsightedness

Myopia, also referred to as nearsightedness, is a visual problem affecting an individual's ability to see objects that are far away. The ability to see objects at a close distance is not impaired with myopia. Myopia is the most common refractive error of the eye, and it currently affects 40% of the US population. The prevalence of myopia is expected to rise to 50% of the world's population by 2050. Myopia occurs if the eyeball is too long or the cornea is too curved. Light entering the eye is not focused correctly, which results in distant objects appearing blurred.

Hold on...the answer is...20.

13 + 7 =

What to look for

There is a significant genetic link in myopia. If one or both biological parents have myopia, their children may experience the same vision problem. Individuals who spend long periods of time reading, working at a computer, or doing other intense close visual work may be more likely to develop myopia.

Myopia first occurs in school-aged children because the eye continues to grow during childhood. Around the age of 20, progression will stop. Adults with health conditions such as diabetes and have increased visual stress may also develop myopia.

What tests tell you

Myopia symptoms include blurry vision when looking at distant objects, frequent squinting to see objects clearly, headaches, and difficulty seeing at night while driving a vehicle. Children with myopia commonly squint, need to sit closer to the television or in front of the classroom, blink excessively, and rub their eyes.

Treatment

Myopia may be corrected with prescription corrective eyeglasses or contact lenses. The prescription is based on the eye examination. Refractive procedures such as LASIK can assist in reducing the refractive error.

Retinal detachment and retinal tears

A retinal tear occurs when the vitreous fluid, which is inside the eye, pulls on the retina causing it to develop tears. Retinal detachment is the sudden separation of the sensory retina from the retinal pigment epithelium. Vitreous fluid accumulates in the space beneath the retina and causes a separation of the retina from the choroidal blood supply. If not treated promptly, the detachment will continue and the retina may lose the ability to function. Depending on the severity of the untreated detachment, it may continue to worsen for hours or years until vision is completely lost.

What to look for

Persons with diabetes who have diabetic retinopathy are most at risk for developing retinal detachment. It is also most common in females. Other risk factors include age, a history of cataract surgery, ocular trauma, severe myopia, and a previous history of retinal detachment. Heredity may play a role in placing a patient at an increased risk.

What tests tell you

Retinal detachment is painless; however, most patients report a sudden loss of vision, which appears as a curtain flailing over the visual field. Often a burst of black spots or floaters, or flashes of light are reported, indicating bleeding and a separation of the retina has occurred.

 Battling illness

Treating retinal detachment

The goal of treatment for retinal detachment and retinal tear is to reattach the retina to the back wall of the eye and seal the tears or holes, which caused the detachment.
• Prompt surgical treatment is necessary to reduce the possible involvement of the macula, which often results in permanent loss of vision.
• If a retinal tear has not detached completely, it can be treated with a laser or cryo-therapy (freezing procedure).
• Retinal tears without symptoms can often be observed without treatment. These low-risk retinal tears can usually heal themselves.

Strabismus (crossed eyes)

Strabismus or crossed eyes is a condition in which both eyes do not focus on the same place at the same time. There are six muscles attached to each eye to control how it moves. The brain sends signals to these muscles to direct movement. If the eye muscle control is poor, one eye may turn in, out, up, or down. Symptoms are not always present, but appear when the person is tired or had excessive eye strain. Poor eye alignment can lead to double vision, poor depth perception, and low vision in the turned eye. Untreated eye turning can lead to reduced vision in one eye, called amblyopia or lazy eye. Strabismus develops in infants and young children under 3 years old.

Causes and risk factors of strabismus
• Family history
• Refractive error—Significant uncorrected farsightedness
• Medical conditions—Down syndrome, cerebral palsy, or those who have suffered a stroke or head injury are at higher risk for developing strabismus.

Treating strabismus

• Eyeglasses or contact lenses.
• Prism lenses—These lenses have a prescription for prism power in them. The prisms alter the light entering the eye and reduce how much turning the eye must do to view objects.
• Vision therapy—Visual activities to improve eye coordination and eye focusing. Vision therapy trains the eyes and brain to work together more effectively. These eye exercises can help correct problems with eye movement, eye focusing, and reinforce the eye–brain connection.
• Eye muscle surgery—Surgery can change the length or position of the muscles around the eye so they appear straight.

Retinoblastoma

Retinoblastoma, a disease of an infant or young child, is the most common primary intraocular cancer. A malignancy arises in the developing retina; tumor formation usually begins because of a mutation in the retinoblastoma tumor suppressor gene RB1. Signs of retinoblastoma include loss of the red reflex of the pupil, white-colored pupil (leukocoria), strabismus, redness, and pain of the affected eye. MRI can visualize the tumor, which is located on the optic nerve. Treatment involves surgical enucleation of the eye and chemotherapy.

Understanding the ear

The ear provides humans with the ability to hear sounds produced in the environment and with a sense of balance. The ear has three main parts: the outer ear, the middle ear, and the inner ear.

Outer (external) ear structures

The outer part of the ear collects sound as it travels through the auricle and the auditory canal to the eardrum.
• Auricle (also called the pinna)—cartilage covered by skin placed on opposite sides of the head.
• External auditory canal (also called the external acoustic meatus or ear canal).

The ear

The following illustration will help you visualize the structures of the ear.

The anatomy of the ear

This figure shows structures of the outer ear, the middle ear, and the inner ear.

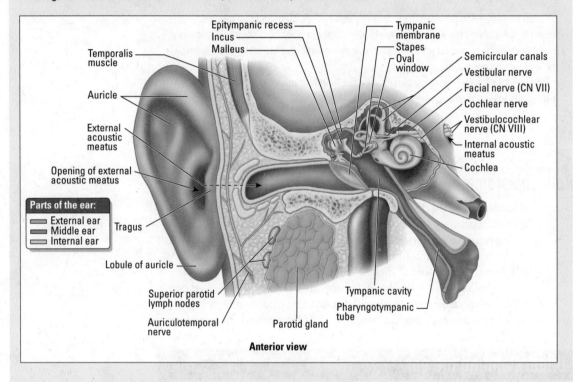

Anterior view

Middle ear structures

- Tympanic membrane (or ear drum).
- Auditory ossicles (three tiny bones that are attached):
  - Malleus (or hammer)—long handle bone attached to the eardrum.
  - Incus (or anvil)—the bridge bone between the malleus and the stapes.
  - Stapes (or stirrup)—the footplate; the smallest bone in the body.
- Eustachian tube (or pharyngotympanic tube).

Inner (internal) ear structures

- Oval window: a membrane-covered opening that connects the middle ear with the inner ear.
- Semicircular canals—filled with fluid; attached to cochlea and nerves; send information on balance and head position to the brain.
- Cochlea—spiral-shaped organ of hearing; transforms sound into signals that get sent to the brain.

How hearing occurs

Sound waves or vibrations pass through the outer, middle, and inner ear and eventually reach the brain for interpretation. As sound waves pass through the outer ear and ear canal, the eardrum vibrates. The vibrations are transmitted to the inner ear by the three tiny bones in the middle ear called the auditory ossicles. The inner ear then transmits the vibrations into electrical impulses to be decoded by the brain. When the vibrations reach the cochlea, the fluid moves, which results in a back and forth motion of tiny hairs (sensory receptors) lining the cochlea. This motion causes the sensory receptors to send a signal along the auditory nerve to the brain to then be interpreted as a type of sound.

What about balance?

The brain also works in response to visual, vestibular, and sensory system messages to produce a sensation of stability. When any of the impulses which the brain receives is disrupted, a sense of balance is disrupted.

The visual system (eyes) contributes to maintaining balance by providing an awareness of the surroundings and the position of the body in relation to the surroundings. The vestibular system (ears) detects circular and linear motion produced through actions such as stopping, starting, or turning. The sensory system contributes to maintaining balance by keeping track of the position of the body to the ground through movement and tension of the muscles and joints. When the brain receives the signals from these three systems, the information is interpreted, and a sensation of stability is produced.

Common disorders of the ear

In this section, you'll find information on some common ear disorders:

- Hearing loss—deafness
- Infections
- Meniere disease

Hearing loss—deafness

Hearing loss is the reduced ability to hear sound. Deafness is the inability to hear sound. There are many causes to both hearing loss and deafness, which can occur at any age. Complications of a virus, nerve damage, or injury caused by a loud noise may contribute to the sudden and complete loss of hearing. Three out of 1,000 babies are born deaf, and almost half of individuals over the age of 60 have hearing loss.

Hearing loss encompasses a wide range of severity with mild hearing problems on one end and profound, complete deafness on the other. Hearing loss can be categorized as conductive hearing loss or sensorineural hearing loss. Conductive hearing loss occurs when something blocks sound waves from reaching the inner ear. Conductive hearing loss commonly occurs in adults aged 60 or over due to cerumen accumulation in the ear canal. With older age also comes some loss of hearing that is a normal physiologic change, termed *presbycusis*. Sensorineural hearing loss occurs from damage to the inner ear or the nerves that send sound to the brain. Sensorineural hearing loss is most likely permanent and causes deafness.

What to look for

Disorders of the ear: A history of chronic ear infections, fluid buildup behind the eardrum, holes in the eardrum, and problems with the middle ear bones can lead to hearing loss.

Genetics: Genetics play a large role in both conductive and sensorineural hearing loss. Half of the children born with profound deafness have a genetic link to sensorineural hearing loss. Presbycusis, also known as age-associated hearing loss, has a genetic component as well. The sensitive hair cells which line the inner ear slowly decay causing this condition.

Occupational and recreational noises: A history of exposure to loud noises for prolonged periods of time such as working in construction, farming, and factory work. Explosive noises such as firearms can cause immediate permanent hearing loss. Other recreational noises such as listening to loud music for prolonged periods of time, playing an instrument in a band, or motorcycling can lead to hearing loss.

Infectious diseases and medical conditions: Infectious diseases like shingles, meningitis, German measles (rubella), or inner ear infections can lead to auditory nerve damage causing sensorineural hearing loss or deafness. Sensorineural hearing loss may also be caused from a stroke or tumors of the auditory nerve or brain. Presbycusis may be caused from circulatory problems or diabetes.

Medications: Some drugs such as antibiotic gentamicin and chemotherapy drugs may damage the inner ear. Tinnitus or hearing loss can be caused from high doses of acetylsalicylic acid, antimalarial drugs, or loop diuretics.

What tests tell you

Symptoms of hearing loss are easy to recognize if it suddenly occurs. Individuals will report a sudden change of hearing level. When hearing loss slowly progresses over time, symptoms may be difficult to recognize. Understanding conversations becomes difficult, the volume on the radio and television increases, and often people will speak louder or ask for something to be repeated.

High-frequency hearing loss is the most common symptom of age-related hearing loss. Those with higher pitched voices may be difficult to understand or tell the difference between similar sounds.

Signs of deafness in a young child or baby include not responding to noises or responding slowly. The ability to speak is severely delayed or does not occur by the expected age.

Battling illness

Treating hearing loss and deafness

The goal of treatment for hearing loss and/or deafness is to increase the ability to hear sounds. The sooner the hearing loss or deafness is diagnosed in infants and young children and treatment begins, the better the chances for speech and language skills development.
• Removable hearing aids amplify sound and make them easier for the inner ear to pick up.
• Analog hearing aids convert sound into electrical signals.
• Digital hearing aids convert sound into a code of numbers, and then change them back into sound.
• Digital hearing aids allows for greater flexibility.
• Surgically implanted hearing devices will send more sound vibrations to the inner ear.
• Middle ear implants are attached to the bones of the middle ear and assist the bones with sound wave

movement. These implants help with sensorineural hearing loss.
• Bone-anchored hearing aids are surgically placed in the bone behind the ear and assist with transmitting sound to the inner ear through the skull. These devices can be used for conductive and/or sensorineural hearing loss.
• Cochlear implants assist when the inner ear has severe damage, and profound deafness results. The cochlear implant bypasses the damaged part of the ear and sends signals directly to the auditory nerve that relays the sound to the brain. A microphone attaches behind the ear and a transmitter beneath the skin. Sound information goes to electrodes, which are placed in the inner ear during surgery.

Infections

The most common problems found with the ear are infections. Ear infections are primarily bacterial or fungal and can be acute or chronic. Ear infections can involve the external, middle, and inner ear.

Otitis externa is the most common ear pain in adults and results from excessive dryness or wetness, which damages the protective waxy lining of the external ear canal. Most often, water remains in the ear canal producing "swimmer's ear."

Otitis media most frequently occurs in children; however, adults can be affected as well. It is common for symptoms to occur suddenly and last for a short period of time. This is known as acute otitis media. Otitis media may also occur after a sudden change in air pressure causing trauma to the middle ear. This is common after air travel or scuba diving. Fluid may also form in the middle ear as a result of otitis media. During acute otitis media, the eustachian tube may swell and can be blocked causing a vacuum to develop. Fluid forms and becomes too thick to drain after the swelling subsides. This is known as serous otitis media. Repeated acute otitis media can lead to chronic otitis media, which then can lead to retraction of the eardrum, scarring and perforation of the eardrum, and even death of the ossicles. This results in conductive hearing loss.

Labyrinthitis (otitis interna)

Labyrinthitis, also known as otitis interna, refers to inner ear inflammation as a result of an infection. Because the inner ear has many structures which work to maintain balance and support hearing, infections may disrupt these functions. Otitis interna affects the labyrinth part of the inner ear known as the vestibule system.

What to look for

There are several known contributors for otitis interna. Individuals who experience a trauma to the head or have a surgical procedure on the ear may develop an inner ear infection, which can lead to inflammation of the inner ear. Viruses and bacterial infections such as the flu, mumps, measles, shingles, and other respiratory infections can lead to otitis interna. Autoimmune conditions can cause the body to react, which can lead to inflammation of the inner ear. Medications, alcohol, drugs, and other toxins can all contribute to otitis interna and potentially cause irreversible hearing loss.

What tests tell you

Nausea and vomiting may occur as the sense of balance may be disrupted and an individual will experience dizziness. Other symptoms include ear pain, a feeling of fullness in the ear, neck pain and stiffness, visual disturbances, headaches, and ear discharge.

Battling illness

Treating labyrinthitis

• Depending on the cause, IV antibiotics may be required if the infection is a result of bacteria.
• Viral infections may be treated with corticosteroids and other antiviral medications.
• Meclizine is a medication often prescribed.
• Assess for hearing permanent hearing loss after symptoms have resided.
• Encourage patients to avoid allergens, which can aggravate and cause irritation and inflammation.
• Discuss smoking cessation and avoiding secondhand cigarette smoke as smoke can irritate the delicate tissue inside the ear, which can cause inflammation leading to labyrinthitis.
• Encourage patients to wear ear protection when participating in contact sports as trauma to the ear can result in labyrinthitis.
• Educate patients on treating cold/flu symptoms to reduce the risk of illness progressing into an infection.

Meniere disease

Meniere disease is an inner ear disorder usually affecting one ear. Meniere disease is considered to be chronic because there is no cure. The disease will cause pressure or pain in the ear, dizziness or vertigo, hearing loss, or a ringing or roaring noise in the ear, also known as tinnitus. Attacks may occur multiple times over several days or may be isolated to every once in a while.

There is no exact cause of Meniere disease. There is an increase in volume and pressure of the innermost fluid of the inner ear, the endolymph, which is found in the labyrinth of the inner ear. A change in the volume and fluid pressure contributes to recurrent attacks of hearing loss, tinnitus, vertigo, and a sensation of fullness. Potential causes or triggers of Meniere disease include trauma, allergy, adrenal–pituitary insufficiency, hypothyroidism, alcohol use, stress, smoking, anxiety, a family history of the disease, recent viral illness, and migraines.

What to look for

Individuals in their 40s and 50s may be at higher risk for developing Meniere disease; however, the disease can occur at any age. Patients who have had a head injury or chronic middle ear infections are at an increased risk of developing Meniere disease. Individuals who experience a higher level of stress and anxiety are at an increased risk of frequent and severe attacks of the disease.

What tests tell you

Symptoms of Meniere disease vary from patient to patient. Symptoms in the early stage may last between 20 minutes and 24 hours and will include episodes of vertigo, a feeling of fullness in the ear, hearing loss that resolves after the episode fades, and tinnitus.

During the middle stage of the disease, vertigo symptoms lessen; however, hearing loss and tinnitus will increase in severity. Often long periods of remission are reported during this stage.

The late stage of Meniere disease is associated with hearing loss and tinnitus, which is progressively worse, and balance is generally affected. Anxiety and depression is often reported during this stage.

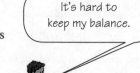

It's hard to keep my balance.

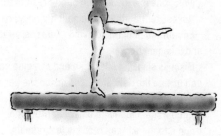

Battling illness

Treating Meniere disease

The goals of treatment for Meniere disease are to decrease the frequency and severity of attacks. Many treatment options involve patients changing their habits, diet, or taking medications to reduce the amount of fluid in the inner ear.
• Patients should be encouraged to reduce intake of sodium-rich foods and beverages as salt can increase water retention.
• Meclizine may be prescribed.
• Tinnitus symptoms are worsened by increased caffeine intake. Encourage patients to decrease or avoid caffeine.
• Because the body's metabolism actively moves and regulates bodily fluids during digestion, eating several smaller meals throughout the day can improve symptoms.
• Encourage smoking cessation as symptoms may be reduced after quitting smoking.
• Patients should be encouraged to reduce stress and anxiety as both have been linked to Meniere disease.

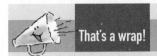

Understanding the sensory system

The sensory system is made up of the visual and auditory components of the body.

The eye

Components of the eye

- The external structure of each eye contains the eyelids and eyelashes, conjunctiva, sclera, cornea, pupil, and iris.
- The internal structures of each eye include the choroid, ciliary body, lens, macula, retina, aqueous humor, vitreous humor, and optic nerve.

How the eye works

- The cornea is responsible for focusing light.
- The iris controls the amount of light reaching the back of the eye by adjusting the pupil size.
- The eye's lens sits behind the pupil, and automatically focuses the light.
- The light, focused by the cornea and lens, reaches the retina, which converts images into electronic signals.
- The optic nerve transmits the electronic signals to the visual cortex of the brain, which controls our sense of sight.

Common disorders of the eye

- Blindness—the inability to see anything, including light.
- Cataracts—clouding of the normally translucent lens of the eye.
- Conjunctivitis—also known as "pinkeye"; an infection or inflammation of the eye.
- Glaucoma—an acute or chronic condition in which an increase in intraocular pressure (IOP) interferes with sight.
- Hordeolum—also known as a "stye," this is a common eye infection that occurs when debris is blocked in the eyelid's sebaceous gland. A painful, pus-filled lump occurs on the under or outer side of the eyelid.
- Macular degeneration—the breakdown of macula cells that leads to vision loss.

- Ocular injuries—trauma involving foreign bodies, open wounds, contusions, and/or burns.
- Refractive errors—hyperopia (farsightedness) and myopia (nearsightedness).
- Retinal detachment and tears—occurs when vitreous fluid inside the eye pulls on the retina, creating a tear. This can be a visual emergency, if not treated promptly.
- Strabismus—also known as "crossed eyes"; a condition in which both eyes do not focus on the same place at the same time.

The ear

Components of the ear

- Outer ear—contains the auricle (pinna), and external auditory canal.
- Middle ear—contains the tympanic membrane (ear drum), auditory ossicles (malleus/hammer, incus/anvil, and stapes/stirrup), and eustachian tube.
- Inner ear—contains the oval window, semicircular canals, cochlea, and auditory tube.

How the ear works

- Sound waves pass through the outer, middle, and inner ear, and reach the brain for interpretation.
- The ears detect circular and linear motion, and contribute to maintaining a sense of balance.

Common disorders of the ear

- Hearing loss—the inability to hear sound; can be caused by ear disorders, genetics, excessive noise, infections or medical conditions, and/or medications.
- Infections—the most common problem associated with the ear. These can be bacterial or fungal, and acute or chronic.
- Meniere disease—this chronic condition usually affects one ear. It is characterized by pressure or pain in the ear, dizziness or vertigo, hearing loss, and/or a ringing or roaring noise in the ear.

Quick quiz

1. Which of the following conditions most commonly affects the external structures of the eye?
   A. Infections and inflammatory responses
   B. Macular degeneration
   C. Retinal detachment
   D. Presbyopia

Answer: A. Infections and inflammatory responses of the eye are the most common conditions affecting the external structures of the eye.

2. Which are most common types of conjunctivitis? (Select all that apply.)
   A. Allergic
   B. Fungal
   C. Bacterial
   D. Viral

Answer: A, C, and D. The three most common types of conjunctivitis are bacterial, viral, and allergic conjunctivitis.

3. Which eye disorder is characterized by an increase in intraocular pressure (IOP) within the anterior chamber of the eye?
   A. Cataract
   B. Macular degeneration
   C. Glaucoma
   D. Ruptured globe

Answer: C. Glaucoma is characterized by an increase in intraocular pressure (IOP) within the anterior chamber of the eye.

4. What is the most common problem associated with the ear?
   A. Deafness
   B. Infections
   C. Meniere disease
   D. Acoustic neuroma

Answer: B. The most common problems found with the ear are infections. Ear infections are primarily bacterial or fungal and can be acute or chronic.

5. Hearing loss can be categorized as which of the following?
   A. Conductive hearing loss or sensorineural hearing loss
   B. Infectious hearing loss or primary hearing loss
   C. Benign hearing loss or neurological hearing loss
   D. Subjective hearing loss or objective hearing loss

Answer: A. Hearing loss can be categorized as conductive hearing loss or sensorineural hearing loss. Conductive hearing loss occurs when something blocks sound waves from reaching the inner ear. Sensorineural hearing loss occurs from damage to the inner ear or the nerves that send sound to the brain.

Scoring

☆☆☆ If you answered all five items correctly, hurray! You're great—it's plain to see you know your stuff!

☆☆ If you answered four items correctly, right on! Extra, extra, let's hear all about it!

☆ If you answered fewer than three items correctly, "eye" know you will astutely narrow down the answers the next time.

Suggested references

Bielory, L., Delgado, L., Katelaris, C. H., Leonardi, A., Rosario, N., & Vichyanoud, P. (2020). ICON: Diagnosis and management of allergic conjunctivitis. *Annals of Allergy, Asthma & Immunology, 124*(2), 118–134. https://doi.org/10.1016/j.anai.2019.11.014

Centers for Disease Control and Prevention (CDC). (2021a). Hearing loss. https://www.cdc.gov/hearingloss/default.html

Centers for Disease Control and Prevention (CDC). (2021b). Types of hearing loss. https://www.cdc.gov/ncbddd/hearingloss/types.html

Centers for Disease Control and Prevention (CDC). (2022a). Vision loss: A public health problem. https://www.cdc.gov/visionhealth/basic_information/vision_loss.htm

Centers for Disease Control and Prevention (CDC). (2022b). Common eye disorders and diseases. https://www.cdc.gov/visionhealth/basics/ced/fastfacts.htm

Cicinelli, M. V., Buchan, J. C., Nicholson, M., Varadaraj, V., & Khanna, R. C. (2023). Cataracts. *Lancet (London, England), 401*(10374), 377–389. https://doi.org/10.1016/S0140-6736(22)01839-6

Gordon, A. A., Danek, D. J., & Phelps, P. O. (2020). Common inflammatory and infectious conditions of the eyelid. *Disease-a-Month, 66*(10), 101042. https://doi.org/10.1016/j.disamonth.2020.101042

Gordon, A. A., Tran, L. T., & Phelps, P. O. (2020). Eyelid and orbital trauma for the primary care physician. *Disease-a-Month, 66*(10), 101045. https://doi.org/10.1016/j.disamonth.2020.101045

Harb, E. N., & Wildsoet, C. F. (2019). Origins of refractive errors: Environmental and genetic factors. *Annual Review of Vision Science, 5*, 47–72. https://doi.org/10.1146/annurev-vision-091718-015027

Hashmi, M. F., Gurnani, B., & Benson, S. (2022). *Conjunctivitis*. In *StatPearls*. StatPearls Publishing. https://www.ncbi.nlm.nih.gov/books/NBK541034/

Hogan, C. J., & Tadi, P. (2022). *Ear examination*. In *StatPearls*. StatPearls Publishing. https://www.ncbi.nlm.nih.gov/books/NBK556014/

Hoskin, J. L. (2022). Ménière's disease: New guidelines, subtypes, imaging, and more. *Current Opinion in Neurology, 35*(1), 90–97. https://doi.org/10.1097/WCO.0000000000001021

Jackson, E. A., & Geer, K. (2023, February). Acute otitis externa: Rapid evidence review. *American Family Physician, 107*(2), 145–151.

Jain, S. (2022, March). Diplopia: Diagnosis and management. *Clinical Medicine, 22*(2), 104–106. https://doi.org/10.7861/clinmed.2022-0045.

McGinley, T. C. Jr. (2022). Adult eye conditions: Common eye conditions. *FP Essentials, 519*, 11–18.

Norris, T. (2025). *Porth's pathophysiology: Concepts of altered health states*, 11th ed. Wolters Kluwer.

Peeler, C. E., & Gonzalez, E. (2022). Retinoblastoma. *The New England Journal of Medicine, 386*(25), 2412. https://doi.org/10.1056/NEJMicm2118356

Pflugfelder, S. C., & Stern, M. E. (2020). The cornea in keratoconjunctivitis sicca. *Experimental Eye Research, 201*, 108295. https://doi.org/10.1016/j.exer.2020.108295

Schmidt, C. H., Volpe, N. J., & Bryar, P. J. (2021, May). Eye disease in medical practice: What you should know and why you should know it. *Medical Clinics of North America, 105*(3), 397–407. https://doi.org/10.1016/j.mcna.2021.02.001.

Shah, S. M., & Khanna, C. L. (2020). Ophthalmic emergencies for the clinician. *Mayo Clinic Proceedings, 95*(5), 1050–1058. https://doi.org/10.1016/j.mayocp.2020.03.018

Stein, J. D., Khawaja, A. P., & Weizer, J. S. (2021). Glaucoma in adults-screening, diagnosis, and management: A review. *JAMA, 325*(2), 164–174. https://doi.org/10.1001/jama.2020.21899

Strayer, D., Saffitz, J., & Rubin, E. (2020). *Rubin's pathology: Mechanisms of disease*, 8th ed. Wolters Kluwer.

Szmuilowicz, J., & Young, R. (2019). Infections of the ear. *Emergency Medicine Clinics of North America, 37*(1), 1–9. https://doi.org/10.1016/j.emc.2018.09.001

Chapter 13

Reproductive system*

Just the facts

In this chapter, you'll learn:

♦ the structures of the reproductive system

♦ how the reproductive system functions

♦ pathophysiology, signs and symptoms, diagnostic tests, and treatments for common reproductive disorders.

Understanding the reproductive system

The reproductive system is a group of internal and external organs, as well as complex hormonal components, that work together on the critical task of procreation of the human species.

The female reproductive system

The female reproductive system has two major components. They include:

1. the external and internal physical structures
2. the hormonal components that control sexual response, ovulation, and the endometrial cycles

The external female genital structures or vulva include the:

- mons pubis
- labia majora
- labia minora
- clitoris
- vestibular glands
- vaginal vestibule
- vaginal orifice
- urethral opening
- perineum

(See *A close look at the female reproductive system.*)

---

*Note: In this chapter, the term "male" refers to a person assigned male at birth, and the term "female" refers to a person assigned female at birth.

A close look at the female reproductive system

This illustration shows the organs of the female (external and internal) reproductive system.

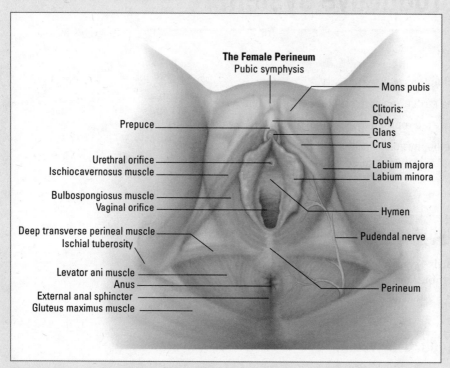

The Female Perineum

- Pubic symphysis
- Mons pubis
- Clitoris:
  - Body
  - Glans
  - Crus
- Prepuce
- Urethral orifice
- Ischiocavernosus muscle
- Labium majora
- Labium minora
- Bulbospongiosus muscle
- Vaginal orifice
- Hymen
- Deep transverse perineal muscle
- Ischial tuberosity
- Pudendal nerve
- Levator ani muscle
- Anus
- External anal sphincter
- Gluteus maximus muscle
- Perineum

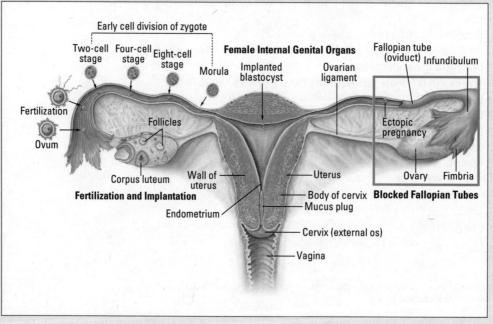

Early cell division of zygote

- Two-cell stage
- Four-cell stage
- Eight-cell stage
- Morula

Female Internal Genital Organs

- Implanted blastocyst
- Ovarian ligament
- Fallopian tube (oviduct)
- Infundibulum
- Fertilization
- Follicles
- Ectopic pregnancy
- Ovum
- Corpus luteum
- Wall of uterus
- Uterus
- Ovary
- Fimbria
- **Fertilization and Implantation**
- **Blocked Fallopian Tubes**
- Endometrium
- Body of cervix
- Mucus plug
- Cervix (external os)
- Vagina

The mons pubis lies over the symphysis pubis and, in the adult female, is covered with pubic hair. The labia majora and minora help protect the inner vulvar structures and are highly vascular. Hair follicles are found only on the majora. The labia minora fuse to form the prepuce (clitoris hood) and frenulum (fold under the clitoris). The clitoris is composed of erectile tissue and increases in size during sexual arousal.

The vaginal vestibule contains the urethra opening (usually below the clitoris), vagina, Skene glands (which lubricate the vagina), and Bartholin glands (which produce clear mucus to lubricate the vaginal opening). The perineum is the area between the anus and fourchette and covers the pelvic structures.

Other external structures that are considered part of the female reproductive system include the breasts. The breasts are mammary glands, which are made of lobes that are divided into lobules or clusters of acini. These acini are lined with epithelial cells that secrete colostrum and milk after birth and connect to ducts. Cooper ligaments separate and support the acini and milk ducts. Each breast has a nipple with openings to the milk ducts and is surrounded by the areola. The areolas contain Montgomery tubercles that secrete a fatty substance that lubricates the nipple. Nodules may develop just before and during menstruation based on the effects of estrogen and progesterone. The breasts function as food production for an infant (milk) and as organs of sexual arousal in the adult female.

The internal female reproductive structures include the:
- vagina
- uterus
- uterine tubes (fallopian tubes)
- ovaries

The vagina is a canal between the bladder and rectum that connects the vulva and uterus. There are folds in the vagina, called *rugae*, found during reproductive years that allow for stretching during childbirth and coitus. The vagina serves as the birth canal following conception, allows menstrual fluid to leave the body, and receives the penis during coitus. The cervix, which is part of the uterus, is found at the upper end of the vagina and dilates during child birth. The uterus (or womb) is a muscular organ and the fundus sits at the top of the uterus, which is where the fallopian tubes (also called *uterine tubes*) enter the uterus. The fallopian tubes provide a passage from the ovaries to the uterus allowing ovum and sperm to move through them. The uterus is the site for reception, implantation, retention, and nutrition for the fertilized ovum and later the fetus during pregnancy, as well as cyclic menstruation. There are two ovaries that are on each side of the uterus below and behind the uterine tubes. During reproductive years (after menarche and before menopause), the ovaries produce ovum (ovulation), and they yield estrogen, progesterone, and androgen hormones.

Hypothalamic–pituitary and ovulation cycles

Estrogen and progesterone are the major hormones in the female reproductive system (see *Hormonal components of the female reproductive system*). Low blood levels of these hormones stimulate the hypothalamus to secrete gonadotropin-releasing hormone (GnRH), which causes the anterior pituitary to secrete follicle-stimulating hormone (FSH). FSH stimulates the production of estrogen. Low levels of estrogen stimulate release of luteinizing hormone (LH) from the anterior pituitary, which stimulates the release of the ovum. Before the ovum is released, follicles begin to develop. After the release of the ovum, these follicles mature into a corpus luteum. If fertilization and implantation of the ovum does not occur, progesterone and estrogen levels decline and the corpus luteum degenerates, and menstruation occurs. The cycle then starts again.

The endometrial/menstrual cycle

The endometrial/menstrual cycle consists of the growing and shedding of the uterine walls and consists of four phases. The proliferative phase occurs when there is rapid growth of the endometrial surface of the uterus. The secretory phase starts with the day of ovulation to the around 3 days before bleeding menstruation occurs. Because large amounts of progesterone are present, the endometrial lining becomes very vascular and thick awaiting implantation of the fertilized ovum. If implantation does not occur, there is a reduction of estrogen and progesterone levels, causing the uterine arteries to spasm, and blockage of the blood supply to the endometrium ensues. This is the ischemic (premenstrual) phase. Necrosis develops, the large endometrial lining sloughs off, and menstruation (or the menstrual phase) begins.

Hormonal components of the female reproductive system

There are three cycles that effect the female reproductive system:
• Hypothalamic–pituitary cycle
• Ovarian cycle
• Endometrial/menstrual cycle

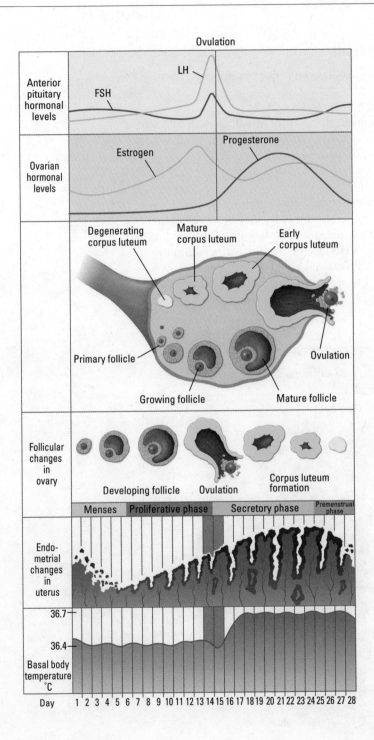

The male reproductive system

The male reproductive system has two major components. They include:

1. the external and internal physical structures
2. the hormonal components that control sexual response and semen production

The external male reproductive structures consist of the:

- penis
- scrotum (testicles)

(See *A close look at the male reproductive system*.)

The penis is a long shaft with a bulbous-shaped tip called the *glans penis*, which may be or may not have foreskin. During sexual arousal, the penis becomes erect as the erectile tissues within the shaft become engorged with arterial blood and compress the veins. The scrotum is a pouch-like sac located behind the penis that holds and protects the testicles, epididymis, and the spermatic cord.

A close look at the male reproductive system

This illustration shows the organs of the male (external and internal) reproductive system.

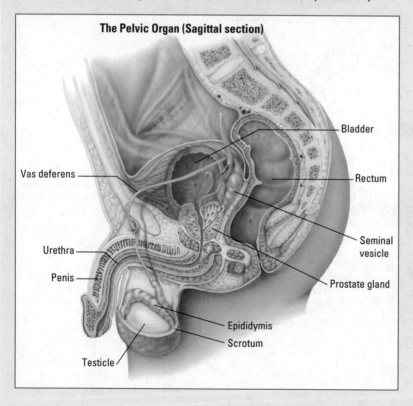

The Pelvic Organ (Sagittal section)

- Vas deferens
- Urethra
- Penis
- Testicle
- Epididymis
- Scrotum
- Bladder
- Rectum
- Seminal vesicle
- Prostate gland

The cremaster and dartos muscles bring the scrotum away from the body in heat and toward the body in cooler temperatures. The scrotum is connected to the body by the inguinal canal.

The internal male reproductive structures include the:
- epididymis
- vas deferens
- accessory glands (seminal vesicles, the prostate gland, and bulbo-urethral glands)

The epididymis is a mass of tightly coiled tubes that lay against the testicles that act as a storage and maturation site for sperm. The vas deferens or sperm duct is a tube that connects the epididymis to the pelvic cavity and carries the sperm to the ejaculatory duct in the penis, which leads to the outside of the body.

The three accessory glands all provide fluids that nourish the sperm cells and lubricate the duct system. The seminal vesicles are located behind the bladder and join with the vas deferens to become the ejaculatory duct. The prostate is a small, glandular organ that surrounds the urethra. The bulbourethral glands (also known as Cowper glands) are below the prostate and add fluid to the ejaculate that occurs with erection and expulsion of semen.

Testosterone is primarily secreted by the testicles but is also secreted in small amounts by ovaries and the adrenal glands. This hormone in males causes the maturation of the male sex organs, spermatogenesis, increased libido, and male secondary sex characteristics such as facial, axillary and pubic hair, and deepening voice.

Reproductive disorders

The disorders discussed in this section include:
- fibroadenomas
- endometriosis
- uterine leiomyoma (fibroids)
- pelvic organ prolapse
- polycystic ovary syndrome (PCOS)
- vaginal candidiasis (VC)
- cervical cancer
- other human papillomavirus (HPV)-associated cancers
  - These include HPV-induced anorectal, penile, vulvar, and oropharyngeal cancers.
- endometrial cancer
- ovarian cancer
- breast cancer
- benign prostatic hyperplasia (BPH)
- prostatitis
- prostate cancer
- testicular cancer
- sexually transmitted infections (STIs)

Fibroadenomas

Fibroadenomas are benign, painless tumors of the female breast that often occur during the childbearing years. Glandular tissue and connective tissue form a compact, firm, well-defined lump. Fibroadenomas are very rare in males as the cause is considered to be hormone specific in females.

Prevention

The incidence of fibroadenomas is lower in females who:
- have a higher intake of fruits and vegetables
- participate in moderate exercise
- have multiple live births
- do not use or use fewer oral contraceptives

What tests tell you

These tests are used to diagnose fibroadenomas:
- Clinical examination and palpation of breast tissue and lump.
- Diagnostic mammography revealing a breast mass with smooth, round edges, distinct from the surrounding breast tissue.
- Breast ultrasonography confirms the breast lump especially in dense breast tissue. This test may be ordered before the mammography if the patient is less than 30 years old. Ultrasound helps further assess the lump to determine if it is solid (fibroadenoma) vs. fluid filled (cyst).
- Fine needle aspiration may be used to collect a sample of the tissue for laboratory analysis; a thin needle may be inserted into the lump or a core needle biopsy may be used, where ultrasound is used to help guide needle insertion.

Battling illness

Treating fibroadenomas

A "wait-and-see" approach is a common treatment for fibroadenomas as they are noncancerous, painless tumors. Slow growth rates are considered safe and treatment may not be necessary. Other treatment options include:
- acetaminophen and nonsteroidal anti-inflammatory drugs and athletic bras can help relieve symptoms
- treatment with vitamin E and evening primrose oil to relieve symptoms of fibrocystic changes have also been used recently
- high-intensity ultrasound
- cryoablation (extremely cold temperatures [to destroy the enlarged cells], which are then reabsorbed by the body)
- surgical excision

Endometriosis

Endometriosis is usually a chronic condition that occurs when the tissue that normally grows inside the uterus grows outside the uterus on surrounding internal structures such as the ovaries, and uterine (fallopian) tubes. The endometrial tissue continues to act like uterus tissue by thickening, breaking down, and bleeding in response to hormonal influences. The tissue becomes trapped, which usually causes pain, especially during menstruation. However, some people do not have symptoms.

Endometriosis occurs in reproductive females in their 30s or 40s but can start in adolescence. Although it can be debilitating, it rarely causes death.

How it happens

The cause of endometriosis is not completely clear. Some theories include:

- retrograde menstruation, where endometrial tissue exits the uterus during menstrual flow through the uterine tubes and attaches itself to other surfaces in the abdominal cavity. However, this does not explain all cases, and not all people who have retrograde menstruation develop endometriosis
- embryonic cell transformation, where cells with the potential to become endometrial tissue are found in the wrong place during embryonic development
- autoimmune component, where the immune system does not recognize and destroys the endometrial tissue outside the uterus
- surgical scar implantation, where endometrial cells may implant following a cesarean birth or hysterectomy along the surgical incision
- endometrial cell transport, where endometrial cells are transported through the blood or lymphatic system to other parts of the body

Getting complicated

When endometriosis obstructs the uterine tube, the sperm and ovum cannot unite, or the sperm and ovum can be damaged by the endometrial tissue. This is caused by adhesions that may form around the uterus or uterine tubes. People with endometriosis have a higher incidence of ovarian cancer and adenocarcinoma.

What to look for

The most common symptom is pelvic pain that usually occurs during menstruation, called *dysmenorrhea*. Other symptoms include:

- pain with intercourse
- pain with bowel movements or urination, usually during menstruation

- excessive bleeding during periods called *menorrhagia* or bleeding between periods called *menometrorrhagia*
- infertility
- fatigue, diarrhea, constipation, bloating, or nausea, usually during menstrual periods

What tests tell you

Although healthcare providers may feel endometrial growths during a pelvic examination, diagnosis cannot be confirmed by pelvic examination. Tests to determine endometriosis diagnosis include:

- pelvic ultrasound to identify endometriomas (cysts from endometriosis)
- laparoscopy is the "gold standard" diagnostic procedure for endometriosis; it allows visualization and biopsy of the lesions

---

Battling illness

Treating endometriosis

Treatment for endometriosis is usually pharmacological or surgical in nature.

Drug therapy
Drug therapy usually starts conservatively. These medications include:
• Nonsteroidal anti-inflammatory drugs (NSAIDs) like ibuprofen, or naproxen, which can decrease pain associated with menstruation.
• Hormone therapy which can assist with reducing pain during menstruation, slowing endometrial growth, and preventing further implantation.
• Hormonal contraceptives can reduce menstrual flow and duration, which can reduce pain.
• Gonadotropin-releasing hormone (GnRH) agonists and antagonists can cause the endometrial tissue to shrink. These medications do induce artificial menopause.

Low-dose estrogen or progesterone may be prescribed in conjunction to reduce the side effects associated with menopause such as vaginal dryness and hot flashes.
• Progestin-only contraceptives, as found in some IUDs or Depo-Provera, can stop menstrual periods and the growth of endometrial implants.

Surgery
During laparoscopy, the surgeon may remove endometric tissue, especially if the patient is trying to become pregnant or is having severe pain from endometriosis. However, conservative surgery has no guarantee that the endometriosis will not return. In severe cases, a hysterectomy may be performed, but if the ovaries remain, the estrogen produced by them still may stimulate any remaining endometriosis.

Uterine leiomyoma (fibroids)

A uterine leiomyoma (also called a *fibroid*) is a tumor of the smooth muscle that is usually benign, and most commonly found in the uterus.

Many females develop fibroid tumors; however, in some cases, fibroids do not cause symptoms, and people are unaware they have them. Risk factors for developing fibroids include:

- heredity and early menstruation
- ethnicity (risk is greater in African American females)
- environmental factors such as obesity, vitamin D deficiency, high red meat intake, alcohol intake, and low green vegetable, fruit, and dairy intake

How it happens

Although researchers are still studying the cause of leiomyoma, possible causes include:

- genetic changes in that the genes in fibroids are different from the normal uterine muscle cells
- hormones of estrogen and progesterone can promote the growth of fibroids so after menopause fibroids may decrease
- growth factors that help maintain tissues like insulin-like growth factor may promote growth of fibroids

What to look for

Although leiomyoma is not life threatening, symptoms can greatly affect activities of daily living. These symptoms may include:

- heavy or prolonged menstrual bleeding
- frequent urination or difficulty emptying the bladder
- constipation
- pelvic pressure/pain
- back or leg pain

What tests tell you

Leiomyoma can be found on a routine pelvic examination; however, other tests are used to confirm diagnosis. Those tests may include:

- ultrasound either transabdominal or transvaginal
- magnetic resonance imaging (MRI)
- hysterosonography and hysterosalpingography
- hysteroscopy
- complete blood count (CBC)

Treating uterine leiomyoma

There are many treatment options for uterine leiomyomas.

But just wait...
Because fibroids are usually not cancerous, don't interfere with pregnancy, and may shrink on their own, sometimes the treatment by the healthcare provider is "watchful waiting." If the fibroids cause symptoms, treatment options are explored.

Drug therapy
Drug therapy does not eliminate uterine fibroids. However, it may shrink them. Drugs are commonly used to regulate the menstrual cycle, decrease menstrual bleeding, and reduce pelvic pressure. These drugs include:
• Gonadotropin-releasing hormone (GnRH) agonists. These drugs block estrogen and progesterone production, which stops menstruation and induces menopause. This can shrink the fibroids and may improve anemia associated with prolonged menstruation. However, this should not be used as a long-term therapy because bone loss can occur.
• Progestin-releasing intrauterine device (IUD). An IUD can help to relieve heavy bleeding caused by fibroids, but it does not shrink the fibroids. This therapy may be another option if the patient does not want to become pregnant.
• Tranexamic acid. This nonhormonal drug can be used to reduce heavy menstrual periods, possibly decreasing anemia.
• Oral contraceptives (OCs). OCs are hormones commonly referred to as birth control pills, because they work to prevent pregnancy. However, they are also used to regulate menstruation and to control bleeding associated with fibroids.
• Nonsteroidal anti-inflammatory drugs (NSAIDs). Drugs from this category are nonhormonal and are used primarily to reduce the pain associated with menstruation.
• Vitamins and iron. B vitamins and iron are used as a supplement to reduce anemia that can occur with heavy menstrual bleeding.

MRI-guided focused ultrasound surgery
Focused ultrasound surgery (FUS) is a noninvasive treatment option where fibroids that are found during an MRI equipped with a high-energy ultrasound transducer can be destroyed by sound waves and heat. This treatment option is generally limited to specialized clinics.
Other procedures that may be used include:
• uterine artery embolization, which cuts off blood flow to the fibroid(s)
• myolysis, which is a laparoscopic procedure that uses an electric current or laser to destroy fibroids. Cryomyolysis has the same effect only by freezing the fibroids
• laparoscopic or robotic myomectomy surgery for removal of fibroids
• endometrial ablation, which uses heat to destroy the lining of the uterus; however, this permanently ends menstruation
• abdominal myomectomy, which is abdominal surgery to remove very large and deep fibroids
• hysterectomy, which is a surgical procedure, used as a last resort removing the uterus and therefore the fibroids

Pelvic organ prolapse

When the muscles and the ligaments in a woman's pelvis loosen, or weaken, the organs in the pelvis can slip out of place creating a bulge (usually in the vagina), which is called a *prolapse*. This usually occurs over time, long after childbirth, a hysterectomy, and menopause.

How it happens and what to look for...

As the muscles/ligaments weaken, bulging occurs in the vagina. People who experience pelvic organ prolapse do not usually experience pain and may not have any symptoms. If symptoms do occur, they may include:

- painful intercourse
- a feeling as if something is coming out of the vagina
- urinary concerns, like leaking of urine, or chronic urge to urinate
- low back pain
- feeling of pressure or fullness in the pelvic area

What tests tell you

Besides a pelvic examination by a healthcare provider to determine the type of prolapse and possibly replace the prolapse, other tests that may be done depend on symptoms and problems that the patient is experiencing including:

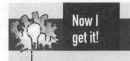

Pelvic organ prolapse

Over time, due to muscle/ligament weakening in the pelvis, the pelvic organs can prolapse into the vagina.

Battling illness

Treating pelvic organ prolapse

Treatment for pelvic organ prolapse will depend on how severe symptoms are.

Just wait and see...
- If quality of life is not impeded, the healthcare provider will monitor the prolapse and no treatment may be used.

Drug therapy
- Topical estrogen therapy may be used for vaginal dryness that can occur due to the prolapse.

Physical therapy
- Pelvic floor exercises with biofeedback may be used to strengthen the pelvic muscles.

Pessaries
- Use of a silicone device, called a *pessary*, may be placed in the vagina to hold the pelvic organs in place.

Surgery
Depending on the location of the prolapse, there are different surgical procedures. A posterior prolapse involves the rectum and is called a *rectocele*. The bulge is reduced by securing the connective tissue between the vagina and rectum. An anterior prolapse encompasses the bladder and is called a *cystocele*. The bulge is reduced by securing the connective tissue between the vagina and the bladder and putting the bladder back in its proper position. A uterine prolapse is specific to the uterus and usually requires removal of the uterus (hysterectomy). A vaginal vault prolapse, or *enterocele*, occurs at the apex of the vagina and can involve the bladder, rectum, and small bowel. An enterocele is surgically repaired by returning all organs to their respective, correct anatomical location.

Prevention of pelvic organ prolapse includes:
- smoking cessation
- weight loss
- treatment for conditions that cause strain to the pelvic floor like constipation or chronic cough
- strengthen core and pelvic floor muscles

- bladder function tests, which may be done to determine if the bladder is leaking, how it empties, and if there is bladder damage
- pelvic floor strength tests, which determine the strength of sphincter and pelvic floor muscles, as well as the strength of ligaments that support the vaginal walls, uterus, rectum, urethra, and bladder
- MRI, which is used in complex cases for a 3D image
- ultrasound, also used in complex cases, to view kidneys, bladder, and muscles around the anus

Polycystic ovary syndrome

PCOS occurs in females when there is an endocrine imbalance and high levels of estrogen, testosterone, and LH with decreasing secretion of FSH.

How it happens

Although not completely understood, PCOS is thought to be caused by a combination of heredity and environmental factors. Numerous follicles (polycystic) develop on the ovaries, which produce excess estrogen, causing the ovaries to enlarge and fail to regularly release eggs.

What to look for

Females with PCOS may have infrequent or prolonged menstrual periods and excessive male hormone levels. PCOS is usually diagnosed in adolescence when symptoms appear. Other symptoms may include:

- acne
- obesity
- hirsutism (excessive hair growth in male pattern, such as the face, chest, and back)
- amenorrhea

Getting complicated

If obesity is not controlled, complications can occur. Complications can include:

- infertility
- hyperinsulinemia
- nonalcoholic fatty liver disease
- cardiovascular disease
- sleep apnea
- abnormal uterine bleeding
- endometrial cancer
- depression, anxiety, and eating disorders
- miscarriage or premature birth

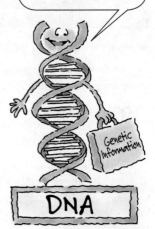

PCOS is thought to be caused by a combination of heredity and environmental factors in females in their reproductive years.

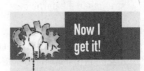

Now I get it!

PCOS can be complicated, but keeping a healthy weight can reduce associated complications.

What tests tell you

Although there are no definitive tests to diagnose PCOS, the following tests may be combined to help make the diagnosis of PCOS:

- Pelvic examination to inspect reproductive organs for masses, growths, and other abnormalities
- Blood test to analyze hormone levels, glucose levels, and cholesterol/triglyceride levels
- Transvaginal ultrasound to view the ovaries and the lining of the uterus
- Screening for depression and anxiety
- Screening for obstructive sleep apnea

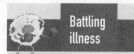

Battling illness

Treating PCOS

Treatment is individualized and is often based on symptoms, fertility needs, and prevention of complications. Treatments may include:
- lifestyle changes to reduce weight, decrease hyperlipidemia, and decrease hyperglycemia and hyperinsulinemia
- a combination of oral contraceptives, antiandrogen agents, and insulin sensitizers
- hormonal therapy to regulate menstruation, decrease androgen production, and decrease abnormal bleeding
- if fertility is desired, drugs such as clomiphene may facilitate ovulation

Vaginal candidiasis

VC, also called *candida vulvovaginitis*, is common; approximately 70% to 75% of females will have VC at least once in their lifetime. In premenopausal, pregnant, asymptomatic, and healthy females, *Candida albicans* (also referred to as yeast) is the predominant species that causes the infection. Candida overgrowth is usually due to a disturbance in the balance of normal flora that is in the vaginal canal. The presence of lactobacilli in the vaginal canal suppresses overgrowth of candida. The diagnosis of VC is based on clinical symptoms and microscopic detection of pseudohyphae, which is characteristic of candida. Candidiasis is *not* considered an STI.

Risk factors for VC include:
- recent antibiotic treatment
- recent corticosteroid treatment
- uncontrolled diabetes mellitus
- hormonal imbalances
- use of antidiabetic SGLT2 inhibitors (e.g., dapagliflozin and canagliflozin)
- tight undergarments made of synthetic fabric (noncotton)

Symptoms of VC:
- itching of the perineal area
- redness of vulva and vaginal canal
- white discharge

Diagnosis requires a pelvic examination and microscopic examination of vaginal discharge with saline or 10% potassium hydroxide solution using microscopy. This shows the characteristic pseudohyphae of candida.

Treatment

VC can be treated locally with topical imidazole derivatives (e.g., terconazole, butoconazole, tioconazole). Vaginal suppositories and creams are available, with dosages and preparations for a treatment duration from 1 to 3 days to 6 to 7 days. Taking oral probiotics or eating yogurt with active cultures is recommended to restore the lactobacilli, which protect against yeast accumulation, in the vaginal canal.

Cervical cancer

Cancer of the cervix is a neoplastic change in the epithelium of the cervix. These changes are called *cervical intraepithelial neoplasia* (CIN). There are degrees of CIN with progression to carcinoma in situ (CIS) as the cervical epithelium is replaced with abnormal cells. This cancer is the third most common reproductive cancer and is progressive in nature.

Cancer but healthy

Preinvasive cancer conditions can exist for years before development of invasive problems. Most cervical cancers are limited to the cervix, originating in the transformational zone, which is the area between the endocervical glands and the squamous epithelium, and are highly treatable. The average of onset is between 40 and 50 years of age.

How it happens

Although other viruses can lead to cervical cancer, HPV—especially types 16 and 18—presents a significant cause. Risk factors for contracting a virus that can lead to cervical cancer include:

- failure to obtain HPV vaccine before initial sexual activity
- early age of initial coitus (younger than 20 years)
- multiple sex partners (more than two over a person's lifetime)
- a sexual partner with a history of multiple sexual partners

It gets complicated

- Invasive cervical cancer invades into the lymph or vascular systems leading to metastasis to the pelvis or other parts of the body.

What to look for

Most of the time, cervical cancer has no symptoms; however, abnormal bleeding especially postcoital is a classic symptom of invasive cancer. Other late signs include back pain, leg pain, anemia, rectal bleeding, and hematuria.

What tests tell you

The most widely used method of detection of cervical cancer is the Pap test as it can detect early cervical changes with 90% reliability. Currently, the guidelines for having a Pap test are:

- begin Pap test screening at 21 years of age
- continue to have a Pap test every 3 years between ages 21 and 29 (if test is negative)

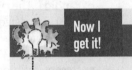

Now I get it!

When abnormal cells penetrate the membrane, cervical cancer develops. Reducing risk factors can reduce exposure to viruses that can lead to cervical cancer.

Prevention is the key!

- Reduce risk factors
- Get the HPV vaccine
- Have a Pap test and HPV testing

- have a Pap test and HPV test every 5 years between ages 30 and 65 or every 3 years with Pap test alone (if test is negative)
- stop Pap testing in people 65 or over or in those who have no cervix (total hysterectomy), if the patient has had three or more consecutive negative Pap tests or more than two consecutive negative HPV and Pap tests within the past 10 years with the most recent test occurring within 5 years

Pap test results and classifications

If the Pap testing is positive, recommendations can include immediate colposcopy, repeat cytology at 6 and 12 months, or HPV testing and referral for colposcopy.

- A colposcopy is used to magnify examination of the cervix.
- A biopsy or removal of a piece of the cervix for study can be done during the colposcopy. This procedure is outpatient and does not require anesthesia.
- Conization or cone biopsy of the cervix can be used to diagnose and treat cervical cancer. The procedure removes the abnormal tissue while preserving childbearing capacity. This procedure is only effective if the cancer is noninvasive.

 Battling illness

Treating cervical cancer

Treatment of cervical cancer is divided into preinvasive and invasive cancer

Preinvasive lesion treatments include:
• Cryosurgery, which freezes the abnormal cells allowing the area to slough off and regenerate normal tissue.
• Laser ablation, which uses a beam of light to heat the abnormal cervical cell area.
• Loop electrosurgical excision procedure (LEEP), which uses a wire electrode that excises and cauterizes the abnormal cell site.

Once staging is done (which determines the invasiveness of the cancer), a treatment plan is developed, which can include surgery, radiation therapy, and chemotherapy.

Invasive cancer treatments include:
• For microinvasive cancer (no lymphatic or vascular involvement), conization or hysterectomy is done depending on future childbearing wishes of the patient.
• Early-stage invasive cancer care includes hysterectomy or chemotherapy and radiation therapy.
• Later stages of invasive cancer care include a radical hysterectomy, radiation therapy (both internal and external), and chemotherapy.

Other HPV-associated cancers

An *HPV-associated cancer* is a specific cellular type of cancer that is diagnosed in a part of the body where HPV is often found. These parts of the body include the cervix, vagina, vulva, penis, anus, rectum, and oropharynx (back of the throat, including the base of the tongue and tonsils). The most virulent strains of the many HPV strains are HPV16 and 18. HPV-associated cancers usually take years before they become apparent and symptomatic.

Usually, HPV resolves by itself within 2 years and does not cause health problems. It is thought that the immune system fights off HPV naturally. However, when HPV stays in the body for many years, it can cause carcinomas of the cervix and squamous cell carcinomas of the vagina, vulva, penis, anus, rectum, and oropharynx. It is not known why HPV goes away in most people but causes cancer in some people.

HPV is thought to be responsible for more than 90% of anal and cervical cancers, about 70% of vaginal and vulvar cancers, and 60% of penile cancers. Also, recent studies show that about 60% to 70% of cancers of the oropharynx may be linked to HPV. For this reason, it is highly recommended that preteens, adolescents, and young adults aged 9 to 26 obtain the HPV vaccine. Because HPV is transmitted mainly through sexual activity, the HPV vaccine is most effective when administered before a preteen, adolescent, or young adult has their first sexual experience. Recently, U.S. health officials have expanded the recommended age range for people receiving the HPV vaccine to protect against several types of cancer to people in their mid-40s.

Endometrial cancer

Endometrial cancer is a neoplasm that usually develops from endometrial hyperplasia. The tumor usually starts in the fundus of the uterus, which can then spread to the myometrium and cervix, as well as other reproductive organs. This cancer is the most common reproductive malignancy, seen more in premenopausal and postmenopausal females between the ages of 50 and 65. The rate of this cancer is slightly higher in White females. The following gene mutations are commonly found in endometrial and ovarian cancer: *PTEN, PIK3CA, KRAS, FBXW7, CTNNB1, BRAF,* and *TP53*.

How it happens
Most endometrial cancers are slow growing adenocarcinomas. Risk factors associated with development of endometrial cancer include:
- obesity
- nulliparity
- infertility
- late onset of menopause
- diabetes mellitus
- hypertension
- PCOS
- family history of ovarian or breast disease; certain genetic mutations are associated with endometrial and ovarian cancer
- hormonal imbalances

It gets complicated
Metastasis can occur through the lymphatic system or through the blood to the lungs, brain, and liver.

What to look for
The cardinal sign of endometrial cancer is uterine bleeding, which is abnormal because most females who develop this are postmenopausal. Late signs may include:
- low back pain
- lower pelvic pain
- uterine enlargement or mass
- mucosanguineous vaginal discharge

What tests tell you
A diagnosis of endometrial cancer is made by the following:
- Pap test. This test only identifies about one-third of the cases.
- PapSEEK, a test that is currently under development, can identify endometrial cancer prior to development of symptoms. This test finds endometrial cell DNA that is shed from the uterine lining and migrates to the endocervical mucosa, where it can be collected by the Pap smear technique.
- Endometrial biopsy or fractional curettage (scrapings from the endocervix and endometrium). This procedure has the most accurate results.
- Tests to determine metastasis may include liver and renal function tests, chest x-ray, computed tomography (CT), MRI, bone scans, and biopsy of possibly cancerous tissue.
- Staging of the cancer is based on the results of the biopsy; histological examination.

Treating endometrial cancer

• The primary goal of treatment for endometrial cancer is to rid the body of the cancer through medical or surgical management.

Stage I
When the cancer is limited to the uterus, a total abdominal hysterectomy (TAH) and bilateral salpingo-oophorectomy (BSO) are done. Radiation is sometimes used, but it does not improve survival rates or reduce metastasis. Radiation alone may be used if the patient is a poor surgical risk.

Stage II
A radical hysterectomy (which includes excision of parametrical tissue laterally and uterosacral ligaments posteriorly, BSO, and pelvic node dissection) is performed. Lymph nodes are tested, and if positive, radiation is done postoperatively.

Stage III
If the tumor invades outside the uterus, a radical hysterectomy is performed (as described above), and radiation may be done externally or internally by placing the radiation source in the uterine cavity. Chemotherapy may be used as well. Multiagent platinum-based chemotherapy regimens include carboplatin/paclitaxel, cisplatin/doxorubicin, cisplatin/doxorubicin/paclitaxel, or carboplatin/docetaxel.

Stage IV
All of the treatments discussed above are done with longer lengths of time for the radiation and chemotherapy. Recurrence is common.

Drug therapy
• Progestational therapy (medroxyprogesterone acetate and megestrol acetate) may be effective for recurrent cancers.
• Antiestrogens (tamoxifen, raloxifene, and aromatase inhibitors) have shown some effectiveness with endometrial cancer.
• Specific types of pharmacologic-targeted therapy such as monoclonal antibody type agents; trastuzumab and pembrolizumab can be added to chemotherapeutic agents above.

Ovarian cancer

Ovarian cancer is the second most common cancer found in the female reproductive system. Ovarian cancer causes more deaths than any other female reproductive cancer. This cancer is usually diagnosed in late stages because there is no screening test, and symptoms are vague. Over 70% of ovarian cancers are not diagnosed until the disease has progressed to stage III or IV. Although ovarian cancer can be diagnosed at any age, it is more common in people over 50, and 50% of ovarian cancers occur in those over age 63. Females from North America or who are of Northern European descent have a higher rate of ovarian cancer. Ovarian cancers are often linked to mutations of the tumor-suppressing genes *BRCA1*, *BRCA2*, and *p53*.

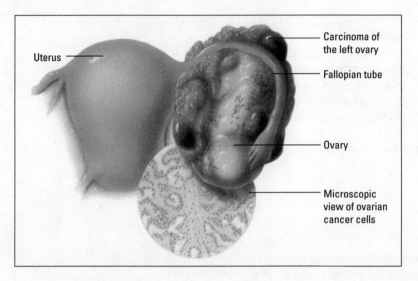

Uterus

Carcinoma of the left ovary

Fallopian tube

Ovary

Microscopic view of ovarian cancer cells

How it happens

The cause of ovarian cancer is unknown, but there are risk factors for development, which include:

- nulliparity
- infertility
- previous breast cancer
- *BRCA1*, *BRCA2*, *P53* gene mutations
- smoking
- endometriosis
- family history of ovarian or breast cancer
- hereditary nonpolyposis colorectal cancer (HNPCC) (Lynch syndrome)
- use of postmenopausal estrogen (hormone replacement)
- studies have shown that the more ovulatory cycles a female completes, the higher the risk of ovarian cancer.

What to look for

Although difficult to distinguish from other problems or changes in the middle-aged woman, there are some early warning signs that ovarian cancer may be present. These signs can include:

- abdominal bloating and noticeable increase in abdominal girth
- pelvic or abdominal pain
- feeling full quickly when eating
- urinary frequency or urgency

However, early diagnosis of ovarian cancer is still uncommon as current screening methods have not proven reliable. Although the elevated levels of the cancer antigen 125 (CA125) has been used historically as a tumor marker for ovarian cancer, it lacks specificity and sensitivity. For example, it can be elevated in people who do not have ovarian cancer, and it may not be elevated in up to 50% of patients with early stages of ovarian cancer. As such, the CA125 marker is no longer a recommended method of screening for ovarian cancer.

Tumors of any size can be a problem; tumor size does not indicate severity.

Symptoms of late stages of ovarian cancer include:
- pelvic pain
- anemia
- general weakness
- malnutrition

What tests tell you

Although there are no specific screening tests for ovarian cancer, routine pelvic examination continues to be the only method used to detect early disease. Ovarian enlargement should be further evaluated by laparoscopy or laparotomy. If a tumor is detected, a biopsy is done to assess malignancy.

Battling illness

Treating ovarian cancer

Just like other cancers, staging is determined by location of the disease. However, since ovarian cancer is usually found in late stages, treatment is usually a combination of surgical and medical management.

Surgical therapy
Surgery removes the tumor, the ovary and tube (if the cancer is limited to one ovary and childbearing is desired), or radical hysterectomy. Cytoreductive surgery (the debulking of the poorly vascularized large tumors) may be done with the goal of removing as much of the tumor as possible.

Medical therapy
Chemotherapy is the mainstay of medical management. Radiation has been used in early-stage ovarian cancer treatment and can also be used as a palliative measure for advanced disease.

Breast cancer

Breast cancer is the second leading cause of cancer death in females, especially those between the ages of 45 and 55. Although it is considered a breast cancer, it is also a systemic disease because it can easily transfer to other places in the body. Although the majority of breast cancer is found in females over the age of 50, breast cancer can also be found also in males, most commonly in older males (the average age of male breast cancer is 67).

Looking up…

The prognosis for breast cancer is good when found early. Early detection is improving due to the push for screening by the American Cancer Society.

How it happens

There are multiple risk factors that can lead to breast cancer. Determining risk factors also helps to determine who needs more surveillance. Intrinsic risk factors (risks that are within the body) for breast cancer include:

- sex (female)
- late age of menarche
- menopause
- first pregnancy after age 40
- fibrocystic disease
- high-density breast tissue
- past breast cancer
- having genetic mutation of *BRCA1* or *BRCA2*. Genetic testing can identify some females who have inherited mutations in the *BRCA1* or *BRCA2* tumor suppressor genes as well as in other less common gene mutations such as *PALB2*, *ATM*, or *CHEK2*.

Extrinsic risk factors (risks outside the body) for breast cancer include:

- obesity especially in childbearing females (increased circulating estrogen)
- lack of exercise
- moderate to high alcohol consumption
- diet high in saturated fats
- use of oral contraception or hormone replacement postmenopause if used more than 10 years

Screening guidelines

Screening for breast cancer continues to evolve. Monthly self-breast evaluation is no longer a standard recommendation because research does not suggest an early detection benefit or overall survival difference. Clinical breast examination by healthcare providers has also been shown to be unreliable. Currently, screening mammography is still the gold standard, with digital mammography better able to detect abnormalities than standard mammography. Screening mammography guidelines are different from one leading agency to another. One group (U.S. Preventive Services Task Force) recommends a baseline mammography in the average risk females at age 50, with mammograms every 2 years after that. Another group (American Cancer Society) recommends a baseline mammography

Now I get it!

Mammography screening is the gold standard for detecting breast cancer.

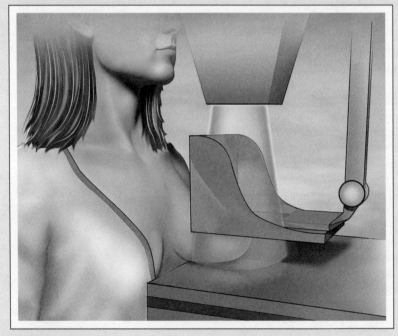

(Shutterstock/ilusmedical)

at age 40 with annual mammograms after that. Mammography is better at detecting cancer in patients over 50. Ultrasound can also be used as an adjunct to mammography because it can distinguish between cysts and solid masses. If a screening mammogram identifies something warranting further inspection, a diagnostic mammogram is performed. Mammograms can detect calcifications; where macrocalcifications are a sign of aging and benign, microcalcifications can be concerning and may warrant biopsy.

Getting complicated

The size of the tumor and nodal involvement determine the prognosis for long-term survival. Staging is determined based on tumor size, location, nodal involvement, and metastasis, which also helps determine treatment.

Emotional support is important...

Emotional support after diagnosis and throughout care options is important to help clarify and validate feelings. Fears related to body image, treatment, and negative outcomes are a big concern for patients with a breast cancer diagnosis.

What to look for

Most breast cancer is painless. Detection of a lump or thickening in the breast, found through mammography, self, or partner detection, is usually the first sign of a problem. Nipple retraction, skin dimpling or skin changes to the nipple, redness with edema, and pitting of the skin are suggestive of more advanced breast cancer.

What tests tell you

Besides mammography (discussed above), other tests used to detect and help with diagnosing and staging (I to IV) are:
- MRI
- ultrasound-guided needle breast biopsy

After tumor removal and biopsy of tissue, breast cancer can be categorized into three groups:
- breast cancer expressing hormone receptor (estrogen receptor [ER$^+$] or progesterone receptor [PR$^+$])
- breast cancer expressing human epidermal receptor 2 (HER2$^+$)
- triple-negative breast cancer (ER$^-$, PR$^-$, HER2$^-$)

Treatment approaches are based on these molecular characteristics of the cancer.

Treating breast cancer

The goals of treatment for breast cancer are to contain, prevent spread, and remove the cancer so that it does not reoccur.

Surgery

There are several approaches to surgery for breast cancer depending on the staging. Patient needs must also be considered as treatment options often affect self-image and a common goal of treatment is important. Surgical treatment may include:
• Lumpectomy, which is the removal of just the tumor itself (and a small amount of healthy tissue around the tumor) and is considered a breast-conserving surgery.
• Segmental mastectomy (partial mastectomy), which is wide excision and quadrantectomy which removes the tumor and a large amount of healthy tissue.
• Mastectomy, which is the removal of the breast (one or both), including the nipple and areola. There are several types of mastectomy, which include total simple, modified, radical skin-sparing, nipple-sparing, and preventive/prophylactic mastectomies. A preventative mastectomy may be suggested for those who have many risk factors, especially genetic risks.
• Oophorectomy, which is surgical removal of the ovaries, may be an option for high-risk individuals.
• Breast reconstruction, which is used to achieve symmetry and preservation of body image.

Types of radiation
• Accelerated breast radiation, which delivers a larger dose of radiation over a 3-week period using an external beam.
• Brachytherapy, which is when a deflated balloon, is inserted into the lumpectomy space and filled with saline and left in place until margins are clear. A balloon with radiation replaces the saline balloon, which allows for a shorter completion time of radiation therapy as most local reoccurrences of cancer happen at or near the original site.
• Partial breast radiation is done usually at the time of surgery and used for small, less aggressive tumors.

Chemotherapy and hormonal therapy

Adjuvant chemotherapy is also used to treat breast cancer based on risk of recurrence testing. There may be a combination of chemotherapy and hormonal therapy as well. Hormonal therapy is based on a receptor assay testing. There are several hormonal therapy drugs including:
• Tamoxifen, which mimics progesterone and estrogen. This drug attaches to the hormone receptors on cancer cells and does not let the cancer cell grow.
• Raloxifene hydrochloride, serves as an agonist and antagonist to estrogen receptor sites. It is also used to treat and prevent osteoporosis.
• Letrozole, which inhibits the conversion of androgens to estrogen.

Benign prostatic hyperplasia

BPH is another name for an enlarged prostate gland. Enlargement of the prostate gland occurs as a natural physiologic change in older adult men, usually after age 60. Excessive cellular tissue grows within the gland and surrounds the urethra. This can cause compression on the urethra, creating difficulty in urination.

How it happens

The cells of the prostate increase in number (hyperplasia), which results in formation of large nodules. As the nodules increase, they push on the urethra resulting in narrowing. This increases the resistance of flow of urine from the bladder. The resistance to urine flow makes the bladder work harder during voiding. BPH, the most common benign tumor found in males, happens more frequently in older males, especially those age 60 and older.

Getting complicated

When the bladder has to work harder to push the urine through the urethra, problems such as hypertrophy, instability, or atony of the bladder muscle can occur. If left untreated, obstruction of the bladder can occur, which can lead to recurrent urinary tract infections, bladder stones, and chronic kidney disease and failure.

What to look for

BPH is a chronic problem that has mild symptoms at first but can progressively become more serious. Common symptoms include:
- nocturia
- dribbling at the end of urinary stream
- incontinence of urine
- urgency to urinate
- painful urination
- weak, narrowed urinary stream
- straining to urinate
- incomplete bladder emptying
- slowed or delayed urinary stream

What tests tell you

BPH diagnosis is based on clinical findings of a history of lower urinary tract symptoms, a digital rectal examination, and exclusion of other causes.
- Urinalysis is done to evaluate for urinary tract infection, glucose in the urine, and protein in the urine, which can be signs of diabetes or kidney disease.
- Prostate-specific antigen (PSA) is a necessary blood test to rule out prostate cancer. If the PSA is high, more tests will be necessary. (See *Prostate cancer*.)
- A digital rectal examination finding of a symmetric and smooth but enlarged prostate.
- Screening questionnaires can be used to help with quantifying the severity of urinary tract symptoms.

Is it really BPH?

It is important to rule out illnesses with similar symptoms such as bladder infection, bladder cancer, urethral stricture, urethral calculi (stones), chronic prostatitis, neurogenic bladder, and prostate cancer. Some medications can also increase urination problems and should be considered such as decongestants with pseudoephedrine, calcium channel blockers, and medications with anticholinergic properties such as loop diuretics or thiazides.

Treating BPH

Some people have minimal symptoms and do not require treatment. Those who experience worse symptoms require treatment; depending on the severity of symptoms, treatment can vary from lifestyle changes to surgery. Lifestyle changes include:
• increasing physical activity
• decreasing fluid intake before sleep
• moderating alcohol and caffeine intake
• establishing a voiding schedule
• avoiding medications with anticholinergic properties
• voiding in the sitting position

Use of alpha blockers, 5α-reductase inhibitors, and or antimuscarinic medications can assist with symptoms or reduction of prostate size. Phosphodiesterase-5 inhibitors may be used when erectile dysfunction occurs with BPH. A transurethral resection of prostate (TURP) is commonly performed if pharmacologic treatment is insufficient.

Prostatitis

Prostatitis is the inflammation and distension of the prostate gland (which produces semen that transports and nourishes sperm). It can affect males of all ages, most commonly those under 50. Although prostatitis is the most common urologic diagnosis in males, acute prostatitis is an infrequent occurrence.

How it happens

There are multiple forms of prostatitis:
• Acute
• Chronic
• Chronic prostatitis/chronic pelvic pain syndrome (CPPS)
• Asymptomatic

Prostatitis is either caused by an infection or inflammation that presents with varying clinical features. Sometimes, the cause can't be identified, but acute prostatitis is often triggered by a bacterial infection, usually from the urine, or by an STI. If the bacteria are not destroyed, reoccurrence can occur and the problem can become chronic. Nerve damage in the lower urinary tract (which is caused by surgery or trauma) could also contribute to prostatitis. The asymptomatic form is usually found during a workup for infertility or a laboratory finding of an elevated PSA.

Prostatitis promoters

Risk factors for developing prostatitis include:
• being a young or middle-aged male
• having an STI (e.g., chlamydia or gonorrhea)
• previous prostate biopsy

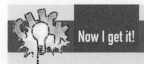

Now I get it!

Prostatitis is different from BPH because with prostatitis, the prostate is not just enlarged but inflamed and tends to happen at a younger age than BPH.

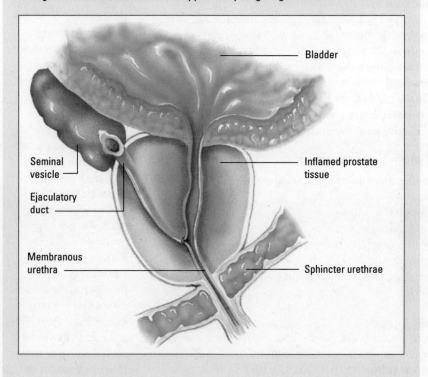

- having pelvic trauma
- having a urinary catheter
- having HIV/AIDS
- bladder or urethral infection (urinary tract infection)

Getting complicated

Possible complications of prostatitis can include:
- semen abnormalities and infertility (especially with chronic prostatitis)
- epididymitis
- bacteremia
- prostatic abscess
- renal damage
- pyelonephritis

What to look for

Although the signs and symptoms of prostatitis depend on whether it is acute or chronic, acute symptoms may include:
- fever, chills, and malaise
- arthralgias, myalgias
- low abdominal and back pain
- perineal/prostatic pain
- obstructive urinary tract symptoms (frequency, urgency, nocturia, dysuria, hesitancy, weak stream, and incomplete voiding)
- spontaneous urethral discharge

For chronic prostatitis, the patient usually does not have systemic symptoms. However, symptoms may include:
- recurrent urinary tract infections
- intermittent obstructive urinary tract symptoms (see above)
- pelvic pain, ejaculatory pain, erectile dysfunction (CPPS patients)

It can be embarrassing, but on physical examination...

The healthcare provider may find the following on physical examination for acute prostatitis:
- suprapubic abdominal tenderness
- enlarged tender bladder
- tender, nodular, hot, boggy, or normal-feeling prostate gland on digital rectal examination.

For chronic prostatitis, examination findings may be normal between acute episodes.

What tests tell you

Tests are done to rule out other conditions and to determine the type of prostatitis (acute or chronic). These tests include:
- urinalysis and urine culture to check for infection
- CBC with differential to check for infection and PSA to check for other prostate problems
- ultrasound or CT scan of the urinary tract and prostate to give a visual image
- massage of prostate with prostate fluid culture

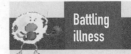
Battling illness

Treating prostatitis

Drug therapy
If a bacterial infection is the cause, antibiotics are prescribed. The type (oral or IV) and length of time the antibiotics need to be taken depend on the severity of symptoms and whether the prostatitis is acute or chronic.

Alpha blockers may be used to relax the bladder and muscle fibers, which can ease symptoms and pain. Nonsteroidal anti-inflammatory drugs (NASIDs) may be used to reduce pain and inflammation. Biofeedback and acupuncture show some research evidence of helping with chronic prostatitis.

Prostate cancer

The prostate produces semen and transports and nourishes sperm. About 1 in 8 males will be diagnosed with prostate cancer during their lifetime. About 6 cases in 10 cases are diagnosed in males who are 65 or older, and the disease is infrequent in males under 40. The average age of diagnosis is 66. Prostate cancer is the second leading cause of cancer death in American males, behind only lung cancer. About 1 male in 41 will die of prostate cancer.

How it happens

Although the cause of prostate cancer is not clear, the majority of prostate cancers are adenocarcinomas. Mutations of abnormal cells start in the prostate and can eventually (but not always) metastasize to other parts of the body.

Screening is the question

Prostate cancer incidence rates are increasing, so screening for prostate cancer is crucial. Currently, some recommendations have screening start with males in their 50s (or sooner if there are risk factors). Risk factors include:

- age: as a person ages, their risk of having prostate cancer increases
- ethnicity: non-Hispanic African American males have the highest risk for contracting prostate cancer
- family history: having two or more close relatives diagnosed before age 55, prostate cancer in three generations on the same side of the family, or three or more first-degree relatives with prostate cancer
- Inherited gene mutations: mutations of the *BRCA1* or *BRCA2* gene (associated with breast, ovarian, and prostate cancer), or mutation of the *APC* gene associated with HNPCC, also called *Lynch syndrome*
- obesity
- smoking
- chronic prostatitis
- agent orange exposure: veterans exposed to this herbicide in war are at higher risk

What to look for

Although most prostate cancer in the United States is found through screening, there are symptoms of prostate cancer. These symptoms include:

- decreased urinary stream
- urgency
- hesitancy
- nocturia
- incomplete bladder emptying
  Signs of metastasis include:
- back pain
- pathologic vertebral fractures

What tests tell you

Screening tests available for prostate cancer include:

- PSA blood test, which is a protein produced by the prostate gland. There are many reasons for fluctuations in these levels so other diagnostic testing may be done if findings are above normal ranges.

- digital rectal examination (DRE), which may reveal a hard, bumpy, or enlarged prostate.
- needle biopsy or transrectal biopsy is done to detect cancer. A score is then assigned to the cancer based on histology review, which guides treatment.

Battling illness

Treating prostate cancer

The goal of treatment for prostate cancer is to use the least invasive treatment for the best outcomes.

Surgery
Removal of the prostate gland (radical prostatectomy) is a treatment for more advanced prostate cancer.

Radiation therapy
There are different types of radiation therapy for prostate cancer. This can be a good choice for those patients who cannot have surgery. External beam radiation therapy (EBRT), brachytherapy, and radiopharmaceutical therapy are all types of radiation therapy that can be used for prostate cancer.

Hormone therapy
This treatment is usually reserved for advanced prostate cancer or for patients with early-stage prostate cancer to help shrink the tumors before radiation therapy. These hormone therapies can include:

- luteinizing hormone-releasing hormone (LHRH) agonist to stop testicles from receiving information to make testosterone
- antiandrogens may be given to keep testosterone from reaching the cancer cells
- orchiectomy, which removes the testicles and reduces testosterone levels in the body. However, this treatment has disadvantages including depression, loss of libido, less reversible impotency, hot flashes, and osteoporosis.

Cryosurgery and biological therapy
Cryosurgery is a surgical technique under investigation at the present time for treatment for prostate cancer. It involves destruction of the prostate cancer cells by intermittent freezing of the prostate. Biological therapy or immunotherapy uses the patient's immune system/cells to fight the prostate cancer. Currently, this therapy is only used in advanced or recurrent cancer.

Testicular cancer

Testicular cancer is cancer that occurs in the testicles, which produce the male sex hormones and sperm for reproduction. This cancer is considered rare (only 1% of all cancers in men), although it is the most common cancer in males between the ages of 15 and 35 years of age.

How it happens
The cause of testicular cancer is not clear, but like most cancers, it is the abnormal growth of abnormal cells that accumulate to form a tumor. There are risk factors for development of testicular cancer. These risk factors include:

- ethnicity: White males are more likely to have testicular cancer than African-American males
- age: although this cancer can occur at any age, it is more likely to affect males in their teens, 20s, and early 30s
- family history: if family members have had this cancer, the patient is at higher risk for development
- abnormal testicle development: if a patient has a condition that causes abnormal testicle development, like Klinefelter syndrome, this can increase the risk of testicular cancer
- cryptorchidism (undescended testicle): if a person had this problem as a child, there is a higher risk of testicular cancer

Getting complicated

As with most cancer, the worst complication is metastasis to other parts of the body. When testicular cancer has metastasized, it usually goes to the liver and lungs.

What to look for

Signs and symptoms of testicular cancer include:
- pain or discomfort in a testicle or the scrotum
- a sudden collection of fluid in the scrotum
- a dull ache in the abdomen or groin
- a lump or enlargement in either testicle
- a feeling of heaviness in the scrotum
- back pain
- enlargement or tenderness of the breasts

Men may find a lump themselves unintentionally or while doing a self-testicular examination. A healthcare provider may detect a lump during a routine physical examination. However, no studies have found that doing routine screenings (such as self-examination or periodic clinical examination) for asymptomatic males improve health outcomes unless a patient has had testicular cancer before or has cryptorchidism or surgically corrected cryptorchidism.

What tests tell you

These tests are used to diagnose testicular cancer:
- Ultrasound, which helps determine if a lump is solid or fluid filled and whether the lump is inside or outside the testicle.
- Blood tests include chemistry profile, CBC, and serum tumor markers. These tests help determine the type of cancer, which can help determine treatment.
- CT scan is done to look at the abdomen, chest, and pelvis for possible metastases.

Treating testicular cancer

Treatment is based on the type of cancer that is found. There are two cancer types:

• Seminoma, which is not as aggressive
• Nonseminoma, which can spread rapidly

Staging of the cancer is also done similar to other types of cancers.

Surgery

A radical inguinal orchiectomy removes the testicle(s) that has (have) the cancer. A prosthetic, saline-filled testicle can also be placed. In early stages, this surgery may be the only treatment needed. Histologic evaluation will be done on the tumor to confirm diagnosis. A retroperitoneal lymph node dissection may also be performed if lymph node involvement is suspected, but there can be a high rate of nerve damage, which can cause problems with ejaculation.

Radiation therapy

This treatment option is usually only for those patients who have seminoma-type cancer but can be recommended after the removal of the testicle.

Chemotherapy

This may be suggested before or after surgery or it may be the only treatment given depending on the staging. However, it can lead to infertility, so discussion about cryopreservation of sperm should be done with the patient.

Sexually transmitted infections

STIs are infections that are primarily passed through sexual contact. Because STIs are often asymptomatic until they cause complications, they present major public health problems. In the United States, approximately 20 million people are affected by an STI annually, with 1 in 5 people having an STI.

How it happens

Prevention is key to stopping STIs. Strategies include abstinence from all sexual activity, staying in a long-term monogamous relationship, limiting the number of sexual partners, proper condom use, and vaccines (for males and females) for HPV. The cycle of STIs continues because many are asymptomatic, and unprotected sex spreads the infection.

Getting complicated

Complications of untreated STIs can lead to infertility, chronic pelvic pain, cervical cancer, vaginal or vulvar cancer, anorectal cancer, oropharyngeal or penile cancer, chronic infection with hepatitis viruses, and HIV. Screenings for STIs are recommended but different groups have different recommendations, which make it difficult sometimes for healthcare professionals to follow.

If one infection is found...

Many times, if one STI is diagnosed, there are others. If one STI is found, it is recommended that screening be done for other infections, including screening for HIV, hepatitis B, and C.

What to look for
The STIs chart provides a summary of the most common infections.

Sexually transmitted infections

Type	*Chlamydia trachomatis*	Gonorrhea	*Trichomonas vaginalis*
Symptoms	Usually no symptoms or minimal symptoms **In females:** • Cervicitis **In males:** • Urethritis	Usually no symptoms or minimal symptoms **In females:** • Cervicitis **In males:** • Urethritis	**In females:** Discharge may be yellowish to greenish, frothy, mucopurulent, copious, or malodorous; pruritus, dysuria, and dyspareunia **In males:** Usually no symptoms; can have pruritus or burning after sexual intercourse
Complications	Pelvic inflammatory disease (PID), infertility, chronic pelvic pain, ectopic pregnancy, epididymitis	PID, infertility, chronic pelvic pain, endocarditis, meningitis	
Tests	**Males:** NAAT[a] on urine **Females:** Vaginal swab	**Males:** NAAT[a] on urine **Females:** Vaginal swab	**Males:** NAAT[a] on urine **Females:** Vaginal swab
Treatment	Single-dose antibiotic azithromycin or ceftriaxone when coinfected with gonorrhea	High antibiotic resistance. Injection of ceftriaxone appears to be reliable. May give azithromycin too.	Metronidazole or tinidazole single oral dose
Screening	Recommended for high-risk populations	Recommended for high-risk populations	Recommended for high-risk populations

[a]Nucleic acid amplification testing.

(Continued)

Sexually transmitted infections *(continued)*

Syphilis	Human papillomavirus (HPV)	*Mycoplasma genitalium*	Herpes simplex (II) virus
Early symptoms Chancre, usually in genital area; usually painless papule General lymphadenopathy **Late symptoms** Can have no symptoms; CNS, cardiac, and lymphatic problems	**In males and females:** Sometimes no symptoms External genital warts found on the genital or groin areas. The warts vary in size and presentation. The warts typically have no symptoms but may be pruritic.	Common cause of nongono-coccal urethritis (urethral discharge) in males and cervicitis (purulent or muco-purulent cervical discharge) in females	**In males and females:** Primary infection is highly variable ranging from severe painful genital ulcers, and systemic symptoms, to no symptoms Recurrent infection is common but usually less severe
Untreated syphilis can lead to late symptoms up to 25 years after inoculation	Cervical cancer from specific types, and head and neck cancers from genital warts	PID in females and urethritis in males	Proctitis and meningitis
Initial testing Rapid plasma regain, Venereal Disease Research Laboratory, toluidine red unheated serum test	Warts are diagnosed on physical examination.	**Males:** NAAT[a] on urine **Females:** Vaginal swab	Viral culture, direct fluorescence antibody and type-specific serologic tests
Penicillin G or doxycycline	See cervical cancer; warts usually regress after 4 months even without treatment. No single therapy recommended; podophyllotoxin or imiquimod medications are used.	Azithromycin 1 g ×1	Acyclovir, famciclovir, or penciclovir Recurrent therapy may include episodic or daily antiviral therapy
Not usually done because patients usually have visible symptoms (chancre)	Vaccine for prevention and regular Pap screenings (see cervical cancer)	Not routinely recommended	Recommended for high-risk populations or symptomatic individuals

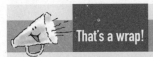

That's a wrap!

Reproductive system review

Understanding the reproductive system
• The reproductive system is a group of internal and external organs, as well as complex hormonal components, that work together to assist with procreation.
• The external female reproductive system includes the mons pubis, labia majora and minora, clitoris, vestibular glands (also called *Bartholin glands*), vaginal vestibule, vaginal orifice, perineum, and the urethral opening.
• The internal female reproductive structures include the vagina, uterus, uterine tubes (fallopian tubes), and ovaries.
• There are three cycles that effect the female reproductive system:
  – Hypothalamic–pituitary cycle
  – Ovarian cycle
  – Endometrial cycle
• The external male reproductive structures consist of the penis and scrotum (testicles).
• The internal male reproductive structures include the
  – epididymis
  – vas deferens
  – accessory glands (seminal vesicles, the prostate gland, and bulbourethral glands)

Reproductive disorders
• Fibroadenomas: benign, painless tumors of the female breast that often occur during the childbearing years
• Endometriosis: a condition where tissue that normally grows inside the uterus grows outside the uterus on surrounding internal structures
• Leiomyoma: (also called a *fibroid*) a tumor of the smooth muscle in the uterus
• Pelvic organ prolapse: occurs when the muscles or the ligaments in a woman's pelvis weaken and the organs in the pelvis slip out of place
• Polycystic ovary syndrome: numerous follicles develop on the ovaries, which produce excess estrogen causing the ovaries to enlarge and fail to regularly release eggs
• Breast cancer: second leading cause of cancer death in females
• Cervical cancer: neoplastic change in the epithelium of the cervix
• Endometrial cancer: neoplasm that usually develops from endometrial hyperplasia; most common reproductive malignancy
• Ovarian cancer: causes more deaths than any other female reproductive cancer
• BPH: noncancerous enlargement of the prostate gland
• Prostate cancer: occurs in the prostate (which produces semen and transports and nourishes sperm); one of the most common types of cancer in males
  – Testicular cancer: occurs in the testicles, which produce the male sex hormones and sperm for reproduction
  – Sexually transmitted infections (STIs): complications of untreated STIs can lead to infertility, chronic pelvic pain, cervical cancer, chronic infection with hepatitis viruses, and HIV

Quick quiz

1. Low levels of estrogen and progesterone stimulate the hypothalamus to secrete:
    A. luteinizing hormone.
    B. follicle-stimulating hormone.
    C. testosterone.
    D. gonadotropin-releasing hormone.

Answer: D. Low levels of estrogen and progesterone stimulate the hypothalamus to secrete gonadotropin-releasing hormone, which causes the anterior pituitary to secret follicle-stimulating hormone.

2. The _____ acts as a storage and maturation site for sperm
   A. Prostate gland
   B. Epididymis
   C. Vas deferens
   D. Penis

Answer: B. The epididymis is a mass of tightly coiled tubes that lay against the testicles and function as a storage and maturation site for sperm.

3. Which of the following is true about uterine leiomyoma?
   A. Most fibroids are benign.
   B. It is more common in Hispanic or White females.
   C. Light menstrual bleeding is a sign of fibroids.
   D. Leiomyoma cannot be found on physical examination.

Answer: A. Leiomyomas are tumors of the smooth muscle that are usually benign, are mostly commonly found in the uterus but can be found in any part of the body where smooth muscle is found.

4. Which of the following is not considered a sexually transmitted infection (STI)?
   A. Candidiasis
   B. *Chlamydia trachomatis*
   C. *Mycoplasma genitalium*
   D. *Trichomonas vaginalis*

Answer: A. Candidiasis or a yeast infection causes vulvar or vaginal pruritus but is not sexually transmitted. Use of antibiotics or change in pH of the genital area can lead to a yeast infection.

Scoring

☆☆☆ If you answered all four items correctly, excellent! When it comes to understanding the reproductive system, you're on the right track.

☆☆ If you answered three items correctly, relax and enjoy! Your performance on this test will reproduce.

☆ If you answered fewer than three items correctly, don't worry. Reproducing is not always easy on the first try. Baby steps!

Suggested references

Abou Zahr, R., Chalhoub, K., Matta, I., Horani, S., Bedoyan, Z., El Hachem, G., Ghantous, I., & Jabbour, M. (2019). Classic testicular seminoma in men aged 50 Years or over: A case report and review of the literature. *Case Reports in Urology, 2019*, 4391015. https://doi.org/10.1155/2019/4391015

Al Wattar, B. H., Fisher, M., Bevington, L., Talaulikar, V., Davies, M., Conway, G., & Yasmin, E. (2021). Clinical practice guidelines on the diagnosis and management of polycystic ovary syndrome: A systematic review and quality assessment study. *The Journal of Clinical Endocrinology and Metabolism, 106*(8), 2436–2446.

American Cancer Society. (2023a). *Prostate cancer.* https://www.cancer.org/cancer/prostate-cancer.html

American Cancer Society. (2023b). *What is endometrial cancer?* https://www.cancer.org/cancer/endometrial-cancer/about/what-is-endometrial-cancer.html

American Cancer Society. (2023c). *What is ovarian cancer?* https://www.cancer.org/cancer/ovarian-cancer/about/what-is-ovarian-cancer.html

American Cancer Society. (2023d). *Key statistics for ovarian cancer.* https://www.cancer.org/cancer/ovarian-cancer/about/key-statistics.html

American Cancer Society. (2023e). *What is breast cancer?* https://www.cancer.org/cancer/breast-cancer/about/what-is-breast-cancer.html

American Cancer Society. (2023f). *What causes breast cancer?* https://www.cancer.org/cancer/breast-cancer/about/how-does-breast-cancer-form.html

American Cancer Society. (2023g). *What is testicular cancer.* https://www.cancer.org/cancer/testicular-cancer/about/what-is-testicular-cancer.html

Barzaman, K., Karami, J., Zarei, Z., Hosseinzadeh, A., Kazemi, M. H., Moradi-Kalbolandi, S., Safari, E., & Farahmand, L. (2020). Breast cancer: Biology, biomarkers, and treatments. *International Immunopharmacology, 84,* 106535. https://doi.org/10.1016/j.intimp.2020.106535

Cai, Y., Wang, B., Xu, W., Liu, K., Gao, Y., Guo, C., Chen, J., Kamal, M. A., & Yuan, C. (2021). Endometrial cancer: Genetic, metabolic characteristics, therapeutic strategies and nanomedicine. *Current Medicinal Chemistry, 28*(42), 8755–8781. https://doi.org/10.2174/0929867328666210705144456

Carlsson, S. V., & Vickers, A. J. (2020). Screening for prostate cancer. *Medical Clinics of North America, 104*(6), 1051–1062. https://doi.org/10.1016/j.mcna.2020.08.007

Centers for Disease Control and Prevention (CDC). (2021). *Human papilloma virus (HPV) vaccination: What Everyone should know.* https://www.cdc.gov/vaccines/vpd/hpv/public/index.html

Centers for Disease Control and Prevention (CDC). (2022). *HPV and cancer.* https://www.cdc.gov/cancer/hpv/statistics/cases.htm

Collins, S., & Lewicky-Gaupp, C. (2022). Pelvic organ prolapse. *Gastroenterology Clinics of North America, 51*(1), 177–193. https://doi.org/10.1016/j.gtc.2021.10.011

Corey, B., Smania, M. A., Spotts, H., & Andersen, M. (2020). Young women with breast cancer: Treatment, care, and nursing implications. *Clinical Journal of Oncology Nursing, 24*(2), 139–147. https://doi.org/10.1188/20.CJON.139-147

Desai, P., & Aggarwal, A. (2021). Breast cancer in women over 65 years- a review of screening and treatment options. *Clinics Geriatric Medicine, 37*(4), 611–623. https://doi.org/10.1016/j.cger.2021.05.007

Devlin, C. M., Simms, M. S., & Maitland, N. J. (2021). Benign prostatic hyperplasia—What do we know? *BJU International, 127*(4), 389–399. https://doi.org/10.1111/bju.15229

El Sabeh, M., & Borahay, M. A. (2021). The future of uterine fibroid management: A more preventive and personalized paradigm. *Reproductive Sciences, 28*(11), 3285–3288. https://doi.org/10.1007/s43032-021-00618-y

Erickson, L. A., & Chen, B. (2020). Fibroadenoma of the breast. *Mayo Clinic Proceedings*, *95*(11), 2573–2574. https://doi.org/10.1016/j.mayocp.2020.08.040

Farr, A., Effendy, I., Frey Tirri, B., Hof, H., Mayser, P., Petricevic, L., Ruhnke, M., Schaller, M., Schaefer, A. P. A., Sustr, V., Willinger, B., & Mendling, W. (2021). Guideline: Vulvovaginal candidosis (AWMF 015/072, level S2k). *Mycoses*, *64*(6), 583–602. https://doi.org/10.1111/myc.13248

Jackson, T., Carmichael, C., Lovett, K., Scott, M., Shakya, S., & Sotak, M. (2022). Approach to the patient with a palpable breast mass. *JAAPA: Official Journal of the American Academy of Physician Assistants*, *35*(10), 22–28. https://doi.org/10.1097/01.JAA.0000873772.13779.01

Jafarzadeh, L., Ranjbar, M., Nazari, T., Naeimi Eshkaleti, M., Aghaei Gharehbolagh, S., Sobel, J. D., & Mahmoudi, S. (2022). Vulvovaginal candidiasis: An overview of mycological, clinical, and immunological aspects. *Journal of Obstetrics Gynaecology Research*, *48*(7), 1546–1560. https://doi.org/10.1111/jog.15267

Lam, J. C., Lang, R., & Stokes, W. (2023). How I manage bacterial prostatitis. *Clinical Microbiology and Infection*, *29*(1), 32–37. https://doi.org/10.1016/j.cmi.2022.05.035

Mahoney, D. E., & Pierce, J. D. (2022). Ovarian cancer symptom clusters: Use of the NIH symptom science model for precision in symptom recognition and management. *Clinical Journal of Oncology Nursing*, *26*(5), 533–542. https://doi.org/10.1188/22.CJON.533-542

Makker, V., MacKay, H., Ray-Coquard, I., Levine, D. A., Westin, S. N., Aoki, D., & Oaknin, A. (2021). Endometrial cancer. *Nature Review Disease Primers*, *7*(1), 88. https://doi.org/10.1038/s41572-021-00324-8

Marnach, M. L., Wygant, J. N., & Casey, P. M. (2022). Evaluation and management of vaginitis. *Mayo Clinic Proceedings*, *97*(2), 347–358. https://doi.org/10.1016/j.mayocp.2021.09.022

Menon, U., Karpinskyj, C., & Gentry-Maharaj, A. (2018). Ovarian cancer prevention and screening. *Obstetrics Gynecology*, *131*(5), 909–927. https://doi.org/10.1097/AOG.0000000000002580

Norris, T. (2025). *Porth's pathophysiology: Concepts of altered health States*, 11th ed. Wolters Kluwer.

Penny, S. M. (2020). Ovarian cancer: An overview. *Radiologic Technology*, *91*(6), 561–575.

Pleasant, V. (2022). Benign breast disease. *Clinical Obstetrics and Gynecology*, *65*(3), 448–460. https://doi.org/10.1097/GRF.0000000000000719

Prostate cancer. (2021). *Nature Reviews. Disease Primers*, *7*(1), 8. https://doi.org/10.1038/s41572-021-00249-2

Raju, R., & Linder, B. J. (2021). Evaluation and management of pelvic organ prolapse. *Mayo Clinic Proceedings*, *96*(12), 3122–3129. https://doi.org/10.1016/j.mayocp.2021.09.005

Ren, W., Chen, M., Qiao, Y., & Zhao, F. (2022). Global guidelines for breast cancer screening: A systematic review. *Breast (Edinburgh, Scotland)*, *64*, 85–99. https://doi.org/10.1016/j.breast.2022.04.003

Sadeghi, H. M., Adeli, I., Calina, D., Docea, A. O., Mousavi, T., Daniali, M., Nikfar, S., Tsatsakis, A., & Abdollahi, M. (2022). Polycystic ovary syndrome: A comprehensive review of pathogenesis, management, and drug repurposing. *International Journal of Molecular Science*, *23*(2), 583. https://doi.org/10.3390/ijms23020583

Sekhoacha, M., Riet, K., Motloung, P., Gumenku, L., Adegoke, A., & Mashele, S. (2022). Prostate cancer review: Genetics, diagnosis, treatment options, and alternative approaches. *Molecules (Basel, Switzerland)*, *27*(17), 5730. https://doi.org/10.3390/molecules27175730

Stewart, C., Ralyea, C., & Lockwood, S. (2019). Ovarian cancer: An integrated review. *Seminars in Oncology Nursing*, *35*(2), 151–156. https://doi.org/10.1016/j.soncn.2019.02.00

Su, Z. T., Zenilman, J. M., Sfanos, K. S., & Herati, A. S. (2020). Management of chronic bacterial prostatitis. *Current Urology Reports*, *21*(7), 29. https://doi.org/10.1007/s11934-020-00978-z

Taylor, H. S., Kotlyar, A. M., & Flores, V. A. (2021). Endometriosis is a chronic systemic disease: Clinical challenges and novel innovations. *Lancet (London, England)*, *397*(10276), 839–852. https://doi.org/10.1016/S0140-6736(21)00389-5

Ulin, M., Ali, M., Chaudhry, Z. T., Al-Hendy, A., & Yang, Q. (2020). Uterine fibroids in menopause and perimenopause. *Menopause (New York, N.Y.)*, *27*(2), 238–242. https://doi.org/10.1097/GME.0000000000001438

Wasim, S., Lee, S. Y., & Kim, J. (2022). Complexities of prostate cancer. *International Journal of Molecular Science*, *23*(22), 14257. https://doi.org/10.3390/ijms232214257

Yang, Q., Ciebiera, M., Bariani, M. V., Ali, M., Elkafas, H., Boyer, T. G., & Al-Hendy, A. (2022). Comprehensive review of uterine fibroids: Developmental origin, pathogenesis, and treatment. *Endocrine Reviews*, *43*(4), 678–719. https://doi.org/10.1210/endrev/bnab039

Yen, T. T., Wang, T. L., Fader, A. N., Shih, I. M., & Gaillard, S. (2020). Molecular classification and emerging targeted therapy in endometrial cancer. *International Journal of Gynecological Pathology*, *39*(1), 26–35. https://doi.org/10.1097/PGP.0000000000000585

Appendices and index

Practice makes perfect   **496**

Glossary   **533**

Index   **539**

Questions

1. What intracellular structure (organelle) is responsible for producing cellular energy?
    A.   Ribosome
    B.   Mitochondrion
    C.   Golgi apparatus
    D.   Nucleus

2. The cell's primary response to adverse stimuli and threats to cellular integrity is:
    A.   cellular adaptation.
    B.   cellular regeneration.
    C.   sending nerve signals to the central nervous system.
    D.   cellular death.

3. Which endocrine gland is central to maintaining homeostasis by
means of regulating other glands?
    A.   Thyroid
    B.   Pituitary
    C.   Adrenal
    D.   Parathyroid

4. In the fight-or-flight response, the rush of adrenaline is associated with what kind of behavior?
    A.   Aggression and panic
    B.   Crying and sadness
    C.   Withdrawal and depression
    D.   Panic and withdrawal

5. The prodromal stage of a disease occurs when:
    A.   the disease reaches its full intensity.
    B.   the body regains health and homeostasis.
    C.   signs and symptoms are mild and nonspecific.
    D.   the patient progresses toward recovery.

6. A carcinoma is a cancer that derives from what kind of tissue?
    A.   Glandular
    B.   Liver
    C.   Bone marrow
    D.   Epithelium

---

[*]Note: In this appendix, the term "male" refers to a person assigned male at birth, and the term "female"
refers to a person assigned female at birth.

7. When instructing a patient on performing breast self-examination, which area of the breast should you teach as the one in which the majority of tumors arise?
   A. Upper outer quadrant
   B. Lower inner quadrant
   C. Areolar area
   D. Upper inner quadrant

8. A 60-year-old patient tells you that she fears the rectal examination portion of her annual gynecologic checkup. What teaching will you provide regarding the importance of the rectal examination?
   A. "Colorectal cancer is the most common cause of death in females older than age 60."
   B. "The rectal examination is important for identifying most polyps."
   C. "The rectal examination is a way to check for occult blood in feces."
   D. "The rectal examination is the best way to detect colon cancer."

9. A patient at increased risk for malignant melanoma asks how to perform a self-check for this disease. Which nursing response is appropriate?
   A. Check existing moles for changes, such as enlargement or discoloration.
   B. Have yearly examinations performed by a health care provider.
   C. Report new moles located on the abdomen.
   D. Contact the health care provider if a nevus develops.

10. Which cancer should you monitor for in a patient with a history of infectious mononucleosis?
    A. Multiple myeloma
    B. Leukemia
    C. Malignant melanoma
    D. Hodgkin disease

11. Which term indicates cell-damaging proteins derived from bacteria?
    A. Erythrogenic toxins
    B. Exotoxins
    C. Neurotoxins
    D. Endotoxins

12. Which teaching will the nurse provide to a patient who is newly pregnant and has cats for pets?
    A. "Be sure that they're tested and vaccinated against feline leukemia."
    B. "Have someone else change the litter."
    C. "Avoid contact with the cats during the summer flea season."
    D. "Avoid being scratched by the cats."

13. What's the most likely cause of diarrhea in an 84-year-old patient who, 3 to 4 days earlier, consumed a supplemental drink to which a raw egg had been added for protein supplementation?
    A. Toxoplasmosis
    B. Typhoid fever
    C. Salmonellosis
    D. Botulism

14. A student comes to the student health clinic reporting a terrible sore throat and fever. The prescribed antibiotics haven't helped after 1 week. What other disease should the student be tested for?
    A. Hodgkin disease
    B. Rubella
    C. Infectious mononucleosis
    D. Leukemia

15. The caregiver of a 12-year-old patient reports that the child isn't getting enough sleep, as evidenced by dark circles underneath the eyes. The nurse will further assess for which symptoms?
    A. Bruises and darkened areas elsewhere on body
    B. Periods of altered states of consciousness such as staring off into space
    C. Drug use
    D. Headaches and nasal congestion due to allergies

16. A hospital employee with a history of severe reactions to bee stings comes to the emergency department after being stung by a bee while working outside. Which medication should be given immediately?
    A. Epinephrine
    B. Aminophylline
    C. Diphenhydramine
    D. Methylprednisolone

17. Which test would be used initially to determine the presence of human immunodeficiency virus (HIV) infection in a 26-year-old woman with a history of intravenous drug use and herpes simplex infection?
    A. White blood cell (WBC) count
    B. Erythrocyte sedimentation rate
    C. Enzyme-linked immunosorbent assay (ELISA)
    D. Serum beta microglobulin

18. A 38-year-old woman comes to the office reporting morning stiffness and pain affecting the small joints of her hands and feet. The symptoms have progressively worsened over several months, and she isn't aware of having fever, rash, or other symptoms. Which disorder should be further investigated?
    A. Systemic lupus erythematosus (SLE)
    B. Rheumatoid arthritis (RA)
    C. Osteoarthritis
    D. Lyme disease

19. Which part of the immune system is responsible for rejecting organ transplants?
    A. Humoral
    B. Complement system
    C. Autoimmunity
    D. Cell-mediated

20. The caretaker of a 24-year-old patient with Down syndrome notices that the patient has begun to urinate frequently and in large amounts. The assessment data alert the nurse to the development of which disease, common in adults with Down syndrome?
    A. Diabetes mellitus (DM)
    B. Diabetes insipidus (DI)
    C. Rheumatoid arthritis (RA)
    D. Syndrome of inappropriate antidiuretic hormone (SIADH)

21. A patient whose son has hemophilia is pregnant. The fetus has been determined to be female. Which statement by the nurse is accurate regarding the chances that the child will be born with hemophilia?
    A. "There is a 25% chance that the child will have hemophilia."
    B. "The child isn't at risk for the disease."
    C. "It is unusual for two children of the same biological parents to develop the disease."
    D. "The child will most likely have hemophilia."

22. A patient with sickle cell trait is married to someone who also has the trait. The patient asks the nurse what the chances are that one of their children will have sickle cell anemia. What is the best nursing response?
    A. Each child has a 1 in 2 chance.
    B. Each child has a 1 in 4 chance.
    C. Each child has a 1 in 8 chance.
    D. Each child will have sickle cell disease.

23. A pregnant person has learned that a neonate is given a blood test that requires taking blood from the heel. They report that they do not want this done to their baby. Which nursing response regarding the purpose of the test for phenylketonuria (PKU) may alleviate the patient's anxiety?
    A. PKU is most common in people of African descent.
    B. The test shows whether the child will contract the disease later in life.
    C. Testing for PKU is mandatory in the state.
    D. PKU affects infants in the first few months of life, causing devastating irreversible damage.

24. Which signs and symptoms will the nurse anticipate in a patient with Addison disease?
    A. Darkening skin and a craving for salty food
    B. A craving for sweet foods and other carbohydrates
    C. Excessive thirst and urination
    D. Buffalo hump and thinning scalp hair

25. Which assessment would be most informative when Graves disease is suspected?
    A. Checking the patient's reflexes
    B. Doing a urinalysis
    C. Checking for Romberg sign
    D. Checking urine specific gravity

26. What does the nurse suspect in a female patient who takes prednisone for chronic asthma, reports fragile skin that bruises easily, has a lump on the back of the neck, and has a round, swollen face?
    A. Cushing syndrome
    B. Addison disease
    C. Hyperthyroidism
    D. Graves disease

27. A patient complains of heat intolerance, weight loss, and nervousness for the last month. Which may be the cause of these problems?
    A. Hashimoto disease
    B. Menopause
    C. Graves disease
    D. Cushing disease

28. A patient reports of burning pain in the feet and lower legs. What disease will the nurse ask about during the assessment?
    A. Hashimoto disease
    B. Diabetes insipidus
    C. Cushing disease
    D. Diabetes mellitus

29. A 73-year-old patient with a history of chronic obstructive pulmonary disease (COPD) is admitted with respiratory failure. The patient is intubated and placed on mechanical ventilation. Which process is interrupted when oxygen is delivered directly to the lower airways?
   A. Gas exchange
   B. Humidifying and warming of air
   C. Conversion of oxygen to carbon dioxide
   D. Reflex bronchospasm

30. The results of a ventilation-perfusion scan (V/Q scan) indicate a high V/Q ratio. What problem does this reflect?
   A. Decreased alveolar perfusion
   B. Increased alveolar perfusion
   C. Pulmonary edema
   D. Decreased ventilation

31. A patient with chronic obstructive pulmonary disease (COPD) has a sudden onset of unilateral pleuritic chest pain that worsens with coughing. The patient has severe shortness of breath and chest wall movement is asymmetrical. Which assessment finding is most significant in establishing a diagnosis?
   A. Crackles in both lung bases
   B. Significantly decreased breath sounds on the symptomatic side
   C. Expiratory wheezing
   D. Rhonchi scattered throughout both lung fields

32. How is cor pulmonale best described?
   A. Left-sided heart failure
   B. Pulmonary hypertension
   C. Ventilation-perfusion (V/Q) mismatch
   D. Right ventricular failure

33. A 76-year-old patient is admitted with a history of heart failure and now presents with pulmonary edema. What pathophysiologic process is occurring?
   A. Perfusion to the lungs is interrupted by a pulmonary embolus.
   B. Increased hydrostatic pressure in the capillaries causes fluid to leak into the alveoli, collapsing them.
   C. Increased hydrostatic pressure in the capillaries causes fluid to leak into the interstitial spaces.
   D. Fluid accumulates in the lung interstitium, alveolar spaces, and small airways.

34. What is the best method to assess for pulsus paradoxus?
    A. Check for central venous pressure elevation greater than 15 mm Hg above normal.
    B. Auscultate for muffled heart sounds on inspiration.
    C. Measure blood pressure at rest and again while the patient slowly inspires to check if the systolic pressure drops more than 10 mm Hg during inspiration.
    D. Check the electrocardiogram (ECG) for reduced amplitude.

35. When myocardial cells are hypoxic, they signal the body to produce epinephrine and norepinephrine, which cause the heart to beat stronger and faster (thus increasing blood flow to the cells). Why is this compensatory mechanism sometimes harmful?
    A. It actually increases oxygen demand in the heart.
    B. It depletes the myocardial cells of calcium.
    C. It diverts blood to the extremities.
    D. It decreases contractility of the heart.

36. The nurse is obtaining a throat culture on an 8-year-old child who has fever, purulent tonsilar drainage, and difficulty swallowing. What bacteria does the nurse suspect?
    A. *Staphylococcus aureus*
    B. Group A beta-hemolytic streptococci
    C. *Clostridium perfringens*
    D. *Pseudomonas aeruginosa*

37. A patient with chronic heart failure caused by pulmonic stenosis begins to have symptoms of abdominal pain and distention. On examination, the patient is found to have an enlarged liver. What does the nurse suspect as the likely cause of these findings?
    A. Cirrhosis
    B. Hepatic vein engorgement
    C. Hepatitis
    D. Ascites

38. A patient with a history of chronic renal failure develops left-sided chest pain that begins in the sternum and radiates to the neck. It worsens with deep inspiration and eases when sitting upright and leaning forward. On assessment, the nurse notes that the heart sounds are muffled. Which condition does the nurse suspect as causing these symptoms?
    A. Pneumonia
    B. Cardiac tamponade
    C. Myocardial infarction
    D. Pericarditis

39. A 30-year-old woman presents with a recent onset of blurred vision, loss of sensation in the lower legs, and difficulty speaking clearly. The symptoms come and go unpredictably, but they have been occurring for several months. What's the most likely cause of these symptoms?
    A. Multiple sclerosis
    B. Myasthenia gravis
    C. Aneurysm
    D. Guillain-Barré syndrome

40. Which portion of the neurologic system causes the heart to pound and dry mouth when faced with a scary situation?
    A. Somatic
    B. Extrapyramidal
    C. Pyramidal
    D. Autonomic

41. What brain neurotransmitter is deficient in patients who have Alzheimer disease?
    A. Dopamine
    B. Serotonin
    C. Norepinephrine
    D. Acetylcholine

42. What is the most common cause of stroke in middle-aged and older adults?
    A. Aneurysm
    B. Thrombosis
    C. Embolism
    D. Hypertension

43. A patient is experiencing hallucinations and vertigo. Which seizure disorder is the patient most likely to be experiencing?
    A. Absence seizure
    B. Parietal lobe sensory seizure
    C. Jacksonian seizure
    D. Grand mal seizure

44. A patient who has chronic renal failure has been diagnosed with anemia. The nurse knows that anemia is caused by which of the following?
    A. Loss of albumin lost through impaired kidney function
    B. Bleeding rapidly from the damaged kidneys
    C. A lack of erythropoietin due to a lack of kidney response
    D. A sudden loss of blood from the hemodialysis treatments

45. A patient has an increase in white blood cell precursor cells in the bone marrow. Which condition is the most likely cause?
    A. Leukemia
    B. Polycythemia
    C. Thrombocytopenia
    D. Multiple myeloma

46. A patient who was diagnosed with an acute myocardial infarction has an intra-aortic balloon pump in place. The patient developed thrombocytopenia. Which condition is the most likely cause?
    A. Malnutrition
    B. Platelet destruction
    C. Internal hemorrhage
    D. Disseminated intravascular coagulation (DIC)

47. A patient develops petechiae and an oral blood blister. Thrombocytopenia is suspected and a platelet count is obtained. Which assessment finding is significant for the diagnosis of thrombocytopenia?
    A. 400,000/mm^3
    B. 90,000/mm^3
    C. 500,000/mm^3
    D. 150,000/mm^3

48. A patient diagnosed with disseminated intravascular coagulation (DIC) is receiving anticoagulants. Which teaching should the nurse provide to the patient regarding the purpose of the anticoagulants?
    A. "They prevent emboli formation that may occur as a result of increased clotting factors seen in DIC."
    B. "They combat clot formation in the small blood vessels."
    C. "They prevent clot formation that may develop as blood pools beneath the skin."
    D. "They combat thrombus formation that may occur because the patient requires bed rest."

49. A woman who is obese, consumes a high-cholesterol diet, and is receiving hormone replacement therapy (HRT). This patient carries an increased risk for what disorder?
    A. Appendicitis
    B. Cirrhosis
    C. Pancreatitis
    D. Cholecystitis

50. What hepatic tissue changes have taken place in a patient newly diagnosed with cirrhosis?
    A. Hepatic cells are distended and misshapen.
    B. Hepatic blood vessels are destroyed.
    C. Fibrous tissue replaces normal hepatic cells.
    D. Hepatic cells begin to die.

51. A patient who has a history of alcohol misuse and gastric ulcers comes to the emergency department with severe, persistent, piercing abdominal pain in the midepigastic region that radiates into the back. What is the most likely cause of the patient's pain?
    A. Perforated gastric ulcer
    B. Pancreatitis
    C. Appendicitis
    D. Cholecystitis

52. A patient presents to the emergency department reporting severe midepigastric pain. Pancreatitis is suspected. Which laboratory tests help to confirm the diagnosis?
   A. White blood cell (WBC) count and hemoglobin level
   B. Serum amylase and lipase levels
   C. Serum lipid and trypsin levels
   D. Total serum bilirubin and indirect bilirubin levels

53. A patient is diagnosed with peptic ulcer disease caused by *Helicobacter pylori* infection. The patient asks how bacteria can cause an ulcer. Which nursing response is appropriate?
   A. Bacteria colonize the mucous lining.
   B. Bacteria cause regurgitation of duodenal contents into the stomach.
   C. Bacteria release an enzyme that destroys the stomach's mucous lining.
   D. Bacteria cause persistent inflammation of the stomach.

54. A patient has been diagnosed with chronic renal failure. What percent of the patient's renal tissue is probably nonfunctional?
   A. Less than 24%
   B. 25% to 49%
   C. 50% to 74%
   D. 75% or greater

55. A patient is recovering from septic shock. Upon assessment, the nurse notes a blood pressure of 110/82 and urinary output of 100 milliliters per 8 hours. Which statement by the nurse to the patient is accurate regarding the urine output?
   A. "You have an acid–base imbalance."
   B. "You are experiencing blood loss."
   C. "Oliguria, which is low urine output, occurs in acute tubular necrosis."
   D. "The amount of urine indicates dehydration."

56. A patient has been diagnosed with acute bacterial prostatitis. Which is a common cause of bacterial prostatitis?
   A. An ascending infection of the urinary tract
   B. Lymphatic migration of pathogenic bacteria
   C. Prostatic hyperplasia
   D. An infection in the patient's blood

57. A patient presents with acute, severe pain in the lower back, radiating to the side and pubic region. Renal calculi are suspected. What test is most likely performed to confirm the diagnosis?
   A. Computed tomography (CT) scan of the abdomen
   B. Magnetic resonance imaging (MRI) of the pelvis
   C. Cystoscopy of the bladder
   D. X-ray of abdomen

58. An athlete is most likely to experience injury in which type of joint?
   A. Synarthrosis
   B. Amphiarthrosis
   C. Diarthrosis
   D. None of these

59. A patient who takes furosemide twice per day reports pain in the right great toe. Which substance is the cause of the pain?
   A. Calcium pyrophosphate
   B. Sodium urate
   C. Ammonia sulfate
   D. Sodium bicarbonate

60. A patient reports progressively worsening pain in one knee that is more severe in the morning. This pain is most likely caused by which disorder?
   A. Rheumatoid arthritis (RA)
   B. Systemic lupus erythematosus (SLE)
   C. Gouty arthritis
   D. Osteoarthritis

61. A patient is admitted with difficulty breathing. On admission, the patient's arterial blood gas (ABG) results are pH 7.25, $Paco_2$ 70 mm Hg, Pao_2 52 mm Hg, and HCO_3^- 32 mEq/L. Which acid–base imbalance is this patient exhibiting?
   A. Metabolic acidosis
   B. Metabolic alkalosis
   C. Respiratory acidosis
   D. Respiratory alkalosis

62. A patient comes to the emergency department with a history of vomiting for the past 5 days. An arterial blood gas (ABG) analysis obtained on admission reveals the following:

05/30/24	0530	Laboratory called with ABG results: pH = 7.5,
		$Paco_2$ = 48 mm Hg, HCO_3 = 39 mEq/L, and
		Pao_2 = 110 mm Hg. Dr. Riggins notified of ABG results.
		Louise Reynolds, RN

These ABG results reveal which acid–base imbalance?
   A. Respiratory acidosis
   B. Respiratory alkalosis
   C. Metabolic acidosis
   D. Metabolic alkalosis

63. Which condition can results in metabolic acidosis?
    A. Central nervous system (CNS) depression from drugs
    B. Renal disease
    C. Gram-negative bacteremia
    D. Asphyxia

64. A patient presents with partial pressure of arterial carbon dioxide ($PaCO_2$) above 50 mm Hg and partial pressure of arterial oxygen (PaO_2) below 50 mm Hg. The assessment data alert the nurse to the development of which disease in a patient with normal lung tissue?
    A. Acute respiratory failure
    B. Severe acute respiratory syndrome
    C. Asthma
    D. Cor pulmonale

65. Which is thought to contribute to diverticular disease in developed countries?
    A. Low intake of dietary protein
    B. High intake of dietary fiber
    C. High dietary intake of saturated fat
    D. Low intake of dietary fiber

66. Which type of gastrointestinal disease would cause LLQ abdominal pain, constipation alternating with diarrhea, and abdominal distension?
    A. Diverticulitis
    B. Cholecystitis
    C. Appendicitis
    D. Pancreatitis

67. Which statement best describes the pathophysiology of gastroesophageal reflux disease (GERD)?
    A. The sphincter doesn't remain closed, and the pressure in the stomach pushes the stomach contents into the esophagus.
    B. The mucosa takes on a "cobblestone" appearance.
    C. A defect in the diaphragm permits a portion of the stomach to pass through the esophageal hiatus into the chest cavity.
    D. *Helicobacter pylori* bacteria release a toxin that destroys the stomach's mucous lining.

68. Which laboratory test helps distinguish esophagitis from cardiac disorders?
    A. Esophageal manometry
    B. Barium swallow
    C. Acid perfusion test
    D. Upper GI series

69. Which disorder occurs more commonly in persons with diabetes mellitus?
    A. Osteoarthritis
    B. Osteomyelitis
    C. Osteomalacia
    D. Osteoporosis

70. What's the most common causative organism in osteomyelitis?
    A. *Staphylococcus aureus*
    B. *Streptococcus pyogenes*
    C. *Pseudomonas aeruginosa*
    D. *Proteus vulgaris*

71. Pulmonary embolism generally results from an obstruction of the pulmonary arterial bed caused by:
    A. sickle cell disease.
    B. foreign substance.
    C. heart valve growth.
    D. dislodged thrombi originating in the leg veins or pelvis.

72. Which signs and symptoms does the nurse anticipate in a patient who has been diagnosed with severe acute respiratory syndrome (SARS)? **Select all that apply.**
    A. High fever
    B. Chills
    C. Sudden onset of chest pain
    D. Dry cough
    E. Shortness of breath
    F. Neck stiffness

73. When rhabdomyolysis occurs, which substances are released from necrotic muscle fibers into the circulation? **Select all that apply.**
    A. Myoglobin
    B. Sodium
    C. Creatine kinase (CK)
    D. Urate
    E. Potassium
    F. Calcium

74. Replication and duplication of deoxyribonucleic acid (DNA) occur during four phases of mitosis. Which illustration shows anaphase?

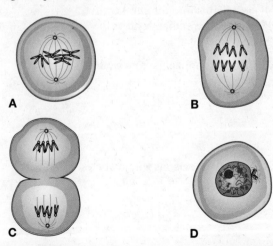

A

B

C

D

75. Which of the following is the BEST test for diagnosis of myocardial infarction?
    A. Myoglobin level
    B. ECG changes
    C. Troponin level
    D. CPK elevation

76. In gastroesophageal reflux disease, the lower esophageal sphincter (LES) doesn't remain closed because of deficient lower esophageal pressure. Place an "X" over the LES.

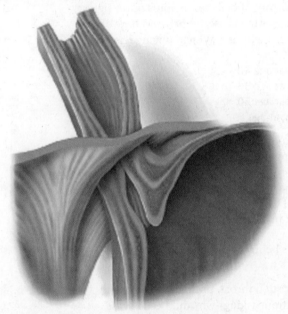

77. A patient is hospitalized for observation after a head injury now having tonic-clonic seizures and has been ordered an immediate injection of 15 mg/kg phenytoin IV. The patient's weight on admission was 176 lb. In grams, what total dose of phenytoin should be administered by slow IV infusion? Record your answer using one decimal place. _____ g

78. Which disorder should the nurse suspect when a patient presents with thin skin, GI disturbances, bone loss, hyperglycemia, and a rounded face?
    A. Hypothyroidism
    B. Addison disease
    C. Diabetes insipidus
    D. Cushing syndrome

79. A patient is diagnosed with Addison disease and asks the nurse, "What caused this to happen?" Which nursing response is appropriate?
   A. It is from too much glucocorticoids.
   B. The thyroid hormone is being overproduced.
   C. Your adrenal gland has been attacked by your immune system.
   D. The cause is from an insufficient antidiuretic hormone production.

80. A patient with no family history of diabetes mellitus or no signs/symptoms of diabetes mellitus asks the nurse, "When and how often should I be screened for diabetes mellitus?" Which nursing response is appropriate?
   A. Every 5 years starting at age 40
   B. Every 3 years starting at age 35
   C. Every 2 years starting at age 50
   D. Every 10 years starting at age 55

81. A patient is diagnosed with diabetes insipidus and asks the nurse, "What caused this to happen?" Which nursing response is appropriate?
   A. "The thyroid hormone is being overproduced."
   B. "It is from a release of too much glucocorticoids."
   C. "The cause is from an insufficient antidiuretic hormone production."
   D. "Your adrenal gland is being grossly attacked by your immune system."

82. A patient, being treated for strep throat, presents to the health clinic with a vaginal yeast infection, asking "why did I get a yeast infection?" Which nursing response is appropriate?
   A. "Strep throat causes other types of infections in the body."
   B. "The yeast infection was a result of mycotoxin release from fungi."
   C. "Antibiotic treatment kills normal body flora allowing fungus to grow."
   D. "It is a coincidence and doesn't have anything to do with strep throat."

83. When assessing a patient at risk for infection, which factors should the nurse assess? **Select all that apply.**
   A. Nutritional status
   B. Who lives in the patient's home
   C. Serum potassium level
   D. Bowel movement regularity

84. A patient has bilateral conjunctivitis. Which is appropriate for the nurse to teach the patient?
    A.   "Avoid getting water in or around the eyes."
    B.   "Gently rub or massage the eyes twice daily."
    C.   "Wash your hands after caring for your eyes."
    D.   "Carry a tissue to wipe both eyes when drainage occurs."

85. A nurse is caring for a patient who has been diagnosed with labyrinthitis. Which actions should the nurse take to prevent possible complications? **Select all that apply.**
    A.   Assess hearing.
    B.   Provide low-fat diet.
    C.   Administer IV antibiotics.
    D.   Discuss smoking cessation.
    E.   Assist the patient when getting out of bed.

86. The nurse is caring for a patient with a bleeding disorder. Which product should the nurse prepare to administer to replace clotting factors?
    A.   Platelets
    B.   Albumin
    C.   Cryoprecipitate
    D.   Packed red blood cells

87. A patient with disseminated intravascular coagulation asks the nurse "What is happening to me?" Which statement by the nurse is appropriate?
    A.   "There aren't enough red blood cells in your body to stop the bleeding."
    B.   "The clotting factors in your body have been used up, causing you to bleed."
    C.   "Your high blood pressure is causing you to bleed uncontrollably."
    D.   "Disseminated intravascular coagulation is a very rare disease that can only be cured with antibiotics."

88. The nurse is caring for a patient with a clotting disorder. Which lab value should the nurse monitor?
    A.   Iodine
    B.   Sodium
    C.   Calcium
    D.   Phosphorous

89. A student nurse asks the instructor, "How will I know if the treatments for neutropenia have been effective?" The nursing instructor should direct the student to look at which assessment data?
    A.   Energy level
    B.   Temperature
    C.   Urine output
    D.   Hematocrit level

90. Which type of epileptic seizure has signs and symptoms that include a glassy stare, aimless wandering, and no memory of actions during the seizure?
   A. Grand mal seizure
   B. Complex partial seizure
   C. Generalized tonic-clonic seizure
   D. Jacksonian seizure

91. Which neurologic disorder is characterized by progressive degeneration of the cerebral cortex?
   A. Alzheimer disease
   B. Epilepsy
   C. Guillain-Barré syndrome
   D. Myasthenia gravis

92. In patients with celiac disease, which food item must be avoided in the gluten-free diet? **Select all that apply**.
   A. Barley
   B. Rice
   C. Rye
   D. Wheat

93. The nurse is teaching a patient about modifiable risk factors for colon cancer. Which factors should be included? **Select all that apply**.
   A. Excessive alcohol intake
   B. Smoking
   C. Age
   D. Irritable bowel diseases
   E. Obesity

94. Which factors contribute to Virchow triad? **Select all that apply**.
   A. Long-term use of antibiotics
   B. Hypercoagulability
   C. Massage
   D. Venous stasis
   E. Venous endothelial injury
   F. Wearing compression stockings

95. Which parameters are used in the diagnosis of stage 1 hypertension?
   A. Sustained systolic BP greater than or equal to 140 mm Hg or a diastolic BP greater than or equal to 90 mm Hg
   B. Sustained systolic BP of 130 mm Hg to 139 mm Hg or a diastolic BP of 80 mm to 89 mm Hg
   C. One-time systolic BP of 150 mm Hg and diastolic BP of 90 mm Hg
   D. Sustained systolic BP of 120 mm Hg to 129 mm Hg or a diastolic BP of less than 80 mm Hg

96. Which of the following patients does the nurse recognize as most susceptible to respiratory syncytial virus (RSV)?
    A. A 1-year-old
    B. A 7-year-old
    C. A 24-year-old
    D. A 39-year-old

97. The health care provider discusses ordering a novel oral anticoagulant for a patient who is at risk for pulmonary embolism. Which medication does the nurse anticipate will be ordered?
    A. Heparin
    B. Enoxaparin
    C. Alteplase
    D. Apixaban

98. Which is the most accurate measurement of glomerular filtration?
    A. Blood pressure
    B. Intake and output
    C. Creatinine clearance
    D. BUN

99. What is the cause of prerenal failure?
    A. Bilateral obstruction of urine outflow
    B. Conditions that diminish blood flow to the kidneys
    C. Damage to the kidneys themselves
    D. Damage to the filtering systems of the kidneys

100. Which is the main complication of benign prostatic hyperplasia?
    A. Urinary obstruction
    B. Renal calculi
    C. Prostatitis
    D. UTI

101. When do the kidneys secrete erythropoietin?
    A. Renin is secreted in response to a decrease in extracellular fluid volume.
    B. Calcium levels are insufficient.
    C. Vitamin D becomes inactive.
    D. The oxygen supply in the blood circulating through the tissue drops.

102. Which factor can contribute to the formation of renal calculi?
    A. Hypocalcemia
    B. Changes in urine pH
    C. Hypothyroidism
    D. Hypophosphatemia

103. After contraction of HIV, when does HIV antibody usually first appear in the bloodstream?
   A. Immediately after HIV exposure
   B. 10 to 15 days after HIV exposure
   C. 2 weeks to 6 months after HIV exposure
   D. 1 to 2 years after HIV exposure

104. Which immunoglobulin is responsible for the hypersensitivity reaction?
   A. IgA
   B. IgG
   C. IgE
   D. IgM

105. Which type of rhinitis is caused by excessive use of nasal sprays or drops?
   A. Allergic rhinitis
   B. Chronic vasomotor rhinitis
   C. Infectious rhinitis
   D. Rhinitis medicamentosa

106. Which is the most common anaphylaxis-causing antigen?
   A. Bee sting
   B. Penicillin
   C. Shellfish
   D. Nuts

107. The nurse notices that a patient has several 2-cm vesicles, all filled with serous fluid. How does the nurse document this finding?
   A. Bulla
   B. Cyst
   C. Nodule
   D. Plaque

108. A patient having an allergic reaction is noted to have transient, elevated, irregularly shaped areas of local swelling on the skin. How does the nurse identify these lesions?
   A. Vesicle
   B. Macule
   C. Wheal
   D. Lichenification

Answers

1. B. Adenosine triphosphate, which is the energy that fuels cellular activity, is made in the mitochondria. The ribosome is a submicroscopic ribonucleic acid–containing particle in the cytoplasm of a cell, sometimes closely associated with endoplasmic reticulum and the site of cellular protein synthesis. The Golgi apparatus is a lamellar membranous structure near the nucleus of almost all cells. It contains a curved parallel series of flattened saccules that are often expanded at their ends. In secretory cells, the apparatus concentrates and packages the secretory product. The nucleus is the structure within a cell that contains the chromosomes. It's responsible for the cell's metabolism, growth, and reproduction. CN: Physiological integrity; CNS: Physiological adaptation; CL: Remembering

2. A. When cellular integrity is threatened, the cell reacts by drawing on its reserves to keep functioning and adapting through changes. Cellular regeneration pertains to cellular repair or regrowth. Sending nerve signals to the central nervous system is the responsibility of an afferent sensory nerve. Cellular death is cessation of cellular function. CN: Physiological integrity; CNS: Physiological adaptation; CL: Remembering

3. B. The pituitary gland regulates the function of other glands and is commonly referred to as the "master" gland. The thyroid gland contains active substances such as thyroxine and triiodothyronine. The adrenal gland is a double gland composed of the outer cortex and an inner medulla. The adrenal medulla is controlled by the sympathetic nervous system and functions in conjunction with it. The cortex secretes a group of hormones that vary in quantity and quality. The parathyroids are located close to the thyroid gland and secrete a hormone, parathormone, that regulates calcium and phosphorus metabolism. CN: Physiological integrity; CNS: Physiological adaptation; CL: Remembering

4. A. The release of adrenaline is associated with panic and aggression. Crying and sadness aren't associated with the rush of adrenaline. Withdrawal and depression are behaviors that are associated with a slowing down of responses. Panic and withdrawal is incorrect because withdrawal doesn't correlate with an automatic fight-or-flight response. CN: Physiological integrity; CNS: Physiological adaptation; CL: Remembering

5. C. The prodromal stage is an early phase of disease, when signs and symptoms have begun to appear but are mild and not fully expressed. Thus, the disease hasn't reached its full intensity, the body hasn't regained health and homeostasis, nor has the patient begun to recover from illness. CN: Physiological integrity; CNS: Physiological adaptation; CL: Remembering

6. D. Most cancers derive from epithelial cells and are called *carcinomas*. *Glandular* pertains to, or of, the nature of a gland. The liver is

the largest organ in the body. Bone marrow is the soft tissue occupying the medullary cavities of the sternum, long bones, some haversian canals, and spaces between the trabeculae of cancellous or spongy bone. CN: Physiological integrity; CNS: Physiological adaptation; CL: Remembering

7.   A. About 50% of breast cancers are located in the upper outer quadrant of the breast (not the lower inner quadrant nor the upper inner quadrant). The areolar area and nipple area are the second most common sites for tumors to arise. CN: Physiological integrity; CNS: Reduction of risk potential; CL: Understanding

8.   C. The rectal examination provides a stool sample for performing an occult blood test of feces, which is the simplest and most important screening examination for colorectal cancer. Colorectal cancer is the fourth most common cause of death from cancer in the United States. The rectal examination also helps in determining whether there are masses in the pelvic region. More extensive examinations are needed for diagnosis of polyps. Proctoscopy is necessary to detect colon cancer. CN: Physiological integrity; CNS: Physiological adaptation; CL: Application

9.   A. Because most melanomas arise from existing moles, the patient should be most concerned about checking these moles for enlargement or discoloration. Yearly examinations by the health care provider isn't the best answer, as existing moles can change any time. This would delay diagnosis and intervention, which could lead to a poor outcome. All moles should be monitored for changes in appearance or size, scaliness, oozing, bleeding, itchiness, tenderness, or pain. Development of a nevus (mole) doesn't increase the risk for developing malignant melanoma. CN: Physiological integrity; CNS: Reduction of risk potential; CL: Application

10. D. Although the exact cause of Hodgkin disease is unknown, it's believed to involve a virus because many patients with Hodgkin disease have had infectious mononucleosis. Multiple myeloma is a neoplastic disease characterized by the infiltration of bone and bone marrow by myeloma cells forming multiple tumor masses that lead to pathological fractures. The condition is usually progressive and fatal. Leukemia is a malignancy of the blood-forming cells in the bone marrow. In most patients, the cause is unknown. Malignant melanoma is a malignant, darkly pigmented mole or tumor of the skin. Etiology includes excessive exposure to the sun; heredity may also be a factor. CN: Health promotion and maintenance; CNS: None; CL: Understanding

11. D. Endotoxins are released when the bacterial cell wall decomposes. Erythrogenic toxins pertain to the development of red blood cells. Exotoxins are poisonous substances produced by certain bacteria, including staphylococci, streptococci, and tetanus bacteria. Neurotoxins are substances that attack nerve cells. CN: Physiological integrity; CNS: Physiological adaptation; CL: Remembering

12. B. *Toxoplasma gondii* is commonly found in cat feces and therefore the cat litter; it can cause serious birth defects if the disease is contracted by a person early in pregnancy. Feline leukemia, contact with cats during the summer flea season, and scratches from cats have not been shown to affect the developing human fetus. CN: Physiological integrity; CNS: Reduction of risk potential; CL: Application

13. C. Salmonellosis commonly follows ingestion of inadequately processed foods, especially chicken, turkey, and duck. Toxoplasmosis is a disease caused by infection with the protozoan *Toxoplasma gondii*. The organism is found in many mammals and birds. Diarrhea isn't a symptom. Typhoid fever is an acute infectious disease caused by *Salmonella typhi* found in infected water or milk supplies. Early symptoms include headache, weakness, indefinite pains, and nosebleed. Botulism is a severe form of food poisoning from foods containing the botulinus toxins produced by *Clostridium botulinum* bacteria, which are found in soil and in the intestinal tract of domestic animals. It's usually associated with improperly canned or preserved foods, especially meats (such as ham and sausage) and nonacidic vegetables (such as string beans). CN: Physiological integrity; CNS: Reduction of risk potential; CL: Understanding

14. C. Infectious mononucleosis usually presents as a sore throat and fever along with fatigue in young adults. Hodgkin disease is a malignancy that usually begins in lymph nodes of the supraclavicular, high cervical, or mediastinal area. Rubella is a highly infectious, febrile, viral disease common in children; slight sore throat, lymphadenopathy, and rash are the main symptoms. Clinical findings of leukemia include fatigue, lethargy, and fever; bone and joint pain may also be present. CN: Safe, effective care environment; CNS: Reduction of risk potential; CL: Understanding

15. D. Allergic "shiners" (which are dark circles around the eyes), headaches, and nasal congestion are typical symptoms of allergic rhinitis commonly found in young children and adolescents. Bruises and darkened areas other than near the eyes aren't symptoms of allergic rhinitis. Periods of altered states of consciousness, such as staring off into space, are symptomatic of seizure activity, specifically petit mal seizures. Drug use would likely produce physiologic and behavioral changes well beyond those discussed in this question. CN: Physiological integrity; CNS: Reduction of risk potential; CL: Application

16. A. The single most important medication for this patient is IM or subcutaneous epinephrine. Aminophylline is used to treat asthma that hasn't responded to epinephrine. It's also used as a stimulant to the respiratory center and heart muscle and as a diuretic. Diphenhydramine is an antihistamine. Methylprednisolone is an adrenal corticosteroid. CN: Physiological integrity; CNS: Reduction of risk potential; CL: Understanding

17. C. ELISA is ordered because it's highly sensitive to viral antibodies. However, the test is nonspecific, and it's necessary to follow up with additional, more specific tests to make sure that the infection is caused by HIV. WBC count measures the number of white blood cells; white blood cells are leukocytes. Erythrocyte sedimentation rate measures the rate at which erythrocytes settle out of unclotted blood in an hour. The test is based on the fact that inflammatory processes cause an alteration in blood proteins. Serum beta microglobulin measures beta globulins present in blood plasma or serum, the fraction of the blood serum with which antibodies are associated. CN: Physiological integrity; CNS: Reduction of risk potential; CL: Analysis

18. B. RA usually attacks small, peripheral joints in females ages 35 to 50. Patients with SLE present with a wide diversity of symptoms, but polyarthralgia, polyarthritis, glomerulonephritis, fever, malaise, normocytic anemia, and vasculitis of the hands and feet causing peripheral neuropathy are most common. Osteoarthritis is a type of arthritis marked by progressive cartilage deterioration in synovial joints and vertebrae. Lyme disease is a multisystem disorder caused by the tick-transmitted spirochete *Borrelia burgdorferi*. The patient has a skin lesion, flulike symptoms, and headache. CN: Physiological integrity; CNS: Reduction of risk potential; CL: Analysis

19. D. Cell-mediated immunity is responsible for destroying cells targeted as foreign to the body. Humoral immunity is acquired immunity in which the role of circulating antibody is predominant. Complement system pertains to a group of proteins in the blood that play a vital role in the body's immune defenses through a cascade of alterations. Auto-immunity is the body's tolerance of the antigens present on its own cells. CN: Physiological integrity; CNS: Reduction of risk potential; CL: Remembering

20. A. Adults with Down syndrome have a high incidence of DM. DI is characterized by polyuria and polydipsia caused by inadequate secretion of antidiuretic hormone from the hypothalamus or its release by the posterior pituitary gland. RA is a form of arthritis, the cause of which is unknown, although infection, hypersensitivity, hormone imbalance, and psychological stress have been suggested as possible causes. SIADH isn't associated with Down syndrome. CN: Physiological integrity; CNS: Reduction of risk potential; CL: Analysis

21. B. The child isn't at risk for hemophilia because an X-linked chromosomal abnormality causes it. The daughter may carry the trait but won't have the disease; classic hemophilia is hereditary and is limited to males. It's always transmitted through the female to the second generation. CN: Physiological integrity; CNS: Reduction of risk potential; CL: Analysis

22. B. Because sickle cell trait is an autosomal recessive gene, one normal gene will suppress the trait. Thus, there's a 1 in 4 chance that each biological parent's sickle cell gene will be passed on to the child, who would then have the disease. CN: Physiological integrity; CNS: Reduction of risk potential; CL: Understanding

23. D. PKU affects infants in the first few months of life, causing devastating irreversible cerebral damage very quickly. By the time an untreated child begins to show signs of arrested brain development, usually at about 4 months, the damage is significant. Persons with PKU are usually blue-eyed and blond, the skin being excessively sensitive to light. The disorder can be detected at or shortly after birth. The test is required by law in several (not all) states, and the facts presented in this question did not address where the patient lived. CN: Physiological integrity; CNS: Reduction of risk potential; CL: Application

24. A. Darkening skin coloration and a craving for salty foods are most specific to Addison disease. Addison disease is the lack of hormones secreted by the adrenal gland. The lack of cortisol causes the pituitary to secrete excessive ACTH, which causes skin cells to darken (ACTH and melanin-secreting hormone (MSH) are similar in structure). The lack of aldosterone causes a lack of sodium and therefore a craving for salt. A craving for sweet foods and other carbohydrates would suggest premenstrual syndrome. Excessive thirst and urination are indicative of diabetes mellitus. Buffalo hump and thinning scalp hair are more indicative of Cushing syndrome. CN: Physiological integrity; CNS: Physiological adaptation; CL: Understanding

25. A. A patient with hyperthyroidism has hyperactive reflexes; therefore, you should check the patient's reflexes. Urinalysis isn't a diagnostic test for Graves disease. Romberg sign is used to test for cerebellar disease. Checking urine specific gravity won't be diagnostic for Graves disease. CN: Physiological integrity; CNS: Reduction of risk potential; CL: Analysis

26. A. The symptoms the patient is exhibiting are those associated with Cushing syndrome and result from the presence of excess glucocorticoid. Addison disease results from deficiency in the secretion of adrenocortical hormones. The symptoms are increased pigmentation of skin and mucous membranes, black freckles over the head and neck, fatigue, nausea, vomiting, diarrhea, abdominal discomfort, and hypoglycemia. Hyperthyroidism is marked by overactivity of the thyroid gland, which causes tachycardia, nervousness, weight loss, and anxiety. Graves disease is the most common cause of hyperthyroidism. CN: Physiological integrity; CNS: Physiological adaptation; CL: Analysis

27. C. Graves disease is hyperthyroidism that can cause intolerance to heat, weight loss, and nervousness. Hashimoto thyroiditis commonly causes hypothyroidism, which causes weight gain, cold intolerance, and sluggishness. Menopause causes hot flashes but not weight loss. Cushing disease causes weight gain, hyperglycemia, and hypertension. CN: Physiological integrity; CNS: Physiological adaptation; CL: Understanding

28. D. Diabetes mellitus produces damage to peripheral nerve fibers, causing the patient to lose sensation in the extremities and making the patient susceptible to unrecognized trauma and infections. Hashimoto disease is a form of autoimmune thyroiditis that affects females eight times more often than it does males. Diabetes insipidus is exhibited by

polyuria and polydipsia caused by inadequate secretion of antidiuretic hormone from the hypothalamus or its release by the posterior pituitary gland. Cushing disease results from hypersecretion of the adrenal cortex in which there's excessive production of glucocorticoids. CN: Physiological integrity; CNS: Reduction of risk potential; CL: Analysis

29. B. Normal humidifying and warming that take place in the upper airways are interrupted by mechanical ventilation. Therefore, air is warmed and humidified artificially by the ventilator. Gas exchange occurs with exchange of oxygen and carbon dioxide with inspiration and expiration at the alveolar-capillary membrane. Conversion of oxygen to carbon dioxide occurs in the lung tissues. Reflex bronchospasm occurs sometimes during intubation. CN: Physiological integrity; CNS: Physiological adaptation; CL: Remembering

30. A. When ventilation is greater than perfusion, the blood supply to the alveoli is decreased. Increased alveolar perfusion indicates increased perfusion of air in the pulmonary alveoli that's involved in the pulmonary exchange of gases. Pulmonary edema occurs when blood backs up from the left atrium of the heart into the lungs. Decreased ventilation indicates decreased, inadequate, or ineffective respiratory exchange. CN: Physiological integrity; CNS: Reduction of risk potential; CL: Analysis

31. B. Significantly decreased breath sounds on one side aren't typical of COPD and should alert the nurse to the possibility of spontaneous pneumothorax. Crackles in both lung bases indicate fluid in the lung bases. Expiratory wheezing results from constriction or obstruction of the throat, pharynx, trachea, or bronchi. Rhonchi scattered throughout both lung fields result in a coarse, dry crackle in the bronchial tubes. CN: Physiological integrity; CNS: Reduction of risk potential; CL: Analysis

32. D. Cor pulmonale is defined as right ventricular failure due to a pulmonary disease that causes chronic hypoxia. Left-sided heart failure would indicate congestive heart failure, which is the inability of the heart to pump sufficient blood to ensure normal flow through the circulation. Pulmonary hypertension is hypertension in the pulmonary arteries. V/Q mismatch occurs when there's a pathologic problem that inhibits normal exchange of oxygen and carbon dioxide in the pulmonary alveoli. CN: Physiological integrity; CNS: Physiological adaptation; CL: Remembering

33. C. There's increased hydrostatic pressure in the pulmonary capillaries, causing fluid to leak into the interstitial spaces, thus collapsing the alveoli. Perfusion to the lungs that's interrupted by an obstruction of the pulmonary artery or one of its branches is usually caused by an embolus from the thrombosis in a lower extremity. Increased hydrostatic pressure in the capillaries that causes fluid to leak into the alveoli, collapsing them, indicates heart failure. Fluid that accumulates in the lung interstitium, alveolar spaces, and small airways indicates severe refractory heart failure. CN: Physiological integrity; CNS: Physiological adaptation; CL: Understanding

34. C. You would measure blood pressure at rest and again while slowly the patient inspires to check if the systolic pressure drops more than 10 mm Hg during inspiration. Although the other options are signs of cardiac tamponade, pulsus paradoxus occurs when negative intrathoracic pressure reduces left ventricular filling and stroke volume. Checking to see if central venous pressure is elevated more than 15 mm Hg above normal would indicate heart failure. Auscultating for muffled heart sounds on inspiration isn't the best method of assessment at this time because a quiet heart with faint sounds usually accompanies only severe tamponade and occurs within minutes of the tamponade. Checking the ECG for reduced amplitude in all leads is diagnostic of cardiac tamponade, but may not always be apparent. CN: Physiological integrity; CNS: Reduction of risk potential; CL: Application

35. A. The compensatory mechanism can be harmful because, as epinephrine and norepinephrine make the heart work harder to beat stronger and faster, the heart's oxygen demand increases. Myocardial cells are depleted of potassium (not calcium), due to use of diuretics. The blood isn't diverted to the extremities; the heart perfuses during diastole, so less volume is ejected to the extremities. The contractility of the heart would hopefully be increased. CN: Physiological integrity; CNS: Physiological adaptation; CL: Analysis

36. B. Group A beta-hemolytic streptococcal infections can become systemic, causing rheumatic fever. *Staphylococcus aureus* causes suppurative conditions such as boils, carbuncles, and internal abscesses in humans. *Clostridium perfringens* causes gas gangrene. *Pseudomonas aeruginosa* may cause urinary tract infections, otitis externa, or folliculitis, including inflammation that may follow use of a hot tub. CN: Physiological integrity; CNS: Reduction of risk potential; CL: Understanding

37. B. Patients with chronic heart failure frequently develop symptoms of liver impairment (a late finding) because hepatic venous congestion develops from right-sided heart failure. Cirrhosis is a chronic disease. Symptoms include anorexia; chronic dyspepsia; indigestion; nausea and vomiting; dull, aching abdominal pain; ascites; and jaundice. Hepatitis is marked by gradual onset of general malaise, low-grade fever, anorexia, nausea and vomiting, muscle and joint pain, fatigue, headache, dark urine, and clay-colored stools. Ascites refers to abdominal distention that occurs from cirrhosis. CN: Physiological integrity; CNS: Reduction of risk potential; CL: Understanding

38. D. Chest pain that increases with deep inspiration and is relieved when the patient sits up and leans forward is typically associated with pericarditis. Pneumonia would have decreased or absent breath sounds. In cardiac tamponade, inspiratory heart sounds would be muffled. The chest pain experienced with myocardial infarction isn't positional. CN: Physiological integrity; CNS: Reduction of risk potential; CL: Analysis

39. A. Signs and symptoms of multiple sclerosis may be transient, or they may last for hours or weeks. They may wax and wane with no predictable pattern. In most patients, vision problems and sensory impairment (such as burning, pins and needles, and electrical sensations) are the first signs that something may be wrong. Associated signs and symptoms include poorly articulated speech or scanning speech, and dysphagia. The average age of onset is 18 to 40, and it occurs most commonly in females from higher socioeconomic classes from northern urban areas. Patients with myasthenia gravis find that certain muscles feel weak and tire quickly on exertion. Muscles frequently affected are those of the face, eyelids, larynx, and throat. Drooping of the eyelids and difficulty chewing or swallowing may be the first symptoms. Symptoms of an aneurysm include generalized abdominal pain, low back pain unaffected by movement, and systolic bruit over the aorta. In Guillain-Barré syndrome, paresthesia usually occurs first, followed by muscle weakness and flaccid paralysis that most commonly ascends from the extremities to the head. CN: Physiological integrity; CNS: Reduction of risk potential; CL: Analysis

40. D. The autonomic nervous system controls involuntary body functions, including the fight-or-flight response, which causes the mouth to become dry and the heart to beat faster. Somatic pertains to nonreproductive cells or tissues. Extrapyramidal is outside the pyramidal tracts of the central nervous system. Pyramidal is any part of the body resembling a pyramid. CN: Physiological integrity; CNS: Physiological adaptation; CL: Remembering

41. D. The brains of patients with Alzheimer disease may contain as little as 10% of the normal amount of acetylcholine. Dopamine is altered in Parkinson disease. Serotonin is altered in depression. A disturbance in norepinephrine's metabolism at important brain sites has been implicated in affective disorders. CN: Physiological integrity; CNS: Physiological adaptation; CL: Remembering

42. B. Thrombosis that leads to ischemia of cerebral tissue is the most common cause of stroke in middle-aged and older adult patients. Aneurysm refers to an abnormal dilation of a blood vessel, usually an artery, due to a congenital defect or weakness in the vessel wall. Embolism refers to a mass of undissolved matter present in a blood or lymphatic vessel, brought there by the blood or lymph current. Emboli may be solid, liquid, or gaseous. Hypertension is rarely a direct cause of death. It's more often an indication that there's something wrong, either physically or emotionally, that must be corrected. CN: Physiological integrity; CNS: Reduction of risk potential; CL: Remembering

43. B. Sensory-type seizures cause hallucinations and vertigo, along with the sensations of seeing flashing lights, experiencing déjà vu, and smelling a particular odor. In absence (petit mal) seizure, activity ceases for a few seconds to several minutes. In Jacksonian seizure, movement "marches" from one part of the body to another. Grand mal seizures involve the whole body. CN: Physiological integrity; CNS: Physiological adaptation; CL: Remembering

44. C. In response to tissue oxygen deprivation, the kidneys typically release erythropoietin. Patients with chronic renal failure typically

lack erythropoietin because of the kidney's inability to respond. Loss of albumin through impaired renal tubular filtration wouldn't cause anemia. Bleeding from damaged tubules would result in gross hematuria, which would be recognized quickly. Blood loss from hemodialysis would also be recognized quickly. CN: Physiological integrity; CNS: Physiological adaptation; CL: Application

45. A. In leukemia, immature WBCs are overproduced. The immature WBCs crowd normal WBCs and interfere with their production. Polycythemia is an abnormal increase in the erythrocyte count or in hemoglobin concentration. Thrombocytopenia is a decrease in the number of platelets in circulating blood. Multiple myeloma is a primary malignant tumor of bone marrow. CN: Physiological integrity; CNS: Physiological adaptation; CL: Remembering

46. B. Platelet destruction caused by the intra-aortic balloon pump most likely caused this patient's thrombocytopenia. Malnutrition would have occurred over a long time. Internal hemorrhage would cause a decrease in the complete red blood cell count. DIC involves bleeding from surgical or invasive procedure sites and bleeding gums, cutaneous oozing, petechia, ecchymoses, and hematomas. CN: Physiological integrity; CNS: Reduction of risk potential; CL: Analysis

47. B. A platelet count below $150,000/mm^3$ indicates thrombocytopenia. A platelet count of $400,000/mm^3$ is within the normal range; one of $500,000/mm^3$ is too high, and one of $150,000/mm^3$ is within the normal range. CN: Physiological integrity; CNS: Reduction of risk potential; CL: Analysis

48. B. Anticoagulants are administered to combat clot formation in the small blood vessels, which occurs with DIC. Anticoagulants won't prevent emboli formation that may occur as a result of increased clotting factors seen in DIC. Anticoagulants won't prevent clot formation that may develop as blood pools beneath the skin. Anticoagulants won't prevent thrombus formation that may occur due to bed rest. CN: Physiological integrity; CNS: Reduction of risk potential; CL: Application

49. D. This patient is at risk for developing cholecystitis. These risk factors predispose a person to gallstones: obesity and a high-calorie, high-cholesterol diet; increased estrogen levels from hormonal contraceptives, HRT, or pregnancy; use of clofibrate, an antilipemic drug; diabetes mellitus; ileal disease; blood disorders; liver disease; or pancreatitis. HRT doesn't increase risk for appendicitis, cirrhosis, or pancreatitis. CN: Physiological integrity; CNS: Reduction of risk potential; CL: Analysis

50. C. In a patient with newly diagnosed cirrhosis, normal hepatic cells are typically replaced by fibrous, nonfunctional tissue. In later stages of cirrhosis, hepatic cells become distended and misshapen, blood vessels become destroyed, and the cells begin to die. CN: Physiological integrity; CNS: Physiological adaptation; CL: Remembering

51. B. Acute pancreatitis causes severe, persistent, piercing abdominal pain, usually in the midepigastric region, although it may be generalized or occur in the left upper quadrant radiating to the back. The pain usually begins suddenly after eating a large meal or drinking alcohol. It increases when the patient lies on the back and is relieved when the patient rests on the knees and upper chest. Perforated gastric ulcer causes peritonitis, in which the abdomen becomes rigid and sensitive to touch. Fever, vomiting, and extreme weakness are observed. Appendicitis causes right lower quadrant pain. Cholecystitis causes right upper quadrant pain. CN: Physiological integrity; CNS: Physiological adaptation; CL: Analysis

52. B. Elevated serum amylase and lipase levels are the diagnostic hallmarks that confirm acute pancreatitis. A WBC count usually is ordered to see if infection is present. Hemoglobin measures red blood cell count, which may indicate anemia. Elevated lipid and trypsin levels would appear in stool samples, not serum samples. Total serum bilirubin and indirect bilirubin levels measure liver dysfunction. CN: Physiological integrity; CNS: Reduction of risk potential; CL: Understanding

53. C. H. pylori releases an enzyme (urease) that destroys the stomach's mucous lining, reducing the epithelium's resistance to acid digestion and causing gastritis and ulcer disease. H. pylori doesn't cause bacteria to colonize the mucous lining, cause regurgitation of duodenal contents into the stomach, or cause persistent inflammation of the stomach. CN: Physiological integrity; CNS: Physiological adaptation; CL: Application

54. D. The kidneys can usually maintain homeostasis with just 25% of their normal functioning capacity. When greater than 75% of the functioning capacity is destroyed, signs and symptoms of chronic renal failure occur. CN: Physiological integrity; CNS: Physiological adaptation; CL: Remembering

55. C. Because the patient suffered a lack of blood flow to the kidneys while in septic shock, they're now experiencing acute tubular necrosis. Early-stage acute tubular necrosis may be difficult to identify because the patient's primary disease may obscure the signs and symptoms. The first recognizable effect may be decreased urine output, usually less than 400 mL/24 hours. An acid–base imbalance is associated with acidosis or alkalosis imbalance and isn't the etiology of septic shock. Blood loss leads to anemia and hypovolemia, but isn't the etiology of septic shock. Dehydration leads to hypovolemia and isn't the etiology of septic shock. CN: Physiological integrity; CNS: Physiological adaptation; CL: Analysis

56. A. Acute bacterial prostatitis is usually caused by an ascending infection of the urinary tract. Lymphatic migration of pathogenic bacteria would circulate in the bloodstream. Prostatic hyperplasia is excessive proliferation of normal cells in the normal tissues of the prostate. An infection in the patient's blood wouldn't be specific to prostatitis. CN: Physiological integrity; CNS: Reduction of risk potential; CL: Remembering

57. A. CT scan of the abdomen would produce a precise reconstructed image of the abdomen and would show the kidney stone. MRI of the

pelvis provides soft-tissue images of the central nervous and musculo-skeletal systems. Cystoscopy of the bladder would examine the bladder only with a cystoscope. KUB x-ray is a nonspecific test for kidney stone; it may or may not show the stone. CN: Physiological integrity; CNS: Reduction of risk potential; CL: Analysis

58. C. Athletes are prone to injury of the diarthroses, which include all synovial joints. These joints include the ankle, wrist, knee, hip, and shoulder. Synarthrosis is a type of joint in which the skeletal elements are united by a continuous intervening substance. Movement is absent or limited. Amphiarthrosis is a form of articulation in which the body surfaces are connected by cartilage; mobility is slight but may be exerted in all directions. CN: Physiological integrity; CNS: Reduction of risk potential; CL: Remembering

59. B. Sodium urate forms crystalline deposits in the affected joints. Calcium pyrophosphate, called *pseudogout,* is deposition of calcium phosphate crystals in the joints. Ammonia sulfate is an inorganic chemical compound. Sodium bicarbonate is a white odorless powder, used to treat acidosis. CN: Physiological integrity; CNS: Physiological adaptation; CL: Remembering

60. D. Osteoarthritis pain is worse on initial movement and is commonly most exaggerated in an isolated weight-bearing joint. RA is a generalized disease characterized by a persistent synovitis of peripheral joints. SLE is an idiopathic autoimmune disease characterized primarily by fatigue, fever, migratory arthralgia, weight loss, and sicca syndrome. Gouty arthritis presents with acute painful attacks of swelling joints. CN: Physiological integrity; CNS: Physiological adaptation; CL: Analysis

61. C. This patient is exhibiting signs of respiratory acidosis (excess carbon dioxide retention). It's present when ABG values are pH less than 7.35, HCO_3^- greater than 26 mEq/L (if compensating), and $Paco_2$ greater than 45 mm Hg. Metabolic acidosis is a state in which the blood pH is low (under 7.35), due to increased production of hydrogen (H) by the body or the inability of the body to form bicarbonate (HCO) in the kidney. Metabolic alkalosis depletes the body of H ions leading to an increase of bicarbonate in the body. The pH is high (greater than 7.35). Respiratory alkalosis is a state in which the blood pH is high (greater than 7.35) due to increased levels of carbon dioxide "blown" off by the lungs, which are hyperventilating. CN: Physiological integrity; CNS: Reduction of risk potential; CL: Analysis

62. D. These ABG results reveal metabolic alkalosis. Metabolic alkalosis is present when ABG results show pH greater than 7.45, HCO_3^- greater than 26 mEq/L, and $Paco_2$ greater than 45 mm Hg (if compensating). Respiratory acidosis is diagnosed when pH is less than 7.35 with a $Paco_2$ greater than 45 mm Hg. Respiratory alkalosis is diagnosed when the pH is greater than 7.45 with a $Paco_2$ less than 35 mm Hg. Metabolic acidosis is diagnosed when pH is less than 7.35 and the bicarbonate level (HCO_3^-) is less than 22 mEq/L. CN: Physiological integrity; CNS: Reduction of risk potential; CL: Analysis

63. B. Inadequate excretion of acids as a result of renal disease can cause metabolic acidosis. CNS depression from drugs would cause respiratory acidosis. Gram-negative bacteremia would be associated with respiratory alkalosis. Asphyxia would cause respiratory acidosis. CN: Physiological integrity; CNS: Reduction of risk potential; CL: Remembering

64. A. In patients with essentially normal lung tissue, acute respiratory failure usually presents with $PaCO_2$ above 50 mm Hg and PaO_2 below 50 mm Hg. These limits, however, don't apply to patients with chronic obstructive pulmonary disease (COPD), who usually have a consistently high $PaCO_2$. In patients with COPD, only acute deterioration in arterial blood gas values, with corresponding clinical deterioration, indicates acute respiratory failure. A patient with severe acute respiratory syndrome would have a $PaCO_2$ above 50 mm Hg and a $PaCO_2$ below 50 mm Hg, but the lung tissue wouldn't be essentially normal. A patient with asthma would have a $PaCO_2$ greater than 50 mm Hg and a $PaCO_2$ less than 50 mm Hg, but the lung tissue wouldn't be normal. A patient with cor pulmonale would have decreased perfusion of the heart, which could lead to a $PaCO_2$ below 50 mm Hg, but the lungs are compromised. CN: Physiological integrity; CNS: Physiological adaptation; CL: Analysis

65. D. One factor may be low intake of dietary fiber. High-fiber diets increase stool bulk, thereby decreasing the wall tension in the colon. High wall tension is thought to increase the risk of developing diverticula. Low intake of dietary protein is associated with lower bone mineral density and greater risk of fractures. High intake of dietary fiber increases risk of kidney abnormalities. High dietary intake of saturated fat increases cholesterol. CN: Physiological integrity; CNS: Reduction of risk potential; CL: Remembering

66. A. Diverticulitis presents as severe LLQ abdominal pain and alternating bouts of diarrhea and constipation. Cholecystitis presents as RUQ pain with indigestion, eructation, and flatulence. Appendicitis presents as RLQ pain with constipation. Pancreatitis presents as mid-abdominal pain radiating into the back. CN: Physiological integrity; CNS: Physiological adaptation; CL: Remembering

67. A. In GERD, the sphincter doesn't remain closed (usually due to deficient lower esophageal sphincter [LES] pressure or pressure within the stomach that exceeds LES pressure), and the pressure in the stomach pushes the stomach contents into the esophagus. The high acidity of the stomach contents causes pain and irritation when it enters the esophagus. Mucosa that takes on a "cobblestone" appearance could be related to many conditions other than GERD. A defect in the diaphragm that permits a portion of the stomach to pass through the esophageal hiatus into the chest cavity is a hiatal hernia. Destruction of the stomach's mucous lining by *H. pylori* is consistent with an ulcer. CN: Physiological integrity; CNS: Physiological adaptation; CL: Remembering

68. C. The acid perfusion test confirms esophagitis and distinguishes it from cardiac disorders. Esophageal manometry measures pressure

within the esophagus. Barium swallow is used to determine the cause of painful swallowing. Upper GI series is used to diagnose problems in the esophagus. CN: Physiological integrity; CNS: Reduction of risk potential; CL: Remembering

69. B. Osteomyelitis occurs more commonly in persons with uncontrolled diabetes mellitus as a complication of an acute localized infection. Osteoarthritis occurs more commonly in older adults. Osteomalacia is the adult equivalent of the disease rickets. Osteoporosis occurs more commonly in older adults, particularly females. CN: Physiological integrity; CNS: Reduction of risk potential; CL: Remembering

70. A. While each of these organisms causes osteomyelitis, the most common causative organism is *Staphylococcus aureus*. *Streptococcus pyogenes* is a common bacterium of the skin. *Pseudomonas aeruginosa* is the most common organism in urinary tract, respiratory, skin, bone, and joint infections. *Proteus vulgaris* commonly causes urinary and hospital-acquired infections. CN: Physiological integrity; CNS: Reduction of risk potential; CL: Remembering

71. D. Pulmonary embolism generally results from dislodged thrombi originating in the leg veins or pelvis. In sickle cell disease, the red blood cell changes shape upon deoxygenation. A foreign substance is the "invader" into the body system. A heart valve growth would be "attached" to the heart valve. CN: Physiological integrity; CNS: Reduction of risk potential; CL: Remembering

72. A, B, D, E. SARS begins with a high fever (usually a temperature greater than 100.4° F [38° C]), chills, and achiness. Patients develop respiratory symptoms 4 to 7 days after the onset of fever. Respiratory symptoms can be mild to severe and include dry cough, shortness of breath, hypoxemia, and pneumonia. Some patients develop diarrhea. A sudden onset of chest pain is not associated with SARS. Neck stiffness is associated with meningitis or musculoskeletal conditions. CN: Physiological integrity; CNS: Physiological adaptation; CL: Analysis

73. A, C, D, E. With rhabdomyolysis, myoglobin, CK, urate, and potassium are released from the necrotic muscle fibers into the circulation. Sodium is located in the blood and the space surrounding the cells. Calcium is located mostly in the teeth and bones. CN: Physiological integrity; CNS: Physiological adaptation; CL: Application

74. B. In anaphase, the third phase of cell reproduction, the centromeres separate and pull chromosomes toward the opposite sides of the cell. In prophase (option D), the first stage, chromosomes coil and shorten and then nuclear membrane dissolves. In the second stage, or metaphase (option A), the centromeres divide and pull the chromosomes apart. Then the centromeres align themselves in the middle of the spindle. In the fourth stage, or telophase (option C), the new membrane forms around chromosomes, and the cytoplasm divides. CN: Physiological integrity; CNS: Physiological adaptation; CL: Remembering

75. C. The single best test to confirm myocardial infarction is cardiac troponin level. Cardiac troponins are proteins released from dead myocardial tissue. Myoglobin is released by any kind of muscle damage but is not specific to the heart. Creatinine phosphokinase (CPK) is also released from muscle damage but is not specific to the heart. ECG changes are nonspecific. CN: Physiological integrity; CNS: Physiological adaptation; CL: Analysis

76. The LES is located under the diaphragm. CN: Physiological integrity; CNS: Physiological adaptation; CL: Remembering

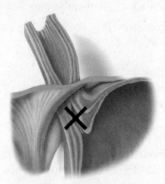

77. 1.2

First, calculate the patient's weight in kilograms by using the conversion factor 1 kg = 2.2 lb:

$$\frac{1 \text{ kg}}{2.2 \text{ lb}} = \frac{X \text{ kg}}{176 \text{ lb}}$$

Cross multiply and divide both sides by 2.2:

$$2.2X = 176$$
$$X = 80$$

Next, determine how many milligrams of phenytoin would be given:

$$1.5 \text{ mg} \times 80 \text{ kg} = 1,200 \text{ mg}$$

Finally, convert milligrams to grams:

$$1,200 \text{ mg} \div 1,000 = 1.2 \text{ g}$$

CN: Physiological integrity; CNS: Pharmacological and parenteral therapies; CL: Application

78. D. Other classic symptoms of Cushing syndrome include susceptibility to infection, male gynecomastia, bruises/petechiae, female amenorrhea/hirsutism, and hypernatremia. Addison disease would typically present with dry skin/mucous membranes, poor coordination, vitiligo, and darkening of skin at hands/elbows/knees. Hypothyroidism would present with energy loss, constipation, weight gain, forgetfulness, and sensitivity to cold. Diabetes insipidus would present with weight loss, weakness, dizziness, and constipation. CN: Physiological integrity; CNS: Physiological adaptation; CL: Understanding

79. C. Addison disease is primarily autoimmune-caused destruction. Glucocorticoid excess would result in Cushing syndrome; thyroid hormone overproduction would result in hyperthyroidism; insufficient antidiuretic hormone production would result in diabetes insipidus. CN: Physiological integrity; CNS: Physiological adaptation; CL: Application

80. B. Asymptomatic healthy adults with NO risk factors should begin routine screening at age 35 and continue screening every 3 years as long as results are normal. Obese/overweight individuals and those with other risk factors such as hypertension, hyperlipidemia, gestational diabetes, first-degree relative with diabetes, and certain ethnicities such as African American, Native American, and Latino should be screened at any age (American Diabetes Association, 2016). CN: Physiological integrity; CNS: Reduction of risk potential; CL: Remembering

81. C. A lack of ADH (antidiuretic hormone) in diabetes insipidus leads to polyuria. Surplus of ADH would result in SIADH. Abnormal insulin secretion is often a characteristic of diabetes type 2 when common cause is underproduction of insulin. Lack of ACTH is often the cause of Addison disease. CN: Physiological integrity; CNS: Physiological adaptation; CL: Application

82. C. Antibiotics are used to kill bacteria that result in infection such as strep throat. Antibiotics destroy normal bacterial flora allowing fungi (yeast) to grow. In pathogenic fungal infections, mycotoxin is released. This is called a mycotic infection. Strep throat is caused by bacteria, which can lead to other strep infections within the body but does not lead to fungal infections. CN: Physiological integrity; CNS: Physiological adaptation; CL: Application

83. A, B. Factors that create a climate for infection include poor nutrition, stress, poor sanitation, crowded living conditions, pollution, dust, medications, and hospitalizations. A serum potassium level provides information on the level of potassium in the blood. Potassium is essential for heart function/muscle contraction. Bowel movement regularity indicates normal or abnormal function of the bowels and possibly the GI system. CN: Physiological integrity; CNS: Physiological adaptation; CL: Understanding

84. C. The nurse should teach a patient who has conjunctivitis to wash hands after caring for the eye(s). The nurse should teach the patient to avoid touching or rubbing the eyes, to cleanse the eyes gently with water and wipe with a tissue or cloth and then dispose of the tissue, and/or to use separate cloths/tissues for each eye. In addition, the patient should change pillowcases at least once daily, replace eye makeup that was used when infected (if applicable), and avoid sharing personal cloths with others. CN: Physiological integrity; CNS: Physiological adaptation; CL: Application

85. A, C, D, E. Patients who present with labyrinthitis have inner ear inflammation as a result of an infection (bacterial or viral). Bacterial infections are treated with antibiotics to prevent further inflammation

and spread of infection to other body areas. The nurse should assess for hearing loss to determine safety risks of the patient. Patients with labyrinthitis may experience impaired balance and dizziness, which requires bed rails raised to prevent a fall. They also will require assistance getting up from the bed to prevent a fall. Diet modifications are not commonly needed for patients with labyrinthitis. CN: Physiological integrity; CNS: Reduction of risk potential; CL: Application

86. C. The nurse should prepare to administer cryoprecipitate to replace the missing clotting factors needed to prevent bleeding. Cryoprecipitate contains fibrinogen, von Willebrand factor, factor VIII, factor XIII, and fibronectin. Albumin is a plasma expander. Packed red blood cells are used to replace red blood cell mass in acute blood loss. Immunoglobulins are commonly administered to patients with immunosuppression or viral infection. CN: Physiological integrity; CNS: Physiological adaptation; CL: Understanding

87. B. In disseminated intravascular coagulation (DIC), increased clotting causes a depletion of the body's clotting factors. Platelets are affected in DIC. The underlying causes of DIC are related to infection, inflammation, or cancer, not high blood pressure. DIC is not a disease but is a condition that arises from clotting factors becoming overactive. Treatment for DIC involves identifying and treating the underlying cause. CN: Physiological integrity; CNS: Physiological adaptation; CL: Application

88. C. Calcium is essential in the clotting cascade and to activate platelets. Iodine is necessary for thyroid function. Phosphorous is required for cell and tissue maturation and repair. Sodium helps to regulate water balance in the body and is necessary for nerve and muscle function. CN: Physiological integrity; CNS: Physiological adaptation; CL: Understanding

89. B. An elevated temperature will indicate the presence of infection. An increased or decreased energy level is not an indication that treatments for neutropenia have been effective. Hematocrit levels measure the amount of red blood cells in the blood; neutropenia affects white blood cells. Urine output is not a direct indicator of infection. CN: Physiological integrity; CNS: Physiological adaptation; CL: Evaluation

90. B. Patients experiencing a complex partial seizure may have symptoms that include a glassy stare, aimless wandering, and no memory of actions during the seizure. These seizures may last from a few seconds to 20 minutes. A grand mal seizure is a type of whole-body, tonic-clonic seizure. Typically, a generalized tonic-clonic seizure begins with a loud cry, caused by air rushing from the lungs through the vocal cords. The patient falls to the ground, losing consciousness. The body stiffens (tonic phase) and then alternates between episodes of muscle spasm and relaxation (clonic phase). Tongue biting, incontinence, labored breathing, apnea, and cyanosis may also occur. A Jacksonian seizure is a simple partial seizure in which one muscle group in the body under-

goes higher tonicity and clonic movements. CN: Physiological integrity; CNS: Physiological Adaptation; CL: Remembering

91. A. Alzheimer disease is caused by progressive degeneration of the cerebral cortex. Epilepsy is a brain disorder characterized by seizures. Guillain-Barré syndrome is a rapidly progressive syndrome that is associated with segmented demyelination of the peripheral nerves. Myasthenia gravis is a condition that produces sporadic, progressive weakness and abnormal fatigue of the voluntary skeletal muscles. CN: Physiological integrity; CNS: Physiological Adaptation; CL: Remembering

92. A, C, D. Celiac disease is an autoimmune disease caused by the ingestion of gluten. Foods that contain gluten include those with wheat, rye, barley, and malt. Rice does not contain gluten and can be included in a celiac diet. CN: Physiological integrity; CNS: Physiological Adaptation; CL: Understanding

93. A, B, E. Common risk factors for colorectal cancer can be divided into modifiable and nonmodifiable categories. Modifiable risk factors include diet (high fat, low fiber), increased consumption of red meat and other processed meats, alcohol intake in large amounts, cigarette smoking, obesity, and sedentary lifestyle. Nonmodifiable risk factors include age greater than 50 years, inflammatory bowel diseases such as Crohn and ulcerative colitis, and type 2 diabetes mellitus CN: Physiological integrity; CNS: Physiological Adaptation; CL: Application

94. B, D, E. Virchow triad includes (1) venous stasis (for example immobility, age), (2) venous endothelial injury (for example trauma, IV medications), and (3) hypercoagulability (oral contraceptives, inherited disorders, pregnancy). CN: Physiological integrity; CNS: Physiological Adaptation; CL: Understanding

95. A. Hypertension is sustained elevation of diastolic or systolic blood pressure. Stage 1 hypertension is a sustained systolic blood pressure of 130 mm Hg to 139 mmHg and/or a diastolic pressure of 80 mm Hg to 89 mmHg. Sustained systolic BP greater than or equal to 140 mm Hg or a diastolic BP greater than or equal to 90 mm Hg is considered stage 2 hypertension. A one-time systolic BP of 150 mm Hg and diastolic BP of 90 mm Hg is not enough evidence to diagnose hypertension; there needs to be sustained high BP. A sustained systolic BP of 120 mm Hg to 129 mm Hg or a diastolic BP less than 80 mm Hg is not hypertension but is considered elevated. CN: Physiological integrity; CNS: Physiological Adaptation; CL: Remembering

96. A. Infants and young children are most susceptible to RSV. It can be a life-threatening condition for children under the age of 2. CN: Physiological integrity; CNS: Physiological Adaptation; CL: Understanding

97. D. Apixaban is a novel oral anticoagulant. The other drugs listed are categorized as heparin or a fibrinolytic. CN: Physiological integrity; CNS: Physiological Adaptation; CL: Understanding

98. C. Creatinine is only filtered by the glomeruli and not reabsorbed by the tubules. CN: Physiological integrity; CNS: Physiological Adaptation; CL: Remembering

99. B. One such condition, prerenal azotemia, accounts for between 40% and 80% of all cases of acute renal failure. Prerenal azotemia is caused by an excess of nitrogen in the bloodstream due to a lack of blood flow to the kidneys. CN: Physiological integrity; CNS: Physiological Adaptation; CL: Understanding

100. A. Depending on the size of the enlarged prostate and resulting complications, the obstruction may be treated surgically or symptomatically. CN: Physiological integrity; CNS: Physiological Adaptation; CL: Understanding

101. D. Erythropoietin is secreted by the kidneys when there's a drop in the oxygen supply in tissue blood. CN: Physiological integrity; CNS: Physiological Adaptation; CL: Remembering

102. B. Urine that's consistently acidic or alkaline provides a favorable medium for stone formation. CN: Physiological integrity; CNS: Physiological Adaptation; CL: Understanding

103. C. Antibodies to HIV develop from 2 weeks to 6 months after exposure to the virus. Testing earlier than 3 months after exposure may give unclear test results because the infected person may not yet have developed antibodies to HIV. Testing 1 to 2 years after HIV exposure would be an excessively prolonged time and would not indicate the first appearance of antibody. CN: Physiological integrity; CNS: Physiological Adaptation; CL: Understanding

104. C. IgE is the immunoglobulin involved in the immediate hypersensitivity reactions of humoral immunity. CN: Physiological integrity; CNS: Physiological Adaptation; CL: Remembering

105. D. Rhinitis medicamentosa can be resolved by discontinuing these medications. CN: Physiological integrity; CNS: Physiological Adaptation; CL: Understanding

106. B. Penicillin is the most common anaphylaxis-causing antigen because of its systemic effects on the body. Other agents are not the most common causing antigen. CN: Physiological integrity; CNS: Physiological Adaptation; CL: Remembering

107. A. Bulla are vesicles that are 1 cm or larger in diameter and are filled with serous fluid. CN: Physiological integrity; CNS: Physiological Adaptation; CL: Understanding

108. C. Wheals are transient, elevated, irregularly shaped areas of localized skin edema. Vesicles are elevated, circumscribed, superficial lesions filled with serous fluid, less than 1 cm in diameter. Macules are flat, nonpalpable circumscribed areas up to 1 cm in diameter. Lichenification is a rough thickening of the epidermis. CN: Physiological integrity; CNS: Physiological Adaptation; CL: Understanding

Glossary*

acute illness: sudden onset of illness having severe symptoms and a short course

agranulocyte: leukocyte (white blood cell) not made up of granules or grains; includes lymphocytes, monocytes, and plasma cells

allele: one of two or more different genes that occupy a corresponding position (locus) on matched chromosomes; allows for different forms of the same inheritable characteristic

allergen: substance that induces an allergy or a hypersensitivity reaction

anaphylaxis: severe allergic reaction to a foreign substance

androgen: steroid sex hormone that promote male secondary sex characteristics, such as facial hair and a low-pitched voice (The two main androgens are androsterone and testosterone.)

anemia: reduction in the number and volume of red blood cells, the amount of hemoglobin, or the volume of packed red cells

aneurysm: sac formed by the dilation of the wall of an artery, a vein, or the heart

angiography: radiographic visualization of blood vessels after injection of radiopaque contrast material

anoxia: absence of oxygen in the tissues

antibody: immunoglobulin molecule that reacts only with the specific antigen that induced its formation in the lymph system

antigen: foreign substance such as bacteria or toxins that induces antibody formation

antitoxin: antibody produced in response to a toxin that's capable of neutralizing the toxin's effects

aqueous humor: a clear, watery fluid, produced in the ciliary body, that fills the area between the lens and cornea

atrophy: decrease in size of a cell, tissue, organ, or body part

autoimmune disorder: disorder in which the body launches an immunologic response against itself

autosome: any chromosome other than the sex chromosomes (Twenty-two of the human chromosome pairs are autosomes.)

bacterium: one-celled microorganism that breaks down dead tissue, has no true nucleus, and reproduces by cell division

baroreceptor: receptor that responds to changes in pressure

benign: not malignant or recurrent; favorable for recovery

biopsy: process of removing tissue from living patients for diagnostic examination

bone marrow: soft organic material filling the cavities of bones

Bowman capsule: contains the glomerulus and acts as a reservoir for glomerular filtrate

bronchiolitis: inflammation of the small airways. It is often associated with respiratory syncytial virus (RSV)

bursa: fluid-filled sac or cavity found in connecting tissue in the vicinity of joints; acts as a cushion

calculus: any abnormal concentration, usually made up of mineral salts, within the body; for example, gallstones and renal calculi

carcinogen: substance that causes cancer

carcinogenesis: the origin, production, or development of cancer

carcinoma: malignant growth made up of epithelial cells that tends to infiltrate surrounding tissues and metastasize

cardiac output: volume of blood ejected from the heart per minute

cartilage: dense connective tissue made up of fibers embedded in a strong, gel-like substance; supports, cushions, and shapes body structures

cataract: the clouding of the normally translucent lens of the eye

cell: smallest living component of an organism; the body's basic building block

cholestasis: stopped or decreased bile flow

chondrocyte: cartilage cell

choroid: the middle layer of the eye between the sclera and the retina

---

*Note: In this glossary, the term "male" refers to a person assigned male at birth, and the term "female" refers to a person assigned female at birth.

chromosome: linear thread in a cell's nucleus that contains deoxyribonucleic acid; occurs in pairs in humans

chronic illness: illness of long duration that includes remission and exacerbation

ciliary body: a circular band of tissue at the front of the choroid that supports the lens

clearance: complete removal of a substance by the kidneys from a specific volume of blood per unit of time

Clostridium difficile: (*C. diff*) is a bacterial infection in the colon associated with antibiotic use that causes colitis, and the patient experiences diarrhea.

coagulant: substance that promotes, accelerates, or permits blood clotting

collagen: main supportive protein of the skin, tendon, bone, cartilage, and connective tissue

colonoscopy: examination of the upper portion of the rectum with an elongated speculum or colonoscope to visualize the colon, remove polyps, or biopsy suspicious growths

compensation: the counterbalancing of any defect in structure or function; measure of how long the heart takes to adapt to increased blood in ventricles

complement system: major mediator of inflammatory response; a functionally related system made up of 20 proteins circulating as functionally inactive molecules

conjunctivitis: an inflammation and redness of the transparent, mucous membrane (conjunctiva) covering the white part of the eye (sclera)

cornea: the transparent, clear layer that is at the front of the eye

cytoplasm: aqueous mass within a cell that contains organelles, is surrounded by the cell membrane, and excludes the nucleus

cytotoxic: destructive to cells

degeneration: nonlethal cell damage occurring in the cell's cytoplasm while the nucleus remains unaffected

demyelination: destruction of a nerve's myelin sheath, which interferes with normal nerve conduction

deoxyribonucleic acid (DNA): complex protein in the cell's nucleus that carries genetic material and is responsible for cellular reproduction

dermis: the layer of the skin beneath the epidermis; contains tough connective tissue, hair follicles, and sweat glands

differentiation: process of cells maturing into specific types

disease: pathologic condition that occurs when the body can't maintain homeostasis

distal: farthest away

diverticulitis: inflammation of one or more diverticula in the muscular layer of the colon

dominant gene: gene that expresses itself even if it's carried on only one homologous (matched) chromosome

dyscrasia: a condition related to a disease, usually referring to an imbalance of component elements (A blood dyscrasia is a disorder of cellular elements of the blood.)

dysphagia: difficulty swallowing

dysplasia: abnormal development of tissue

embolism: sudden obstruction of a blood vessel by foreign substances or a blood clot

endemic: disease of low morbidity that occurs continuously in a particular patient population or geographic area

endochondral ossification: process in which cartilage hardens into bone

endocrine: pertaining to internal hormone secretion by glands (Endocrine glands, including the pineal gland, the islets of Langerhans in the pancreas, the gonads, the thymus, and the adrenal, pituitary, thyroid, and parathyroid glands secrete hormones directly into circulation.)

endogenous: occurring inside the body

epidermis: outermost layer of the skin

erythrocyte: red blood cell; carries oxygen to the tissues and removes carbon dioxide from them

erythropoiesis: production of red blood cells or erythrocytes

estrogen: female sex hormone produced by the ovaries that promotes female secondary sex characteristics, such as enlarged breasts and widened hips; also thought to be responsible for sex drive

etiology: cause of a disease

exacerbation: increase in the severity of a disease or any of its symptoms

exocrine: external or outward secretion of a gland (Exocrine glands discharge through ducts opening on an external or internal surface of the body; they include the liver, the pancreas, the prostate, and the salivary, sebaceous, sweat, gastric, intestinal, mammary, and lacrimal glands.)

exogenous: occurring outside the body

fasciculation: involuntary twitching or contraction of the muscle

fungus: nonphotosynthetic microorganism that reproduces asexually by cell division

glaucoma: an increase in intraocular pressure (IOP) within the anterior chamber of the eye

gland: specialized cell cluster that produces a secretion used in some other body part

glomerulus: a network of twisted capillaries that acts as a filter for the passage of protein-free and red blood cell–free filtrate to the Bowman capsule

glucagon: hormone released during the fasting state that increases blood glucose concentration

granulocyte: any cell containing granules, especially a granular leukocyte (white blood cell)

hematopoiesis: production of red blood cells in the bone marrow

hemoglobin: iron-containing pigment in red blood cells that carries oxygen from the lungs to the tissues

hemolysis: red blood cell destruction

hemorrhage: escape of blood from a ruptured vessel

hemostasis: complex process whereby platelets, plasma, and coagulation factors interact to control bleeding

heterozygous genes: genes having different alleles at the same site (locus) (If each gene in a chromosome pair produces a different effect, the genes are heterozygous.)

homeostasis: dynamic, steady state of internal balance in the body

homologous genes: gene pairs sharing a corresponding structure and position on the chromosome

homozygous genes: genes that have identical alleles for a given trait (When each gene at a corresponding locus produces the same effect, the genes are homozygous.)

hordeolum: an infection of the external structure of the eye

hormone: chemical substance produced in the body that has a specific regulatory effect on the activity of specific cells or organs

host defense system: elaborate network of safeguards that protects the body from infectious organisms and other harmful invaders

hyperplasia: excessive growth of normal cells that causes an increase in the volume of a tissue or organ

hypersensitivity disorder: state in which the body produces an exaggerated immune response to a foreign antigen

hypertension: abnormally high blood pressure

hypotension: abnormally low blood pressure

hypoxia: reduction of oxygen in body tissues to below normal levels

idiopathic: disease with no known cause

immunocompetence: ability of cells to distinguish antigens from substances that belong to the body and to launch an immune response

immunodeficiency disorder: disorder caused by a deficiency of the immune

response due to hypoactivity or decreased numbers of lymphoid cells

immunoglobulin: serum protein synthesized by lymphocytes and plasma cells that has known antibody activity; main component of humoral immune response

immunosurveillance: defense mechanism in which the immune system continuously recognizes abnormal cells as foreign and destroys them (For example, an interruption in immunosurveillance can lead to overproduction of cancer cells.)

insulin: hormone secreted into the blood by the islets of Langerhans of the pancreas; promotes the storage of glucose, among other functions

iris: the pigmented layer of muscular tissue that gives the eye its color and controls the size of the pupil to regulate how much light is entering the eye

ischemia: decreased blood supply to a body organ or tissue

joint: the site of the union of two or more bones; provides motion and flexibility

karyotype: chromosomal arrangement of the cell nucleus

labyrinthitis: also known as otitis interna, refers to inner ear inflammation as a result of an infection

Langerhans cells: a type of dendritic cell that moves to the epidermis from the bone marrow; in cooperation with dermal dendritic cells, starts an immune response

leaflets: cusps in the heart valves that open and close in response to pressure gradients to let blood flow into the chambers

lens: a transparent, round, and biconvex structure whose elasticity allows the curvature to change to adjust its focusing power

leukocyte: white blood cell that protects the body against microorganisms causing disease

leukocytosis: increase in the number of leukocytes in the blood; generally caused by infection

leukopenia: reduction in the number of leukocytes in the blood

ligament: band of fibrous tissue that connects bones or cartilage, strengthens joints, provides stability, and limits or facilitates movement

loop of Henle: a U-shaped nephron tubule located in the medulla and extending from the proximal convoluted tubule to the distal convoluted tubule; site for further concentration of filtrate through reabsorption

lymphedema: chronic swelling of a body part from accumulation of interstitial fluid secondary to obstruction of lymphatic vessels or lymph nodes

lymph node: structure that filters the lymphatic fluid that drains from body tissues and is later returned to the blood as plasma; removes noxious agents from the blood

lymphocyte: leukocyte produced by lymphoid tissue that participates in immunity

macrophage: highly phagocytic cells that are stimulated by inflammation

macula: located near the central portion of the retina, enables the eye to view detailed central vision

macular degeneration: a disorder resulting in the breakdown of cells in the macula and surrounding tissues of the eye

malabsorption: insufficient intestinal absorption of nutrients

malignant: condition that becomes progressively worse and results in death

megakaryocytes: giant bone marrow cells

meiosis: process of cell division by which gametes (egg or sperm) are formed

melanin: dark skin pigment that filters ultraviolet radiation and is produced and dispersed by specialized cells called *melanocytes*

Ménière disease: an inner ear disorder usually affecting one ear

Merkel cells: cells that are responsible for sensation

metastasis: transfer of malignant cells via pathogenic microorganisms or vascular system from one organ or body part to another not directly connected with it

mitosis: ordinary process of cell division in which each chromosome with all its genes reproduces itself exactly

multifactorial disorder: disorder caused by genetic and environmental factors

mycotic infection: an infection caused by fungi that release mycotoxin

myelin: a lipidlike substance surrounding the axon of myelinated nerve fibers that permits normal neurologic conduction

myelitis: inflammation of the spinal cord or bone marrow

necrosis: cell or tissue death

neoplasm: abnormal growth in which cell replication is uncontrolled and progressive

nephron: structural and functional unit of the kidney that forms urine

neuritic plaques: areas of nerve inflammation; found on autopsy examination of the brain tissue of people with Alzheimer disease

neuron: highly specialized conductor cell that receives and transmits electrochemical nerve impulses

nevus: circumscribed, stable malformation of the skin and oral mucosa

nondisjunction: failure of chromosomes to separate properly during cell division; causes an unequal distribution of chromosomes between the two resulting cells

opportunistic infection: infection that strikes people with altered, weakened, immune systems; caused by a microorganism that doesn't usually cause disease but becomes pathogenic under certain conditions

optic nerve: a nerve located at the back of the eye and transmits nerve impulses from the photoreceptors to the brain

organ: body part, made up of tissues, that performs a specific function

organelle: structure of a cell found in the cytoplasm that performs a specific function; for example, the nucleus, mitochondria, and lysosomes

osmolality: concentration of a solution expressed in terms of osmoles of solute per kilogram of solvent

osmoreceptors: specialized neurons located in the thalamus that are stimulated by increased extracellular fluid osmolality to cause release of antidiuretic hormone, thereby helping to control fluid balance

osteoblasts: bone-forming cells whose activity results in bone formation

osteoclasts: giant, multinuclear cells that reabsorb material from previously formed bones, tear down old or excess bone structure, and allow osteoblasts to rebuild new bone

pancytopenia: abnormal depression of all the cellular elements of blood

parasite: single-celled or multicelled organism that depends on a host for food and a protective environment

parenchyma: essential or functional elements of an organ as distinguished from its framework

pathogen: disease-producing agent or microorganism

pathogenesis: origin and development of a disease

perennial: occurring year-round

peristalsis: intestinal contractions, or waves, that propel food toward the stomach and into and through the intestine

phagocyte: cell that ingests microorganisms, other cells, and foreign particles

phagocytosis: engulfing of microorganisms, other cells, and foreign particles by a phagocyte

plasma: liquid part of the blood that carries antibodies and nutrients to tissues and carries wastes away from tissues

platelet: disk-shaped structure in blood that plays a crucial role in blood coagulation

polypeptide chains: chains of amino acids linked by a peptide bond; for example, hemoglobin

proximal: nearest to

primary lesion: lesions that are directly connected to the immediate health problem

pulmonary alveoli: grapelike clusters found at the ends of the respiratory passages in the lungs; sites for the exchange of carbon dioxide and oxygen

pulsus paradoxus: pulse marked by a drop in systolic blood pressure greater than 10 mm Hg during inspiration

pupil: the opening at the center of the iris that permits light to enter the eye

pyrosis: heartburn

recessive gene: gene that doesn't express itself in the presence of its dominant allele (corresponding gene)

remission: abatement of a disease's symptoms

remyelination: healing of demyelinated nerves

renin: enzyme produced by the kidneys in response to an actual or perceived decline in extracellular fluid volume; an important part of blood pressure regulation

resistance: opposition to airflow in the lung tissue, chest wall, or airways

retina: the innermost, light sensitive layer of the eyeball, where images are formed

retinal detachment: the sudden separation of the sensory retina from the retinal pigment epithelium

sarcoma: connective tissue neoplasm formed by proliferation of mesodermal cells

sclera: the "white part of the eye," surrounds the eye to give it its shape

secondary lesion: lesions that result from the primary lesion or develop as the result of a different health problem

sepsis: pathologic state resulting from microorganisms or their poisonous products in the bloodstream

sigmoidoscopy: inspection of the rectum and sigmoid colon through a sigmoidoscope

stasis: stagnation of the normal flow of fluids, such as blood and urine, or within the intestinal mechanism

stenosis: constriction or narrowing of a passage or orifice

stomatitis: inflammation of the mucous membrane of the mouth

stratum corneum: most superficial layer of the epidermis

stratum germinativum: formed by the stratum basale and stratum spinosum

subchondral: below the cartilage

subcutaneous layer: third layer of the skin also known as the hypodermis, consisting of fat cells

surfactant: lipid-type substance that coats the alveoli, allowing them to expand uniformly during inspiration and preventing them from collapsing during expiration

synovial fluid: viscous, lubricating substance secreted by the synovial membrane, which lines the cavity between the bones of free-moving joints

synovitis: inflammation of the synovial membrane

tendon: fibrous cord of connective tissue that attaches the muscle to bone or cartilage and enables bones to move when skeletal muscles contract

thenar: palm of the hand or sole of the foot

thrombolytic: clot dissolving

thrombosis: obstruction in blood vessels

tissue: large group of individual cells that perform a certain function

tophi: clusters of urate crystals surrounded by inflamed tissue; occur in gout

toxin: a poison, produced by animals, certain plants, or pathogenic bacteria

toxoid: toxin treated to destroy its toxicity without destroying its ability to stimulate antibody production

trabeculae: needle-like, bony structures that form a supportive meshwork of interconnecting spaces filled with bone marrow

transferrin: trace protein in blood that binds and transports iron

translocation: alteration of a chromosome by attachment of a fragment to another chromosome or a different portion of the same chromosome

trisomy 21: aberration in which chromosome 21 has three homologous chromosomes per cell instead of two; another name for Down syndrome

tubercle: a tiny, rounded nodule produced by the tuberculosis bacillus

tubules: small tubes; in the kidney, minute, reabsorptive canals that secrete, collect, and conduct urine

urate: salt of uric acid found in urine

uremic frost: white, flaky deposits of urea on the skin of patients with advanced uremia

ureters: tubes that move urine from the kidneys to the bladder before excretion

urinary tract infection: infection anywhere in the urinary tract

urticaria: wheals associated with itching; another name for hives

vasopressor: drug that stimulates contraction of the muscular tissue of the capillaries and arteries

virus: microscopic, infectious agent that contains genetic material and needs a host cell to replicate

vitreous humor: transparent, jelly-like substance, forms the main bulk of the eyeball

V/Q ratio: ratio of ventilation (amount of air in the alveoli) to perfusion (amount of blood in the pulmonary capillaries); expresses the effectiveness of gas exchange

X-linked inheritance: inheritance pattern in which single-gene disorders are passed through sex chromosomes; varies according to whether a male or female carries the gene (Because the male has only one X chromosome, a trait determined by a gene on that chromosome is always expressed in a male.)

Index

Note: Page numbers followed by f indicate figures, t indicate tables, and b indicate boxes.

A

AAAs. *See* Abdominal aortic aneurysms (AAAs)
Abdominal aortic aneurysms (AAAs), 44
    diagnostic tests, 47
    incidence of, 47
    treatments, 46b
Absence seizure, 203b
Acetylcholine, 192
Acid–base imbalances, 98–106, 98b, 99t–100t
Acquired immunodeficiency syndrome (AIDS)
    children, 392–393
    modes of transmission, 387–388
    opportunistic diseases associated with, 388t–392t
    treatment, 393b
ACS. *See* Acute coronary syndrome (ACS)
Acute coronary syndrome (ACS), 43, 55. *See also* Myocardial infarction (MI)
Acute inflammatory demyelinating polyneuropathy (AIDP), 205. *See* Guillain-Barré syndrome (GBS)
Acute kidney injury
    causes of, 345b–346b
    treatment, 348
Acute peripheral facial paresis. *See* Bell palsy
Acute phase, 11
Acute respiratory distress syndrome (ARDS), 137–140
    alveolar changes in, 138f
    diagnostic tests, 140
    differential diagnosis, 140
    signs and symptoms, 139
    treatment, 139b
Acute respiratory failure (ARF), 141–143
    diagnostic tests, 143
    hypoventilation, 141
    hypoxemia, 142
    symptoms, 142
    treatment, 144b
Acute tubular necrosis, 349–353
    complications, 351–352
    disruption, 349–350
    nephrotoxic injury, 350
    toxicity, 350

    treatment, 352–353
AD. *See* Alzheimer disease (AD)
Adaptation, 4–6
Addison disease, 305–309
    adrenal crisis, 306
    crisis, 305, 309
    getting physical, 308–309
    outside influence, 305
    primary report, 305
    secondary disease, 307–308
Adenosine triphosphate (ATP), 2
Adipokines, 54b
Adrenal disorder
    Addison disease, 305–309
    Cushing syndrome. *See* Cushing syndrome
    pheochromocytoma, 313–314
Adrenal glands, 302
Adrenal medulla, 303
AIDP. *See* Acute inflammatory demyelinating polyneuropathy (AIDP)
Air pollution, 54b
Airway resistance, 136
Akinesia, 224
Akinetic seizure, 203b
Aldosterone, 50, 303
Alleles, 26
Allergic conjunctivitis, 431
ALS. *See* Amyotrophic lateral sclerosis (ALS)
Alveoli, 133
Alzheimer disease (AD), 189–195
    brain tissue, 192
    complications, 193
    developments in, 193b
    diagnostic tests, 194–195
    familial, 190
    genes and, 190b
    risk factors, 192
    sporadic, 190
    symptoms of, 193
    tissue changes in, 191f
    treatments, 194b
Amyotrophic lateral sclerosis (ALS), 195–197, 196b
    diagnostic tests, 197
    muscle weakness, 196

    signs and symptoms of, 196
    treatments, 197b
Anaphase, 4
Anaphylaxis, 385f
    anaphylaxis, 384b
    angioedema, 386
    cardiovascular, 386
    definition, 383–384
    gastrointestinal system (GI), 386
    neurologic effects, 386
    reaction, 384
    skin effects, 386
Anemia, 106
    blood loss, 107b
    causes of, 107b
    decreased erythrocyte production, 108t–109t
    diagnosis of, 106b
    increased erythrocyte production, 110t
Aneurysm, 44–47
    dissecting, 45f
Angina, 55
Anginal equivalents, 62
Angioedema, 386
Angiography
    in aneurysm, 47
    in coronary artery disease (CAD), 57
    in cor pulmonale, 152
    in restrictive cardiomyopathy, 66
Angioplasty, 56b
Angiotensin II, 50
Antidiuretic hormone (ADH), 304, 320–323
Apoptosis, 7
Appendicitis, 248–249
Arachnoid mater, 184
ARDS. *See* Acute respiratory distress syndrome (ARDS)
ARF. *See* Acute respiratory failure (ARF)
Arrhythmias, 61b
Arterial blood gas (ABG) analysis
    in cardiogenic shock, 52
Arterial blood gases (ABGs), 136
    in acute respiratory distress syndrome (ARDS), 140
    in acute respiratory failure (ARF), 143
    in asthma, 147
    in chronic bronchitis, 150
    in cor pulmonale, 152

Arterial blood gases (ABGs) *(continued)*
in emphysema, 155
in pneumonia, 161
in pneumothorax, 166
in pulmonary edema, 169
in pulmonary embolism, 173
Arterial pressure, 42
Aseptic viral meningitis, 209, 209b
Aspiration pneumonia, 159, 161
Asthma, 143–148, 145f, 146b
diagnostic tests, 147
environmentally induced, 144
intermittent, 146
mild persistent, 146
moderate persistent, 147
severe persistent, 147
treatment, 148b
Atherectomy, 56b
Atherosclerosis, 53
Atherosclerotic lipid plaque, 44f
Atrophy, 5, 8
Auscultation
myasthenia gravis, 221
in pulmonary embolism, 173
Autonomic nervous system, 189
Autosomal dominant inheritance, 27–28, 28f
Autosomal recessive inheritance, 28–29, 29f
Autosomes, 26
Axons, 183

B

Bacteria, 18–19
Bacterial conjunctivitis, 431
Bacterial meningitis, 208
Bacterial pneumonia, 159
Barium studies, Crohn disease, 259
Basal cell carcinoma (BCC), 412–413
Basophils, 93
Beck's triad, 48
Bedbugs, 413
Bell palsy, 197–199, 198f
diagnostic tests, 199
risk factors, 198
Benign prostatic hyperplasia (BPH),
478–480
Beta-amyloid plaques, 192
Bilirubin, 253
Blasts, 96
Blindness, 428, 429b
Blood, 91
components, 91
plasma, 92
platelets, 94

red blood cells (RBCs), 92–93
white blood cells (WBCs), 93
Blood disorders
acid–base imbalances, 98–106
anemia, 106–110
causes of, 96
disseminated intravascular coagulation
(DIC), 110–113
hemophilia, 113–114
idiopathic thrombocytopenic purpura
(ITP), 114–116
iron deficiency anemia, 116–118
leukemia, 119–120
lymphomas, 120–122
multiple myeloma, 122
primary, 94
qualitative, 94
thrombocytopenia, 122–124
Blood dyscrasias, 94–97, 95f
Borrelia burgdorferi, 198
Brain stem, 186
Breast cancer, 475–478
Breathing, mechanics of, 135–136
Bronchial challenge testing,
in asthma, 147
Bronchogenic carcinomas. *See* Lung
cancer
Bronchopneumonia, 159, 160f
Bronchoscopy
in pneumonia, 161
in tuberculosis, 176
Brudzinski sign, meningitis, 211f
Buffer balancing act, 99–101
Buffer system, 98b
Burns, 413–414

C

CAD. *See* Coronary artery disease (CAD)
Cancer, 21
abnormal cell growth in, 21–23, 22f
causes of, 23–25
classifications, 21–23
early detection of, 21
metastasis in, 22f
Carcinogenesis, 23
Carcinomas, 21
Cardiac catheterization, 85
Cardiac enzyme levels in cardiogenic
shock, 52
Cardiac tamponade, 47–49, 48f
diagnostic tests, 49
features, 48–49
treatment, 49b

Cardiac valves, 41f
Cardiogenic shock, 50–52, 51f
diagnostic tests, 52
tissue perfusion, 51–52
treatment, 52
Cardiomyopathy, 63
dilated, 64
hypertrophic, 64–65
restrictive, 66–67
Cardiovascular disorders, 44
acute coronary syndrome (ACS), 57–63
aneurysm, 44–47, 45f
cardiac tamponade, 47–49, 48f
cardiogenic shock, 50–52, 51f
cardiomyopathy, 63
coronary artery disease (CAD), 53–57
dilated cardiomyopathy, 64
Cardiovascular system, 39
cause of death, 39
oxygen balancing act, 40–42, 40f
risk factors, 42–43
Cataracts, 429–430
C. difficile, 284–285
Celiac disease
complications, 263
diagnosis, 263
symptoms, 263
treating, 262
treatment, 263
Cell
adaptation of, 4–6
aging of, 8
components of, 1–2, 2f
death of, 8
degeneration of, 7–8
division and reproduction of, 3–4, 4f
injury to, 6–7
Cellulitis, 415
Central nervous system (CNS), 136, 142,
183–188
Centromere, 3
Cerebellum, 186
Cerebral angiography, stroke, 232
Cerebrovascular accident (CVA), 226
Cerebrum, 184–185
Cervical cancer, 468–469
Checkpoint, 3
Chemoreceptors, 136
Chest wall compliance, 135
Chest x-ray
in acute respiratory distress syndrome
(ARDS), 140
in acute respiratory failure (ARF), 143

in asthma, 147
in cardiac tamponade, 49
in chronic bronchitis, 150
in cor pulmonale, 152
in emphysema, 155
in heart failure (HF), 75
in hypertension, 80
in meningitis, 212
in myasthenia gravis, 222
in pneumonia, 161
in pneumothorax, 166
in pulmonary edema, 169
in pulmonary embolism, 173
in respiratory acidosis, 105
in restrictive cardiomyopathy, 66
in rheumatic fever, 85
in tuberculosis, 176
Cholecystitis
    complications, 252–253
    foundation stone, 250, 251
    gallstone formation, 251b
    risk factors, 250
    treating, 253
Cholecystokinin (CCK), 246
Choroid, 426
Chromatid, 3, 25
Chromosomal disorders, 32–34, 33f
Chromosomes, 3, 25
    counting, 25
Chronic bronchitis, 148–151. See also
        Chronic obstructive pulmonary
        disease (COPD)
    chronic hypoxia in, 150
    diagnostic tests, 150
    mucus buildup in, 149f
    signs and symptoms of, 150
    treatment, 151b
Chronic hypoxia, 150, 151
Chronic obstructive pulmonary disease
        (COPD), 148, 148b
Chronic renal failure
    body count, 360
    complications, 359–360
    nephron damage, 359
    stages of, 358b
    treatment, 361b
Ciliary body, 426
Cimex lectularius, 413
Cirrhosis
    esophageal and gastric varices,
        256–257
    final act, 256
    hepatitis, 254

nonalcoholic fatty liver disease (NAFLD),
        254
    treating, 258
Clotting cascade, 95f
Colorectal cancer (CRC), 24
    chemotherapy, 292
    early detection, 292
    gastrointestinal system, 293
    modifiable and nonmodifiable risk
        factors, 291
    screening, 291–292
    surgery, 292
    symptoms, 291
    treatment, 292
    tumors, 289–291
    types of, 290f
Complex partial seizure, 203b
Computed tomography (CT)
    in Alzheimer disease (AD), 194
    in aneurysm, 47
    in Bell palsy, 199
    in epilepsy, 204
    in meningitis, 212
    in myasthenia gravis, 222
    in stroke, 232
    in tuberculosis, 176
Conducting airways, 130–133
Conjunctiva, 425
Conjunctivitis, 431–432
Constrictive pericarditis, 80
Convalescence, 11
Cornea, 426
Coronary artery bypass graft (CABG),
        56b
Coronary artery disease (CAD), 53–57
    diagnostic tests, 57
    inflammation and thrombosis, serum
        markers for, 54b
    risk factors, 53
    treatment, 56b
Coronary artery spasms, 54
Cor pulmonale, 151–154, 153f
    diagnostic tests, 152
    in older adults, 151
    symptoms, 152
    treatment, 154b
Corticospinal tract, 188
Cortisol, 303
Creatine kinase (CK), 63
Crohn disease
    biopsy, 261–262
    changes to bowel in, 261b
    colonoscopy, 261

complications, 260
comprehending, 260
sigmoidoscopy, 261
CT. See Computed tomography (CT)
Cushing syndrome, 78
    complications, 311–312
    corticotropin, 310
    sexual/psychological complications,
        312–313
    treatment, 312b
Cyanosis, 142
Cytokinesis, 3

D

D-dimer blood test, in pulmonary embolism,
        173
Deafness, 444–445
Decompensation, cycle of, 51f
Deep vein thrombophlebitis (DVT), 68f
    pulmonary embolus (PE), 67
    treatment, 69
Deep venous thromboembolism, 67
Deficit injury to cell, 7
Dementia, 192
Dendrites, 183
Diabetes insipidus, 320–323
Diabetes mellitus (DM)
    acute danger, 315
    chronic complications, 315–320
    diabetic ketoacidosis (DKA), 318
    hyperosmolar hyperglycemic nonketotic
        syndrome (HHNS), 318
    screening guidelines, 317
    secondary diabetes, 315
    treatment, 319
    type 1 diabetes mellitus (T1DM),
        314, 315
    type 2 diabetes mellitus (T2DM), 314,
        316b
Diabetic ketoacidosis (DKA), 318
DIC. See Disseminated Intravascular
        coagulation (DIC)
Digital subtraction angiography, 232
Dilated cardiomyopathy, 64
Disease
    cause of, 10
    development of, 11
    factors that influence outcome of, 10
    vs. illness, 10–13
    stages of, 11
    stress and, 11–13, 12f
Disjunction, 32
Disorderly conduct, 305

Disseminated intravascular coagulation
  (DIC), 110–113, 111f
  causes of, 110–111
  diagnostic tests, 113
  pathologic processes, 111
  signs and symptoms, 112
  treatment, 112b
Diverticular disease
  chronic diverticulitis, 266
  dietary fiber, highs and lows of, 264
  diverticula domiciles, 264
  diverticular sacs under attack, 264
  diverticulitis of the colon, 265b
  mild diverticulitis, 265
  severe diverticulitis, 266
  treating, 266
Drug therapy, 52b
  in amyotrophic lateral sclerosis (ALS),
    197b
  in epilepsy, 204b
  myocardial infarction (MI), 61b
Dura mater, 184
DVT. See Deep vein thrombophlebitis (DVT)
Dyscrasia, 94
Dysplasia, 6

E
Ear
  anatomy, 442f
  common disorders, 443–448
  deafness, 444–445
  external ear structures, 441, 442f
  hearing loss, 444–445
  infections, 446, 447b
  internal ear structures, 443
  Meniere disease, 447–448
  middle ear structures, 442
  treatment, 448b
Echocardiography
  in cardiogenic shock, 52
  in cor pulmonale, 152
  in myocardial infarction (MI), 63
  in pericarditis, 82
  in rheumatic fever, 85
Edrophonium test, in myasthenia gravis, 222
Ejection fraction, 70
Electrical impulses, in seizures, 202f
Electrocardiography (ECG)
  in acute respiratory failure (ARF), 143
  in cardiac tamponade, 49
  in cardiogenic shock, 52
  in chronic bronchitis, 150
  in coronary artery disease (CAD), 57

in cor pulmonale, 152
in emphysema, 155
in heart failure (HF), 74
in hypertension, 80
in metabolic alkalosis, 106
in myocardial infarction (MI), 63
in pericarditis, 82
in pulmonary edema, 169
in pulmonary embolism, 173
in respiratory alkalosis, 105
in restrictive cardiomyopathy, 66
in rheumatic fever, 85
Electroencephalogram (EEG)
  in Alzheimer disease (AD), 194–195
  in epilepsy, 204
  in meningitis, 212
  in stroke, 233
Electromyography
  in amyotrophic lateral sclerosis (ALS),
    197
  in Guillain-Barré syndrome (GBS), 207
  in myasthenia gravis, 222
Electrophysiologic testing, in Guillain-Barré
    syndrome (GBS), 207
Embolism, 228
Embolus, 67
Emphysema, 154
  air trapping in, 155f
  diagnostic tests, 155
  signs and symptoms of, 155
Endocarditis, 83
Endocrine disorder
  feedback, 301f
  primary vs. secondary, 302
Endocrine disorders, Addison disease,
    305–309
Endocrine glands
  adrenal glands, 302
  adrenal medulla, 303
  aldosterone, 303
  antidiuretic hormone (ADH), 304
  cortisol, 303
  disorderly conduct, 305
  glucagon, 303
  insulin, 303
  pituitary gland, 304
  thyroid gland, 304
  treatment, 304
Endocrine system, hypothalamus, 299–300
Endogenous factors, 7
Endometrial cancer, 470–471, 472b
Endometriosis, 461–462
Endoplasmic reticulum, 2

Endotoxins, 18
Environmentally induced asthma, 144
Eosinophils, 93
Epidural space, 184
Epilepsy, 199–204
  diagnostic tests, 204
  electrical impulses in, 202f
  signs and symptoms of, 201
  treatment of, 204b
Erythema marginatum, 84
Erythrocytes, 91. See Red blood cells (RBCs)
Erythropoiesis, 92
Estrogen, 43
Etiology, 10
Exogenous factors, 7
Exotoxins, 18
Extracorticospinal tract, 188
Extrapyramidal system, 188
Extrinsic causes of disease, 10
Eye
  anatomy, 424f–425f
  aqueous humor, 427
  blindness, 428, 429b
  cataracts, 429–430
  choroid, 426
  ciliary body, 426
  common disorders, 428
  conjunctiva, 425
  conjunctivitis, 431–432
  cornea, 426
  external structures, 425–426
  eyelashes, 425
  eyelids, 425
  glaucoma, 432–434
  hordeolum, 434–435
  internal structures, 426–427
  iris, 426
  lens, 426
  macula, 427
  macular degeneration, 435–436
  ocular trauma, 436, 437b
  optic nerve, 427
  pupil, 426
  refractive errors, 438–439
  retina, 427
  retinal detachment, 439–440
  retinal tears, 439–440
  retinoblastoma, 441
  sclera, 426
  strabismus, 440–441
  vitreous humor, 427
Eyelashes, 425
Eyelids, 425

F

Farsightedness, 439
Feedback mechanisms, homeostasis and, 9–10
Fibroadenomas, 460
Fissure of Rolando, 185f
Fissures, 185f
Forced exhalation of nitric oxide (FeNO) testing, 147
Forced expiratory volume (FEV), 147
Four-alarm inflammation, 398
Free radicals, 54b
Fungi, 19

G

Gastroesophageal reflux disease (GERD)
    complications of, 269
    heartburn, 267
    less LES pressure, 267–269
    treating, 269b
Gastrointestinal system (GI), 241–248
    disorders, 247–248
GBS. *See* Guillain-Barré syndrome (GBS)
Generalized seizures, 203b
Generalized tonic-clonic seizure, 203b
Genes, 25
    Alzheimer disease (AD) and, 190b
    lung cancer, 156
    mutations in, 27
Genetic inheritance
    autosomal dominant, 27–28, 28f
    autosomal recessive, 28–29, 29f
    sex-linked, 30, 30f–31f
Genetics, 25
    alleles, 26
    chromosomes, counting, 25
    different division, 26
    gen XX (or XY), 26–27
    inheritance, 25
    location, 26
    mutation, 27
Glaucoma, 432–434
Glomerulonephritis
    acute situations, 353
    chronic cases, 353–354
    glomerulus, immune complex deposits on, 355f
    Goodpasture disease, 354
    treatment, 355b
    unwelcome lodger, 354
Glucagon, 303
Goiter, 325

Golgi apparatus, 2
Granulocytes, 93
Guillain-Barré syndrome (GBS), 205–207
    diagnostic tests, 207
    peripheral nerve demyelination in, 205, 206f
    phases, 205
    respiratory muscles, 207
    signs and symptoms of, 206
    treatment, 207b

H

Headache phase, 214
Hearing loss, 444–445
Heart failure (HF), 69–75
    causes of, 73
    classification, 72b–73b
    diagnostic tests, 74–75
    ejection fraction, 70
    left-sided, 70b–72b
    right-sided, 70b–72b
    signs and symptoms of, 74
    treatment, 75b
Heart failure with preserved ejection fraction (HFpEF), 73b
Heart failure with reduced ejection fraction (HFrEF), 73b
Hematologic system, 91–125. *See also* Blood disorders
Hemoglobin, 92, 101
Hemophilia A, 113
Hemophilia B, 113
Hemorrhage, 228
Hemorrhagic stroke, 226
Hemostasis, 94
Hepatitis B virus (HBV), 253
Hepatitis C virus (HCV), 253
Herpes simplex virus (HSV), 416
Herpes zoster, 416
Hiatal hernia
    collar loosening, 270–271
    stomach herniation, 271f
High-density lipoprotein (HDL), 53
High-sensitivity C-reactive protein (hs-CRP), 54b
Hodgkin lymphoma, 120t–121t
Homocysteine, 53
Homeostasis, 9
    feedback mechanisms and, 9–10
    structures responsible for maintaining, 9
Homocysteine, 53
Hordeolum, 434–435
Hormones, cancer, 24
Human Genome Project, 26

Human immunodeficiency virus (HIV)
    children, 392–393
    classification, 387
    modes of transmission, 387–388
    opportunistic diseases associated with, 388t–392t
    treatment, 393b
Human papillomavirus (HPV)-associated cancer, 470
Hydrogen ion concentration (pH), 136
Hydronephrosis
    obstruction, instruction on, 355
    renal damage, 357f
    symptoms of, 357–358
Hyperlipidemia, 43
Hyperopia, 438
Hyperosmolar hyperglycemic nonketotic syndrome (HHNS), 318
Hyperplasia, 6, 8
Hypertension, 53, 76–80
    blood vessel damage in, 79f
    complications, 78–79
    development of, 76–77
    diagnostic tests, 79–80
    renin–angiotensin–aldosterone system, 77f
    secondary, 78
    treatment, 80b
    types of, 76
Hyperthyroidism
    Graves disease, 325
    recognizing, 327f
    treatment, 328
    types of, 326
Hypertrophic cardiomyopathy, 64–65
Hypertrophy, 5
Hypocapnia, 101
Hypothalamus, 9, 186, 299–300
Hypothyroidism, 329–332
    myxedema coma, 332f
    organ system, 330–331
    primary, 330
    recognizing, 331f
    secondary, 330
Hypoventilation, 141
Hypoxemia, 130, 137, 142
Hypoxia, 54, 135

I

Idiopathic diseases, 10
Idiopathic thrombocytopenic purpura (ITP), 114–116
Illness *vs.* disease, 10–13

Immune disorders
  allergen, 381
  response, 380
Immune system
  structures of, 377–378
  types of, 378–380
Immunity, 18
Immunoglobulin G (IgG), 114
Immunosuppression, 21
Immunosurveillance, 25
Immunotherapy, 122
Increased intracranial pressure (ICP), 208
Incubation period, 11
Ineffective gas exchange, 135
Infarction, 7
Infection(s), 17
  barriers to, 19–20
  microorganisms that cause, 18–19
  process, 20–21
Infectious injury to cell, 7
Inflammation, 18
Inflammatory injury to cell, 7
Inherited traits, 25
Insulin, 303
Integumentary system
  healthy skin, 407
  layer upon layer, 405–407
  primary lesions, 408–410
  secondary lesions, 410–411
  skin assessment, 411, 412t
  skin disorders. See Skin disorders
  skin lesions, types of, 408–411, 412t
Intermittent asthma, 146
Internal structures, 426–427
Interphase, 3
Intra-aortic balloon pump (IABP), 52b
Intrinsic causes of disease, 10
Iris, 426
Iron (Fe++), 92
Iron deficiency anemia, 116–118, 117b, 118f
Irritable bowel syndrome (IBS), 271
  disturbing pattern, 273, 274f
  stress, 272–273
  treating, 272
Irritant reflex, 132
Ischemia, 7
Ischemic stroke, 226, 229f
ITP. See Idiopathic thrombocytopenic
  purpura (ITP)

J

Jacksonian seizure, 203b
Joints, 399f

K

Keratoconjunctivitis sicca, 432
Kernig sign, meningitis, 211f
Kidney disease, chronic. See Chronic renal
  failure
Kidney infection. See Pyelonephritis
Kidney stones. See Renal calculi
Kyphoscoliosis, 151

L

Laser angioplasty, 56b
Lens, 426
Leukemia, 96
  complications, 119
  diagnosis, 120
  treatments, 120–122
  types of, 119t
Leukocytes, 91
Lobar pneumonia, 160f
Lobes, 185f
Locus, 26
Lou Gehrig disease, 195
Low-density lipoprotein (LDL), 53
Lower airways, 130–132, 131f
Lung cancer, 157t
  diagnosis, 158
  genetics, 156
  non–small cell lung carcinoma, 156–157
  risk factors, 156
  small cell carcinoma, 157
  symptoms of, 157
Lungs, 133–135
  alveoli, 133
  gas exchange, 133
  ineffective gas exchange, 135
  ventilation and perfusion, 134f
  V/Q ratio, 133
Lymphocytes, 18, 93
Lymphomas, 120
  Hodgkin, 120t–121t
  non-Hodgkin, 120t–121t
  treatments, 121–122
Lysosomes, 2
Lysozymes, 20

M

Macrophages, 93
Macula, 427
Macular degeneration, 435–436
Magnetic resonance angiography, in stroke,
  233
Magnetic resonance imaging (MRI)
  in Alzheimer disease (AD), 194

in Bell palsy, 199
in cor pulmonale, 152
in epilepsy, 204
in meningitis, 212
in multiple sclerosis (MS), 218
in stroke, 233
in tuberculosis, 176
Malignant melanoma, 416–417
Marfan syndrome, 45
McBurney point, 249
Medulla oblongata, 9, 186
Megakaryocytes, 123
Meiosis, 26
Meniere disease, 447–448
Meningitis, 208–212
  aseptic viral, 209, 209b
  bacterial, 208
  complications of, 210
  diagnostic tests, 212
  meningeal inflammation in, 210f
  prognosis, 208
  signs and symptoms of, 210–211, 211f
  treatment, 212b
Mesotheliomas, 158
Metabolic acidosis, 101, 104, 105, 140
Metabolic alkalosis, 102, 104–105, 105–106
Metaphase, 3
Metaplasia, 6
Midbrain, 186
Middle ear structures, 442
Migraine, 213–214
  aura, 214
  diagnosis, 214
  management, 214
  pathophysiologic basis, 214
  phases, 214
Mild persistent asthma, 146
Mismatch mayhem, 135
Mitochondrion, 2
Mitosis, 25
  phases of, 3–4, 4f
Moderate persistent asthma, 147
Molds, 19
Monocytes, 93
Monosomy, 32
Mosaicism, 33
Motor neurons, 195–196
Mucociliary system, 132
Multifactorial disorders, 34
Multiple myeloma, 122
Multiple sclerosis (MS), 214–218
  complications of, 217
  diagnostic tests, 218

incidence, 215
myelin breakdown, 216f
signs and symptoms of, 215–217
treatment, 217b
Muscle biopsy, amyotrophic lateral
sclerosis (ALS), 197
Muscle rigidity, 223
Muscle weakness, 196
Myasthenia gravis, 218–222, 219f
diagnostic tests, 222
signs and symptoms of, 220
treatment, 221b
types of crisis, 220b
Mycobacterium tuberculosis, 174, 176
Mycotic infections, 19
Mycotoxin, 19
Myelencephalon, 186
Myocardial infarction (MI), 39, 40f, 58f–59f
cardinal symptom of, 62
complications, 60
diagnostic tests, 63
infarction site, 62
predisposing factors, 60
symptoms of, 63
tissue destruction in, 61b
treatment, 61b
Myocardial perfusion imaging, coronary
artery disease (CAD), 57
Myocarditis, 83
Myoclonic seizure, 203b
Myopia, 438

N
Nearsightedness, 439
Necrosis, 7
Negative feedback mechanisms, 9
Nephrolithiasis. *See* Renal calculi
Nerve cell, 183
Nerve conduction studies, myasthenia
gravis, 222
Neurologic disorders, 189
Alzheimer disease (AD), 189–195
amyotrophic lateral sclerosis (ALS),
195–197
Bell palsy, 197–199
epilepsy, 199–204
Guillain-Barré syndrome (GBS), 205–207
meningitis, 208–212
migraine, 213–214
multiple sclerosis (MS), 214–218
myasthenia gravis, 218–222
Parkinson disease (PD), 222–226
stroke, 226–233

Neurologic system, 183–189
Neuron, 183
Neutropenia, 97
Neutrophils, 93
Nonalcoholic fatty liver disease (NAFLD),
253
Nondisjunction, 32
Nongranular leukocytes, 93
Non-Hodgkin lymphoma, 120t–121t
Non–small cell lung carcinoma, 156–157
NSTEMI, 58
Nuclear ventriculography, in myocardial
infarction (MI), 63

O
Obesity, 53
Ocular trauma, 436, 437b
Ophthalmoscopy, stroke, 233
Opportunistic infections, 21
Optic nerve, 427
Ovarian cancer, 472–474
Oxygen balancing act, 40–42, 40f

P
Pain, appendicitis, 248–249
Pancreas, 246–247
Pancreatic disorder, diabetes mellitus (DM),
314–320
Pancreatitis
acting prematurely, 276–277
complications, 277
pain, 277–279
permanent change for, 276
treating, 278b
Parasites, 19
Parasympathetic nervous system, 189
Parieto-occipital fissure, 185f
Parkinson disease (PD), 222–226
complications of, 225
diagnosis of, 226
neurotransmitter action in, 224f
signs and symptoms of, 224–225
treatments, 225b
Partial seizures, 203b
Partial thromboplastin time (PTT), 113
Pathogenesis, 11
Pectus excavatum, 151
Pediculosis, 417
Pelvic organ prolapse, 464–466
Peptic ulcer
aiding and abetting bacterial infection,
280
common ulcer types and sites, 279

complication, 280
duodenal, 280
dynamic duodenal ulcer, 281
gastric, 280
mucosa, 280
peptic promoters, 280
upper part upsetting, 280
Percutaneous coronary intervention (PCI),
56b
Percutaneous myocardial revascularization
(PMR), 56b
Percutaneous transhepatic
cholangiography, 253
Percutaneous transluminal coronary
angioplasty (PTCA), 56b
Pericardial effusion, 81
Pericarditis, 80–82
causes of, 81
laboratory test, 82
treatment, 82b
Peripheral nerve demyelination, 205, 206f
Peripheral nervous system (PNS), 183,
188–189
Pheochromocytoma, 78, 313–314
Physical injury to cell, 7
Physiologic stressors, 12
Pia mater, 184
Pinkeye. *See* Conjunctivitis
Pituitary disorder
diabetes insipidus, 320–323
syndrome of inappropriate antidiuretic
hormone (SIADH), 323–325
Pituitary gland, 9, 304
Plasma, 91–92
Platelets, 94
disorders, 97
Pneumocystis carinii pneumonia, 21
Pneumonia, 158–163
classification, 159
diagnostic tests, 161
prognosis, 158
signs and symptoms of, 161
types of, 162t–163t
Pneumothorax, 164–167
diagnostic tests, 166
signs and symptoms of, 165–166
spontaneous, 164
traumatic, 164
treatment, 167b
Polycystic ovary syndrome (PCOS), 466–467
Polymerase chain reaction (PCR)
in pneumonia, 161
Pons, 186

Positive feedback mechanisms, 10
Positron emission tomography (PET)
    in Alzheimer disease (AD), 194
    in stroke, 233
Postdrome, 214
Postviral thrombocytopenia, 114
Pregnancy, dilated cardiomyopathy and, 64
Premonitory phase, 214
Pressure injury, 417
Pressure of arterial carbon dioxide ($PaCO_2$), 136
Pressure of arterial oxygen (PaO_2), 136
Prinzmetal angina, 54
Prodromal period, 11
Prodrome, 214
Programmed degeneration, 7
Prophase, 3
Prostate cancer, 482–484
Prostatitis, 480–482
Prothrombin time (PT), 113
Psychological stressors, 12–13
Pulmonary airway, 132f
Pulmonary angiography, pulmonary embolism, 173
Pulmonary arterial vasoconstriction, 151
Pulmonary artery catheterization
    in acute respiratory distress syndrome (ARDS), 140
    in acute respiratory failure (ARF), 143
    in cor pulmonale, 152
    in pulmonary edema, 169
Pulmonary artery pressure (PAP)
    in cardiac tamponade, 49
    in cardiogenic shock, 52
    in heart failure (HF), 75
Pulmonary capillary wedge pressure (PCWP), 52, 55
Pulmonary edema, 71b, 167–170
    development of, 168f
    diagnostic tests, 169
    signs and symptoms of, 169
    treatment, 170b
Pulmonary embolism, 170–173
    diagnostic tests, 173
    symptoms of, 171
    thrombus formation, 171
    treatment, 173b
Pulmonary embolus (PE), 67
Pulmonary function tests
    in asthma, 147
    in chronic bronchitis, 150
    in cor pulmonale, 152
    in emphysema, 155

Pulmonary hypertension, 142, 150
Pulse oximetry
    in acute respiratory distress syndrome (ARDS), 140
    in acute respiratory failure (ARF), 143
    in asthma, 147
    in chronic bronchitis, 150
    in cor pulmonale, 152
    in emphysema, 155
    in pneumonia, 161
    in pneumothorax, 166
    in pulmonary edema, 169
Pump failure, 50, 69
Pupil, 426
Pyelonephritis, 365–369
Pyramidal system, 188

Q

QuantiFERON-TB, 176
Quantitative blood disorders, 94

R

Radiation exposure, tumor development, 23
Rami, 188
Recovery, 11
Recovery phase, 214
Red blood cells (RBCs), 92–93
    disorders, 96
Refractive errors, 438–439
Regurgitation in valvular disease, 41
Remission, 11
Renal calculi, 362–365
Renal disorders
    acute kidney injury, 345–349
    acute tubular necrosis, 349–353
Renal system, 338f
    blood pressure regulation, 343–344
    calcium formation, 344
    fluid and acid–base balance, 339–341
    red blood cells (RBCs) production, 344
    renal labor, 339
    renin-angiotensin-aldosterone system (RAAS), 343–344
    vitamin D regulation, 344
    waste collection, 341–343
Renin–angiotensin–aldosterone system (RAAS), 50, 77f
Reproductive disorders
    benign prostatic hyperplasia (BPH), 478–480
    breast cancer, 475–478
    cervical cancer, 468–469
    endometrial cancer, 470–471, 472b

endometriosis, 461–462
    fibroadenomas, 460
    human papillomavirus (HPV)-associated cancer, 470
    ovarian cancer, 472–474
    pelvic organ prolapse, 464–466
    polycystic ovary syndrome (PCOS), 466–467
    prostate cancer, 482–484
    prostatitis, 480–482
    sexually transmitted infections, 486–487, 487t–488t
    testicular cancer, 484–485
    uterine leiomyoma, 463, 464b
    vaginal candidiasis (VC), 467–468
Reproductive system
    endometrial/menstrual cycle, 456, 457f
    female reproductive system, 453–456, 454f
    hypothalamic–pituitary and ovulation cycles, 456
    male reproductive system, 458–459
Resistance, airway, 136
Respiration, neurochemical control of, 136
Respiratory acidosis, 101, 102–104, 105, 140
Respiratory alkalosis, 101, 104, 105
Respiratory center, 136
Respiratory disorders, 137
    acute respiratory distress syndrome (ARDS), 137–140
    acute respiratory failure (ARF), 141–143
    asthma, 143–148
    chronic bronchitis, 148–151
    cor pulmonale, 151–154
    emphysema, 154–155
    lung cancer, 156–158
    pneumonia, 158–163
    pneumothorax, 164–167
    pulmonary edema, 167–170
    pulmonary embolism, 170–173
    respiratory syncytial virus (RSV), 174
    tuberculosis, 174–176
Respiratory syncytial virus (RSV), 174
Respiratory system
    breathing mechanics and, 135–136
    conducting airways, 130–133
    function of, 129
    gas exchange in, 129
    lower airway in, 130–132, 131f
    lungs in, 133–135
    neurochemical control, 136
    upper airway in, 130, 131f

Restrictive cardiomyopathy, 66–67, 66b
Reticular formation, 186
Reticuloendothelial cells, 93
Retina, 427
Retinal detachment, 439–440
Retinal tears, 439–440
Retinoblastoma, 441
Rheumatic fever, 83–86
    laboratory tests, 85
    treatment, 85b
Rheumatic heart disease (RHD), 83–86
    sequelae of, 84f
    treatment, 85b
Rheumatoid arthritis
    four-alarm inflammation, 398
    joints, 399f
    treatment, 397–398
Rhinitis, allergic
    allergen, 381
    treatment, 383b
    types of, 382b
Ribosomes, 2
Right lower quadrant (RLQ), 249
RSV. *See* Respiratory syncytial virus (RSV)

S

Salmonellosis, 289
Scabies, 418
Sclera, 426
Secondarily generalized seizure, 203b
Secretory immunity, 132
Seizures
    disorder, 199. *See* Epilepsy
    electrical impulses in, 202f
    types of, 203b
Sensory impairment, 232
Sensory seizure, 203b
Sensory system
    ear. *See* Ear
    eye. *See* Eye
Sepsis, 20
Septum, 64–65, 65f
Severe persistent asthma, 147
Sex-linked inheritance, 30, 30f–31f
Sexually transmitted infections, 486–487,
        487t–488t
Single-gene disorders, 27–32, 28f–31f
Single-photon emission computed
        tomography, stroke, 233
Skin disorders
    basal cell carcinoma (BCC), 412–413
    bedbugs, 413
    burns, 413–414

cellulitis, 415
Cimex lectularius, 413
herpes simplex virus (HSV), 416
herpes zoster, 416
malignant melanoma, 416–417
pediculosis, 417
pressure injury, 417
scabies, 418
tinea infections, 418–419
Skin testing, in asthma, 147
Small cell carcinoma, 157
Somatic nervous system, 189
Spinal cord, 187, 187f
Spinal nerves, 188, 188b
Spontaneous pneumothorax, 164–165
Stable angina, 55
Status epilepticus, 201, 201b
ST-elevation myocardial Infarction (STEMI),
        58
Stenosis in valvular disease, 41
Strabismus, 440–441
    causes, 440
    risk factors, 440
    treatment, 441
Stress, disease and, 11–13, 12f
Stroke, 226–233
    causes of, 228
    diagnostic tests, 232–233
    hemorrhagic, 226
    ischemic, 226, 229f
    neurologic deficits in, 230b, 231t
    neurologic examination, 230
    risk factors, 228
    transient ischemic attack (TIA), 227, 227b
    treatment, 233b
Subarachnoid space, 184, 208
Subclinical identification, 8
Sudden unexpected death in epilepsy
        (SUDEP), 201
Sylvian fissure, 185f
Syndrome of inappropriate antidiuretic
        hormone (SIADH)
    causes, 324
    diagnostics, 325
    treatment, 324
Systemic lupus erythematosus (SLE)
    cardiopulmonary effects, 396
    drugs, 395b
    lupus, 395–396
    neurologic effects, 396
    susceptibility, 395
    treatment, 394b
    urinary system effects, 396–397

T

Tachycardia, 142
Targeted therapy, 122
Telophase, 4
Tension pneumothorax, 164, 165f
Testicular cancer, 484–485
Thalamus, 186
Thrombocytes, 91
Thrombocytopathy, 97
Thrombocytopenia, 122–124
Thrombosis, 228
Thyroid disorder, 325
    goiter, 325
    hyperthyroidism, 325–329
    hypothyroidism, 329–332
Thyroid gland, 304
Tinea infections, 418–419
Tissue hypoxemia, 142
Tissue hypoxia, 40
Toxic injury to cell, 7
Transcranial Doppler, in stroke, 233
Transesophageal echocardiography,
        cardiac tamponade, 49
Transient ischemia, 54
Transient ischemic attack (TIA), 227,
        227b
Translocation, 34
Transmyocardial revascularization, 56b
Transthoracic echocardiography, cardiac
        tamponade, 49
Traumatic pneumothorax, 164
Troponin I, 54b
Troponins, 63
Tuberculin skin test, tuberculosis, 176
Tuberculosis, 174–176, 175f
    diagnostic tests, 176
    dissemination, 175
    immune response, 175
    incidence, 174
    transmission, 175
    tubercle formation, 175
Turner syndrome, 32
Type 1 diabetes mellitus (T1DM), 314, 315
Type 2 diabetes mellitus (T2DM), 314, 316b

U

Ulcerative colitis
    colon, looking closer at, 283f
    damage surveying, 281–282
    treating, 284b
Ultrasonography, abdominal aortic
        aneurysms (AAAs), 47

Unstable angina, 55, 57
Upper airways, 130, 131f
Upper motor neurons, 188
Urinalysis, 79
Urinary tract infection (UTI)
    pyelonephritis, 365–369
    treatment, 369
    urosepsis, 365–369
Urosepsis, 365–369
Uterine leiomyoma, 463, 464b

V

Vaginal candidiasis (VC), 467–468
Vagus nerve paralysis, 207
Valvular disease, 41
Variant/Prinzmetal angina, 57
Ventricular arrhythmias, 64
Viral conjunctivitis, 431
Viral hepatitis

clinical stage, 288
complication, 287–288
hepatitis A virus (HAV), 285
hepatitis B virus (HBV), 286
hepatitis C virus (HCV), 286–287
hepatitis D virus (HDV), 287
hepatitis E virus (HEV), 287
prodromal stage, 288
recovery stage, 288
Viral pneumonia, 159
Virchow's triad, 67, 171
Viruses, 18
Vitreous humor, 427
von Willebrand disease, 113
V/Q ratio, 133

W

White blood cells (WBCs), 93
    disorders, 96

X

X-ray. *See also* Chest x-ray
    in abdominal aortic aneurysms (AAAs),
        47
    in cholecystitis, 252
    chronic renal failure, 361
    in cirrhosis, 257
    in meningitis, 212
    in pancreatitis, 278
    in peptic ulcer, 281
    in rheumatoid arthritis, 400
    urinary tract infection, 368

Y

Yeasts, 19

Z

Zona as opportunistic disease, 391t
Zoster as opportunistic disease, 391t